Healing Foods

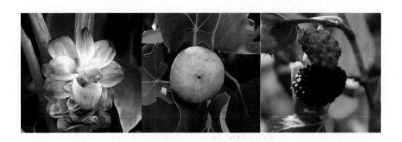

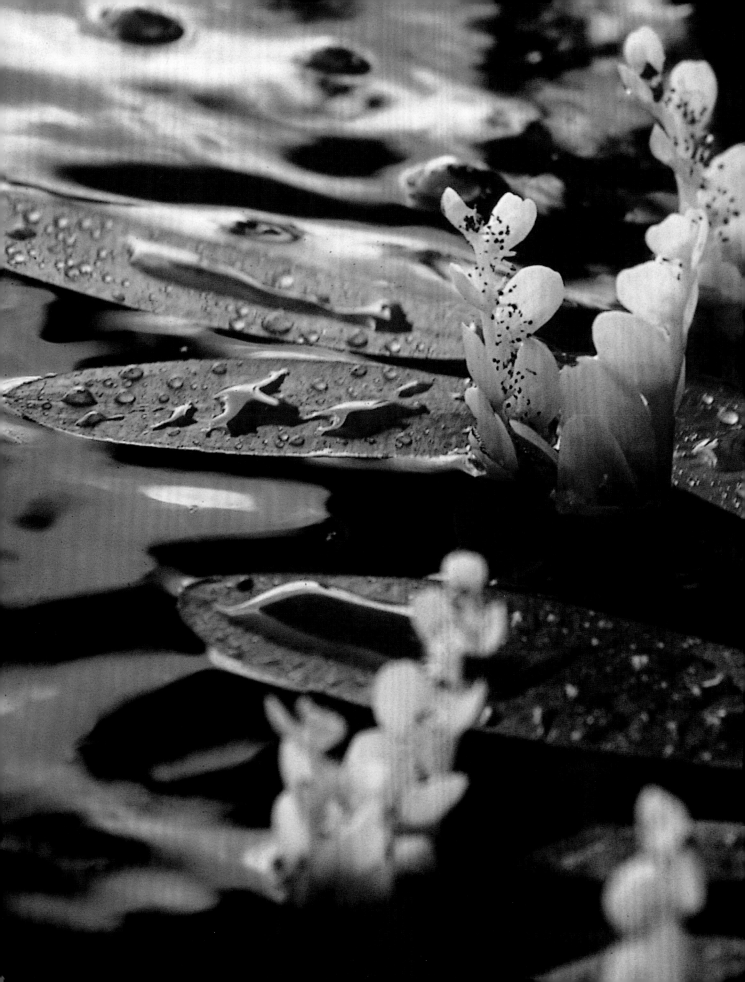

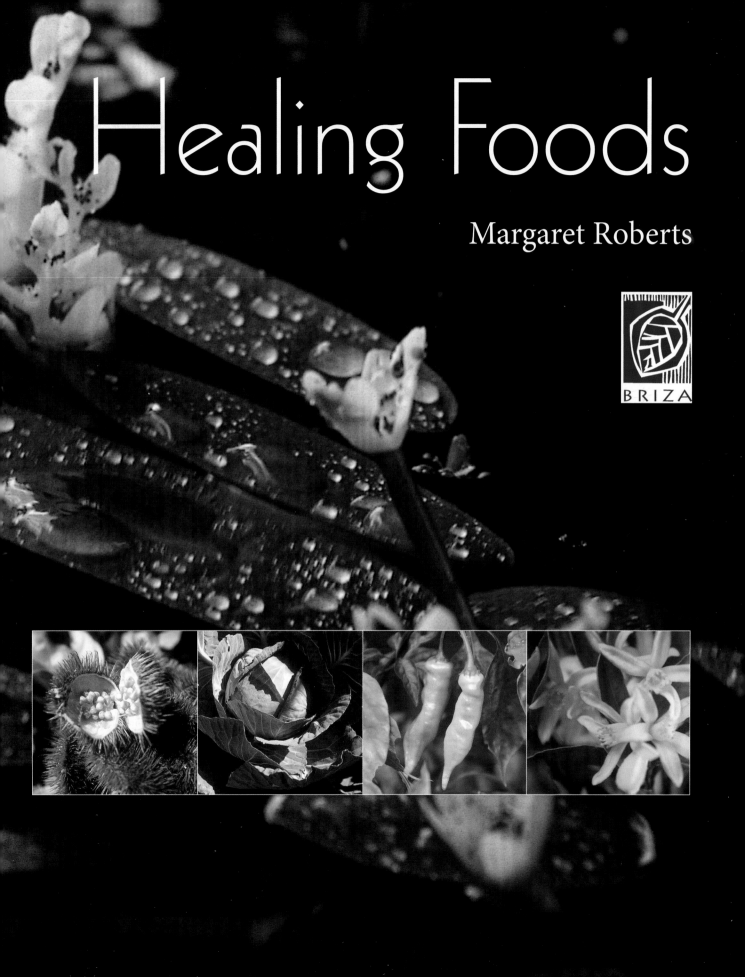

Healing Foods

Margaret Roberts

BRIZA

Published by
BRIZA PUBLICATIONS
CK 1990/011690/23

PO Box 11050
Queenswood 0121
Pretoria
South Africa
www.briza.co.za

First edition, first impression, 2011
First edition, second impression, 2012

ISBN 978 1 875093 86 1

Project manager: Reneé Ferreira
Design and layout: Alicia Arntzen, The Purple Turtle Publishing Services
Front cover photograph: Lizette Jonker
Cover design: Sally Whines, the Departure Lounge
Reproduction: Resolution, Cape Town
Printed and bound by PrintWORKS Global Services (Shenzhen) Company Limited, China

Photo credits: All photographs by Phyllis Green with the exception of the following which are used courtesy of
Ben-Erik van Wyk: Pages 59, 73, 85 (bottom), 86, 89, 93, 94, 109, 110, 112 (top), 132, 143, 146, 151, 159 (main),
161, 164, 165, 176, 179, 188 and 205. Photographs on the front cover and on page 5 (contents page) are used
courtesy of Lizette Jonker.

Contents

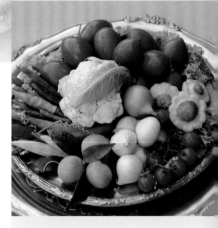

Descriptions of more than 150 vegetables, fruits, herbs, spices and other food plants that
are the building blocks of good health, with information on the plant's history, how to
grow it and how to use it.

An A–Z list of more than 100 common ailments, with suggestions on the danger foods to
avoid and the superfoods, supplements and other therapies to consider as part of a treatment
programme.

Acknowledgements

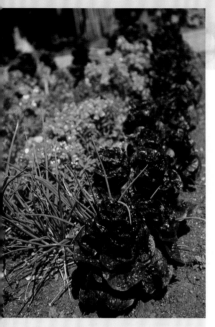

This book has been a long time coming! Perhaps I could say my whole life has shaped it. I think I have been writing it in so many ways – from my childhood with my mother and my grandmother's beautifully creative cooking based on the endless and delicious supply of fruits and vegetables from our suburban garden, to my isolation and necessity to put good meals onto the table in my farm kitchen from the age of 23. In those days there were no convenience foods, fast foods or takeaways, we had to bake our own bread, make our own chicken pies and sustaining soups, custards, jams and pickles.

So my gratitude begins many years ago with my father's vegetable garden, and I am grateful for my sister Suzie's green mealies and green beans and potatoes and tomatoes, for my mother's cleverness in bottling the summer peaches, the abundant apricots and plums, and for the strawberry jam my grandmother made for the home-baked scones and muffins that came from our kitchen, and for the basic and beautiful recipes that I grew up with and that spilled into my life. Later, with those basic recipes, I cooked the same meals for my family, the same divine smells of home-baked bread, rich stews, and the comforting great pot of winter soup simmering on my stove, enveloped the farm.

A way of life, I continued the vegetable gardens thanks to my father's teachings, the filling of the Ball jars of peaches and plums from my garden, just the way my mother and my grandmother did, the bread baking, the biscuit making, filled the valley with scents of deliciousness, and with a thankful heart I blessed my strict grandmother for her precise measurements, and I blessed my beautiful mother for her elegant creativity in making so many feasts with what there was in the garden and on the pantry shelves.

I learnt thrift, creativeness, and those precious baking skills from an early age, and, with my youngest child at my side, from the age of three, I could teach her just the way I was taught to cook a nourishing and simple and delicious meal!

And so I dedicate this book to Sandra, my youngest child, my partner in the Herbal Centre business, and my loyal and loving behind-the-scenes-supporter who cooks with creativity and joyfulness the way my mother did, who has inherited my mother's elegance and beauty in everything she is and does, and who loves cooking and who can make so many delectable and exquisite silk purses out of so many dreary sow's ears! And who can run her restaurant, and create feasts for celebrations, for family Christmases, for cookery classes, and for 400 visitors, with the same perfection that she cooks for an intimate dinner party.

Many of the recipes within these pages are hers, her interest never wavers, she has spurred me on, suggesting exquisite combinations, tastes and refinements, all amidst giving birth to her second baby, Michael, and running her restaurant and creating products for the huge Herbal Centre shop, and being a hands-on mom to Skye and Michael. Sandy does not know about rest, brakes, breaks or ever thinking about herself!

She cooks with her daughter the way I cooked with her! Her kitchen smells of cakes and jams, pies and soups the way my mother's and my farm kitchen did. May this book become her loved reference book the way my mother's books and my early *Cooking with Herbs and Spices* book became for her so long ago – easy to cook from and lots of health-building ideas to grow even more of her own recipes. It is with much loving gratitude that I place it in her capable hands.

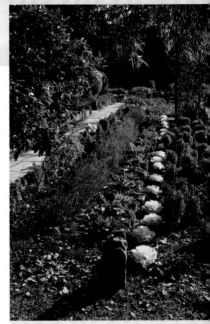

My heartfelt thanks goes to Reneé Ferreira. She has played so great a role in so many of my books. She has the enviable skills and thoroughness of both production and management, as well as the quiet authority that puts her in a league of her own. It is thanks to her that a book such as this emerges from a hurricane of pages, neatly in order and indexed and cross-indexed. It is with such gratefulness that I again have her guiding and steering this book into the place where it belongs.

To Annatjie van Wyk, my most valuable and appreciated clever-at-deciphering friend, who never tires of typing out the hundreds of pages I have written in the small hours. It is with so much gratitude for the long years of friendship we have shared, and your kindness and efficiency in getting the deadlines together for me, for not only the writing of books but for all my endless magazine articles as well. For your kindness, your dear friendliness and your efficiency, and all your e-mails, I can never thank you enough!

To Phyllis Green, one of South Africa's top photographers, who manages miraculously to fit into her busy work schedule a Sunday afternoon's or a public holiday's flurry of photographs to catch up with what is in fruit or flower, my gratitude, my gratefulness and my admiration for your beautiful work knows no bounds. Through the years for so many of my books, you never tire of finding the plants, sometimes travelling great distances, and getting the perfect light and making so fabulous a portfolio of countless medicinal plants, fruits, vegetables and flowers and the rare specialised ones included. Thank you for making this book so special and so different.

To Lizette Jonker for her superb cover photograph and for the photographs used on the contents page – my huge appreciation of the hasty happy Sunday afternoon's urgent photoshoot! To Anton Ungerer for his expert scientific eye on the water section and his valuable input that has changed my thinking, my grateful thanks.

To Alicia Arntzen, for your inspired layout and design for yet another of my books, I am again so thankful for your expertise and creativity in putting so professional a touch onto each page. Thank you for being so big a part of this remarkable team.

To Sally Whines, thank you for your beautiful and inspiring cover design that invites investigation into this book's pages.

To Briza Publishers – I can never thank you enough for extending the deadlines, for being so accommodating, so kind and so considerate to all my unforeseen commitments, and for being so enthusiastic about a book such as this, which is fast becoming so much a way of life. Thank you for supporting my dedication to building wellness.

Finally last, but never least, to the many students at my Building Wellness classes over the last two decades or more, who urged me on to record all I was lecturing on and who changed their way of eating accordingly! It is through you and your questions that I offered more and more, culminating in this book. I hope that it will complement your notes on every lecture.

The charts for healthy eating on our restaurant walls are part of this book – the charts that have fascinated and become a way of life for so many visitors – and we thank the many hundreds of visitors for their interest and feedback on their breakthrough with healthy food that began with these charts. Here they are in book form – easy to use and even more inspiring, I hope.

It has taken a long time for this book to come to fruition and my fervent hope is that it will inspire you, the reader, to eat for health and to build wellness into every day of your life.

Introduction

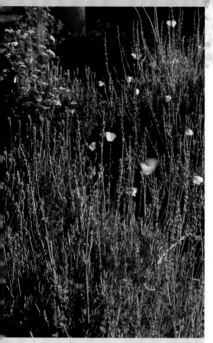

Over 2000 years ago Hippocrates wrote: 'Let your food be your medicine and your medicine be your food. Each one of the substances in a man's diet, acts upon his body and changes it in some way, and upon these changes his whole life depends, whether he be in health, in sickness or convalescent. To be sure, there can be little knowledge more necessary.'

Now, as never before, we have got to really think about these wise words for in our modern fast-paced, rushed, stressed, worry- and fear-filled lives, we are not coping and we are not glowing with that, the most precious state of all things – abundant health and well-being.

And building wellness is what this book is all about. What we are doing to our bodies with our dietary excesses, cravings and imbalances, is a leading cause of illness. Coronary disease, obesity, strokes, cancer, high blood pressure, cholesterol, diabetes, the list is endless, are all associated with the daily diet. What is more worrying is that we allow our children to indulge in the fizzy drinks, the endless sweets, the fast foods, the snack foods so laden with unhealthy fats, sugar, salt, flavourants, colourants and preservatives that they want nothing to do with anything fresh or health building.

I stand appalled in the queues at the tills in the supermarkets as in virtually every trolley I see no fruits or fresh vegetables, no basic health-building foods, but rather a trolley so laden with expensive convenience foods, pre-cooked, instant, tinned, bottled, fast foods. I hear the rudeness, the aggressiveness, the impatience, I see the obesity, the dull eyes, the spotty skin, the dank hair, the hyperactive, badly behaved children, the trolley piled with sweets, tubs of ice-creams, carbonated drinks – which are nothing but bottled 'poison' – and sugary cakes, jams, pies, and piles of red meats awaiting the fry-up and the braai-up, loads of artificially coloured, artificially flavoured, fast and instant foods, topped with boxes of sweetened custards, instant puddings and snacks, packets of refined sugar, piles of white bread and rolls, and I am even more shocked at the huge financial outlay such a trolley entails!

What are we doing to ourselves? What are we teaching our children, starting them off on instant milks, instant baby foods, instant sweetened everything? No wonder picky eaters are the order of the day and most children won't touch a piece of fruit or a fresh salad.

Slowly, far too slowly, with beautiful and inspiring cookbooks that offer so great a variety of home-cooked dishes, people are beginning to take notice, and there is sometimes a willingness to rethink, but often only after a serious diagnosis. A few, far too few, schools are starting to ban tins of carbonated drinks, bars of chocolate and sweets, crisps, snacks and fast foods in their school tuck shops and in the school lunch boxes, and stocking the tuck shops with more wholesome fare – home-baked breads and sandwiches, salads, fresh fruit and freshly squeezed fruit juices.

Each one of us needs to sit up and take notice with speed – there really is no time to be lost – and each one of us needs to take responsibility for our own health. No one can do it for us! Is life too frenetic now for us even to think? Are we just letting it all push us along in the great seething mass of unconscious acceptance? Or do we dig our heels in and say: 'STOP! – I want to change my direction!' We have to ask ourselves: Do I want to feel well, strong, positive, ready for anything? Do I want to get the best out of this life, feeling fit, looking good and knowing I can cope? Do I want to enjoy my spare time building fitness – going for energy-building walks, enjoying a swim or a jog or a run around the block? Do I want to feel good about my body, my life and my way of making things happen?

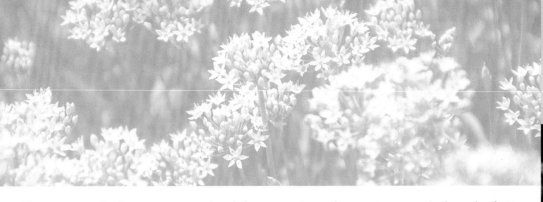

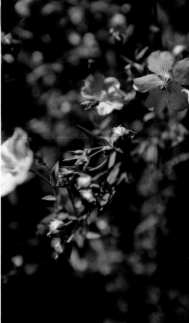

If you answer 'yes' to even a couple of these questions, the rest is easy, simple and effective. Change the way you eat, change the way you think about food, and change the way you shop! Best of all, even in a small way, *grow your own*! Read up everything you possibly can on growing and gardening the organic way. Make it a priority, become aware and ask questions! Start with my book *Companion Planting*, become aware of natural insecticides, become familiar with the garden fork and spade, start with a small patch, but *start*, and start today! We literally have not got time to procrastinate. We need to make the switch to organically grown fruit and vegetables with speed.

This is what this book is all about – just that. With every mouthful of fresh, delicious, organically grown food we can restore and strengthen our over-stressed, over-exhausted bodies. We can change our health around. We can make the greatest difference in our lives by merely changing the way we eat. With this simple step the rewards are so great, so far reaching and so valuable we will become so positive, so energetic, so strong and so well, we will be able to cope with everything, taking the changes and turning the obstacles into opportunities!

May this book be the start of the best days of your life!

Margaret Roberts

The Herbal Centre
De Wildt
North West Province
SOUTH AFRICA

e-mail: margaretroberts@lantic.net
www.margaretroberts.co.za

Healing Foods at a Glance

This first part of the book provides a bird's eye view of the 'superfoods' – the 'healing foods' that build health, restore vitality and help to prevent disease. At the same time, it points out the health hazards associated with many of the 'danger foods' we consume every day – the refined, over-processed, fat- and sugar-laden foods that drain our energy, pile on the kilograms and are often directly associated with life-threatening diseases such as cancer, diabetes, atherosclerosis, high blood pressure and high cholesterol.

The charts for healthy eating that are depicted on our restaurant walls also find a place in this section; they have been expanded and tell you in a nutshell which foods to eat and which foods to avoid to help you cope with, treat and prevent many of the common ailments that are the result of our fast-paced, stressed-out modern lifestyle.

This first part of the book concludes with a quick reference table to the healing foods that are covered in detail in the second part of the book. The table lists the major nutrients and main benefits of the more than 150 food plants that form the backbone of this book.

What are the danger foods?

These are the foods that have been so over-processed that they have little nutritional value left – all the goodness has been removed and replaced by high levels of saturated fats, sugar, salt, additives and preservatives. Danger foods have no health benefits at all – in fact, they are implicated in many modern lifestyle diseases. Below is a basic list of foods that all of us should eliminate from our diets. Note, however, that in the course of this book, and especially in the Ailment Chart at the back of the book, other foods may be listed as potential danger foods because they aggravate or promote certain diseases.

Avoid the following at all costs:

Refined carbohydrates (including white bread, white buns, cakes, sugary biscuits, sugary cereals); refined sugar; artificial sweeteners; sweets and chocolates; fast foods; snack foods; fried foods; processed cold meats; salty snacks and crisps; all processed foods; anything containing artificial colourants, flavourants or preservatives of any kind; tinned foods; long-life foods; sugary desserts; ice-creams; frozen desserts; tinned jams; tinned fruits in syrups; carbonated drinks and flavoured water; foods packaged in plastics and aluminium; instant sauces, instant custards, instant porridges, instant coffee, instant anything!

What are the superfoods?

These are the foods that are so high in nutrients – vitamins, minerals, antioxidants, complex carbohydrates, proteins and dietary fibre – that they actually benefit our health and well-being. Fresh vegetables, fruits and grains, unprocessed and raw wherever possible, need to form the backbone of our daily diet.

Note:

Only the main sources of vitamins and minerals are listed below. Please refer to the Quick Reference table starting on page 41 as well as the detailed descriptions of healing foods in the second part of this book for other sources of vitamins, minerals, antioxidants and the like.

Vitamins

Vitamin A

Vitamin A is a fat-soluble vitamin that is stored in the liver. It is available in two forms: retinol, which is obtained from animal sources or as carotenoids or carotenes (including beta-carotene), which are the yellow or orange pigments found in many plant foods, and which the body converts to vitamin A.

Vitamin A is essential for eye health; skin health; for bone and teeth building; it boosts the immune system; it maintains the health of the mucous membranes that line the respiratory, gastrointestinal and urinary tracts as well as the mucous membranes of the mouth, nose and throat. Vitamin A is a powerful antioxidant and may be helpful in preventing cancer of the lungs and cervix in women.

Deficiency symptoms include mouth ulcers; cracked, dry lips and sores; fever blisters; very dry skin; dry eyes that are sensitive to light; cystitis; thrush; not being able to see well at night.

> **Main Sources:** Apricots, asparagus, carrots, broccoli, peas, cabbage, kale, spinach, pumpkin, peaches, papayas, mangoes, tomatoes, watercress, sweet potatoes, eggs, beef and liver from organically raised cattle.

> ■ **Caution**
> Take care not to overdose! Vitamin A is stored in the liver and too much can overload the liver. Take vitamin A supplements only under your doctor's supervision.

Vitamin B-complex

The B vitamins are a group of water-soluble vitamins that must be replenished on a daily basis, as any excess is lost in the urine. Once thought to be a single vitamin, the B vitamins are actually a group of several distinct vitamins that are often found in the same foods and which work closely together to ensure the proper functioning of almost every process in the body. They play an important role in our metabolism, helping to convert carbohydrates into glucose; they promote growth and development; help to maintain healthy skin, nails and hair; are essential for the correct functioning of the nervous system and for proper digestion; they boost the immune system and reduce the risk of certain cancers and are essential for cardiovascular health.

> **Main Sources:** Avocados, lentils, dried beans, peas, chickpeas, the cabbage family, oats, nuts, sunflower seeds, brown rice, whole grains, leafy green vegetables.

Vitamin B1 (Thiamine)

Vitamin B1 is essential for mental efficiency and a feeling of well-being; it is needed for nerve cells to function normally and energy production (converting food into glucose for the body's cells to use).

> **Main Sources:** It is found particularly in wheat germ, wheat bran and brown rice.

Vitamin B2 (Riboflavin)

Vitamin B2 is essential for good vision, healthy skin; it helps to convert carbohydrates into glucose (the body's energy fuel). It colours the urine bright yellow.

> **Main Sources:** Eggs, milk and dairy products, lean meat, nuts, whole grains, green leafy vegetables.

Vitamin B3 (Niacin)

Vitamin B3 is essential for proper circulation and healthy skin; it helps to reduce cholesterol levels in the blood and is a memory-enhancer.

> **Main Sources:** Nuts and peanuts, lean meat and liver, wholegrain cereals, legumes, asparagus, seeds, milk, green leafy vegetables.

Vitamin B5 (Pantothenic Acid)

The 'anti-stress vitamin', vitamin B5 works with the adrenal glands which respond to stress and helps to maintain a healthy nervous system; it is also involved in cholesterol and hormone synthesis, a vital and complicated role.

> **Main Sources:** Available in most fruits and vegetables, meat, nuts, legumes and grains, it is easily destroyed by food processing and by deep freezing. Just think of how around 50% of it is lost in the milling of wheat and how the cooking of meat destroys 37%! This is one vitamin that may need to be taken in supplement form – your doctor will advise you.

Vitamin B6 (Pyridoxine)

Vitamin B6 helps to maintain a healthy nervous system. It also helps to process amino acids and to produce melatonin and serotonin; helps to alleviate carpal tunnel syndrome and morning sickness during pregnancy and eases premenstrual tension. A lack of vitamin B6 can cause depression.

Main Sources: Brewer's yeast, eggs, chicken, carrots, fish, liver, kidneys, peas, wheat germ, spinach, sunflower seeds, blackstrap molasses, nuts, bananas.

Vitamin B12 (Cobalamin)

Vitamin B12 helps iron to function effectively in the body; along with folic acid it regulates homocysteine levels (a product of the breakdown of an amino acid which, when occurring in excess, is associated with stroke, heart disease, Alzheimer's disease and osteoporosis). It also helps to maintain a healthy nervous system.

Main Sources: Meat, milk, fish and eggs.

Biotin

Biotin assists with the making of new cells, the synthesis of fatty acids, the metabolism of fats and proteins and it plays an important role in the release of energy from food; it also helps to maintain healthy hair, skin, nails, sweat glands and nerve cells.

Main Sources: Bananas, dairy products, eggs, whole grains, oats, beans, poultry, mushrooms, meat, brown rice, lentils, soya beans and fish.

Choline

Choline is essential for maintaining healthy cell membranes and cell function; it helps to break down dietary fats and so helps with weight control; it lowers cholesterol levels and prevents gallstones; it also plays a role in the maintenance of the nervous system, improves memory and learning and helps to fight infections.

Main Sources: Cabbage, cauliflower, whole grains, legumes, wheat germ, wheat grass, sprouts, fish, eggs, meats.

Folic Acid

Also known as folate, it is essential for regulating homocysteine levels, to prevent strokes, osteoporosis, heart disease, Alzheimer's disease and circulatory disorders. It is crucial during pregnancy as it regulates cell formation in the foetus and helps to prevent birth abnormalities such as cleft palate, spina bifida and mental disorders.

Main Sources: Asparagus, peas, split peas, lentils, chickpeas, broccoli, spinach, barley and barley grass, brown rice and Brussels sprouts.

■ Caution

Often some birth control pills as well as a diet high in saturated fats and refined carbohydrates can cause a deficiency in folic acid, so watch this carefully.

Inositol

Inositol helps to maintain healthy cell membranes, especially in the brain, bone marrow, eyes and intestines; promotes healthy hair and lustrous hair growth; lowers blood cholesterol levels and keeps the arteries supple; helps to control oestrogen levels and may prevent breast lumps.

Main Sources: Beans, melons, citrus fruits, whole grains (especially whole wheat), legumes (especially alfalfa), blackstrap molasses, nuts, meat (especially liver) and raisins.

PABA (Para-aminobenzoic Acid)

This B vitamin helps the body to break down and utilise protein; it plays a role in the formation of red blood cells and assists with the manufacture of folic acid in the intestines. PABA is used as an ingredient in sunscreen as it protects the skin against ultraviolet radiation and prevents skin cancer.

Main Sources: Dairy products, whole grains, meats, blackstrap molasses, mushrooms, green leafy vegetables, wheat germ.

Vitamin C (Ascorbic Acid)

This is an essential nutrient for strengthening the immune system and fighting infection; it also helps to build strong bones, teeth and gums and is a superb antioxidant. It clears pollution from the body; it is an excellent de-stressor; it protects against cancer, heart disease and constant colds and 'flu; it aids iron absorption and is valuable for healing wounds, grazes, scratches and for treating allergies.

Deficiency symptoms include fatigue, bruising easily with bruises forming after the slightest bump; tender gums that bleed easily after brushing the teeth; frequent nose bleeds; spotty skin, acne and pimples; kidney stones; frequent colds and 'flu; boils and throat infections.

Main Sources: Raw fruits, especially berries; broccoli; red peppers; oranges; lemons; naartjies; kumquats; sprouted seeds; green leafy vegetables like cabbage, kale and watercress; guavas, tomatoes; kiwifruit; peas; sweet potatoes.

Vitamin D

Vitamin D is essential for the development of healthy bones and teeth: it is necessary for the absorption of calcium and works with phosphorus to prevent bone loss. It also promotes healthy hair and nails; plays a role in fighting 'flu and colds, heart disease, diabetes and cancer; and it maintains and stabilises muscle strength in all ages; it is involved in cell reproduction, enhances the immune system and helps to regulate blood glucose levels.

A deficiency of vitamin D is common with ageing as the body's ability to synthesise and utilise it declines, and it declines further with each passing year.

Commonly known as the 'sunshine vitamin' we have been careful not to be out in the sun because we have been afraid of skin cancer, but a dose of early morning and late afternoon sun and lots of sun in winter whenever you can get out there is vital, especially for the over-sixty-year-olds.

Main Sources: Egg yolks, milk, yoghurt, butter, sardines, salmon, fish liver and fish oil, green vegetables, carob, almonds, sesame seeds, figs, hazelnuts, alfalfa. Spending a mere 15 minutes a day outside with sunlight falling directly on the skin helps the body make vitamin D.

■ Caution

Excessive amounts of vitamin D can result in headaches and kidney stones as well as increased levels of calcium and phosphorus, which are then excreted into the urine.

Vitamin E

This valuable vitamin plays a vital role in the cellular respiration of all the muscles and benefits the cardiovascular system, which increases endurance, strength and stamina. It can reduce the stickiness of the blood, thus preventing blood clots and it regulates the heartbeat. It is a powerful antioxidant. It raises the levels of 'good' HDL cholesterol and at the same time protects the LDL blood cholesterol from free radicals.

Main Sources: Whole grains, sunflower seeds, salmon, mackerel, eggs, avocados, green vegetables, wheat germ oil, pumpkin seeds, almonds, olives, oatmeal, sunflower and other plant-based cooking oils, hazelnuts.

■ Caution

Supplementing with vitamin E must be monitored by your doctor, as it can raise the blood pressure in some individuals and high doses interfere with iron absorption.

Vitamin K

Vitamin K is essential for bone formation and repair as it transports calcium, and also for blood clotting. It is absorbed from the upper intestinal tract with the action of the bile salts, and is also manufactured in the intestine by certain bacteria.

Main Sources: Dark green leafy vegetables, broccoli, Brussels sprouts, cauliflower, cabbage, lucerne and alfalfa sprouts, stinging nettle and asparagus.

■ Caution

Supplementing your diet with vitamin K must be done under your doctor's supervision as it can interfere with the actions of some blood thinners.

Minerals

Minerals occur naturally in the soil in the form of mineral salts. Plants take up the mineral salts through their roots and we obtain these minerals when we eat the plants or when we consume meat, milk or eggs from herbivorous (plant-eating) animals. Minerals are essential to maintain the right balance of fluids in the body; they play an important role in the formation of bones and blood and in healthy nerve function and they keep the muscles, including the heart, healthy and toned. We will only look at the main minerals here:

Calcium

Calcium is essential for the formation of strong bones and teeth and to keep the gums healthy. It also plays a role in regulating the heartbeat, muscle contraction and the transmission of nerve impulses. Our bodies contain about 1,2 kg of calcium and most of it stored in the skeleton. More than 90% of the calcium we take in is deposited in our bones.

A good intake of calcium is vital throughout life – not only is it essential for building strong bones in children but it is also extremely valuable for post-menopausal women, for those with aching arthritic joints, gout and stiffness and for the elderly when the bones start to thin.

Note that the body cannot absorb calcium without the correct dosage of magnesium (see below for sources of magnesium).

Main Sources: Milk and dairy products, eggs, salmon (with bones), sardines and pilchards, and many fruits and vegetables (see table below). The following table states the amount of calcium, in milligrams per 100 g for each of the foods listed. Dieticians urge us to include as many of these fruits and vegetables that we possibly can in our daily diet – and fresh and raw is always first choice!

Plant Source	Calcium (mg / 100 g)	Plant Source	Calcium (mg / 100 g)
Sesame seeds (unhulled)	1 150 mg	Radishes	120 mg
Sesame seeds (hulled)	1 100 mg	Sunflower seeds (hulled)	120 mg
Molasses (unrefined and dark)	684 mg	Beetroot leaves (cooked)	98 mg
Apricots	270 mg	Spinach leaves	92–100 mg
Kale leaves	249 mg	Swiss chard leaves	88 mg
Turnip leaves	248 mg	Endive leaves	85 mg
Almonds	234 mg	Green beans (cooked)	85 mg
Lucerne (fresh, green)	220 mg	Lentils	80 mg
Hazelnuts	208 mg	Lettuce (especially the dark outer leaves)	70 mg
Parsley	205 mg	Peas (cooked)	60 mg
Lucerne (alfalfa) sprouts	200 mg	Soya beans (cooked)	60 mg
Mustard leaves	183 mg	Olives	60 mg
Watercress	150 mg	Raisins (sun-dried)	60 mg
Dandelion leaves	150 mg	Cauliflower (raw)	58 mg

Chickpeas (cooked)	150 mg	Globe artichoke	50 mg
Figs (fresh)	150 mg	Leeks (cooked)	50 mg
Beans (dried)	135 mg	Cabbage leaves	49–52 mg
Pistachio nuts	130 mg	Broccoli	49 mg
Figs (dried)	126 mg	Carrots (raw, grated)	47 mg
Sunflower (seeds and sprouts)	125 mg	Sweet potatoes (cooked)	45 mg
Beetroot leaves (fresh)	120 mg	Oranges	43 mg
Buckwheat leaves (fresh)	120 mg	Squash and pumpkin (cooked)	40–50 mg
Chinese pak choi (raw)	120 mg	Cauliflower (cooked)	40 mg
Peas, young pods and vine tips (raw)	120 mg	Cashew nuts	38 mg

Sardines come in at 550 mg per 100 g!

Iron
Valuable as it carries oxygen from the lungs around the body, for strength, endurance and it boosts the immune system.

Main Sources: Lentils, eggs, chicken, dried beans, sun-dried apricots, figs, prunes, watercress, kale, stinging nettle, kelp and seaweed, parsley, beetroot, amaranth.

Magnesium
It works with calcium to form strong and healthy bones and teeth; it plays an important role in energy production; it prevents cardiovascular disease and helps to keep the arteries healthy; and it is a great calming, strengthening supplement to help disturbed sleep patterns, premenstrual tension, muscle weakness and twitching, and for giving us that get up and go!

Main Sources: Almonds, hazelnuts, millet, seaweed and kelp, sesame seeds, rocket, raw cacao, grapes, avocados, bananas, brown rice, watercress, kale, cabbage, alfalfa sprouts.

Phosphorus
Found in most foods, it is an essential part of every cell in the body and an important mineral for bone and teeth formation, blood clotting, normal heart rhythm, kidney function and to convert food into energy.

Main Sources: Whole grains, wheat and barley grass, millet, oats, sesame seeds, sunflower seeds, fish, poultry.

Potassium
Essential for a strong and healthy nervous system, a strong and regular heartbeat and blood pressure and it works smoothly with sodium to control the water balance of the body.

Main Sources: Whole grains, nuts, pumpkin and squash, nettles, dried peas and beans, apricots (fresh and sun-dried), avocados, dates, brown rice, figs (fresh and sun-dried), lentils, chickpeas, bananas.

Selenium
A valuable antioxidant that protects against ageing, cardiovascular disease and cancer; it works well with vitamin E to strengthen and maintain a healthy liver; it is excellent for healthy skin, hair, general growth, proper thyroid function, and is a valuable fertility supplement.

Main Sources: Asparagus, kelp, wheat germ, sardines, herring, Brazil nuts, broccoli, garlic, onions, whole grains.

Sodium

Sodium is vital for proper water balance in the body and for good muscle function. We all need to think about salt and be careful not to add table salt to our food, as an excess sodium can lead to high blood pressure, swelling, potassium deficiency and liver and kidney damage. Packaged and processed foods are laden with salt and we should avoid these and include the safer herbs and vegetables to ensure the balance of sodium in our bodies is correct. Instead of using salt for cooking, try herbs or a natural form of sodium (see also page 35).

Main Sources: Celery, kelp, cabbage, kale, fish, oats, barley, buckwheat, dried beans, garlic, turnips.

Avoid:

Stock cubes, salty snacks and crisps, ham and other processed meats, ketchups, tinned soups, smoked fish and meats, soy sauce, bacon, sausages.

Zinc

Boosts the immune system, keeps the skin clear, is essential for a healthy reproductive system and for fertility and to fight against free radicals.

Main Sources: Seaweed and kelp, wheat germ, chicken, brown rice, eggs, fish, pumpkin seeds, sesame seeds, poppy seeds, asparagus.

Antioxidants

These are natural compounds that protect the body against free radicals and the effects of oxidation. They include vitamins, flavonoids, amino acids and many other substances. Antioxidants are essential in the diet to protect the heart, provide natural resistance to disease, act as an anti-cancer buffer and keep our defence systems active.

Main Sources: Green tea, onions, apples, broccoli, spinach, carrots, garlic, blueberries, pomegranate, raspberries, lemons, grapefruit, tomatoes. Eat these foods often and raw!

What about the need for supplements?

Once, not such a long time ago, when the soil we grew our foods in was rich in natural nutrients and organic matter, all that we needed for our health was found within that food. I remember going with my father on Saturday afternoons to the local Portuguese vegetable growers who grew rows of glistening beautiful vegetables of every description with an orchard of unsprayed peaches, apricots and plums, to buy what our own productive vegetable garden did not have ripe or ready at that particular time. Everything was picked ripe and fully grown – no premature picking of green tomatoes or unripe avocados, which robs the fruit of essential nutrients. Everything was vine ripened, even their luscious grapes, pomegranates and tomatoes were unsprayed, ripened to perfection and packed with goodness. And what was even more charming, we were allowed to assist in the picking!

Today our fruit is grown on chemically fertilised, depleted soils, chemically sprayed, picked long before it is ripe, irradiated, put into cold storage, artificially ripened and packed in plastic and polystyrene. After a long journey to its final destination – the supermarket where it lies under artificial lighting, smothered in plastic – we can buy it! How can we hope to find all the vitamins and minerals we need for perfect health under such circumstances? Today we also battle to find safe and natural meat, eggs, dairy products, with all the hormones, antibiotics, preservatives and steroids that are pumped into everything. No wonder we are not nearly as well and as healthy as we should be!

Because it is so difficult to find reliable organic, free-range, untreated, natural and safe products, we seriously need to think about supplementing our diets with the nutrients – the vitamins and minerals – that are so lacking in our daily diets. Supplements in the form of vitamins and minerals and specific dietary recommendations, always taken under the supervision of a doctor, are needed in the following cases:

- We have become chronically ill or we are fighting cancer, autoimmune disease, heart disease, or other life-threatening diseases.
- We are over-stressed and exhausted and we have become worn out by excessive worry and anxiety.

- We are exposed to toxins at work or we live in a polluted area, such as the city centre with heavy traffic or in a smoke-filled atmosphere or near factories.
- We travel frequently by air.
- We are not thriving, not able to cope, when despair and depression engulf us and we lose the desire to live.
- Supplements are also useful for athletes who need extra stamina, the elderly who are ageing fast and becoming frail, children with poor appetites, very picky eaters or those who have food allergies.

These are just a few guidelines – there can be many other reasons why supplements are needed. Talk to your doctor.

■ Caution

Be vigilant about over-supplementation. Only take supplements after discussing it with your doctor or a qualified clinical nutritionist or dietician. Never just randomly pick off the pharmacy shelves whatever takes your fancy. Find the right supplements for your personal needs by talking to your doctor and pharmacist, and reading up and becoming informed and alert before you take supplements.

Tissue Salts

Tissue salts are a group of 12 minerals that should be present in the body, in perfect balance, to promote good health and well-being.

The 12 Tissue Salts at a glance

No. 1 – Calc. Fluor.: Elasticity; flexibility; toning; strength and resilience of muscular and connective tissue, bones, tooth enamel and walls of the blood vessels.

No. 2 – Calc. Phos.: A cell builder, tonic, growth developer and supporter. Maintains body functions and aids recuperation. It is needed for blood, connective tissue, teeth and bones.

No. 3 – Calc. Sulph.: Cleanser and blood purifier, it drains tissues and clears suppuration; an eliminator, it works particularly on the liver, blood and bile.

No. 4 – Ferrum Phos.: Oxygen transporter; anti-inflammatory; anti-haemorrhage; helps the formation of red blood corpuscles and strengthens the blood vessels.

No. 5 – Kali. Mur.: A superb tissue salt for children, specifically for childhood diseases; liver function; decongestant; anti-inflammatory; glandular tonic; blood and lymphatic conditioner; a digestive.

No. 6 – Kali. Phos.: A nerve nutrient and natural tranquilliser; lifts the mood and gives emotional balance; pain reliever; important for heart, brain tissue and intracellular fluid.

No. 7 – Kali. Sulph.: Works with Ferrum Phos. to transport oxygen to the cells; supports liver function; good for skin conditions like eczema; normalises and conditions the mucous membranes; clears mucus.

No. 8 – Mag. Phos.: Antispasmodic, natural pain reliever and muscle relaxant, it treats cramps, spasms, bladder stones and stress-related pains and tension.

No. 9 – Nat. Mur.: For heavy emotions, anger, depression, irritability; it also treats a runny nose, hay fever and all mucous membrane conditions.

No. 10 – Nat. Phos.: Antacid and natural acid–alkaline balancer, it treats digestive complaints, arthritic pains and stiffness. Generally this is a mood lifter, system neutraliser and a stress reliever.

No. 11 – Nat. Sulph.: Diuretic and toxin cleanser, it is a liver decongestant, and a regulator of body fluid in the whole metabolism.

No. 12 – Silica: Eliminates toxins from the tissues, clears suppuration, and expels foreign matter from the body; strengthens connective tissue; supports and sustains after excess stress and overwork; improves memory function and helps brain fog, stress, mental exhaustion, slow and difficult thought patterns and absentmindedness.

Note that silica will get rid of foreign objects in the body like splinters, plates, screws, implants and tubes – *so always discuss starting a home treatment with your doctor before you begin*. When in doubt leave out!

Tissue salts combined with herbs

The Margaret Roberts & Fithealth range of natural remedies combines tissue salts and herbs and are worth investigating. The remedies include:

Mood Lifter: Treats nervous conditions, mild depression and lowered vitality. Includes lemon balm, oats, pennywort (*Centella asiatica*) and Tissue Salts No. 2, 4, 6, 9 and 11.

Cope & Calm: Promotes general relaxation, soothes anxiety and assists in alleviating insomnia. Includes valerian root, lemon balm, chamomile and Tissue Salts No. 3, 6 and 12.

Easy Sleep: Promotes rest, relaxation and tranquil sleep. Includes valerian root, chamomile, hops and Tissue Salts No. 2, 4, 6, 8, 9 and 10.

Sinus & Hayfever: Assists in the treatment of sinus congestion, runny nose, sneezing, itching of the nose, postnasal drip, allergic rhinitis and hayfever. Includes Tissue Salts No. 7 and 9, violet, mullein, lemon and pantothenic acid.

Menopause: To alleviate the symptoms associated with menopause such as hot flushes, irritability, nervousness and insomnia; also effective for symptoms of pre-menstrual tension. Includes oat straw, liquorice root, raspberry leaf, sage, fenugreek seed, chamomile and Tissue Salts No. 4, 6, 7, 8 and 12.

Natural Antibiotic: Builds depleted immune systems and fight infections. Includes garlic, chickweed, mullein, burdock, wormwood and Tissue Salts No. 4 and 5.

Cholesterol Control: Treats elevated cholesterol levels. Includes barley grass and barley grains, fenugreek seed, hawthorn berry, parsley, psyllium husk, cayenne pepper and Tissue Salts No. 5 and 12.

Intestinal Cleanser: Cleanses and detoxes the intestinal system with a safe and natural laxative effect. Includes psyllium husk, *Cassia angustifolia*, cramp bark, dandelion root, slippery elm and Tissue Salts No. 4 and 6.

Pain: Assists in alleviating pain and fever associated with colds, inflamed wounds and joints, menstrual cramps, headaches and mild migraines. Includes white willow bark, catnip, feverfew, boneset, vervain and Tissue Salts No. 4, 6 and 8.

For more information, read *Tissue Salts for Healthy Living* (available from www.margaretroberts.co.za).

The following are basic lists of the most familiar foods in the day-to-day diet. I suggest you add in any other foods that you have found to be beneficial.

Pharmacological activity in common foods

Analgesic activity
Chillies (sweet peppers for sensitive stomachs), cinnamon, cloves, coffee, garlic, onions and leeks, ginger, peppermint and some mints like chocolate mint and apple mint.

Antibacterial activity
Apples, bananas, basil (especially 'tulsi' or sacred basil), beetroot, berries (especially blueberries, blackberries, cranberries), Bulgarian yoghurt, the cabbage family (cabbage, kale, broccoli, Brussels sprouts), carrots, celery, chillies (especially cayenne pepper and jalapeño), dill and dill seed, ginger, green tea, honey, horseradish, lemons and limes, linseed (flaxseed) and golden linseed, melons (including watermelon, spanspek and green melon), nutmeg, nuts (especially cashew, pecan and macadamia nuts), olives and olive leaves, the onion family (garlic, onions, spring onions, chives), papaya and papino, plums, radish, sage and thyme (added fresh to food and made into teas).

Anti-cancer activity
Asparagus, barley grains (also barley grass and wheat grass), berries (especially raspberries, strawberries, blackberries, blueberries), brinjal, brown rice, buckwheat, the cabbage family (cabbage, broccoli, kale, Brussels sprouts, cauliflower), carrots, celery, chillies, citrus fruit (especially lemons and limes), cucumber, fennel, fenugreek (fresh leaves and seeds), ginger, green tea, kiwifruit, lentils, mango, melons, mustard greens, oats, olive oil and olive leaves in a tea, the onion family (garlic, onions, chives, leeks), papaya and papino, parsley, parsnip, potatoes and sweet potatoes, pumpkins, squash and marrows, soya beans, thyme (especially fresh), tomatoes, turmeric, turnips and turnip leaves.

Anti-coagulant activity
Amaranth (fresh leaves and seeds), cinnamon powder, cumin seed, fenugreek (fresh leaves and seeds), garlic, onions and spring onions, ginger, grapes (especially red grapes), lettuce, melons and watermelon, rooibos tea and green tea (without sugar and milk), spinach and Swiss chard.

Antioxidant activity
Apricots, asparagus, avocado, beetroot, berries (especially blackberries, blueberries and raspberries), the cabbage family (cabbage, kale, Brussels sprouts, broccoli, cauliflower), carrots, chillies and sweet peppers, garlic and onions (especially red onions), ginger (especially in tea with honey and lemon), grapefruit (especially Star ruby and pink grapefruit juice), grapes (especially red and black grapes), green leafy vegetables (including lettuce, lucerne, watercress, sweet potato vine leaves, pumpkin vine tips and pumpkin courgette flowers), kiwifruit, loquats, oranges, kumquats, persimmons, nuts (especially Brazil nuts, pecan nuts, macadamias), pumpkin and squashes, sesame seeds, spinach, sweet potatoes (especially the yellow ones), tomatoes.

Antiviral activity

Apples, barley grains (make barley water, see recipe on page 135), barley grass and wheat grass juice, berries (especially blueberries, raspberries, cranberries and blackberries), coffee (but only 1 cup of filter coffee per day), dandelion greens, dill and fennel (fresh leaves and seeds), garlic, onions and spring onions, ginger, gooseberries, grapefruit, kumquats, limes, lemons and oranges, grapes (especially red grapes), green tea, linseed (flaxseed), peaches and nectarines, pineapple, plums.

Cholesterol-lowering activity

Almonds, apple, avocado, barley water, green barley grass and barley grains, beans (kidney, haricot, butter and broad beans), beetroot, brown rice, carrots, chickpeas, garlic, onions and spring onions, grapefruit, oats and oat straw tea, olive oil and olive leaf tea, soya beans, walnuts.

Calming sedative activity

Almonds, aniseed, cabbage, broccoli and kale, celery and celery seed, chamomile, cloves, cumin, fennel, garlic and onions, ginger, honey, lettuce, mango, marjoram, mint, oats, parsley, potatoes, sage, watercress.

Combating arthritis, gout and sore joints

Debilitating and painful, arthritis and gout are an inflammation of the joints. Diet plays a major role, both in the cause and treatment of the inflammation, and one of the most effective treatments is to eliminate meat, fish and dairy products entirely from the diet.

The superfoods

Vegetables: Cabbage, carrots, celery, chicory, dandelion, fennel, globe artichoke, Jerusalem artichoke, leeks, nettles, olives, onion, parsley, radish, sweet potatoes, turnips.

Fruit: Apples, bananas, cherries, gooseberries, grapes, lemons, melons, pears, pineapple, plums, raspberries, strawberries.

Grains: Brown rice, buckwheat, millet, rye.

Nuts and seeds: Alfalfa sprouts, mung bean sprouts, sesame seeds, sunflower seeds, walnuts.

The danger foods

Potatoes, brinjals, peppers, chillies and paprika, dairy, wheat, oats, eggs, refined white flour, sugar, processed foods, yeast and meat extracts, chicken, beef, pork, tea and coffee, especially instant coffee, white bread, chocolate, carbonated drinks, especially cola drinks, sardines, mussels, anchovies, herrings, caviar.

These foods are dangerous because they contain purines, which increase uric acid within the body and worsen the pain, heat and swelling of the joints. Make a note of any foods that have agreed with you and those that have not, and eliminate the latter from your diet.

Other recommendations

Drink at least 6 glasses of water spread throughout the day. This is a daily must – the water helps to flush the uric acid from the body and maintains kidney health. Also drink 1 glass of water daily with 2 teaspoons of apple cider vinegar in it.

Building strong bones

Osteoporosis, or thinning of the bones, is a very real problem as the bones become weakened, more fragile and easily fractured. It affects a high percentage of usually post-menopausal women but also a high percentage of men, and the whole skeleton system can be affected. It is something we need to become aware of and look after ourselves accordingly.

This is what we need to look out for:

- High stress levels, especially chronic, continuous stress.
- Lack of, or poor quality sleep.
- Lack of exercise, especially weight-bearing exercise.
- Medications and supplements we are on.
- Early menopause, hormone replacement therapy and hysterectomy.
- What we eat and drink – junk food eats away bone, especially carbonated drinks; how much sugar and saturated and trans fats we consume; how much caffeine and alcohol we take in; a high-protein diet is a risk too; salt is another culprit – too much salt interferes with calcium, preventing the body from assimilating it.

- Chronic dieting, especially fad diets, and whether we are very underweight.
- Poor childhood eating habits.
- How acidic our bodies are.
- Smoking, even passive smoking.
- Not getting enough sun, which is essential for the production of vitamin D. Fear of skin cancer is keeping many of us indoors – wear thin cotton shirts and a hat and go for a daily early morning or late afternoon walk!

The superfoods

Foods rich in calcium – see the list on page 14. Also important is magnesium, which mobilises calcium. For this we need look no further than green leafy vegetables (see also the list on page 14) as well as foods rich in vitamins D and K (see pages 13 and 14).

Vegetables: Beans (fresh and green), broccoli, buckwheat, cabbage, carrots, celeriac, celery, dandelion leaves, green lucerne and alfalfa sprouts, kale, lettuce, oats, rocket, sweet potatoes, turnip greens, watercress.

Fruit: Apples, apricots, figs, oranges, papaya, pineapple, strawberries.

Nuts and seeds: Almonds, hazelnuts, linseed (flaxseed), macadamia nuts, millet, pumpkin seeds, sesame seeds, sunflower seeds. Also pulses – chickpeas, dried beans of all types, lentils, soya beans (always pre-soak dried pulses, discard the water and cook in fresh water).

The danger foods

Avoid sugar, salt, caffeine, alcohol, processed meats (especially ham, sausages and bacon), cakes, sweets and chocolate. Don't eat too much meat. Avoid rhubarb, cranberries, sour plums and spinach as these contain oxalates that can bind calcium.

Other recommendations

Vitamin D and boron are valuable supplements if there is not enough sunlight in the winter months. Get into the sunlight 30 minutes a day! Sunbathing in winter is beneficial.

Talk to your doctor about whether you need supplements: manganese and magnesium, vitamin B12 as it builds bone health, vitamin K and folic acid. If you have coeliac disease or take antidepressants and certain medications, you may need supplements. Discuss this with your doctor.

Do weight-bearing exercise: take daily walks and try skipping, jogging, yoga and aerobics.

Use natural progesterone cream from wild yam to slow down bone loss.

Building brain power

Stress and worry and a changing world take so much from us that we fear we are not coping and often doubt our very actions. We wonder if we are taking leave of our senses – we seem to be unable to think clearly. We seem equally unable to concentrate: dealing with so many external and far too intense stimuli, crisis management and just too much of everything causes our brains to all but shut down! Well, now is the time to really rethink our way of living. We need to look at what we are running around for and what we can eliminate from this over-busy, brain-addling mode of living. Let's start with food!

The danger foods

Without a doubt we need to look carefully at eliminating quick fixes like cups of coffee, tea, sugar, sugary cakes, chocolates, sweets, instant snacks, the all too easily available fast foods, carbonated drinks, alcohol and smoking, which we imagine calms our nerves but which, in the long term, only adds to our distress by harming our health.

Cutting down on red meat and saturated fats and changing to fish and chicken is a valuable step. Wherever possible, look out for organically raised free-range poultry and eggs, vegetables and fruit, and start including lentils, dried beans, peas and nuts in the diet to replace meat a couple of times a week.

The superfoods

Know that every mouthful you take of a superfood will nourish the brain.

Sprouts

Topping the list are sprouts like alfalfa, mung beans, sunflower seeds, buckwheat and flaxseed. Sprouts are packed with vitamins, minerals and enzymes that literally feed the brain cells and sprinkled over salads, stir-fries, grills and bakes are extremely valuable for brain nourishment. See also page 27.

Herb teas

Replace that caffeine fix with herb teas: Pour 1 cup of boiling water over ¼ cup fresh leaves or sprigs of the herb of your choice. Stand 5 minutes, strain and sip slowly. Add a touch of honey and/or a squeeze of lemon juice or a slice of lemon.

Pennywort (*Centella asiatica*) is one of the most valuable herb teas to include in the daily diet. Excellent for exam-time stress and anxiety, and a revitalising, anti-ageing and medicinal herb of note, each one of us needs to include one cup daily of this really amazing herb. It grows easily in both sun and shade and in pots and makes a very undemanding groundcover.

Other herbs to try are rosemary, lemongrass or peppermint. All are brain boosters that focus and stimulate the mind and aid our concentration. Students find peppermint tea excellent for exam-time stress and brain fog.

> ### ■ Caution
> All herbs are strong, effective and powerful. Therefore, 10 days of taking a specific herb is enough, then give it a break for 2–3 days, then resume for another 10 days and give it that important break of 2–3 days before repeating the cycle.

Other brain-boosting foods

Include the following foods in the diet frequently:

- Chickpeas are an almost perfect food – they contain a perfect balance of minerals and protein to stimulate the brain (see also page 99).
- Lentils assist with poor memory, are rich in vitamin B-complex and vitamin C and will help with concentration (see also page 139).
- Millet is a real 'super grain'. An almost complete protein (it contains 8 of the 9 essential amino acids), it unclogs the arteries and helps with concentration. Combine it with a legume – think chickpeas or lentils! – for a complete protein food.
- Broccoli is superb as a capillary toner; it literally gets the circulation moving and provides the spark a sluggish brain needs.
- Sesame seeds are rich in vitamins and minerals and a true get-up-and-go food. Sprinkle them on everything, they will kick-start a lethargic brain into action.
- Oats porridge (not the instant kind but the large-flake, slow-cooked type) with 2 tablespoons milled flaxseed, sesame seeds, almonds, sunflower seeds, pumpkin seeds added, served with soaked seedless raisins, finely chopped pecan nuts or walnuts, is a real superfood for the brain. Mixed with plain Bulgarian yoghurt, a mashed banana and a touch of honey, you have a kick-start to the day that will keep you firing on all cylinders for hours!
- Wheat grass and barley grass are an exceptional brain-boosting, energising and anti-ageing food. I simply cannot do without my daily tot of wheat grass juice. Grow your own wheat and barley grass (see page 29) for a steady supply and juice daily for a brainpower boost.

Body and Mind Turbo Boost

Serves 1

Drink this magic brew daily and you *will* feel the difference. It is literally a turbo boost to the whole body and gives you a sparkling mind. Use a juicer (not a liquidiser) that has a spiral action processor. (I use the Oscar juicer and have never had a moment's trouble even after constant years of use.)

2–3 cups fresh wheat grass and barley grass
2 organically grown apples if possible, or peel the apples (choose hard, crisp apples for the most juice)
2 cups fresh lucerne sprigs (flowers can also be included)
2 organically grown carrots
1 cup fresh parsley
2 sticks celery with leaves

Push through a juice extractor and serve immediately. You can also add fresh beetroot and 1 cup of sprouts.

- Lucerne is alfalfa sprouts in grown-up form and it is packed with vitamins, minerals and enzymes. The young, tender succulent sprigs are delicious in salads and so valuable as a brain tonic we literally need to sit up and take notice. Research indicated that students given fresh lucerne in the daily salad showed increased concentration.
- The daily salad is something we cannot neglect – it is a true superfood for the mentally fatigued. Include the following foods in your daily salad wherever possible (always fresh and organically grown!): alfalfa sprouts; fresh lucerne sprigs; watercress; chopped pineapple; green and red peppers, finely chopped; walnuts or pecan nuts; chickpeas; lettuce; thinly shredded radishes; grated carrots; avocado; sesame seeds; lemon juice; olive oil; a grinding of black pepper and sea salt or Himalayan rock salt. Add other vegetables in season. This is a meal on its own and you will come to crave it.

- Bread is a daily staple, but let rye bread replace white or brown bread, rolls and croissants. Best of all, learn to bake your own bread with brain-boosting sesame seeds, sunflower seeds, flaxseed and pecan nuts added to your home-baked loaf (see also page 35).
- Mental fatigue and brain fog is very often a result of dehydration. To aid concentration and to get those brain cells working, drink plenty of water throughout the day. Just plain water – no juices, no carbonated drinks and no energy drinks! The experts suggest drinking around 6 glasses throughout the day. Keep a jug at your desk or in a place where you can see it frequently (out of sight is so often out of mind!) – sipping even half a glass at intervals will boost those brain cells.
- Tissue Salts No. 2, 6, 11 and 12 are useful to help concentration and clear thinking and to assist in the development of a more positive mental state. Suck 2 tablets of each 3–6 times a day.

Calming children naturally

What is happening to us? Are we creating a bunch of uncontrollable, noisy, impossible little monsters? Why do one in five children today suffer from behavioural problems, ADD, hyperactivity or learning difficulties? Is the age of technology impacting on our children's development and well-being? Have we gone too far? Yes we have. Our children are showing us this in temper tantrums, bad behaviour, aggression and 'heightened alertness'. Cell phones and the flickering screens of TVs and computers keep their developing minds too taut and strained. Researchers are finding growing evidence that cell phones may deplete and suppress the sleep hormone melatonin, and computer games are now proving to be detrimental to a child's development. So let's look at a handful of ways to bring a little balance into the lives of our children.

Food for children

Go back to the basics: lots of fresh fruit, salads, sprouts and vegetables. There should be an absolute minimum intake of 5 fresh fruits and vegetables daily, although 8 are better and 10 are better still. Ideally eat from your own garden – grow your own vegetables, fruit and herbs organically. If this is not feasible, choose organic produce wherever you can. Don't allow fast foods, sugary or salty snack foods, sweets or chocolates.

Cook nourishing stews, soups and casseroles, not in the microwave and without using instant flavourings from packets or bottles. Banish all 'instant' products from the diet of the whole family and reduce salt intake by using herbs like basil, thyme, oregano, coriander and celery to replace some salt (see also page 35).

Get rid of sugar and any foods that contain added sugar. Sugar is one of the modern world's greatest downfalls and winds children up. Dates, raisins, nuts and dried fruit can replace chocolates and sweets, and fresh fruit juices should completely replace fizzy drinks. Don't have bowls of sugar around. Rather use small quantities of honey to sweeten drinks and dishes. And get to know stevia (see page 197). Avoid sugary store-bought cereals and replace with healthy oatmeal porridge (not the instant kind) or make your own muesli.

Wholesome Muesli

8–10 servings

This delicious mixture can be stored safely in the fridge in a sealed container for quick nourishing breakfasts. Ring the changes by adding sliced strawberries, blueberries, banana or papaya. This is like Tiger's milk – it will sustain your child for the day!

4 cups Tiger oats (the large-flake, non-instant kind in the blue box)
2 cups chopped pecan nuts and almonds or cashew nuts (not peanuts as these can start an allergy)
1–2 cups seedless raisins or sultanas (always choose sun-dried fruit)
½ cup sesame seeds
½ cup sunflower seeds
1 cup chopped dried apple rings, or better still add a fresh peeled grated apple as you serve it

Mix everything together and keep in an airtight container in the fridge. Serve with warm milk, plain Bulgarian yoghurt and a dribble of honey.

Energy drinks, carbonated drinks and flavoured water are literally poison for your child! Invest in a juice extractor and juice fresh fruit and vegetables daily. Encourage your children to drink water abundantly. Have jugs of plain, filtered water around and aim at four or five glasses a day. Keep jugs of diluted unsweetened fruit juice in the fridge or fill individual juice bottles with your own juices from your juice extractor. Use a liquidiser or blender to make smoothies for your children and teach them about the goodness in fruit and vegetables. Here are a couple of recipes to try:

Super Smoothie

Serves 1

Sustaining and calming, children will love this delicious smoothie.

½–¾ cup plain Bulgarian yoghurt
a dash of fresh apple juice (about ½ a cup)
1 teaspoon honey

1 banana
½ teaspoon cinnamon

Whirl everything together in a liquidiser and serve at lunchtime or as a mid-afternoon snack.

Health-building 'Jungle Juice'

Serves 1

This vitamin and mineral-rich drink can become a calming ritual to set children up for the school day or give them fuel for the afternoon's activities.

2 carrots, peeled and roughly sliced
1 stick celery
1 medium-sized fresh beetroot peeled and quartered OR
2 handfuls of wheat grass and barley grass to make it a real health booster

1 apple, peeled and cored
1–2 sprigs parsley
½ peeled pineapple

Push through a juice extractor and serve immediately.

Change the fruit and vegetables frequently to keep the child interested, for example carrots, pineapple and peach OR carrots, papaya and apples OR carrots, mango and melon. Children will soon find their favourite combination.

Have a selection of healthy, calming snacks on hand. Homemade cheese straws, thyme fritters or sweetmilk cheese squares are so much more nourishing than crisps or salty snacks. Have bowls of pecan nuts, almonds, sunflower seeds and pumpkin seeds around for easy nibbling. Dried apple rings, dried mango strips, raisins, sultanas, strawberries, kiwifruit and dates will satisfy the sweet tooth. Sun-dry your own fruit (see box) or invest in a home dehydrator to make dried apple rings, peach slices, dried strawberries – the list is endless and they are all chewy and delicious.

Drying Your Own Fruit

Drying fruit when they are in season is easy and very rewarding. Try cored and peeled apples cut into rings, pineapple slices, sliced strawberries, peaches cut into quarters, grapes cut in half and pips removed, apricots halved and pips removed, or sliced figs. Or try making guava or fig rolls. Spread the fruit on stainless steel trays in the sun and cover with a net to keep the insects and the birds away. Turn them frequently to ensure even drying and bring the trays in at night. After 2–3 days the fruit should be dry. Pack into large screw-top jars with greaseproof paper between the layers to keep them form sticking together. I have invested in a dryer and it is always filled with delectable fruits of all kinds, even kiwifruit and star fruit. Loquats remain chewy and litchis are truly delicious. Experiment for taste – for by doing your own drying you'll know they are wholesome with no preservatives, colourants, flavourants, stabilisers or added sugars.

In addition to implementing the above dietary principles and practices, consider too the importance of sitting together at the table as a family and eating healthy, happy meals together. Food is our best medicine. We have to change and change what our children eat. There is no time to lose!

Herbs to calm

The following are simple herb teas that will soothe and calm a restless child. Fresh fruit juice can be added to make the teas more interesting.

Melissa

Melissa, also known as lemon balm, is an amazing herb. It has a refreshing lemon flavour and makes a delicious tea that can be cooled and added to fresh fruit juices. It calms, lowers blood pressure, relieves stress and anxiety, lifts tearful moods, calms tempers and soothes indigestion and colic, especially in children and even tiny babies. It relieves heartburn, quietens hyperactivity, eases panic attacks, nervous irritability, despair, fear and nervousness, and is excellent for 'flu with muscular aches, restless legs, growing pains and headaches. Melissa is safe for tiny babies and little children. This is one herb no mother should ever be without.

> ### Melissa Tea
>
> Pour 1 cup of boiling water over ¼ cup of fresh melissa leaves and sprigs, allow it to stand for 5 minutes and strain. To ease colic give a teaspoon at a time (warm) to a baby every 2–5 minutes. Give ½ a cup to a child from 1 year onwards. Add a tablespoon (or 2 or 3) to the baby's bottle and give ¼ of a cup to babies under 1 at any time. They take teaspoons of warmed tea quite happily.

Chamomile

Chamomile (*Matricaria recutita*) is a much-loved, calming herb that has been used since the 14th century. Chamomile is soothing and acts like a natural aspirin in the body for a feverish cold and for tension, headaches and restlessness. It is worth growing your own and it does well in the cooler months. I love to use fresh chamomile flowers, but as it is a quick annual I dry my organically grown chamomile for summer use. Never be without it, this is a superbly helpful herb.

> ### Chamomile Tea
>
> To make chamomile tea, add 1 tablespoon of flowers to 1 cup of boiling water, let it stand for 5 minutes, strain and add the cooled tea to juice or bottles for babies. In the case of hyperactivity, anxiety and insomnia, ¼ cup of chamomile tea immediately calms and soothes the restless child, and babies easily take teaspoons at a time.

Herbs for bath time

I grow rose-scented geranium and lavender under the bedroom windows. To make soothing, calming additions of these herbs for the bedtime bath, fill a large bowl with 4 cups of fresh leaves and sprigs of rose geranium (do the same with lavender flowers and leafy sprigs using *Lavandula intermedia* var. *Margaret Roberts*, as I have found this variety safest for the skin). Pour at least 2 litres of boiling water over the herbs. Leave this to cool, then strain and add it to the bath. Alternatively you can tie a bunch of fresh sprigs of either rose geranium or lavender in a cotton cloth and hang it under the hot water tap. Let the hot water release the soothing oils and use the whole bundle with soap to wash yourself.

Like chamomile and melissa, rose petals are soothing and calming. These herbs all make beautiful soaps and bath additions. Use them fresh, organically grown and frequently in the bath to soothe and calm that restless little child.

Tissue salts

I call these precious minerals 'coping salts'! I could not have raised my three very active children and managed my own busy life without the calming influence of these easy-to-take minerals. Get to know them. There are 12 and they are available from your pharmacy (see also page 17).

For erratic wild behaviour I recommend No. 1, No. 2 and No. 6. One tablet of each sucked every 2 hours, or even every hour, will soon settle and calm an unruly child.

No. 6 is excellent for hyperactivity, autism, dyslexia, anxiety and frenetic behaviour and can be safely taken daily. It is a natural tranquilliser and one tablet of No. 6 taken even 3 times a day – sucked, not just swallowed – will have a wonderfully soothing effect on the child. By the way, No. 6 also helps with night terrors, tearfulness, tempers, insomnia and bad moods!

Take one tablet of No. 6 and one of No. 8, for prolonged stress, burnout, hyperactivity, and for lack of concentration (and take some yourself to help you cope!).

For bedwetting and nightmares take No. 8 with No. 2 and No. 12, and for restless sleep Numbers 2, 4, 6, 8 and 10 are a wonderfully soothing combination and can be crushed and mixed into warm milk.

No. 2 is a superb salt for children who cannot follow the teacher at school, who lose concentration and who show moody anger and aggressiveness, and with No. 8 you will see a quieter happier and more tolerant child. The usual dose is to suck one tablet 3 times a day.

Other recommendations

Remove all electronic equipment from your child's bedroom, especially cell phones, TVs, computers and computer games. Line curtains with light-blocking fabric to create an atmosphere of quiet and peace. Should your child fear the dark, find a soft night light for the passage.

Create a bedtime ritual. Sit with your child in the dark and say prayers together quietly. At bedtime play soft classical music with a beat slower than a heartbeat. Remember and sing the lullabies your grandparents sang to you.

Read your child a story at the end of each day, in a quiet calm voice, choosing stories that are uplifting, encouraging and have happy endings. Find a book of poetry and let your child experience the beauty of words. Take your child to the library, share books with friends and help them build up their own libraries.

Talk to your child. Always reassure your child calmly and lovingly. Make eye contact, touch and stroke your child, hold him and smooth his hair, tell him you love him. Share information that is peaceful and happy. Encourage your child to tell you about her day.

Share family meals in quiet and peace with no TV, radio or shouting. Share family history, stories and ideas.

Preventing cancer

Our lives have become frenetic. The pace we live in daily runs us ragged. Life deals blows, shocks in ever-increasing waves, becoming almost too much to bear. Fast living, fast foods, microwaves, cell phones and computers all add to the relentless pace, and we all become candidates for the dread diseases. We need to stop and rethink our way of life! Let's look at creating peace and calm – even a small measure of it. Take up tai chi or yoga, listen to gentle music, and change the way you eat and how you think. There is no time to lose!

The superfoods

Vegetables: Asparagus, beetroot, cabbage family, carrots, endives, garlic, horseradish, lettuce, mustard, potatoes (baked), radishes, sweet peppers (all colours), sweet potatoes, turnips and turnip tops, watercress.

Fruit: All citrus fruits, all the berries, apples, apricots, fruit salad plant, peaches, persimmons, spanspek.

Grains and pulses: All the beans (butter beans, haricot beans, hyacinth beans and jugo beans), barley grass, brown rice, buckwheat, chickpeas, lentils, millet, wheat grass and whole wheat.

Seeds and nuts: Almonds, hazelnuts, macadamia nuts, pecans, sesame seeds, sunflower seeds, walnuts.

Herbs and spices: Chamomile, cloves, fennel, parsley, rosemary, sage, tarragon, thyme, violets, ginger.

The danger foods

Animal protein (because most meat today is contaminated with chemicals, hormones, tenderisers, antibiotics, even pesticide residues); char-grilled steaks and barbequed meats that have been burned at the edges; processed, smoked and salted meats like bacon, ham and salami; pickles; coal tar dyes in foods; chemical colourants such as tartrazine; stabilisers; emulsifiers; artificial flavourants; rancid fats and oils; anything mouldy (beware of stored peanuts and rancid nuts and mould on the nuts); saturated fats; refined sugar; artificial sweeteners; alcohol; caffeine; carbonated drinks. Beware of over-heated oils that burn the food, and coated, non-stick pans.

Other recommendations

Eat raw foods in abundance – salads and fruit salads should be a mainstay of your diet.
Wheat grass juice or barley grass juice with carrot, celery, beetroot, parsley, apple, is a *daily must have* – enough to fill at least ½ a glass (see also page 29).

Speak to your doctor about a vitamin and mineral supplement: vitamin A + beta-carotene, vitamin C, vitamin E, selenium and coenzyme Q10.

Convalescence

If you are recovering from a long and serious illness or from fatigue, shock, grief, major surgery, fighting against viral and bacterial infection or need to restore a weakened immune system, this should be mandatory.

The superfoods

Vegetables: Asparagus, avocados, barley, beetroot (always fresh), buckwheat leaves, carrots, celery, garlic, green beans, lettuce (home-grown if possible), millet, oats, onions and spring onions, parsnips, pumpkin and squash, spinach and Swiss chard, sprouts (sprout your own alfalfa, chickpea, buckwheat and mung bean seeds), su-su, tomatoes (home-grown if possible), turnips and turnip greens.

Fruit: Apples, apricots, blackberries, dates, kiwifruit, lemons, mangoes, melons, oranges, pineapple, raspberries.

Herbs and spices: Cinnamon, echinacea, fenugreek, mint, parsley, rosemary, sage, thyme.

Nuts and seeds: Almonds, chestnuts, sesame seeds.

Other foods: Plain Bulgarian yoghurt, free-range eggs, free-range chicken, homemade vegetable soups with lentils, home-baked brown bread (see recipe on page 38), chickpeas, dried beans, daily salads and fruit salads, wheat and barley grass juice (see page 29).

The danger foods

Sugar, sugar, sugar – avoid it in every way; fried foods, fast foods, instant foods, especially instant soups, sauces, custards and breakfast cereals. Replace sugar with fresh or dried stevia (not stevia powder) or a little honey. Replace instant cereals with oats porridge (the non-instant, large flake kind – like Tiger Oats, in the blue box), sprinkled with this special ground seed mix. Serve with plain Bulgarian yoghurt and a touch of honey or chopped dates.

Ground Seed Mix

Place small quantities of almonds, sesame seeds, sunflower seeds, pumpkin seeds and flaxseed in a seed grinder and grind into a powder. Store in a screw-top jar in the fridge and sprinkle onto the oats porridge (about 1–2 tablespoons, and mix it in well).

Dealing with digestive ailments

It has been said, over the ages, that 'correct eating is the best treatment for all digestive problems'! We cannot hope to ease heartburn, digestive discomfort, flatulence, burning colic, tummy rumblings, nausea, dyspepsia, chronic constipation, irritable bowel syndrome, even diarrhoea, unless we look carefully at what we often so thoughtlessly stuff into our mouths. We constantly assault our digestive systems with junk food – no wonder we no longer know what it feels like to be truly well and full of life! To get back to that point, we need to look carefully at the following superfoods and eliminate all the junk from our diets.

The superfoods

Vegetables: Barley, buckwheat, carrots, celery, chicory, dandelion, globe artichokes, maize, millet, oats, potatoes, rye, spinach, stinging nettles, sweet potatoes.

Fruit: Apples, bananas, blackberries, grapes, lemons, mangoes, melons, papaya and papino, pears, pineapple, raspberries.

Hint

Prunes are excellent for constipation. Take 5–7 prunes and soak them in warm water overnight. The next morning, eat these along with the water in which they were soaked, with yoghurt and papaya.

Seeds and nuts: Almonds, flaxseed, sesame seeds, sunflower seeds, walnuts.

Herbs: Anise, caraway, chamomile, cumin, dill, fennel, melissa, peppermint, spearmint. These herbs can all be made into a soothing tea by using ¼ cup fresh herb, or 1–2 teaspoons seeds, pour over this 1 cup of boiling water, stand 5 minutes, strain and sip slowly.

Other foods: Brown rice, extra virgin olive oil, plain Bulgarian yoghurt, spices like cinnamon, cardamom, allspice, cassia, nutmeg and ginger.

The danger foods

Banish coffee, tea, fizzy drinks, refined sugar and refined white flour from your diet. Replace white bread with rye bread and learn to bake your own brown bread (see recipe on page 38). Red meats and processed meats (especially pork, ham, bacon and salami), hamburgers, pâtés and meat pies are often the culprits. Eliminate these too.

Avoid acidic foods such as pickles, relishes, vinegars, olives in vinegar, even orange juice, oranges and grapefruit; also avoid artificial flavourings and colourants, preservatives, stabilisers, monosodium glutamate, fried foods, fast foods and all foods high in fat, including chips, pastries, cakes, doughnuts, packets of crisps and cheesy snacks.

One of the worst culprits for digestive problems is alcohol – even a sip of wine can upset everything! So avoid all alcoholic drinks as well as all carbonated drinks. Replace with a glass of water with a slice of lemon in it. Lemon is a traditional gastric treatment.

Digestive Ease Seeds

Mix together 1 teaspoon each of caraway seed, anise seed, fennel seed, dill seed and celery seed. Keep in a little tin in your pocket and take a pinch of these precious seeds every now and then to ease digestive tension. Chew them slowly or add 1 teaspoon to a cup of boiling water, stand 5 minutes, strain and sip slowly.

Fighting fatigue and loss of energy

Is life going too fast? Are you too tired to cope? Do you go to bed tired and wake up tired? Feel like you are not catching up with anything? A change in diet can reverse these symptoms amazingly!

Note

Firstly establish that there is no serious underlying illness or chronic fatigue syndrome (see page 218) causing this debilitating lack of energy, and that it is not just a string of late nights, not enough sleep or the simple need for a break or too much stress and tension that is sapping your energy.

The superfoods

Vegetables: Asparagus, beetroot, broccoli, cabbage, carrots, celery, chickpeas, chicory and endive, dandelion, horseradish, kale, lentils, lettuce, onions, soya, spinach, stinging nettle, Swiss chard, tomatoes.

Fruit: Apples, apricots (fresh and sun-dried), bananas (eat with honey and cinnamon), blackberries, dates, figs (fresh and sun-dried), grapes, lemons, oranges, peaches, pears, plums, raspberries, strawberries.

Grains: Barley grass, buckwheat, maize, millet, oats, wheat sprouts, wheat grass.

Nuts and seeds: Almonds (as a snack these are invaluable), flaxseed, pecan nuts, pumpkin seeds, sesame seeds, sunflower seeds, walnuts.

Herbs: Basil, coriander, fenugreek, lemongrass, marjoram, mint (also peppermint), oregano, parsley, red clover, rosemary, sage, thyme.

A Note on Herbal Teas

Make your favourite herb into a refreshing tea by pouring 1 cup of boiling water over ¼ cup fresh herb. Stand 5 minutes, strain and sip slowly. Sweeten, if liked, with a touch of honey.

Note that it is always best to use one herb at a time. Only take 1 cup of a specific herb a day, but have lots of different ones throughout the day.

These herb teas are refreshing and revitalising and are available fresh from your garden:

- *Lemongrass is an energy booster and a superb digestive.*
- *Marjoram is an excellent muscle tension reducer and digestive.*
- *Mint is a tension releaser and helps to unwind and give back lost stamina.*
- *Parsley is a superb detoxifier and a good diuretic.*
- *Rosemary is for clear thinking and vitality.*
- *Sage clears sore throats and promotes memory retention and clear thinking.*
- *Thyme is an antiviral, antibacterial cleansing herb.*

Other energy-giving foods: Barley grass juice, wheat grass juice, cinnamon, fresh stevia for sweetening, sprouted seeds – alfalfa, mung beans and wheat especially.

Sprouting your own seeds

Very close to being the perfect food, fresh organic sprouts are packed with energy, vitamins, minerals, amino acids and enzymes and are a literal life force! Favourites are mung beans, alfalfa (lucerne), buckwheat, linseed (flaxseed), chickpeas, fenugreek, red clover, lentils, sunflower seeds, wheat, mustard and cress. Sprinkle them over salads, stir-fries, grills and open sandwiches.

Set up trays of wet cotton wool sprinkled with seeds and kept moist, or large Ball jars with a muslin square over the mouth held in place by an elastic band, ¼ filled with seeds that can be rinsed and drained by shaking the jar and turning it upside down at least twice a day. It is worth buying a sprouting kit, consisting of small, stacked draining trays, available at health shops. Search out organic seeds available at health shops or order from the Margaret Roberts Herbal Centre – we can post anywhere.

The danger foods

Eliminate all of the following from the diet: refined carbohydrates, including white sugar, white bread, biscuits, cakes and anything made with white flour; sweets, chocolates and ice-cream; instant foods – instant coffee, instant puddings, instant commercial breakfast cereals (these can interfere with the absorption of several minerals, including iron and magnesium); all processed foods, salty snacks and crisps.

Avoid caffeine in any form, as it inhibits the uptake of iron. Caffeine is present in tea, coffee, chocolate, chocolate drinks, cola drinks as well as the so-called high-energy drinks.

Steer clear of alcohol – it is more destructive of nutrients to the brain and to the liver than any other substance!

Avoid all carbonated drinks, all sports drinks, all energy drinks, all tinned drinks. These are all exceptionally high in sugar. Replace with water.

Quick Energy Boost

If the need for something sweet is paramount, these are the natural sugars that stop that shaky feeling: dates, dried apple rings, cashew nuts, almonds, pecan nuts, sunflower seeds, raisins.

Or try the following recipe, which I have taught for many years and which can be adjusted, changed and even added to, and this is where things can become interesting:

In a liquidiser whiz:

1 peeled and quartered apple	2 small bananas
½ cup almonds	1 dessert spoon wheat germ flakes
1 cup grape juice	2 teaspoons honey
a handful of alfalfa sprouts, and very importantly,	1–2 teaspoons of powdered cinnamon

Drink it down slowly and you'll literally feel the burst of energy. Add any of the fruits and nuts or sprouts from the lists above to make your own 'rocket fuel'.

Other recommendations

No matter how desperate you are for a chocolate fix, don't! The sugar boost is short lived and drops you down deeper into the spiral of chronic fatigue. Have energy-boosting snacks on hand like almonds, cashew nuts, walnuts, sunflower seeds, pumpkin seeds, sun-dried fruits and so on (avoid salted peanuts).

Eat regularly, choose high-quality foods – including lots of salads – and become familiar with the glycaemic index (see page 29) to make sure you include foods that release their energy slowly in every meal.

Drink energy-building herb teas like mint tea, rosemary tea, lemongrass tea and rooibos tea with lemon and a touch of honey.

Raw food should be a major part of your diet. The daily salad is essential – become creative. Set up a small salad garden for daily pickings: beetroot, cherry tomatoes, spinach, lettuces of all kinds, radishes, watercress in flooded pots in late winter, turnips (baby turnips are delicious, grated fresh into salads, as are the young and tender leaves), spring onions, and so on. Fresh lemon juice with a little olive oil should be the only dressing.

Keep a lunch box of fresh fruits, home-baked (if possible) whole-wheat or rye bread, sandwiches with tomatoes and salad leaves and plain low-fat cream cheese spread on them.

An energy-boosting snack that you'll begin to love is cooked chickpeas with a touch of salt and chopped fresh mint that has been mixed into a little apple cider vinegar or fresh lemon juice.

Grind up a seed mix in a grinder for sprinkling onto oats or millet porridge for breakfast (see also page 26).

Sprout your own seeds, including alfalfa, buckwheat, sunflower, chickpea, green pea and mung bean sprouts (see page 27).

Grow your own wheat grass and barley grass for smoothies and home-pressed juices like wheat grass and barley grass with fresh carrots, beetroot, celery, parsley and apple.

Try to drink at least 6 glasses of water, just plain water, throughout the day.

Avoid all commercial high-energy drinks, which are high in glucose and caffeine. They give a quick boost, followed by a sudden and dramatic let down that leaves one feeling as though the plug had been pulled out. Replace these with wheat grass juice and carrot juice.

Speak to your doctor about a good daily multivitamin supplement.

The glycaemic index

To reduce the amount of sugar and refined carbohydrates in our diet this list will be of great benefit – the higher the count the less we should consume:

White bread	100	Couscous	61
Mealie meal	100	Baked beans	60
Weet Bix	100	Sweetcorn	60
Puffed wheat	100	Ryvita	59
Cornflakes	100	Haricot beans	59
Puffed rice	100	Basmati rice	58
Baked potato	100	Bananas	55
Mashed potato	100	Papaya	55
Honey	100	Mango	55
Sugar	100	Melons	55
Dates	99	All deciduous fruits like apples, pears, plums and all citrus fruits	55
Cooked carrots	85	Whole-wheat bread with seed toppings or seeds added into the dough	55
Instant rice	85	All Bran flakes	54
Doughnuts	85	Pro Nutro	54
Instant oats	85	Raw peas	48
Rice cakes	81	Raw carrots	48
White rice	80	Oats (whole)	47
Boiled potato	80	Sweet potato	46
Pumpkin	75	Chickpeas	46
Potato chips (deep-fried)	75	Lentils	46
Baby potatoes, boiled with skins	70	Whole-wheat pasta	40
Bran muffins	70	Fructose	22
Brown rice	66	Barley	22
Green peas	65	Soya beans	21
Beetroot	64		

The Wonders of Wheat and Barley Grass

In order to reap the full potential of these two superfoods they can be grown in organic compost-filled trays. The seeds are soaked for about an hour, then are sprinkled over the surface of the moist compost and covered with a light layer of compost and kept moist. At this stage keep them out of full sun and never let them dry out. Within 3 to 4 days (or 5 to 6 days in winter), the little sprouts will begin to grow. Let them develop and pull them up any time after they are 2 cm high. You can eat the whole seedling in salads, in stir-fries, sprinkled over grills and sandwiches, or you can let your wheat grass grow and cut it for juicing.

Wheat grass sprouts are an antioxidant powerhouse and a potent anti-ageing food; they also increase stamina and endurance quickly and effectively, and have become a favourite health food virtually all over the world.

Barley grass can be grown the same way as the wheat grass and a juice extractor becomes one of the most important pieces of equipment you could ever possess. Try one of these pick-me-ups the next time your energy flags:

In a juice extractor push through:

1 cup of alfalfa sprouts or 2 cups of lucerne greens　　　　*2 cups of buckwheat sprouts, leaves or flowers*
2 cups pineapple chunks　　　　*1 cup celery*
2 apples, peeled and quartered　　　　*2 cups of fresh wheat grass*
2 cups of fresh barley grass　　　　*add ½ cup water if it's too thick*

Sip slowly. This serves 1 and during exam times or times of intense stress this will provide an instant energy burst.

A quick and easy wheat and barley grass drink for everyday is just this:

In a juice extractor push through 1 carrot, 1 beetroot, 1 peeled apple (or any other fruit of your choice – try pineapple, strawberries, raspberries, peach or plum), 1 stick celery and a handful or two of wheat or barley grass. Drink it right away.

Protecting your heart and circulation

The heart is a muscle that pumps about 10 000 litres of blood around the body per day in its complex circulatory system. By making changes to our diet to assist this vital organ, we can improve and maintain heart health considerably. Become familiar with the superfoods and even more familiar with the danger foods. It is up to you to make the difference.

The superfoods

Vegetables: Barley, broccoli, buckwheat, cabbage, carrots, celery, chicory, chillies, garlic, globe artichoke, green peppers, leeks, oats, onions, potatoes, pumpkin and squash, tomatoes, turnips, watercress.

Fruit: Apples, cherries, grapes, lemons, melons, pineapple, plums.

Nuts, seeds and pulses: All dried beans, almonds, chickpeas, sesame seeds, sunflower seeds, walnuts.

Herbs: Chervil, coriander, dandelion, fenugreek, marjoram, thyme.

Other foods: Olive oil, oily fish like mackerel and sardines, sprouts (see page 27), wheat grass and barley grass juice (see page 29).

The danger foods

Cut out saturated fats: trim meat of all fat; avoid animal-based fats like lard, processed meats, salami, ham, sausages, meat pies, pastries, tinned meats, bacon, fast foods, fried chips, burgers and hard margarines (they contain hydrogenated fats, which are linked to cancer, heart disease and obesity). Use butter and margarine spreads sparingly. Replace high-fat cheese with cottage cheese. Eat eggs only twice a week.

Avoid caffeine – coffee, tea, chocolate, cola drinks, sports drinks and high-energy drinks – as well as excess alcohol. Research suggests that a small glass of red wine occasionally may actually benefit the heart. More than that will definitely *not* benefit your health and think of how that small indulgence could over-burden the liver!

Refined sugar (sucrose) actually raises cholesterol levels and blood pressure in some people. Sweets, chocolates, cakes, biscuits and sugary drinks are a serious danger to the heart and are linked to atherosclerosis. A small amount of unrefined sugar (brown sugar or blackstrap molasses) and honey, which have beneficial trace elements, can be taken occasionally. Better still, get to know and to grow stevia and use it fresh or dried.

Excess salt is dangerous and a known cause of raised blood pressure. Avoid crisps, salted nuts, salty and deep-fried snacks, stock cubes, commercial pickles, chutneys and condiments, processed meats, tinned foods, and put away the saltshaker. Replace table salt with your own herb mixes like celery, oregano, thyme, coriander, fenugreek, caraway seeds. Dry and store in a grinder, grind over food to lessen the salt. Make your own pickles and chutneys.

> ■ **Caution**
> Polyunsaturated fats eaten in excess without sufficient vitamin E can endanger the heart.

Building the immune system

The most intricate of all the systems in the body, the immune system is locked in continuous battle against great armies of viruses, bacteria, pathogens, poisons and pollutants. The battle rages constantly and by watching our diets we can assist the body in the fight. Correct eating, good supplements, lessening the sugar and managing stress, is a good start!

The superfoods

Vegetables: Artichokes, asparagus, avocado, beetroot (leaves included), cabbage family (dark green leaves included, and especially broccoli), carrots, celery, chillies and sweet peppers, dandelion, garlic, horseradish, nettles, onions and leeks, pumpkins, soya beans (green), spinach, sweet potatoes, turnips and their leaves, watercress.

Fruit: Apples, apricots, bananas, citrus fruits, dates, figs, kiwifruit, papaya and papino, pears, pineapple, raspberries, strawberries.

Herbs and spices: Caraway, chives and garlic chives, cinnamon, echinacea, elderberry, fenugreek, ginger, parsley, peppermint, rosemary, sage, thyme.

Nuts, seeds and pulses: Alfalfa sprouts, almonds, cashew nuts, hazelnuts, lentils, mung bean sprouts, pumpkin seeds, sesame seeds, sunflower seeds, walnuts.

Grains: Barley, brown rice, buckwheat, millet, oats, wheat (whole-wheat).

The danger foods

Avoid tea, coffee, sweetened carbonated drinks, sugar in all its many forms, white bread, cakes, sweets, biscuits, sweet snacks, any refined carbohydrates, alcohol in any form, instant commercial breakfast cereals (these can interfere with the absorption of several minerals like iron and magnesium) and all processed and instant foods.

Replace with *fresh*, raw foods wherever possible – choose from the list of superfoods above and also include smoothies and juices like wheat grass and barley grass with fresh carrots, beetroot, celery, parsley and apples (see also page 29).

Try to drink at least 6 glasses of water, just plain water, throughout the day.

Relief from respiratory ailments

Both acute and chronic coughs, colds, 'flu, bronchitis, sinusitis, sore throats, earache, blocked nose, asthma, hay fever, catarrh, even emphysema can be eased by concentrating on eliminating mucus-producing foods, learning deep breathing exercises, opening up rooms that are badly ventilated, avoiding polluted, smoke-filled areas and by sleeping in a well-aired space. A stuffy, stagnant atmosphere affects the mucous membranes of the nose, throat and sinuses, making it a perfect breeding-ground for bacteria. The good news is that eating with care, and drinking lots of water, can change any of the above ailments with astonishing results.

The superfoods

Vegetables: Asparagus, barley grass, black-eyed beans, cabbage, carrots, celery, fennel, garlic, horseradish, kale, leeks, lettuce, onions, peas, radishes, turnips, watercress, wheat grass.

Fruit: Apples, blackberries, dates, figs, lemons, pineapple, raspberries, rose hips.

Herbs and spices: Aniseed, cayenne pepper, chervil, cloves, echinacea, elderflower and elderberry, fenugreek leaves and seeds, ginger, mint, oregano, parsley, rosemary, sage, thyme, turmeric.

Danger foods

Dairy products, sugar, chocolate, ice-cream, pastries, cakes, sugary buns, biscuits, jams, syrups, pork sausages, pies, sugary and carbonated drinks, white flour, anything containing artificial colourings and flavourants, anything with preservatives (these are particularly harmful to people with asthma and hay fever), salty snacks, crisps, fast foods, tea, coffee (especially instant coffee).

Other recommendations

Replace tea, coffee, hot chocolate drinks and carbonated, sugary drinks with lots of plain water or a tea made with thinly sliced fresh ginger with lemon and a touch of honey.

Simply steamed or raw salads and fruits and simply cooked foods are vital in keeping the respiratory system in good working order.

Take regular long walks with deep breathing in a clean atmosphere far from busy roads.

If you eliminate dairy products, except plain Bulgarian yoghurt, talk to your doctor about supplementing calcium and vitamin D.

Facing up to skin problems

The all-embracing words 'skin problems' include eczema, psoriasis, acne, oily skin, extra dry skin, pimples, rashes, blackheads and large pores. Junk food, so beloved by teenagers, will aggravate skin problems, as will stress, anxiety, environmental pollution, lack of exercise, menstruation, menopause, and even pregnancy.

The superfoods

Vegetables: Avocado, beetroot, broccoli, carrots, celery, chickpeas, chicory, cucumber, dandelion, kale, lettuce, lucerne, mung beans, nettle, peas, spinach, sweet peppers, watercress.

Fruit: Apricots, blackberries, grapes, kiwifruit, lemons, melon, nectarines, oranges, papaya, peaches, pineapple, plums, prunes, strawberries, watermelon.

Nuts, seeds and grains: Barley grass, buckwheat, millet, oats, pumpkin seeds, rye, sprouted seeds, walnuts, wheat grass.

Herbs: Basil, fennel, parsley, thyme.

The danger foods

Stay away from chocolates, sweets, chips, fast foods, cakes, biscuits, rolls, sugary buns, carbonated sweet drinks, instant coffee, sugar in any form! Cut down on alcohol, dairy products, meat and animal fats. Instant coffee, even filter coffee, has over 60 different chemicals, none of which will do any good to the skin!

Other recommendations

The best favour you can do for your skin is to drink plenty of good fresh water – at least six glasses a day! In one of those glasses mix in 2 teaspoons of apple cider vinegar and sip it slowly.

Deep and careful cleansing is vital daily – there are many hints for homemade face masks, toners, and cleansers in the second part of this book – take a look at apricot, oats, lemon, kiwifruit, elder, quince and papaya to mention but a few.

Be sure the bowel works well daily (see also page 221) and work out a good menu using the superfoods.

Let's look at sugar

We all know sugar is a danger food, but we keep craving it. It is an addiction, we have come to realise, but we still want it, buy it and have a 'need' for it! This is what sugar does to our bodies:

- It causes lack of energy, fatigue and loss of purpose. It is one of the main causes of anxiety, depression, despair and a sense of hopelessness.
- It compromises the immune system – frequent 'flu, coughs and colds are a clear sign of this.
- It is one of the causes of nasal congestion, sinus attacks and hay fever and it increases the severity of asthma attacks.
- It makes our bodies excessively acidic, which affects everything!
- It interferes with our ability to concentrate, heightens hyperactivity, bad behaviour and restlessness in children *and* in adults, it triggers emotional outbursts, crying fits, temper tantrums and dare we say it, rudeness, road rage and short fuses!
- It easily sends a child into a state of confusion, unable to concentrate or focus or even listen! (Do a few tests to prove this if you are in any doubt!)
- Sugar is a contributing cause of heart disease, it raises cholesterol levels and it is considered to be a carcinogen.
- It is a common cause of migraines (one of the worst culprits is carbonated sugary drinks) and it affects the eyes – weakening the eyesight and the ability to adjust to strong light.
- It interferes with the digestive processes and increases the severity and level of discomfort of bowel disease (Crohn's disease is one serious example), stomach ulcers and gallstones.
- It interferes with the body's ability to process calcium and magnesium, so it could be said that it contributes to osteoporosis. It certainly affects the joints, contributing to arthritis and stiffness.
- It feeds yeast infections like candida, and is one of the main causes of tooth decay.
- It speeds up the ageing process and is a major cause of obesity.

What, you may well ask, are we to do then?

Get to know and use stevia, it is the best sugar substitute there is (see also page 197). I grow it in more and more abundance – and being 'Mrs Natural' I don't use the processed stevia powders, tablets, syrups or liquids, only the fresh or dried leaves. Stevia is perfectly safe for diabetics and children. Please *do not* substitute with artificial sweeteners – be wary of chemically processed sweeteners of any kind.

A New Danger Food: High Fructose Corn Syrup

'Corn syrup', as it was known long ago, is a glucose syrup derived from 'corn' (maize). Widely used as a sweetener in prepared foods in the food industry, it consists mainly of glucose but has maltose, dextrins and water added. It is listed as 'cariogenic', which means it causes tooth cavities.

A new addition to the ever-growing list of sweeteners is 'high fructose corn syrup', often listed as HFCS on food labels. It is basically a corn syrup that has undergone processing to convert some of the glucose into fructose to produce an intensely sweet taste. Stable and easy to use, it retains moisture, does not crystallise and blends beautifully when mixed with other glucoses and synthetic chemical sweeteners! It is also cheaper to use, so today's manufacturers of processed foods are thrilled with it and use it in everything from sauces to dips, ice-creams and custards to ketchup, soft drinks and juices to jams, sweets to salad dressings, the list goes on and on! In fact, it is even to be found in savoury spreads and fast foods.

But the news is not good for consumers. Until recently, fructose was considered to be 'safer' for diabetics, satisfying the sweet tooth and not as harmful as sugar. We were assured that it could even be beneficial to the diabetic! However, today's research finds this to be completely the opposite. Highly processed fructose is metabolised into fat in the liver whereas glucose does not metabolise into fat, and high fructose corn syrup is believed to induce insulin resistance and high levels of fat in the liver. It is implicated in many health problems and even life-threatening diseases: it is believed to alter the magnesium balance, which in turn makes the bones porous and fragile; it is blamed for increased rates of obesity and diabetes; it raises both the blood pressure and blood cholesterol, which increases the risk of a heart attack. Where does it end?

So read the labels and avoid corn syrup and especially high fructose corn syrup. This is a dangerous addition to the diet and for the diabetic it is pure poison. Shun all processed foods, fast foods and packaged foods, as you can be sure high fructose corn syrup is among the list of ingredients!

Let's get to know fats and oils

Fats and oils in some form are needed by the body to build and maintain wellness, but not all fats are created equal. So let us distinguish the good from the bad!

The 'good' fats

Monounsaturated fatty acids

These protect against heart disease, give flexibility to aching joints and, interestingly, they do not increase the weight.

Main Sources: Olive oil, especially extra virgin olive oil; sunflower seeds; avocados; cashews; peanuts and peanut oil (these come with a caution as a serious allergen!); pistachios; pumpkin seeds; walnuts and walnut oil; canola oil.

Polyunsaturated fatty acids

These are the good fats, *but* once the oils are heated the high temperature transforms them into toxic trans fats. So using cooking oil to fry and re-fry food is not good!

Main Sources: Soya oil; organic unheated sunflower oil and grape seed oil are the best (interestingly, grape seed oil is the least likely to form trans fats); flaxseed oil; sunflower seeds; sesame oil; oily fish.

Omega-3 fatty acids

They are polyunsaturated and have beneficial properties in reducing the risk of heart disease and strokes; treating inflammatory ailments like arthritis; improving the skin, hair and nails; and lowering high blood pressure.

Deficiency symptoms include vision impairment, abnormal thirst, dry skin and hair, acne, migraine, excessive earwax and stiff joints.

Main Sources: Oily fish like mackerel, sardines, trout, salmon, tuna, anchovy, herring, as well as white fish; flaxseed and flaxseed oil; leafy green vegetables like spinach, lettuce, cabbage, broccoli and kale, cauliflower leaves, rape leaves, chicory and endive leaves, dandelion leaves; beetroot; whole wheat, sprouted wheat and wheat grass juice; nuts, especially walnuts, almonds and macadamias; pumpkin seeds.

The 'bad' fats

Saturated fatty acids

These fats raise the level of 'bad' cholesterol in the blood – the LDL cholesterol – which in turn increases the risk of heart disease. Linked to both heart disease and cancer (cancer of the small intestine, as well as breast, colorectal, prostate and ovarian cancer), we should have these only occasionally and our milk should be low fat or fat free.

> **Main Sources:** Red meat and animal fat: pork, beef, mutton, especially fried fatty meat; dairy products: full cream milk, butter, cream, cream cheese, hard cheeses; vegetable shortening; palm kernel oil.

Omega-6 fatty acids

These are polyunsaturated fats, but you need to eat twice the quantity of omega-3 fat to reap the benefit of these fats.

> **Main Sources:** Sunflower and soya cooking oils, mayonnaises, meats, margarines, salad dressings, fried chips, hamburgers, pastries, peanuts, poultry, sesame oil.

Trans fats

Also called hydrogenated fats, trans fats are made by a chemical process during which a liquid fat (like vegetable oil) is converted into a solid fat. It is widely used in the food manufacturing industry because it has a high melting point, a creamy, smooth texture and can be reused several times for deep-frying; these fats improve the taste and extend the shelf life of processed foods. No wonder food manufacturers love them! They are bad news for consumers though: there is a strong link between trans fats and heart disease, cancer and obesity. One more reason to avoid processed and fast foods at all costs!

> **Main Sources:** Processed foods, fast foods, meats, pastries, doughnuts, bought biscuits, blocks of margarine, deep-fried foods, re-used cooking oil, and perhaps the worst is chips, deep-fried and saturated in oil.

Let's look at salt

Probably the world's most treasured taste from the beginning of time, salt is obtained from the sea, or from salt lakes fed by inland brine springs, or from underground seams of rock salt which need to be mined. Prehistoric communities established their domain around salt lakes and the earliest of records showed salt to be a precious commodity. Sodium chloride – a white crystalline powder or flake or crystal – became a treasure so great the voyages of discovery began with salt as the greatest prize. The first great classical writers like Pliny the Elder, Herodotus and Hippocrates wrote about the precious brine springs, the salt rivers, the salt lakes, and to this day salt remains our favourite taste, even more than sugar!

Our ancestors quickly learned to use salt as a preservative, especially for meat, and salt pickling was the preferred method to store food for the winter. Salt is a stable inorganic mineral and can be stored indefinitely but it does absorb moisture in damp weather. In humid, damp climates a few grains of rice added to the salt will help to keep it dry.

The different types of salt

Sea salt contains sodium, magnesium and calcium and is made by the evaporation of seawater. Also sometimes known as bay salt, it is gathered from the edges of flat pans as the tide goes out and the evaporation of seawater leaves an easy-to-gather crusty edge of salt crystals. One of the most loved sea salts comes from Maldon, in Essex, England, where the beautifully white salt flakes are still packed and exported all over the world.

South Africa's own Khoisan salt is dried at St Helena Bay on the West Coast through a unique seawater filter made of shell beds, which adds calcium to its other trace minerals. Natural, unrefined with the flavour of pure unpolluted seawater, this salt is fast becoming a local favourite.

Sea salt needs to be well sealed and stored in airtight containers and can be crushed in a mortar or ground in a pepper grinder if the crystals are large. Sea salt is considered to have a saltier taste than rock salt, so a little goes a long way. Look out for non-iodated sea salt at health shops or from our kitchens at the Herbal Centre.

Kitchen salt is the finely milled or sometimes fairly coarse milled free-running salt. It usually has magnesium carbonate or aluminium added to it to aid the flow of the salt. These fine-milled salts are the most easily found salt on the supermarket shelf but can also be found in bricks or blocks or unrefined in huge blocks at farmers' co-ops for cattle licks. Refined salts consist of mainly sodium, so look for coarse, unrefined salts and crush as you need them.

Himalayan salt crystals are an incredibly ancient rock salt, 250 million years old, and contain many of the trace elements that are needed by the body to maintain a perfect balance and which build up vitality, reduce exhaustion and mental fatigue, and are so needed for the stress-filled lives we lead. It has an intense flavour and a little goes a long way.

Kosher salt has the same levels of sodium that most salts have, but it is a highly purified salt that forms large crystals. 'Kosher' is a term that confirms a food or substance is accepted by Jewish dietary laws, so this salt will only be found in specific food shops or delicatessens.

Black lava sea salt is a specialised, almost black salt that can be found occasionally in specialist shops. Also high in sodium but with a different flavour, it is possibly from a source of sea salt where volcanic lava cools into the sea and the salt crystals form on it. Not much is known about it, but for the gourmet cook the search should be interesting.

A word of caution
Salt has a downside in that those suffering from high blood pressure, even mild hypertension, or fluid retention have been warned by their doctors to reduce or even delete the salt in their diets. The dietary blueprint for people suffering from hypertension states:

3–4 servings grains (for example wholegrain bread, brown rice, whole-wheat pasta)
4 servings vegetables (especially leafy greens)
4 servings fruit (especially apples and berries)
1–2 servings low fat dairy (for example Bulgarian yoghurt)
Only 1 serving low fat meat or poultry
And all salt free (replace salt with fresh lemon juice, herbs or a homemade salt substitute – see recipe)

Salt-Free Flavouring

Use your own organically grown herbs wherever possible.

2 tablespoons dried thyme	*2 tablespoons coriander seed*
2 tablespoons celery seed	*2 tablespoons cumin seed*
1 tablespoon caraway seed	*1 tablespoon oregano leaves*
1–2 tablespoons black peppercorns	
2 tablespoons lemon zest (from the Caffea lime, if you have it, or from any organically grown lemon)	

Mix well. Crush in a mortar or grind in a pepper grinder and use lavishly over savoury dishes.

Let's look at bread

Bread making is not just for the experts – it is a fascinating and worthwhile real labour of love to bake your own bread, and everyone benefits. 'I haven't got the time' is what I hear everyone say, but just give a thought to what goes into the bread we live on, our daily bread, and become familiar with stabilisers, preservatives, 'long life' additives, anti-caking agents, and so on, and then consider the plain, pure ingredients that go into your own loaf, and that has to be a good thing!

When my children were small I baked two loaves of whole-wheat brown bread every day. It was part of my very full and very busy daily workload. I ran a huge pottery and craft studio as well as a vegetable garden on an isolated farm, and the children's school was many kilometres away, so every minute counted. Yet I got so organised with my simple farm loaves it just became part of my daily routine, like feeding the chickens and watering the vegetable garden.

The secret is to have a warm place in which to let the dough rise, and this, on a cold winter morning, was in the warming drawer of my stove, the tins on a tray, well covered with oiled greaseproof paper and then carefully wrapped with kitchen towels and a thick old woven cotton tablecloth. I learned early on how long the dough took to rise to the top of the tin so that I could quickly pop it into the hot awaiting oven. On a summer morning I took it out to the warm stone steps outside the kitchen door and tucked its towels and the old tablecloth snugly around it, allowing the morning sun to warm it to its required height in the tins.

As the children grew bigger, three loaves were needed as all the school lunch boxes were filled with sandwiches made from these loaves, and today, looking back on it, I can still feel the satisfaction of knowing my family was well fed from our organically home-grown wheat milled at the nearby mill, butter and cheese made from our Friesland cows' rich milk and tomatoes and lettuce grown in my organic vegetable garden.

Basic ingredients

High-gluten flours

White bread flour is available at most supermarkets, and brown bread flour is there too. These have extra gluten in them for the added stretch in kneading. Additives are present in most flours to prolong their shelf life, but for beginners these flours are worth experimenting with. Some health shops stock pure flours and if you are lucky enough to live near a mill, as I was, you can still today buy a pure freshly ground flour. I found brown bread flour to be my best, and *Nutty Wheat* added to white bread flour also made a good loaf.

Whole-wheat flour, sometimes called wholemeal flour or *Nutty Wheat*, contains bran and wheat germ and is milled from the whole-wheat kernel. This is the most nutritious of breads and has a nutty, coarser, denser texture. The bran inhibits the action of the gluten and so it will take longer to rise or can be mixed half and half with brown bread flour.

Brown bread flour is lighter than whole-wheat flour and rises faster, and other flours like white bread flour or rye flour can be added. It has gluten in it and it kneads well and forms a good base to which other flours can be added. Keep a bread-baking notebook, for this will become a fascinating record of the mixtures you bake and their keeping qualities.

Refined white flour has the valuable wheat kernel and the bran and the wheat germ removed. So a true health loaf is based on brown flour with whole-wheat flour added and is infinitely better for our health.

Low-gluten flours

As more and more people find they are gluten intolerant or can only digest low-gluten flours, this list will become important and worth experimenting with.

Rye flour is most often mixed with other flours (check the labels when you shop for rye bread: it will state 50% rye flour with 50% wheat flour, etc.). On its own in a 100% rye loaf it inhibits gluten development. It has a strong and distinctive flavour and for arthritic and rheumatic ailments rye bread is really the only bread to eat.

Spelt flour – an ancient wheat grain – was one of the first stone-ground flours to be baked into a 'cake' or 'flat bread'. Low in gluten and high in protein, it is useful for those who are wheat intolerant, if you can find it in health shops. It needs to be baked quickly to keep the loaf as light as possible.

Millet flour is low in gluten, high in protein, and also has good levels of vitamins and minerals, once ground. It makes a slightly sweet loaf and is worth experimenting with. Whole millet seeds can be added to the mix.

Gluten-free flours

For anyone with wheat intolerance, coeliac disease or allergies, the following list is invaluable and can replace all gluten-rich flour, and it is so worth experimenting, mixing together and trying out breads, cakes, biscuits, flat breads, soda breads, buns and rusks with these fascinating flours.

Chickpea flour (also sometimes called gram flour) is made from ground chickpeas, the almost perfect food, and tastes rich and delicious. I mix it with potato flour, half and half, or with mealie meal flour, to make a delicious pancake or fritter fried in a little sunflower oil over low heat.

Brown rice flour is milled from wholegrain rice and is an excellent thickener with a sweet, nutty taste. Mix it with buckwheat flour and mealie meal flour and use it in biscuits and flat breads.

Potato flour is an excellent thickener and very useful for adding moistness to breads and fritters and for mixing with other flours.

Buckwheat flour is a real health boost, as buckwheat is a very valuable food rich in rutin. Added to cake and bread mixes it gives a delicious nuttiness and is completely gluten free.

Quinoa (pronounced 'keen-wa') is not really a grain but a seed. The ripe, dehusked seeds can be bought at health shops. I have never been successful in growing it, so I have not included the amazing history and advantages of quinoa in this book. It contains many health-building vitamins, minerals and 8 of the 9 essential amino acids, making it an almost complete protein, and has been the treasured crop of the Incas since the early centuries. It belongs to the *Chenopodium* genus – *Chenopodium quinoa* – and is a leafy annual. The seeds are cooked like rice for a chewy meal or ground into flour. It is gluten free and can be added to other gluten-free flours for a rich and chewy loaf. You may also find quinoa in some breakfast cereals, pastas and puffed grains. Used as far back as 5000 BC, it was eventually replaced by other grains but in the 1970s it suddenly made a comeback as a health food of note! Since the mid-1970s I've tried to grow it in South Africa but have never been successful. An American horticulturalist visiting the Herbal Centre gardens suggested Africa is too hot and too dry for quinoa but I keep trying!

Home grinders and milling

Stone milling is an ideal start to bread-making and today there are small mills that can be bought from health shops to grind your own flours and seed to make that perfect loaf, should you want to add extra ingredients or grind the flours to a certain consistency.

Yeast

My mother and grandmother baked bread with little blocks of moist yeast neatly wrapped in shiny foil. Living on a distant farm I found tins of dried yeast, which I kept in the fridge, were my only answer and later, when a dried yeast sachet was available, I found this to be the perfect amount for one loaf and I buy those for the sheer convenience.

Yeast is the most important ingredient of all. Dried and moist yeast need to be mixed into a little warm (tepid) water with 2 teaspoons of sugar and kept warm while it starts its frothing action. It takes a short while to 'wake up', as my grandmother said, so I always begin with this while I prepare all my other ingredients.

Once it froths and bubbles vigorously it can be added into the mixture of flour and warm water – always keep everything warm. On a cold winter morning I even warm my big mixing bowl in the warming drawer of the stove, filled with the flour, before beginning. But beware – heat kills the yeast action – so use only warm, not hot, water and while warming the bowl and the flour test with your hand for just a gentle warmth.

Don't store opened sachets of yeast. Yeast needs to be used with 12 hours of opening and buying just what you need is best. Always check the sell-by date on yeast!

For yeast-free diets (candida sufferers take note) many delicious loaves can be made with baking powder or 'baking soda' – such as the soda bread on page 39.

Sugar

Just a teaspoon or two is needed to activate the yeast. The ratio is usually 1 teaspoon of sugar to a 500 g loaf. Don't add extra sugar to your bread recipe for although a little sugar activates the yeast, too much sugar can impair its activity. The yeast feeds on the sugar, followed by the starches in the flour, to produce a fermentation process during which a gas (carbon dioxide) is released. These bubbles produce those little pockets of 'air' that actually cause the loaf to rise and give the bread its light, airy texture.

Salt

Usually about 1 teaspoon of salt per loaf is the standard measure. The salt acts as a flavour enhancer, but for a salt-free diet the salt can replaced with a small amount of herbs or spices like caraway seeds, anise seeds, celery seeds, fennel or dill seeds, crushed coriander seeds or any combination of these.

Water

Always use warm water to mix into the flour and *never hot water*. If it is either too hot or too cold, it will destroy the yeast action. I use a steel jug as it helps to retain the heat and on a bitter winter morning I use a thermos filled with warm water and add it to the warmed flour.

Do not use carbonated or bottled water. Tap water is considered best and if you are in doubt, boil the tap water first and let it cool to a pleasant warmth before using it.

Other additions

You can enhance your loaf by adding seeds like sesame seeds, poppy seeds, sunflower seeds, pumpkin seeds, flaxseed, and so on, but only do this once the flours have been well mixed and the yeast is incorporated. Oil, butter or eggs can also be added to enrich the loaf, but there may be a delay in the rising time. Keep a notebook on this, as you can create delicious and interesting variations to your daily bread once you have mastered the basic yeast and flour method.

Techniques

Some recipes call for kneading and this is an exciting process that stretches the gluten so the bread rises beautifully. Have a clean, floured surface for this – I have a much-loved huge big wooden kitchen table that is the perfect kneading height for me and I keep it scrupulously clean for the bread making. Follow the recipe instructions and enjoy the process. I put a prayer into every twist of the dough!

Bread machines are a fairly recent invention and for the busy working mother this is a great help, but you really need to read the instructions carefully to familiarise yourself with programme selections, sizes, degrees of baking and all the rest. There are timers, delay timers, crust makers and a heap of clever technology that can defeat you if you start in a rush. But persist – it is such an achievement and you'll be thrilled with your delicious healthy home-baked bread! Recipes can be adapted to suit the machine.

Recipes

Farmhouse Brown Bread

This is a heavy loaf that does not rise above the level of the tin and is at its most delicious if eaten on the same day it is baked, but it also keeps well in the fridge stored in a plastic bag and slices well for sandwiches on the next day.

2 cups brown bread flour
1 sachet dried yeast
2 teaspoons sea salt

1 cup Nutty Wheat
2 teaspoons brown sugar
warm water in a jug

Mix the sugar and yeast into about ½ cup of warm water.

Mix the Nutty Wheat into the brown flour with the salt.

As soon as the yeast becomes active and rises, its frothiness filling the cup, add it to the flour mixture with some warm water, adding in the warm water gradually, little by little, stirring well and continuously. The dough needs to be slack but not runny, and as this loaf needs no kneading it is soft and sticky.

Turn into a well-oiled loaf tin, medium size, or 2 smaller tins. (I usually line the base of the tin with an oiled strip of greaseproof paper to enable its easy removal once it is baked.)

Cover the tin with oiled cling film and set on a tray covered with a double layer of kitchen towels – it needs warmth in which to rise – and then finally cover with a thick blanket or cloth, tucked in all around. Place it in a warm spot and wait for it to rise. This can take anything from half an hour to over an hour. Check carefully – it needs to rise to the level of the tin.

Bake at 180 °C for approximately 40 minutes or until the loaf sounds hollow when knocked and it has a brown crust. (After 30 minutes test by inserting a skewer – if it comes out clean it is done.)

Remove from the tin by sliding a knife around the sides. Cover with a clean tea towel and cool on a wire rack.

Ciabatta

Serve it the way the Italians do – thickly sliced with cheeses, cold meats and thick soups. The big bubbles made by the yeast are part of its airy light deliciousness and that is why ciabatta bread is never kneaded. Make it three times and you'll become a pro!

You need to start the previous evening:

1¼ cups white bread flour
½ sachet dried yeast

½ teaspoon castor sugar
⅔ cups warm water

Mix everything into a big warm bowl to make a smooth dough. Cover with cling film and kitchen towels and leave in a warm place to rise overnight. This is known as the 'starter'.

The next morning:

3½ cups white bread flour
the rest of the packet of dried yeast
1 tablespoon milk powder
About 1 cup of warm water

1 teaspoon salt
1 teaspoon castor sugar
2 tablespoons olive oil

Mix all the dry ingredients and oil together with the starter dough from the night before. Then gradually add the warm water to make a smooth, soft dough.

Return to the large warm bowl and cover well. Leave to rise for about two hours – it needs to double or triple its size. The more it rises the lighter the loaf.

Grease a large baking tray and sprinkle with flour. Turn out the dough into two mounds and pull them into a flattish loaf shape with floured hands, about 25 cm in length. Lightly sprinkle with flour, cover lightly with tea towels and leave to rise again in a warm place for about 45 minutes.

Bake at 220 °C for about 20 minutes – the loaves will turn golden and sound hollow. Carefully run a long palette knife under the loaves to loosen them and cool on a wire rack.

Focaccia

Delicious served warm with soup. Tear the loaf to pieces rather than slice it.

4½ cups brown bread flour
1 teaspoon salt
3 tablespoons olive oil
sprigs of fresh rosemary
about 2 teaspoons coarse sea salt

1 teaspoon sugar
2 teaspoons yeast
about 1½ cups warm water added slowly
black olives, cut in half and stones removed

In a warm mixing bowl combine the flour, sugar, salt and yeast. Mix well, add the olive oil and the warm water until the dough is smooth and elastic. Knead on a well-floured surface for 5 minutes.

Return the dough to the warm bowl, cover with oiled cling film and kitchen towels and leave it in a warm place to rise until it has doubled in size – about an hour. Then once again knead the dough on a well-floured surface.

Cut in half and gently press and pull the dough out into a rough circle – about 20 cm in diameter – and place on a floured baking tray. Press in the olives and the rosemary sprigs. Sprinkle with the coarse salt and leave it to rise in a warm place, uncovered, for about 20 minutes.

Drizzle with a little extra olive oil and bake at 200 °C for about 15 minutes or until the flat loaves become lightly browned.

Quick Irish Soda Bread

This has been a family standby for generations and it fills many a hungry tummy with great satisfaction. Delicious with soup or hearty stews, we keep a special pan for making it that needs to be well oiled.

4 cups cake flour
about 2 cups warm milk or buttermilk
sunflower cooking oil (about ½ a cup)

1 teaspoon salt
4 teaspoons baking powder

Combine the flour, salt, milk and baking powder in a large bowl and mix to a slack dough.

Have a large stainless steel frying pan ready on the top of the stove (*not* a Teflon-coated one) that is well oiled with sunflower cooking oil. Make sure it is fully coated (about ½ a cup of oil) and heated to medium heat.

Gently pour in the soft dough, tilting the pan to level it. Don't leave it! Stand over it, tilting and shaking the pan gently. With a spatula, lift the edges and add a little extra oil if needed. The idea is to keep the bread loose in the pan. It takes about 10 minutes.

As the edges harden and the dough thickens, place a well-oiled plate over the top and turn the pan over, re-oil the pan and slide the bread back into the pan, its upper side now getting a chance to cook. Shake the pan gently and keep moving it around until the loaf sounds hollow when you knock it.

Slide it onto a thick clean kitchen towel and cover it. Serve hot, sliced and spread with butter, with soup or with homemade marmalade and cream cheese for breakfast. It is an excellent standby when visitors suddenly arrive for a meal, as it can be served with cheese and fig jam as deliciously as it can be served with sausages and grilled tomatoes!

The secret of making soda bread is the warm oiled pan and a medium heat, and never taking your eyes off it. Practice makes perfect, and Sandy has made this since she was 14, and makes it absolutely perfect every time!

Let's look at yoghurt

The scope of this book is plant-based healing foods, but so many questions are asked about yoghurt that I feel strongly it needs to find its place within these pages.

This cherished fermented product is thought to have originated on the slopes of Mount Elbrus in the Caucasus Mountains between the Black Sea and the Caspian Sea. Some believe it to have originated in Bulgaria, which lies on the Balkan Peninsula with Greece and Turkey forming its eastern border and the western border formed by Siberia. So famous this little country became for its treasured and extraordinary yoghurt that the bacillus found in the Bulgarian yoghurt was named after Bulgaria – *Lactobacillus bulgaricus*. The Turks gave the thickened milk the name 'yoghurmak' which means 'to thicken'. An ancient legend tells of the beginning of 'yogurut', a name that was introduced in the 8th century, and in the 11th century was changed to 'yogurt' and that name has remained ever since.

Yoghurt is rich in protein, calcium, riboflavin, potassium, phosphorus, selenium and the valuable vitamin B12, as well as biotin, pantothenic acid and zinc. Yoghurt in the diet enhances the digestion of lactose where there is a low level of lactase in the digestive system and where there is difficulty in digesting lactose.

The live cultures in Bulgarian yoghurt help to maintain the good microflora balance within the intestine, and these live cultures actually suppress harmful bacteria. This helps to ease diarrhoea and neutralises harmful bacteria after a course of antibiotics and during infectious diseases. Research has shown that 1 cup of Bulgarian yoghurt a day lowers blood cholesterol, and if taken every day for 8 months to 1 year it prevents an increase of 'bad' cholesterol (LDL or low-density lipoprotein). Bulgarian yoghurt has shown excellent anti-cancer activity, as well as enhancing the immune system activity. It has been shown that Bulgarian yoghurt eaten daily helps to detoxify the body, removing environmental toxins, meat carcinogens, excess oestrogen and fat-soluble toxins and that it reduces liver stress and impairment.

Include Bulgarian yoghurt in the diet 3 to 5 times a week in cases where there is toxic overload, low immunity and even arteriosclerosis – you will see steady and positive results, and it is delicious!

Let's look at water

Water is vital to keep our brains and our bodies in perfect working order. It is the main component of blood and essential for delivering nutrients and oxygen to the cells and transporting toxins from the cells to the kidneys for elimination through the urine. With too little water, toxic build-up becomes a problem and can manifest as many different disease types.

Nutrients and essential vitamins, minerals and enzymes are dissolved and carried in water to all parts of the body including the brain – our cells maintain vitality only when the body is properly hydrated by having sufficient good quality water intake. During exercise the heart beats faster, the lungs exhale and inhale at a faster rate – and heat is produced – this heat is absorbed by water and is presented to the surface of the skin. Perspiration takes place, cooling the body down. Exercise increases the amount of water lost, so it is essential to replace it before, during and after exercise.

If we do not drink enough water we risk becoming dehydrated as water is lost through urination, breathing, and perspiration. Even mild dehydration will result in reduced brain power, fatigue, lassitude, weakness, muscle cramps, nausea and headaches.

A simple test to see if you are dehydrated is to pinch the skin on your hand. If the skin does not immediately return to its former smoothness, you are dehydrated and should immediately drink water. The colour of your urine is also an indicator – dark-coloured urine is also a sign of dehydration. Discuss this with your doctor.

How much water do we need?

We need to drink at least 8 glasses of water each day (or a daily minimum of 1,5 litres per 50 kg body weight). Teas, juices or flavoured water are not to be confused as an alternative to water intake – pure and plain water is vital. Don't be fooled by the hype around added minerals and synthetic vitamins. You do not need minerals in water: you get those from fresh and organically grown fruits, vegetables and grains.

Don't wait until you feel thirsty – place a jug of water and a glass on your desk or in a place where you can see it to remind you that every 2 hours you need to drink a glass!

The benefits of drinking water

Sufficient daily intake (determined by body weight) will:
- Flush toxins out via the kidneys
- Tone and revitalise the liver
- Boost brain power
- Alleviate headaches
- Lower high blood pressure
- Assist in weight loss
- Prevent premature ageing
- Tone and revitalise the skin, especially problem skins and wrinkles
- Ease psoriasis and chronic eczema
- Improve digestion
- Ease constipation
- Soothe stomach ulcers
- Decrease the size of kidney stones and gallstones
- Ease the pain and discomfort of hiatus hernia
- Reduce the mineral deposits in arthritic joints and ease rheumatic pain, stiffness and inflammation.

A word of caution

Diuretics, which are present in alcohol and in high-caffeine drinks, draw water out of your cells and flush it out during urination. Studies have shown that if you drink 2 glasses of water followed by 2 glasses of beer, cola or coffee, you end up with a net intake of less than 1 glass of water! Not only are the beers, colas and coffees not putting water into your body, they are actually robbing your body of water, setting in motion the dehydration process resulting in headaches, dizziness, distress, palpitations, irritability, dry mouth and tongue and many serious internal effects that strip you of vitality.

Drinking bottled water is on the whole not healthy – the plastic containers can leach chemicals (in particular bisphenol A or BPA) into the water, especially in a hot dry climate. Convenient though it is to have the lightweight bottle in a pocket, we need to be 100% certain the plastic bottle is safe! If in doubt, use your own BPA-free container or, better still, use a stainless steel water bottle.

As a minimum, one should at least filter the tap water to get rid of the harmful chlorine and heavy metals (a KDF / carbon filter is cost effective and easy to install). If this is not possible, boil the tap water, cool it down and then drink it. Recent indications are that almost all tap water and many bottled waters are severely affected by environmental factors and radiation, but there are products and technologies available that can restore the quality of filtered or distilled or bottled water to ensure proper hydration. It would be wise to investigate how you can improve the quality of your drinking water – after all, your body consists of over 70% water and it is clear that we need to spend a lot more effort in this area of our well-being – water is a miracle liquid.

If you use a carbon-based home filter, make sure the cartridges are replaced regularly – this optimises efficacy and reduces the risk of microbial contamination. Note that borehole water needs to be tested as our water sources are badly contaminated.

The home steam-distiller

There are endless arguments, opinions and discussions around the purifying of water – from carbon filtering to spring water, to borehole water, to the pH of water and to the great debate around bottled water. What emerges clearly is that home steam-distilled water is one of the best and safest ways of sourcing water for daily consumption. (Note that this does **not** apply to the distilled water that can be bought in plastic containers from the hardware store or garage!) But having said this, I have also learned that plain distilled water is not ideal for proper hydration and suggest you investigate ways to improve the quality and properties of this distilled water for optimum benefit. New water treatments are promising solutions.

The concept of distilled water thrills me because it actually clears fluoride, bacteria, pesticides, viruses and hormones from the tap water. So should we not be sitting up and taking notice?

Even on distant farms borehole water can be heavily contaminated with pesticides, chemicals, contamination from human and animal waste, hormones and inorganic minerals. Put that same water through a steam distiller and have the distilled water tested. It will emerge pure and uncontaminated by chemicals and pesticides. Pure water is essential to health and vitality and should be top on the list of things to do concerning your health.

Quick Guide to Healing Foods

Food Plant	Major Nutrients	Main Benefits
Acerola See also page 146	Vitamins A, B1, B2, B3 & C, iron, phosphorus and calcium.	Good source of natural ascorbic acid (vitamin C); boosts immune system; treats coughs, colds, 'flu, sore throats.
Agave See also page 59	Rich in potassium, phosphorus, magnesium, vitamins A, B & E and amino acids.	Juice from the stem, leaves and roots is taken to treat rheumatism, scurvy and venereal disease. It lowers fevers, eases constipation and digestive upsets and treats jaundice and dysentery. External application for rashes, burns, grazes.
Air Potato See also page 119	Vitamin C, B-complex, iron, potassium, phosphorus, magnesium, carbohydrates.	Excellent for convalescents and invalids, children who do not thrive; treats irritable bowel syndrome, bedwetting, nerve pain, diarrhoea; warmed and applied externally as a dressing over boils, eczema, suppurating sores, infected wounds and abscesses; used as poultice over arthritic joints.
Almond See also page 173	Vitamins E, B2, B3, folic acid, calcium, potassium, magnesium, phosphorus, protein, zinc.	Excellent source of antioxidants; fights heart disease; lowers cholesterol; anticancer activity; alkalising food; builds bones, endurance.

Food Plant	Major Nutrients	Main Benefits
Amaranth See also page 63	High in protein, lysine, methionine, amino acids, vitamins B2, B3, B5, B6, C & E, folic acid, iron, copper, calcium, manganese, magnesium, zinc, rich in phytosterols, a low GI food.	Blood builder; excellent for anaemia; gives energy, strength, endurance; treats chronic and intermittent diarrhoea, coughs, colds, stomach ulcers, heavy menstrual bleeding, mouth ulcers; lowers cholesterol; excellent for type 2 diabetes.
Annatto See also page 79	Contains bixa, a safe and reliable natural food colouring; carotenoids; antioxidants.	Gives ultraviolet protection; diuretic and purgative; young shoots made into a tea for fevers, dysentery, hepatitis, skin ailments, heartburn, headaches, epilepsy, malaria, throat and stomach ailments, cancer, diabetes, kidney stones, kidney ailments.
Apple See also page 147	Vitamins A, B, C & K, calcium, magnesium, phosphorus, potassium, pectin, dietary fibre.	Reactivates beneficial bacteria in the digestive system; reduces cholesterol; detoxifies; eases chest ailments; eases both constipation and diarrhoea; tonic, keeps liver toned, fights irradiation in the body; flushes kidneys; helps anaemia, obesity, insomnia; clears catarrh, sinus headaches, halitosis, tuberculosis, asthma, gallstones, nausea, worms.
Apricot See also page 170	Vitamins A, B, C, beta-carotene, iron, calcium, phosphorus, potassium.	Prevents night blindness; combats infections; good for chest ailments, catarrh, sinusitis, toxaemia, anaemia, acne, skin rashes, bites, stings, diarrhoea, constipation and overweight. Potent antioxidant.
Asparagus See also page 74	Vitamins A, C, B1, B2, B3, B6 and K, folic acid, potassium, phosphorus, iron.	Restorative; flushes kidneys; treats cystitis, rheumatism, gout, arthritis, oedema, heart ailments; superb detoxifier and diuretic.
Avocado See also page 162	Vitamins B3, B6, E, K, folic acid, beta-carotene, iron, copper, potassium, phosphorus, monounsaturated fatty acids (oleic & linoleic acid).	A perfect food, rich in valuable oils, easily digested; prevents anaemia; blood builder; excellent cholesterol-lowering food; leaves used for coughs, colds, bronchitis and to lower blood pressure. *Caution:* Do not use leaves if pregnant!
Banana See also page 154	Vitamins A, B & C, potassium, iron, calcium, magnesium, phosphorus, fructose, dietary fibre.	Normalises bowel function; soothes stomach ulcers; stabilises blood pressure; protects the body from stress and tension which could result in a stroke; protects against heart disease; strengthens arterial walls; controls fluid balance in the body; regulates heart functions; eaten with cinnamon and honey, it will disperse phlegm.
Baobab See also page 58	Vitamin C & some B vitamins, copper, iron, potassium, tartaric acid. The oil contains omega 3, 6 & 9 fatty acids, palmitic acid, linoleic acid, oleic acid and is rich in vitamin D.	Clears the system of toxins. Oil has anti-ageing properties; excellent for slow-healing ulcers, wounds, stretch marks, sunspots; moisturising and skin softening – used for dry, cracked skin, psoriasis and eczema.
Barley See also page 135	Vitamins C, K & B-complex, especially B3, folic acid, potassium, phosphorus, zinc, magnesium, manganese, calcium.	Superb natural cholesterol treatment; used to treat asthma (releases tension from the lungs), stomach ulcers, diarrhoea; prevents hair and nail loss, tooth decay; strengthens the gums; prevents kidney stones; a detoxifier of note.
Beans See also page 164	Vitamins A, B, C and E, folic acid, calcium, phosphorus, magnesium, potassium, iron, amino acids, protein, dietary fibre, carbohydrates.	An important survival food; highly nourishing, both the leaves and seeds (beans) are eaten. Acts as a tonic to the whole system; energy booster; builds muscle tone, stamina, strength and endurance; treats tuberculosis, pneumonia, malnutrition, emaciation, anaemia; strengthens the veins, soothes haemorrhoids; lowers high cholesterol; boosts immune system; convalescent tonic and for children who do not thrive; tonic against fear, doubt and fatigue.
Beetroot See also page 78	Calcium, magnesium, iron, phosphorus, manganese, potassium, folic acid, vitamins A, C & B6, beta-carotene.	Raw beetroot grated with apple is an excellent internal cleanser; eliminates kidney stones; blood builder; treats jaundice and diverticulitis; prevents and treats colon and stomach cancer; clears pockets of acidity; clears blood of toxins.

Food Plant	Major Nutrients	Main Benefits
Bitter Melon See also page 151	Vitamins A, B5, C & E, folic acid, zinc, potassium, magnesium, manganese, copper, antiviral compounds.	Tea of the leaves treats diabetes, haemorrhoids, scanty menstruation; tea and the fruit in the diet treat leukaemia, asthma, coughs, skin diseases, scabies, bronchitis, breast cancer; can possibly halt the AIDS virus. *Caution:* Avoid during pregnancy.
Blackberry See also page 182	Vitamins A, B, C & E, beta-carotene, calcium, magnesium, phosphorus, iron.	Treats throat infections, snakebite, kidney and bladder infections; dissolves kidney stones; excellent hair tonic; made into a syrup with honey for mouth infections.
Blueberry See also page 204	Vitamins A, C, E & K, beta-carotene, calcium, manganese, phosphorus, anthocyanosides.	Excellent for diarrhoea, urinary tract infections, poor circulation, atherosclerosis, varicose veins, haemorrhoids, eye degeneration, menstrual disorders, constipation, anaemia, inflammatory conditions, acne, problem skin, dysentery.
Brazil Nut See also page 77	Selenium, chromium, polyunsaturated fats, vitamins A, C, D & E, phosphorus and magnesium.	A tonic food; lowers cancer risk; crushed nuts are taken with warm water for stomach ache; oil is used as skin moisturiser, for cracked lips, heels, for healing creams and hair care. *Caution:* Brazil nuts are high in oxalates and those with a tendency to kidney stones should avoid them.
Brinjal See also page 191	Vitamins C & B3, folic acid, beta-carotene, potassium, calcium, phosphorus, iron, nasunin (an antioxidant).	Nasunin is a potent antioxidant and free radical scavenger; it protects cell membranes from damage, purifies the blood, lowers cholesterol and repairs arteries that have been damaged by cholesterol build-up; it also helps to remove excess iron in the body by binding with it, and so lowers the risk of heart disease. Brinjal is an energy-building and tonic food; it eases the pain of arthritic joints and protects the joints against free radical damage.
Broccoli See also page 82	Vitamins A, C, B6, E & K, folic acid, calcium, magnesium, potassium, phosphorus, lutein.	Prevents and treats cancers: breast, colon, lung, oesophagus, larynx, stomach, prostate; fights irradiation; protects smokers; prevents age-related illnesses, eye degeneration, toxaemia, high blood pressure, obesity, constipation, kidney ailments.
Buckwheat See also page 124	Vitamins B, A & E, magnesium, manganese, copper, iron, phosphorus, potassium, zinc, selenium, amino acids.	A tonic food; controls bleeding, dilates the blood vessels, lowers blood pressure; treats winter chilblains and poor circulation, varicose veins and bruising. *Caution:* An allergen in sensitive people, it may cause light-sensitive dermatitis if consumed daily; may irritate the mucous membranes of the mouth and throat.
Burdock See also page 70	Contains carbohydrates, vitamins A & E, folic acid, potassium, magnesium, lignans and arctiin, a smooth muscle relaxant.	A true detoxifier, it eliminates heavy metals from the body; clears congested lungs; antiseptic; anti-tumour, anti-cancer remedy; clears gout, kidney stones; alleviates symptoms of mumps and measles; eases muscular aches, swollen joints, arthritis, coughs, colds, 'flu, stomach disorders; lowers blood sugar levels. Lotion made of leaves is used for psoriasis and eczema.
Cabbage Family See also page 84	Vitamins C, E & K, folic acid, beta-carotene, calcium, magnesium, phosphorus, some iodine, boron, potassium.	Natural antibiotic; cancer fighting; detoxifies the liver, regenerates cells in the digestive tract; lowers rate of cancer of colon, breast, lung and prostate; fresh cabbage juice excellent for duodenal, peptic and stomach ulcers.
Cacao Tree See also page 201	Vitamins A, B1, B2, B3, B5, C & E, magnesium, calcium, iron, zinc, copper, potassium, manganese, arginine (an amino acid), flavonoids, proanthocyanidins.	Mood lifter; anti-depressant; rich in antioxidants, 70% dark chocolate benefits the cardiovascular system; arginine helps nitric oxide dilate the arteries, which prevents platelets from aggregating.
Calabash See also page 138	Vitamins C, D & E, potassium, iron, zinc.	For nursing mothers calabash soup is excellent, also for children and the elderly to strengthen the bones and for energy. Young vine tips, steamed, are a delicious energy-boosting vegetable.

Food Plant	Major Nutrients	Main Benefits
Cardoon See also page 115	Vitamins A, B & C, iron, phosphorus, potassium, magnesium.	A tonic plant with diuretic and purgative properties; clears acidity; treats liver and kidney ailments; flushes out toxins; lowers high cholesterol; blood cleanser; clears acne, pimples and oiliness; good for diabetics.
Carob See also page 97	Contains vitamins A & B-complex, calcium, phosphorus, copper, magnesium, iron, pectin, fructose and protein.	Excellent digestive – make crushed pods into a drink for fatigue, convalescence and diarrhoea. Excellent baby food ground to a soft meal. Good chocolate substitute – naturally sweet, and caffeine and oxalate free. Carob flour is used in pharmaceutical and health food products. A natural thickener.
Carrot See also page 118	Vitamins A, B6, C, E, K & G, beta-carotene, calcium, phosphorus, magnesium, potassium, selenium, zinc.	Eating fresh carrots treats toxaemia, high blood pressure, asthma, acne and skin ailments, bladder and kidney problems, constipation, sinusitis and catarrh, painful menstruation, obesity, improves eyesight and sense of smell. Carrot juice taken daily will prevent infections of throat, tonsils, eyes, lungs and sinuses. Increases breast milk in nursing mothers.
Cashew Nut See also page 64	Iron, phosphorus, calcium, vitamins A, D, E & K.	Cashew nut butter is a body builder, eaten to treat emaciation, lack of energy, vitality, for children who do not thrive, teeth and gum ailments, for the elderly. Can be made into a nourishing drink or soup for the aged. Traditionally, cashew wine is taken for coughs, colds and bronchitis.
Cassava See also page 149	Vitamins C & B3, iron, magnesium, calcium, potassium, phosphorus, carbohydrates.	A valuable food source, both roots and leaves are eaten; root used as a porridge for cramps, colic, diarrhoea, and eaten with milk for insomnia; builds muscles, bones, endurance; mashed warmed root used as a poultice over sprains, swellings, arthritis, headaches, toothache.
Cauliflower See also page 83	Vitamins C, B3, B5, folic acid, iron, potassium, fibre.	Immune system booster; treats coughs, colds, bronchitis, pneumonia; antibiotic properties; increases the action of enzymes; cancer prevention, eliminates carcinogens.
Celery See also page 67	Beta-carotene, folic acid, vitamins B1, B2, B3, B6 & C, potassium, natural sodium, calcium, coumarins.	Blood purifier; lessens the need for salt; bone builder; lowers blood pressure; diuretic, cleanses kidneys and bladder, flushes out urates, clears cystitis; reduces acidity for arthritis; anti-cancer; anti-convulsant; tones the vascular system; excellent digestive. Prevents calcium deposits.
Cherry See also page 171	Vitamins A & C, copper, manganese, calcium, phosphorus; contains perillyl alcohol, which is a cancer cell inhibitor with potent antioxidant activity.	Juice is used to treat gout, arthritis, rheumatism, and swollen, painful joints. Tea of leaves and fruit is an antispasmodic and natural antibiotic to bring down fevers and to ease pain, discomfort and headaches.
Chestnut See also page 96	Rich in vitamins C, B1, B2, B6, folic acid, manganese, magnesium, copper.	Sustaining staple food in Europe; energy boosting; builds immune system; leaves made into a tea for coughs, colds and a gargle for sore throats.
Chickpea See also page 99	Vitamins A, C, B1, B2, B6, folic acid, beta-carotene, magnesium, calcium, manganese, zinc, potassium, phosphorus and absorbable iron.	An almost perfect food for malnutrition caused by protein deficiency; lowers cholesterol; assists kidney function, flushing toxins from the body; gives vitality, energy, a positive outlook, shiny eyes, shiny hair; clears skin problems; cleanses whole digestive system. Valuable snack food.
Chicory See also page 100	Vitamins A & C, folic acid, carotenes, inulin (a sugar safe for diabetics) and bitter compounds.	Blood purifier; natural laxative; digestive tonic; diuretic; eases insomnia; a healthy substitute for coffee.
Chilli Pepper, Bell Pepper & Paprika See also page 90	High in vitamins C, A & E, B6, K, beta-carotene, folic acid, lycopene, amino acids, capsaicin (in chillies – responsible for the heat factor).	Chillies are an endorphin trigger. Boosts immune system, treats winter coughs, colds, 'flu and sore throats; outstanding antioxidant activity, giving protection against heart disease and cancer; protects eyes against formation of cataracts, high cholesterol and blood clot formation; helps irregular heartbeat. Paprika is used for washing wounds, scratches and grazes.

Food Plant	Major Nutrients	Main Benefits
Cinnamon See also page 101	A spice rich in cinnamaldehyde found in the essential oil.	A circulatory stimulant, natural antibiotic and diuretic; treats insomnia, arthritis, diarrhoea, heart ailments, menstrual problems, peptic ulcers, muscle spasms, flatulence, travel sickness; excellent for type 2 diabetes; fights fungal (yeast) and bacterial infections, including *Candida* and *E. coli.*
Coconut See also page 106	Calcium, zinc, selenium, phosphorus, magnesium, potassium, iron, copper. Coconut oil is rich in medium chain fatty acids – a healthy saturated fat that does not raise blood cholesterol.	Roots are used for dysentery, colic, diarrhoea; ash from burned stem is an antiseptic and tooth and mouth cleanser; flowers are used for bladder infections, fever, as a diuretic; fibres are used to treat fever, tapeworm, inflamed throat; sap from trunk is a mild laxative; coconut oil has immune-boosting and anti-cancer properties. Coconut oil, coconut butter, coconut flesh are used in cooking.
Coffee See also page 107	Some B-vitamins, potassium; rich in antioxidants; a cup of filter coffee contains 100–150 g of caffeine.	Rich in antioxidants, moderate intake may reduce the risk of diabetes, cirrhosis of the liver, heart disease and certain cancers. *Caution:* Caffeine is a stimulant that excites the nervous centres of the brain; it is addictive and may cause indigestion, irritability and insomnia.
Coriander See also page 110	Rich in vitamins A & C, calcium, phosphorus and magnesium.	A tonic plant; the leaves and flowers make a calming tea, face lotion and medicinal brew. Used in seasonings, salts and rubs. Excellent digestive: chewing a few seeds relieves flatulence, colic, heartburn, bloating, gripes and hiccups. Clears acne, pimples, oily spotty skin; eases tension, anxiety, temper tantrums, nervous upsets, bad moods, helpless crying, shakiness after upsets.
Cranberry See also page 205	Vitamin C, beta-carotene, copper, iron, zinc, potassium, manganese, high levels of anthocyanidins and phenols.	Treats urinary tract infections, cystitis, genital herpes; prevents kidney stone formation; builds good HDL cholesterol; protects against *E. coli* infections; high antioxidant activity. Add dried cranberries to pear juice for best effect. *Caution:* Do not eat cranberries if you are on Warfarin.
Cucumber See also page 111	Silica, potassium, magnesium, folic acid, beta-carotene, vitamins A & C.	Excellent diuretic; laxative; dissolves uric acid; prevents kidney stones and stiffness in the joints; regulates blood pressure; eases digestion; flushes out toxins and removes acidity; cosmetic cleanser and toner.
Custard Apple See also page 66	Rich in vitamins, especially C, A & D, magnesium, phosphorus, potassium.	Mashed skin and fruit makes a softening scrub for problem skin, dry cracked heels, dry calluses, rashes, scratches and grazes. Leaves boiled in water excellent wash for cracked dry skin, poultice of boiled leaves for painful aching feet and cracked heels.
Dandelion See also page 200	Vitamins A, B6 & C, copper, magnesium, manganese, iron, inulin, digestive bacteria (*Bifidobacterium* & *Lactobacillis*, which are natural protective antibiotics).	Prevents congestion of liver; treats hepatitis, jaundice, gallstones; direct effect on bladder, diuretic; builds bones and teeth; balances digestive tract, especially beneficial after taking antibiotics; raises 'good' (HDL) blood cholesterol; assists with weight loss; inulin helps to regulate blood sugar levels.
Date Palm See also page 167	Vitamins A, B, C & D, folic acid, beta-carotene, calcium, magnesium, phosphorus, potassium, iron, selenium, zinc, beta-d-glucan (an antioxidant).	Treats diarrhoea, dysentery, stomach upsets, chest ailments, asthma, coughs and pleurisy. Beta-d-glucan decreases the body's absorption of cholesterol. Laxative, anti-cancer as it protects against free radicals. Natural sweetener.
Elder See also page 186	Vitamins A, B & C, beta-carotene, calcium, iron, potassium, phosphorus, magnesium.	Berries are used for coughs, colds, 'flu, bronchitis, anaemia, insomnia, anxiety, mouth infections, epilepsy, neuralgia, kidney ailments; flowers are used in face creams and lotions for problem skin.

Food Plant	Major Nutrients	Main Benefits
Enset See also page 121	Rich in starch, calcium, magnesium, phosphorus, vitamins A, C, D & E.	Hot mashed corms are used as a poultice over boils or to cleanse a suppurating wound. A, energy-boosting staple food: leaf sheaths and corms are made into a starchy porridge; fermented leaf bases are high in water, used to make flat breads; young corms eaten like potatoes.
Feijoa See also page 125	Vitamins C and B, folic acid, calcium, iron, magnesium, potassium, manganese, iodine.	Crushed flowers and leaves are used in a lotion for sunburn, rashes, grazes, insect bites, mild burns, itchy and inflamed skin; used in a tea for thyroid conditions; slices of fresh fruit used as a poultice for bites, infected grazes, wounds.
Fennel See also page 127	Vitamin C, A & D, folic acid, potassium, iron, magnesium, manganese, phosphorus, dietary fibre.	Fennel roots, seeds, leaves all valuable for the whole body. Excellent diuretic; has anti-cancer benefits; anti-inflammatory scrub to clear toxins from the skin; treats heartburn, respiratory ailments, constipation; phytoestrogens make fennel a useful menopause treatment and for excessive facial hairiness in women; fennel tea is an excellent slimming aid.
Fenugreek See also page 202	Vitamins B, C, D & E, potassium, calcium, magnesium, phosphorus, manganese, proteins.	Leaves, pods, flowers and seeds rich in nutrients; anti-diabetic; lowers blood cholesterol; helpful with anorexia, stabilises and encourages weight gain in the undernourished; paste of crushed seeds used for abscesses, boils, ulcers, suppurating sores, insect bites; skin cleansing and rejuvenating properties; increases breast milk production and makes an excellent baby food. *Caution:* Do not eat if pregnant as it induces labour.
Fig See also page 126	Vitamins A & C, beta-carotene, calcium, potassium, phosphorus.	Nature's perfect laxative; restores energy, vitality, well-being; clears toxins; builds bones – excellent for growing children; mixed with honey to make an effective cough and cold remedy.
Fruit Salad Plant See also page 192	Vitamins A & C, calcium, iron.	Beauty treatment for problem skin when cooked and mashed as a mask, scrub or soap; used as a cleansing poultice over infected scratches, grazes, scrapes.
Garland Chrysanthemum See also page 98	Vitamins A, C & D, phosphorus, copper, potassium, iron.	A well-established 'health food' in Chinese cuisine. Valuable for blood cleansing and to ease the digestion. Considered to be an energy booster and for winter ailments it is added to soups and stews.
Garlic See also page 62	Vitamins B6 & C, phosphorus, calcium, iron, copper, potassium, manganese, selenium.	Protects against heart disease, atherosclerosis, boosts immune system, lowers high blood pressure and high cholesterol, improves circulation, protects against cancer, 'flu, bronchitis, candida, diabetes, tuberculosis. A fabulous natural antibiotic.
Ginger See also page 208	Calcium, magnesium, phosphorus, potassium, active enzymes.	Neutralises gastro-intestinal hormones, toxins and acids; treats 'flu, bronchitis, sore throats, coughs, colds; helpful for nervous exhaustion, nausea from chemotherapy, diarrhoea, motion sickness, morning sickness; benefits peripheral circulation; carminative, soothes digestive tract, relieves colic, flatulence; releases spasm; lowers high cholesterol; relieves rheumatoid and osteoarthritis pains.
Globe Artichoke See also page 116	Vitamins A, B & C, iron, phosphorus, potassium, magnesium, manganese.	Boosts immune system; excellent for over-acidity, rheumatism, glandular disorders, anaemia, diarrhoea; lowers high cholesterol; improves arterial functioning; beneficial for diabetics; keeps liver and gall bladder healthy; acts as a tonic.
Gooseberry See also page 168	Vitamins B, C & E, beta-carotene, potassium, magnesium, phosphorus.	Fruits are an excellent diuretic and a laxative and reduce fever, treat kidney and bladder disorders; leaves warmed in hot water make a soothing poultice for sprains, strains, arthritic and rheumatic pain and for backache.
Granadilla See also page 160	Vitamins A, C & B, phosphorus and potassium.	Poultice of leaves used for sprains, bruises, varicosities and swollen ankles; treats scurvy, chest and bladder ailments.

Food Plant	Major Nutrients	Main Benefits
Grape See also page 206	Vitamins B, C & K, calcium, iron, magnesium, phosphorus, potassium, manganese, copper, flavonoids, resveratrol (an antioxidant).	Organic grapes valuable for cancers, overloaded liver, chronic congestion, overweight, sluggish metabolism, uneven menstruation, symptoms of menopause, high cholesterol, bladder and kidney ailments; good diuretic; stimulate poor circulation; have an anti-inflammatory action;
Grapefruit See also page 104	Vitamins A, B & C, folic acid, beta-carotene, potassium, lycopene (an excellent antioxidant), flavonoids.	Acts as a tonic to the whole body; fights macular degeneration; lowers cholesterol; contains naringen, a flavonoid that promotes the elimination of old blood cells. *Caution:* Can interact with prescribed medications.
Guava See also page 175	Vitamins C & A, niacin, phosphorus, dietary fibre, pectin, antioxidants.	A superb health food high in vitamins C and A and antioxidants; reduces risk of heart disease; ripe guavas are high in pectin, which helps to lower high blood cholesterol; lowers high blood pressure; a traditional treatment for diabetes.
Horseradish See also page 71	Vitamin C, D & E, copper, sulphur, iron, calcium, magnesium and phosphorus.	Antiseptic, antibiotic, diuretic, expectorant; used for chest ailments, coughs, colds, 'flu, fevers, rheumatism, pain relief; treatment for scurvy, tuberculosis, urinary tract infections; energy-boosting properties; good digestive; poultice for gout, arthritis, aching muscles, sprains, stiff joints, neuralgia, tonic for circulation. *Caution:* Take care on sensitive skins; use sparingly – very powerful!
Jaboticaba See also page 155	Vitamins C, D & E, beta-carotene (in skins), calcium, potassium, phosphorus, magnesium, fructose.	Seeds used for bladder and kidney ailments; skins and fruit flesh are excellent digestives; juice is sweet and rich in natural fructose; energy boosting. Dried skins can be added to spice mixes with coriander and ginger for colour.
Jackfruit See also page 72	Vitamins A & C, beta-carotene, iron, potassium, zinc, manganese, calcium, phosphorus, magnesium, dietary fibre.	Boosts energy levels; wards off colds and 'flu; a general tonic, also excellent for children; builds strong bones and teeth; promotes shining long hair.
Jerusalem Artichoke See also page 133	Potassium, sulphur, phosphorus, chlorine, calcium, iron, magnesium, vitamin C & E; rich in carbohydrates.	A famine food, it makes a nutritious soup or stew; excellent food for diabetics; traditionally used as poultice over sprains, wounds, arthritic joints; opens blocked nose and ears; clears catarrh.
Kiwifruit See also page 57	Vitamins C, A & E, potassium, magnesium, phosphorus, copper and dietary fibre. Contains actinic acid and bromic acid, which tenderise other foods.	Respiratory ailments, reduces incidence of coughs, colds, wheezing, night coughing, shortness of breath. Excellent tonic fruit, mashed pulp is a superb beauty treatment for clearing and softening the skin. *Caution:* Those with kidney stones should avoid kiwifruit as it contains oxalates.
Kumquat See also page 128	Vitamins C & A, calcium, iron, magnesium, phosphorus, potassium, dietary fibre.	Preserved in honey or brandy to make a traditional cough and cold remedy; ancient traditional medicine for digestive disorders, skin conditions, kidney and bladder ailments. Made into chutneys and jams and candied to make a delicious sweetmeat.
Leek See also page 60	A natural antibiotic, rich in vitamins A, C, K and B6, folic acid, iron, manganese, dietary fibre.	Taken through the ages for strength, vitality, courage and endurance; fights coughs, colds, 'flu, chest ailments, pneumonia, bronchitis; improves the voice and eases sore throat, laryngitis; boosts immune system, fights cancer, chronic and degenerative disease; clears toxins from the liver, pancreas and kidneys; lowers cholesterol levels.
Lemon See also page 103	Rich in vitamins A, C, B6, folic acid, potassium, calcium, magnesium, phosphorus and limonene (an antioxidant).	One of the world's most valuable fruits for cleansing and detoxifying externally and internally. Treats coughs, colds, 'flu, bronchitis; detoxifies; anti-cancer properties; limonene is being tested to remove gallstones and as an anti-cancer treatment. Excellent beauty treatment: cleanses and tones the skin; lightens freckles; closes pores, clears the skin of pimples, oiliness; brightens the hair; rejuvenates the scalp; softens and heals calluses and cracked heels; strengthens nails and repairs damaged cuticles.

Food Plant	Major Nutrients	Main Benefits
Lentil See also page 139	Vitamins A, B & C, calcium, iron, phosphorus, potassium, protein, dietary fibre.	Staple food to replace meat. Excellent for the heart; body builder; energy booster; helpful for low blood pressure, anaemia, emaciation, ulcerated stomach, ulcerated digestive tract; lowers high blood cholesterol; stabilises blood sugar (the protein and fibre content prevents spikes in blood sugar levels after a meal); reduces risk of breast cancer.
Lettuce See also page 137	Vitamins A, B, C & E, phosphorus, potassium, calcium, iron.	Used to treat anaemia, insomnia, constipation, obesity, catarrh, tuberculosis, gout, circulation problems, urinary tract ailments, arthritis, rheumatism, acne, skin problems, nervousness, high stress levels, anxiety; valuable salad ingredient and slimming food.
Linseed See also page 141	Vitamins A, B, D & E, manganese, magnesium, potassium, phosphorus, iron, copper, omega-3 fatty acids, alpha-linolenic acid, phytoestrogens (lignans).	Restores general health, boosting energy and vitality; reduces risk of heart disease and cancer; lowers high blood cholesterol; fights and prevents prostate cancer; used as a poultice over inflamed joints to ease pain; lowers risk of breast cancer; stems yield fibre for weaving linen.
Litchi See also page 142	Vitamin C, phosphorus, calcium, iron, carbohydrates, fruit sugars.	Used both fresh and dried as a health and energy booster.
Loquat See also page 122	Vitamins A & C, folic acid, beta-carotene, calcium, iron, phosphorus, selenium, fruit sugars.	Made into a syrup for coughs and colds, a liqueur as an after-dinner digestive, candied loquats for coughs; loquats cooked in syrup with grated ginger excellent as a cough and cold remedy.
Lovage See also page 140	Rich in digestive and volatile oils and flavourants.	Deodorising, sedative, anti-convulsing and anti-microbial action; a soothing and warming tonic herb that clears the skin, eases rheumatism and bronchitis and removes mucus and catarrh; diuretic, soothes urinary tract infections; clears congested chest. Maggi sauce, first made in Switzerland in 1885, remains a legendary condiment.
Lucerne See also page 150	Vitamins A, B, E, D & K, calcium, iron, magnesium, silica, potassium, chlorine, manganese.	A health-building green tonic; leaves, flowers, young shoots and sprouts are used; builds strength, energy, wellness, vitality; detoxifies, reduces inflammation; protects against cardiovascular disease, osteoporosis; eases menopausal symptoms; lowers high blood cholesterol, high antioxidant activity. *Caution:* Eat leaves fresh and unwilted to avoid bloating. Contraindicated in lupus and autoimmune disease.
Macadamia Nut See also page 145	Vitamins B1, B3 & E, zinc, copper, iron, phosphorus, magnesium, rich in antioxidants.	Cholesterol-lowering activity; long storage life; superb cooking oil, low-level polyunsaturated fat and the oil is stable at high temperatures. Macadamia oil has 4–5 times the amount of vitamin E that olive oil has.
Maize See also page 207	Vitamins A, B1, B2, B3 & B6, beta-carotene, calcium, potassium, phosphorus, magnesium, iron, zinc, manganese, selenium, lutein.	Excellent energy-boosting food; good for brain, bones, nervous system, eczema, psoriasis and skin cancer; protects against macular degeneration; yellow maize shows excellent anti-cancer activity (including skin cancer) due to high beta-carotene levels; popcorn is a healthy snack for children, and for arthritis and rheumatism.
Mango See also page 148	Vitamins A, B, C, E, K, folic acid, beta-carotene, magnesium, potassium, copper, digestive enzymes similar to papain, soluble fibre.	Anti-cancer effect; protects against traveller's diarrhoea, anaemia; treats excessive menstruation, muscle cramps, stress, heart palpitations; good for diabetics – has low glucose response; soluble fibre shifts cholesterol build-up; flowers are used in lotions and oils.
Marula See also page 187	Vitamin C, beta-carotene, calcium, magnesium, phosphorus, potassium, protein (inner nut), oil (skin and seeds).	Inner bark boiled and mashed is an excellent poultice over ulcers, wounds, grazes and smallpox pustules; bark rich in tannin: made into a tea to treat dysentery, gonorrhoea, malaria, diarrhoea; oil used as a skin softener and moisturiser, excellent for cracked heels and lips.

Food Plant	Major Nutrients	Main Benefits
Melokhia See also page 109	Rich in vitamins A, C & E, iron, magnesium, calcium and potassium.	Sustainable and drought resistant, a true survival food! Leaves are cooked as a spinach; excellent in soups and stews to build endurance; used as poultices for wounds, sprains, strains and broken bones; helpful for osteoporosis; excellent for children who fail to thrive. Important fibre crop: used as a substitute for sisal and hemp; makes superb ropes and strings; used for brooms and as a building material.
Melon See also page 102	Vitamin B & C, beta-carotene, calcium, magnesium, potassium, phosphorus, antioxidants.	Refreshes and rehydrates – a 'cooling' food; maintains blood pressure levels; flushes kidneys and bladder; diuretic; excellent skin cleanser and astringent; good for problem skin; used as poultice over wounds.
Millet See also page 159	Vitamins A & B-complex, selenium, zinc, iron, potassium, manganese, dietary fibre.	Energy giving; eases gout, as it is low in purines; excellent source of fibre, good laxative; highly alkaline food; low allergenic food.
Moringa See also page 152	Vitamins C, B & E, calcium, iron, potassium, phosphorus, manganese. Seeds are rich in valuable 'oil of ben'.	Both leaves and tender green pods are eaten; excellent general tonic, excellent for fatigue, failure to thrive in children; stabilises blood pressure; prevents and clears infections of throat, chest, lungs and skin; strengthens heart; eases and soothes stomach ailments; juice of flowers and leaves used for skin ailments, rashes, pimples, and as a poultice for strains, sprains, headache; muscle relaxant; water purifier.
Mulberry See also page 153	Vitamin C, beta-carotene, magnesium, phosphorus, calcium, potassium, resveratrol (an antioxidant).	Tonic activity in the blood, reduces build up of plaque in the arteries; anti-cancer activity; reduces inflammation; reduces risk of atherosclerosis; a much-loved tonic food – known as a spring tonic as it is one of the first fruits to ripen in spring.
Mustard See also page 80	Rich in vitamins B1, B2, B6, C & E, folic acid, calcium, manganese, copper, phosphorus, potassium, magnesium, iron.	Strong preservative; leaves and stems used for respiratory ailments, chilblains, coughs; powdered seeds used as poultice for bruises, sprains, joint pains; discourages moulds and bacteria; excellent for menopause as it protects against osteoporosis, breast cancer, heart disease.
Nastergal See also page 193	Vitamin C, beta-carotene, calcium, magnesium, potassium, phosphorus, iron, amino acids, enzymes.	Tea of fresh leaves taken for fevers, convulsions, malaria, headaches, dysentery, diarrhoea, as a sedative, wash for skin ulcers, infected bites, stomach ulcers; leaves used as poultice for haemorrhoids, varicose veins, bruises, severe strains; leaves eaten as spinach are blood cleansing, revitalising and strengthening. Berries crushed into honey are excellent for sore throats and coughs; tea of berries taken as a general tonic, to clear blocked sinuses and to treat liver, kidney, heart and chest ailments, tuberculosis and eye problems. *Caution:* Green berries are very poisonous. Use only the ripe berries.
Niger See also page 131	Vitamins A, B & E, calcium, potassium, silica, linoleic and oleic fatty acids.	Seed contains 'noog oil', which has low rancidity; an unsaturated vegetable fat; eating the seeds or residue seed cake enriches the milk in dairy cows; rough leaves are added to the compost heap because of high silica content; a valuable health ingredient in chutneys and sauces.
Oats See also page 75	Rich in vitamins B1, B2, D & E and beta-carotene, magnesium, calcium, dietary fibre, high in polyunsaturated fatty acids.	Body-building cereal, staple food of great value. Beneficial for stress, multiple sclerosis, recurring colds and 'flu, thyroid deficiency, lack of energy, menopause symptoms, over-tired or over-excited children; binds cholesterol; excellent for diabetics. Oat straw tea is used for osteoporosis; relieves grief, depression, despair and anxiety; also as a cleansing and soothing beauty aid and to soothe sunburn.

Food Plant	Major Nutrients	Main Benefits
Okra See also page 56	Excellent source of folic acid, vitamins A & C, magnesium, potassium, iron, calcium, phosphorus, thiamine, riboflavin, niacin, zinc and dietary fibre.	Gelatinous vegetable, healthy snack, considered a tonic. Gives texture to a dish. Brush whole pods with olive oil and roast for a delicious snack.
Olive See also page 156	Fruit is rich in calcium, magnesium, potassium and most vitamins; oil is high in monounsaturated fats; leaves and fruit contain olearopein, which has strong antibacterial and antibiotic properties.	Olive leaf tea eases dizziness, disorientation, feelings of helplessness and despair, cystitis, high fever; boosts the immune system, excellent for ME, chronic fatigue syndrome and multiple sclerosis; excellent diuretic; helps to lower high blood pressure and improve the whole circulatory system; valuable for diabetics; poultice of fresh leaves crushed into a little oil is used for aching muscles, slow-healing wounds, infected grazes and rashes.
Onion See also page 61	Vitamins C, B1, B6 & K, folic acid, organic sulphur, phosphorus, calcium, high pectin content, flavonoids, volatile oils.	Natural antibiotic. Lowers high blood cholesterol; stabilises blood sugar levels; cleanses and tones the kidneys; treats asthma; prevents clot formation; relaxes muscle spasms, especially in the bronchi; breaks the disease pattern of cancers, atherosclerosis and diabetes, may even have the ability to arrest tumour growth.
Orange See also page 105	Vitamin C, B1, B2, B6, folic acid, beta-carotene, potassium, calcium, flavonoids.	Boosts immune system; protects the lens of the eye, the adrenal glands and the connective tissue of the whole body; cleansing, stimulating, digestive, internal antiseptic, antiviral; fights cancer. Oil extracted from the skin treats and tones reproductive organs, bladder and kidney ailments. Contains the flavonoid hesperidin, which lowers high blood pressure and high cholesterol. Neroli oil from the orange blossom is a calming, quietening oil.
Pachira Nut See also page 158	Vitamins A & E, proteins, amino acids, unsaturated fats.	Ancient beauty treatment, excellent for dry, cracked skin; benefits whole cardiovascular system; poultice from the pounded nut used for cuts, grazes, infected insect bites.
Papaya See also page 92	Vitamins C, E & A, calcium, magnesium, beta-carotene, antioxidants, dietary fibre, papain.	Cleanses, clears, detoxifies; eat fresh papaya for bloatedness, bowel discomfort, colic, heartburn; natural laxative; eat a few seeds for arthritic inflamed joints, gout and rheumatism; wrap a warmed leaf over aching joints, burns, scratches and grazes; inside of the skin makes a fabulous beauty treatment for acne spots, oiliness, coarseness, dry flaky skin, sunburn, scalp problems; milky stems and juice have ability to take away warts and dry calluses.
Parsley See also page 163	Vitamins A, C & B, folic acid, beta-carotene, iron, calcium, magnesium, potassium; rich in chlorophyll; contains valuable volatile oils.	A fabulous health food; should always be eaten with fried foods as it reduces coagulants in the veins! Brightens complexion, clears the skin, heals acne, pimples and keeps the elasticity of the skin; deodoriser, freshens the breath; inhibits cancer; cleanser and diuretic for bladder and kidneys, clears kidney stones; a stable alkalising food.
Parsnip See also page 161	Vitamins C, B & E, folic acid, potassium, phosphorus, calcium, magnesium.	Superb detoxifier and support to the bladder, kidneys and spleen; excellent toner for bowel; energy boosting and restorative.
Peach & Nectarine See also page 174	Vitamins A, B, & C, carotenes, magnesium, calcium, phosphorus, potassium, manganese, flavonoids (lycopene and lutein).	Made into syrups for coughs and colds; tea from leaves and twigs treats bladder ailments, gout, poor eyesight and earache; peaches help eliminate toxins, soothe stomach ulcers and colitis; easily digestible, excellent laxative and colon cleanser; kidney and bladder cleanser; has an alkalising effect on the whole body; lycopene and lutein help to prevent macular degeneration of the eyes. *Caution:* Those with a tendency to kidney stones should limit their intake of peaches.

Food Plant	Major Nutrients	Main Benefits
Peanut See also page 69	Vitamins B1, B3 & E, folic acid, magnesium, phosphorus, manganese, monounsaturated fats, protein.	Protects the cardiovascular system; lowers high cholesterol and maintains the 'good' (HDL) cholesterol. *Caution:* Peanuts are a dangerous allergenic. Never eat rancid peanuts with mould on them, as they can introduce carcinogenic aflatoxins into the body. Avoid salted peanuts.
Pear See also page 177	Vitamins A, B & C, folic acid, beta-carotene, calcium, magnesium, phosphorus, potassium, iodine, pectin, dietary fibre.	Excellent for kidney ailments, even severe malfunctioning of the kidneys; lowers high cholesterol; tones and regulates the bowel; removes toxins from the body; excellent baby food; promotes a pure complexion, shining eyes, shining hair and a happy disposition.
Peas See also page 169	Vitamins B, C & K, folic acid, carotenes, phosphorus, potassium, zinc, magnesium, manganese, iron, amino acids, protein.	Excellent health food for the liver, cleanses and tones the liver; eases stomach ailments, improves digestion; acts as a tonic for the whole system and boosts the immune system; good energy booster.
Pecan Nut See also page 94	Rich in the amino acid arginine, monounsaturated fatty acids and vitamin E. Also contains B-vitamins, calcium, iron, magnesium, phosphorus, manganese, zinc and copper.	Boosts the immune system; heals wounds; clears suppuration; stimulates insulin secretion; relaxes walls of blood vessels to ease circulation; detoxifies liver and kidneys; lowers high cholesterol.
Persimmon See also page 120	Rich in beta-carotene, vitamins A & C, iron, magnesium, potassium, calcium, phosphorus, copper, manganese.	Boosts the immune system; warmed fruit cut in half is an excellent poultice over grazes, cuts, rashes, infected scrapes.
Pigeon Pea See also page 88	Rich in protein, amino acids, vitamins A, B, C, D & E, potassium, phosphorus, calcium, magnesium, iron.	A staple food that is packed with energy-boosting properties. Pulp of cooked mashed peas is an excellent poultice over infected cuts, wounds, rashes and grazes, and to bring boils and abscesses to a head. Chlorophyll in the young sprigs, leaves and tendrils acts as a tonic.
Pineapple See also page 65	Contains bromelian, an excellent digestive aid. Also contains sulphur, protein, digestive enzymes which reduce inflammatory conditions. Rich in vitamins A, C & B6, beta-carotene, calcium, iron and phosphorus.	Clears mucus in pneumonia, bronchitis, acute sinusitis, throat infections; eases arthritis, gout, joint swellings and rebuilds the body after injury and post-operatively. A protective fruit for the digestive system.
Plum See also page 172	Vitamins C, A & E, folic acid, beta-carotene, calcium, potassium, iron.	Excellent food for the brain, the nerves and blood; helps to lower cholesterol; excellent natural laxative (think of prunes) and colon cleanser; circulatory diseases benefit from including fresh plums in the diet (and prunes during the winter).
Pomegranate See also page 176	Vitamins A, B, C & E, potassium, calcium, phosphorus, enzymes, amino acids.	Traditional treatment for diarrhoea, dysentery, stomach cramps, colic, digestive disturbances, infertility and to clear parasites from the body; juice is a general tonic; clears oily problem skin, blackheads and spots; strengthens nails; used as a foot scrub for aching feet, calluses and corns; leaves used as poultices for painful feet, sore back and stiff shoulders.
Potato See also page 194	Vitamins C & B, iron, calcium, potassium, complex carbohydrates, dietary fibre, lysine (an amino acid).	Staple food; tonic; energy booster; fresh skins are used over burns, also as a poultice over wounds; has pain-relieving properties.
Prickly Pear See also page 157	Vitamin C & some B-vitamins; calcium, magnesium, phosphorus, iron, copper.	Important famine food; mashed fruit brings down temperature, fevers and is safe for children; use mashed over grazes, cuts, scrapes, burns; fruits eaten for vitality, energy, 'flu, coughs, colds.
Pumpkins & Squashes See also page 112	Vitamins A, B-complex, C & E, beta-carotene, calcium, iron, magnesium, phosphorus, zinc, potassium, copper, manganese and dietary fibre.	A spinach from vine tips is cleansing and revitalising; ripe pumpkin makes a nourishing baby food; hot poultice of flesh used for abscesses, boils and suppurating wounds; used to treat worms; zinc-rich seeds promote prostate health.

Food Plant	Major Nutrients	Main Benefits
Quince See also page 114	Vitamin C, beta-carotene, potassium, phosphorus, calcium, iron, copper, magnesium, pectin, dietary fibre.	Traditional remedy for stomach ailments, diarrhoea, dysentery, digestive ailments, kidney and bladder ailments and coughs; used as a wash for wounds, a scrub for problem skins, cleanser and hair treatment.
Radish See also page 178	Vitamin C, folic acid, calcium, copper, potassium.	A tonic for the whole body; boosts the immune system; builds resistance to chest ailments; acts as a diuretic, expectorant and digestive; relieves flatulence, colic and heartburn; excellent for the liver, with cleansing and tonic effects.
Rape See also page 81	Vitamins C, B1, B2, B6 & E, beta-carotene, manganese, iron, copper, calcium, potassium, phosphorus, lutein, zeaxanthin. Rapeseed oil is rich in omega-3 fatty acids.	Good for osteoporosis: rape contains three times more calcium than phosphorus, which is a beneficial ratio. Anti-cancer properties; lutein and zeaxanthin are immune boosters.
Raspberry See also page 183	Vitamins A, B, C & E, beta-carotene, calcium, magnesium, iron, potassium, phosphorus, anthocyanins, ellagic acid.	A tonic food; laxative action; eliminates toxins; clears phlegm; relieves menstrual cramps; tones the kidneys and bladder; ellagic acid is a cancer fighter; raspberry leaf tea traditionally used for coughs and colds, and as a mouthwash and gargle for mouth ulcers, gum ailments and throat infections; also used for eye ailments, as a wound wash and for soldier's diarrhoea. *Caution:* Do not take raspberry leaf tea late in pregnancy.
Rhubarb See also page 179	Vitamins C & K, folic acid.	Treats 'flu, coughs, colds; rhubarb syrup is a traditional remedy for constipation; leaves make an excellent insect-repelling spray. *Caution:* Only the stems are eaten. They are high in oxalates and eating too much can interfere with the absorption of iron and calcium in the body.
Rocket See also page 123	Vitamins A and C, folic acid, calcium, iron. Seeds contain an excellent oil, called 'Jamba oil', used for cooking and medicinal purposes and as a lubricant.	An immune booster; used to treat digestive and circulatory disorders; leaves used as a compress over bruises and sprains; seeds pounded with honey are an ancient remedy for coughs, colds, 'flu, mucus, blocked nose; petals used to treat skin ailments and to refine the skin.
Rooibos Tea See also page 73	Excellent source of several vitamins, minerals, amino acids. Rooibos is a true health tea, flushing the body as gentle detox.	Retards ageing; improves digestion; relaxes muscle spasms; assists with colic in babies; relieves allergic reactions; contains a natural fluoride that retards tooth decay; excellent for eczema and psoriasis; kidney and bladder tonic, good for cystitis, kidney stones, slow or burning urine, over-indulgence, diarrhoea.
Rose Apple See also page 198	Vitamins A, C & E, calcium, phosphorus, potassium, magnesium.	Treats rheumatism, colds, 'flu, sore throats, ear and sinus infections, chronic coughs, bronchitis; boosts immune system; combined with lemon and honey it is a safe cough mixture for children; excellent in jams, jellies, syrups.
Rose Hip See also page 181	Vitamins C, D & E, beta-carotene, calcium, magnesium, potassium, zinc, phosphorus, fructose, enzymes, lycopene.	Syrup a traditional remedy for coughs and colds, 'flu, bronchitis; made into a syrup or warming drink that is especially valuable for babies and young children; rose hip oil valuable as a skin softener for cracked heels and cracked lips.
Rosella See also page 134	Vitamins C, B, D, & E, potassium, iron, calcium, several amino acids.	Useful for winter coughs and colds, bronchitis, chronic chest ailments, 'flu; cooled tea is an excellent lotion for skin problems, oily hair, dandruff, acne and as a wash for insect bites, rashes, grazes and sunburn; tea of the calyxes used for tuberculosis, chest ailments. Valuable natural food colouring (used as a substitute for tartrazine); used in cosmetics and medicines; excellent health drink.
Rye See also page 188	Vitamins B, E & K, calcium, iron, phosphorus, zinc, potassium, magnesium, manganese, copper, selenium.	An energy food and a de-stressor; it soothes the digestive tract, stomach, arthritis, stiffness, swollen joints; rye cooked like rice cleanses the liver, removes arthritic stiffness. Look for 100% rye bread or bake your own!

Food Plant	Major Nutrients	Main Benefits
Safflower See also page 93	High in polyunsaturated fatty acids; an excellent cooking oil that is gaining importance as a cholesterol-lowering oil.	Flowers used as a substitute for the expensive saffron. Tea of flowering tips lowers blood pressure and high cholesterol; improves circulation and stimulates the heart; reduces pain; reduces inflammatory conditions like arthritis, sore joints, shoulder pains; flowers make an excellent poultice over bruises and sprains. *Caution:* A uterine stimulant – do not take if pregnant.
Sesame See also page 190	Vitamins E, B1 & B2, copper, iron, magnesium, calcium, phosphorus, zinc, mono- and polyunsaturated fats, sesamin (an antioxidant).	Used for constipation, to remove worms, to aid digestion, to stimulate breast milk production, to improve blood circulation, to strengthen the heart, to lower blood pressure and to cleanse the kidneys; sesamin displays excellent antioxidant effects, lowers cholesterol and cleanses the liver of toxins; taken as a medicine the root is said to cure tinnitus, and blurred vision due to anaemia. Sesame oil is used in cooking and also in cosmetics to moisturise, to soften the skin and is superb for falling dry hair and cracked skin.
Sorghum See also page 195	B-complex vitamins (especially B1, B2 and B3), calcium, iron, phosphorus, potassium, antioxidants.	Excellent for gluten-intolerant diets and coeliac disease; inhibits cancer (breast, colon, lung, pancreatic cancer) and reduces tumour growth; protects against cardiovascular disease; reduces cholesterol; strengthens collagen in the skin and blood vessels; helpful for autism, mood swings and poor eating habits in children.
Sorrel See also page 184	Vitamins C & A, magnesium, potassium.	Blood-building, blood-cleansing properties; its astringent properties stop bleeding and clear infection in cuts and grazes; clears skin rashes, infections, acne; leaves are very nutritious; sorrel juice is a natural way of removing stains on linen. *Caution:* High in oxalates, so be cautious if you have arthritis or kidney problems of any kind.
Soya Bean See also page 130	Vitamins B1, B2, B6, C & E, beta-carotene, phosphorus, calcium, iron, omega-3 fatty acids, complete protein (contains 22 health-building amino acids), polyunsaturated fats, isoflavones.	Exceptionally high in nutritional value and therapeutic properties, known as the 'meat of the earth'. Soya has an alkaline effect on the body; it benefits the nervous system, circulatory system; relieves symptoms of menopause – mimics oestrogen; regulates and treats the bowels; dissolves gallstones; lowers high cholesterol; acts as a general tonic; tones muscles; stimulates liver and kidneys; reverses the effect of wrong eating and over-medication; excellent for diabetics.
Spinach & Swiss Chard See also page 196	Vitamins A, B, C & K, folic acid, beta-carotene, iron, calcium, magnesium, zinc, potassium, phosphorus, manganese, chlorophyll, lutein (an antioxidant), rich in flavonoids.	Spinach is an alkaline food that clears acidity; boosts health, strength, energy; restores vitality; builds up the immune system, restores bone health, valuable for treating cancer of the colon and digestive tract, regulates blood pressure; maintains bone health (vitamin K activates osteocalcin which anchors calcium in the bone); lutein promotes healthy eyesight, prevents macular degeneration.
Star Fruit See also page 76	Vitamins A, B1, B2, B3 & C, iron, phosphorus, calcium, potassium, carotenoids.	Ideal slimmers' fruit, and to treat coughs, colds, 'flu, bronchitis. Used as a poultice over boils, infected wounds, rashes, grazes. Juice used for sunburn and as an application for acne, oily skin and problem skin.
Stevia See also page 197	A low calorie sweetener that does not affect blood sugar levels, its active ingredient, stevicide, is not utilised or absorbed by the body.	A completely natural, safe sweetener: stevicide is 300 times sweeter than sugar; safe for diabetics; strengthens the heart and the whole cardiovascular system; lowers high blood pressure, high blood sugar and high cholesterol levels; soothes and tightens bleeding gums.

Food Plant	Major Nutrients	Main Benefits
Strawberry See also page 129	Vitamins C, B1, B5, B6, B7 & K, beta-carotene, folic acid, potassium, iodine, manganese, flavonoids.	Ancient remedy for headaches, backaches, to strengthen the gums, and as a lotion for the face; anti-cancer and antiviral activity; the high flavonoid content protects against cancer, inflammation, heart disease, arthritis, asthma; anti-ageing.
Sugar Cane See also page 185	Blackstrap molasses is the preferred way of eating sugar: contains sucrose, glucose, fructose, traces of B-vitamins, calcium, magnesium, phosphorus, silicon, iron and potassium.	Sugar is a natural preservative and a source of energy. Valuable in jam, jellies, syrups and sweet sauces. *Caution:* Beware of too much sugar in the diet! Refined sugar promotes obesity and rots the teeth and for diabetics it is life threatening.
Sunflower See also page 132	Vitamins E, B1, B5, B6, folic acid, calcium, copper, zinc, iron, phosphorus, mono- and polyunsaturated fats. Seeds are an excellent source of protein.	A tonic plant; the leaves, seeds and petals are all valuable. Treats bronchial infections, tuberculosis, malaria; oil lowers cholesterol (oil contains more vitamin E than any other oil); sprouted seeds have anti-cancer, anti-inflammatory and anti-allergenic properties; seeds are an energy booster and bone builder in children; oil used commercially in margarine, mayonnaise, cheese, ice-cream.
Su-Su See also page 189	Vitamins B, C & K, folic acid, magnesium, potassium, zinc, copper, manganese, dietary fibre, some protein.	Fresh fruit slices are used over wounds, minor burns, rashes, grazes, sunburn, insect bites; baked hot su-su over a boil brings it to a head; young leaves and vine tips are a valuable mineral-rich vegetable.
Sweet Lupin See also page 143	Vitamins B, C, D & E, protein, lecithin. Seeds yield an excellent edible oil rich in unsaturated fatty acids, including linoleic acid.	Excellent vermifuge, ridding the body of parasites; lupin flour is an excellent beauty mask for problem oily skins; energy booster – cooked seeds make a valuable snack; caffeine-free coffee substitute. *Caution:* Boil the seeds well before eating to release the bitter alkaloids.
Sweet Potato See also page 136	Leaves and tubers are rich in vitamins A, B, C & E, folic acid, carotenes, phosphorus, copper, potassium, manganese, enzymes, unique proteins.	Staple food. Antioxidant and tonic food; stabilises blood sugar levels; improves circulation; gentle digestive; excellent detoxifier – binds heavy metals and waste products for elimination; ancient treatment for ulcers, poor circulation, coughs, colds; juice used for bites and stings; made into poultice for boils, acne, arthritic joints; source of ethanol and starch.
Tamarind See also page 199	Vitamins A, C & some B-vitamins, calcium, phosphorus, iron.	A tonic plant with anti-ageing properties; tea of the pods and young leaves treats fevers, eases the digestive system, acts as a safe and gentle laxative and has strong antiseptic properties; syrup of tamarind treats asthma, catarrh, jaundice, liver ailments, dysentery, morning sickness and nausea.
Taro See also page 108	Rich in vitamin C and some B-vitamins, iron, phosphorus, potassium, calcium, magnesium.	An energy-giving staple food and traditional medicine. Pounded cooked tubers are used as a poultice over bruises, sprains, arthritic joints and swellings. Warmed leaves are used to treat backache. Pain reliever.
Tea See also page 89	Both green and black tea contain calcium, magnesium, iron, fluoride, vitamins C, D & K. High in polyphenols.	Green tea inhibits the growth of cancer cells, particularly breast and prostate cancer. Tea, weak and black, eases diarrhoea, upset tummies and rumbling indigestion. *Caution:* Green tea can interfere with the blood thinner Warfarin.
Tomato See also page 144	Vitamin C, folic acid, beta-carotene, calcium, magnesium, phosphorus. Tomatoes are rich in lycopene, a powerful and protective antioxidant.	Excellent liver and blood cleanser; builds the blood; prevents the risk of cancer (breast, skin, colon and prostate); lowers risk of heart disease, cataracts and macular degeneration by neutralising the free radicals before they damage the cells.
Tree Tomato See also page 117	Vitamins C, A, B6 & E, beta-carotene, phosphorus, calcium.	Boosts immune system, traditional remedy for coughs, colds, bronchitis, congestion of the lungs and nasal passages, and 'flu symptoms.

Food Plant	Major Nutrients	Main Benefits
Turmeric See also page 113	Rich in rare oils, beta-carotene, enzymes, phosphorus, copper and magnesium.	Excellent anti-inflammatory; extracts from rhizomes significantly reduce allergic reactions; tubers made into a paste cleanse and disinfect the skin and clears ulcers; Ayurvedic medicine for treating respiratory ailments; tea of powdered root treats uterine tumours, digestive ailments, liver ailments, menstrual and circulatory problems.
Turnip See also page 87	Rich in vitamins C, E & B-complex, especially B6, folic acid, copper, calcium, manganese, potassium, magnesium, dietary fibre.	Tonic; blood-warming in winter; boosts stamina and endurance; leaves and the root taken for coughs, colds, bronchitis, excess phlegm, aches and pains of old age and as an anti-ager. *Caution:* The leaves contain oxalates, so those with kidney stones should eat the leaves only once or twice a week.
Waterblommetjie See also page 68	Vitamin C, A, D, E & B-vitamins, folic acid, calcium, potassium, magnesium, copper, phosphorus. Rhizomes contain starch.	Juice from the stems used for light burns, scratches, grazes, rashes, insect bites, cuts, sunburn, chafing, hot itchiness. Crushed stems make an excellent poultice over arthritic or swollen rheumatic joints, sprains, strains and bruises. Stems preserved in vinegar are a traditional remedy for rheumatism.
Watercress See also page 180	Vitamin C, folic acid, beta-carotene, calcium, magnesium, phosphorus, potassium, iron, iodine, amino acids.	A superb tonic food; clears toxins and acts as a digestive; blood purifier; wards off chest colds, sore throats, 'flu, bronchitis; prevents scurvy; treats respiratory ailments, catarrh, chronic sinusitis, blocked nose, postnasal drip, wet coughs; reduces phlegm; treats blood disorders, anaemia, liver problems, bladder ailments; breaks up kidney stones, clears bladder stones; acts as a safe diuretic; high iodine content stimulates the thyroid.
Wheat See also page 203	Vitamins E, B1, B2, B5 & B6, folic acid, carotenoids, calcium, iron, magnesium, copper, phosphorus, zinc, manganese, enzymes, chlorophyll, proteins, peptides.	Wheat grass repairs DNA; rebuilds the blood; is an excellent anti-acidic treatment; cleanses an overloaded liver; heals wounds, scratches, grazes, infections; stimulates enzyme activity; rejuvenates and revitalises; neutralises toxins and eliminates parasites. Wheat sprouts, whole wheat and cracked wheat reduce the incidence of colon and breast cancer and promote regular bowel function.
White Sapote See also page 95	Rich in vitamin C, some B-vitamins, calcium, phosphorus, a little iron, potassium, magnesium, several amino acids, high in fructose.	Seeds ground to a powder are an excellent natural sedative; considered to be an excellent tonic fruit, energy boosting. Constantly bears fruits – even in the cold months.

On the following pages we look at each of these plants in more detail, with information on the origin and history of the plant, advice on how to grow it, and suggestions for its use. I have trialled all these plants over the years, and most of them can be grown successfully under local conditions, even in a suburban garden! There are a few exceptions – plants that need very specific growing conditions – but I have included them in these pages anyway because they are so important for building health.

I want to encourage you to plant at least a few of these plants in your garden, and I urge you to save your own seeds. Hybridised seeds and genetically modified foods are becoming commonplace, and as these foods are not labelled as such, we simply do not know what the implications are for our health in the long term. We have established a seed bank at the Herbal Centre, and seed saving has, and needs to still, become a way of life for all of us. A fascinating seed collection can be easily established, well labelled and dated, and stored in glass jars with a screw-top lid.

Our own 'Heritage Seed Collection' has become a landmark of ever-growing importance that we can post all over the country. Keep seed saving in mind and see our website, www.margaretroberts.co.za, for more information.

Okra

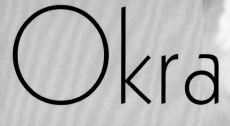

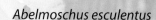

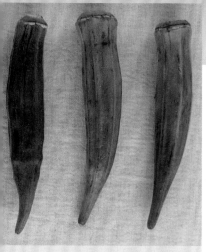

Fried Okra

Fry whole young pods in olive oil in a skillet well covered with a lid to steam or cook it at the same time. Turn very gently to lightly brown the pods. Drain on kitchen paper and serve with a sweet chilli sauce or a squeeze of fresh lemon juice.

A strange and not very well known vegetable, okra is the rigid green immature pod of a hibiscus plant that is indigenous to tropical West Africa, probably from Abyssinia (now Ethiopia) through to the Sudan, but little is recorded about its ancient history. The first recordings were in 1216 by a Spanish Moor who visited Egypt. Taken by the slave trade into Egypt and Arabia it is still popular in Arab dishes today, and its spread into the Mediterranean area and North Africa and the Caribbean on to Southeast Asia was quick. For the *tajine* – a North African stew – okra remains a valuable ingredient and as a quick annual it is grown extensively, crop after crop, all through the year in these hot countries.

Growing Okra

Sow seed directly where it is to grow. Dig a deep furrow and fill with old compost. Dig in the compost thoroughly and flood with water. Space the seed 30 cm apart, press them in 1 cm deep, cover with leaves to keep the moisture in, and water daily. Every 3 weeks from early spring onwards, sow a new row in a different place to ensure a continuous supply of fresh young pods and pick daily. The younger the pod the less slimy it is and the more flavour it has. Commercial growers pick the pods when they are 3–5 days old. The bush, which reaches about 75 cm, will bear usually only one flush of pods, which ripen within a few days of each other.

Using Okra

One of the few vegetables to give a gelatinous texture to the dish, okra is a much-loved ingredient in Creole cookery, and 'gumbo', its common name, is a tasty stew that is served frequently. In the marketplaces tiny three-day-old pods are sold alongside slightly larger ones as one of the most popular of ingredients, bought fresh daily. Traditional dishes handed down from grandmothers remain part of the culture, and hot mashed okra pods are used extensively as a poultice over wounds, slow-healing sores and for sprains, swellings and arthritic joints – traditionally used in rolled up calico and placed over the area.

Okra can be sliced, boiled whole, baked, fried, used in soups, stews and casseroles, and is much enjoyed with chicken and fish, or even served cold in a salad. Usually the whole pod, young and tender, stem intact, and not in any way punctured, is served as an accompaniment to rich fried fish and meat dishes. The leaves are edible and are full of vitamins and minerals, and can be quickly boiled to make a tasty spinach with lemon juice.

The typical yellow hibiscus type flower can also be eaten in a stir-fry, or fresh in salads, or dipped into lemon juice, then into sugar and dried in the sun for festive food decorations, usually served with iced sorbets made with fresh fruit juices.

Dried okra and canned okra in tomato sauce are available in certain delicatessens and in Greek and Middle Eastern food stores, and fried pods in tomato sauce are sometimes available at street markets.

Hint

To help reduce the viscosity, soak the whole pods in vinegar for at least 2 hours. Dry the pods well before frying.

Health Note

Okra is an excellent source of folic acid, vitamins C and A, magnesium, potassium, dietary fibre, iron, calcium, phosphorus, thiamine, riboflavin, niacin and zinc.

Kiwifruit

Actinidia deliciosa

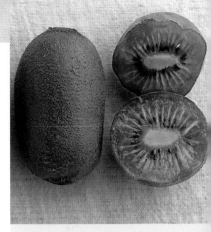

Sometimes known as the Chinese gooseberry, this extraordinary vine, which originates in China, has only fairly recently been introduced to Western countries where it is grown on a small commercial scale. California and New Zealand have the biggest plantings and it continues to grow in popularity.

The climate in Italy is excellent for the growing of kiwifruit, which they export worldwide, and in parts of South Africa it too is becoming a crop to be considered, as it is a sturdy perennial. It was the New Zealanders who named the Chinese gooseberry the 'kiwifruit', so laying a claim to it – and most people know it only as that, 'kiwifruit' – but never forget, it is an ancient Chinese indigenous vine that grows naturally along the outskirts of the Yangtze valley forests and it has been used as a medicine and a food in its native land for centuries!

Growing Kiwifruit

Tough, sturdy and vigorous, this fascinating vine is a deciduous climber which reaches around 8–10 m in length, and it needs both male and female vines to produce its unique oval hairy fruits. The stems and shoots are also thick with reddish brown hairs, and the plant climbs by twining and not by the means of tendrils as many other climbers do. With its fairly large, heart-shaped leaves this vine will make an attractive feature in any garden and will quickly cover a trellis or arbour. The creamy white, honey-scented, nectar-rich, male and female flowers are borne on separate plants.

Plant the male and female plants separately, at least 2 m apart, in well-dug, richly composted holes in full sun. The roots are shallow and spread, so mulching with rich organic matter is vital and substantial dams need to be made around it to conserve water and to keep it from drying out. Drip irrigation works perfectly for kiwi vines. A frost-free, sheltered site is essential, with strong wind protection. Plant in winter and prune to tidy up each winter to encourage young new shoots once the vines are well established and productive. It takes 4–5 years for a vine to become productive – so tie up and train the stems in preparation for its fruiting from the beginning.

Remember to gather the fallen leaves every autumn for a mineral-rich addition to your compost heap!

Using Kiwifruit

Kiwi is a health food of growing importance. It has been found to be excellent in treating respiratory ailments and children in Italy were found to have fewer respiratory ailments, coughs and colds. The more they ate kiwifruit the healthier they became – and this included wheezing, shortness of breath and night coughing. However, kiwi contains high levels of oxalates, so those who suffer from kidney stones should limit their consumption of kiwifruit.

Kiwi is simply glorious in ice-cream, in mousses or added at the last minute to fruit salads, green salads and stir-fries. Add thin, peeled slices to plain yoghurt with almonds, finely chopped, and honey for a delicious breakfast dish.

Health Note

Kiwifruit is an excellent source of vitamins C, A and E, dietary fibre, potassium, magnesium, phosphorus and copper.

All Green Salad

Add slices of kiwifruit to celery, lettuce, avocado, rocket and green pepper. Serve with a little olive oil and lemon juice, and taste the magic of it.

Kiwifruit Face Scrub

Mix ½ cup good aqueous cream with ½ cup peeled mashed kiwifruit to remove heavy make up. Or use thin peeled slices of kiwifruit as a face scrub to refresh and tighten the skin the way the Chinese do. You'll be surprised how soft and clean the skin feels.

Hints

Ripening the kiwifruit is essential to get the full refreshing and delicious benefit from it. Place the fruit in a brown paper bag with either a banana or an apple or a pear. Tie it up and leave it for a couple of days to speed up its ripening process. Very ripe kiwifruit can be refrigerated.

Peeled, sliced kiwifruit can be used as a meat tenderiser, placed under and over the meat and left to absorb the juices in the fridge at least 3 hours before cooking. Kiwi contains actinic acid and bromic acid, which quickly 'tenderise' the other fruits and vegetables it comes into proximity with – so add it last when using in a salad!

Baobab

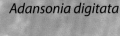

Adansonia digitata

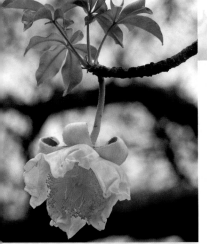

Baobab Lemonade

½–1 cup sieved fruit pulp
4 cups warm water
½–1 cup sugar
ice cubes
½–1 cup lemon juice
lemon slices

Mix the first five ingredients together well, stirring vigorously. Lastly add the lemon slices and refrigerate. Serve with crushed ice.

Mabuyu

The locals sell these mabuyu baobab sweets at Fort Jesus in Mombassa.

seeds and pulp from one or two large baobab fruits (you will need about 1 cup pulp, sieved out of the fibres)
1 tablespoon beetroot juice (taken from the cooking water in which fresh beetroots have been simmered – this is to give it the typical red colour)
1 cup water
1 cup sugar

Mash the pulp, remove the seeds and keep them aside. Boil up the sugar, water and beetroot juice until it thickens (about 15 minutes). Stir in the pulp and add the seeds. Reduce the heat and stir frequently so as to keep the seeds separate. When the mixture has thickened, pour out onto an oiled tray, cool and before it sets hard, cut into small sweets. Only serve to people with very good teeth!

The mighty, breathtakingly impressive baobab is the most extraordinary tree in the world! Its massive trunk of more than 20 metres in circumference is often hollowed out and used for all sorts of storage and even living spaces. But most valuable of all, the hollow trunk can hold well over 1 000 litres of water within it and that, in our hot and dry country, is like gold! Thought perhaps to be the longest living tree in the world, some specimens in Africa are thought to be around 3 000 years old. Wherever it grows it is a valuable source of food, of medicine and even of income to the local people. The entire tree is utilised as food, medicine and a rich and extraordinary oil is found within the seeds. The baobab's great silent presence is both calming and inspiring, and its magnificence is unsurpassed.

Ancient legends tell of the power of the baobab pod: collected under the shade of the great branches, and hung over the doorway of the home, or in the rafters, it would ensure health, wealth and protection to all who entered the house. But commercially picked pods, offered for sale, had no such powers. The home owner had to find it himself, under the shade of this magnificent tree!

Growing the Baobab

Easily propagated from its unique, almost heart-shaped seeds, enshrouded in huge hard-shelled pods. The thick outer shell around the seed is difficult to remove, so soak it thoroughly before planting, at least for 5 hours. Plant individually in extra large bags and keep them moist. Remember, they thrive only in tropical, frost-free areas with dry heat. Do not over-water the emerging seedlings, and once they reach 30 cm and the thickness of a pencil, move them out into the sun to strengthen daily. Plant in a large hole, 1 m wide and 1 m deep, and fill it with compost mixed with sandy loam. As this will be its final growing place, be sure it is not near buildings, roads, pylons or electric substations. Remember its enormous size once it reaches maturity! Water once a week until it reaches 1 m in height, then only occasionally.

Using the Baobab

Rich in nutrients, the young leaves can be cooked to make a spinach-type dish that is energy-rich and clears the system of toxins. The dry, powdery pulp inside the hard pods is acidic and easily dissolved in the mouth and can be made into a pleasant drink. The heart-shaped seeds contained in the pulp are edible, cooked or raw, and they contain an exquisite golden oil. The oil is rich in vitamin D, the omega-3, 6 and 9 fatty acids, oleic acid, palmitic acid and linoleic acid, and is excellent as a moisturiser for treating skin complaints, psoriasis, eczema, skin cancers, diabetic ulcers and slow-healing leg ulcers and wounds. In bath and cosmetic products it is superb – for stretch marks, sunspots, ageing and dry skin, baobab oil literally rejuvenates. It is easily absorbed by the skin and can be rubbed directly onto the area, massaged in and it leaves no oily residue. Add it to creams, to lotions, to the bath, and to your hair conditioner for lustrous shining hair.

Health Note

The leaves and fruit pulp contain vitamin C and some of the B vitamins, copper, iron, potassium, tartaric acid and uronic acid. The oil is rich in omega-3, 6 & 9 fatty acids, palmitic acid, linoleic acid, oleic acid and also contains vitamin D.

Agave

Tequila plant ▪ Century plant

Agave americana

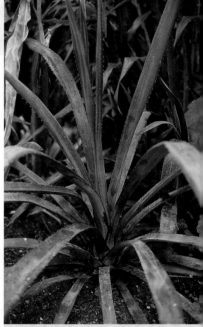

This extraordinary genus consists of around 300 species of perennial and succulent plants that survive in the arid regions of mainly South and Central America. They vary greatly and their swan song, the often huge and spectacular flower spike, heralds the end of their life. It is the sweet juice from this flowering stem that is fermented into the popular drink 'tequila'. Two of the best-known agaves are *Agave americana marginata* and *Agave sisalana*, which are grown in vast tracts of land for their valuable sisal – sometimes it is known as the sisal plant. The medicinal and food uses of the agaves were registered, researched and developed extensively by the 'German East Africa Company', which introduced the plants to Tanganyika (now Tanzania) around 1893 – both for medicine and for sisal. Used as ancient barriers and fences, the Native Americans and the Mexicans were the first to use the agaves medicinally.

Growing Agave

A popular pot plant in cold countries, the agave has spread to the rest of the world as a useful crop and as an effective stock barrier in arid regions. A tough and resilient survivor plant, it literally grows where nothing else does, and it can survive freezing temperatures up to –5 °C! Propagation is by seed, collected from the towering giant flowering spike, or from offsets that grow clustered under the parent plant. Leave the offsets to dry off for 3–4 days before planting. Planted in full sun, literally in any soil, the agave will thrive. Start it off in a compost-filled moist hole and water only once a week until it is established. Thereafter the occasional watering will keep it healthy and productive. Some varieties take 5–20 years to produce their flowering spike, and those with the grey-green leaves, the sisal agaves, are the hardiest of all. Their thorny leaf margins and sharp spikes at the end of the great thick leaves make them a marvellous barrier. Plant them 3 m apart – they do well in sandy soil.

Using Agave

Medicinally the whole plant, leaves, roots and the sap from the flowering stem, have been taken for centuries to treat rheumatism, scurvy, venereal diseases and to lower fevers by increasing perspiration. In Mexico, ancient uses include hormonal treatment, digestive ailments, flatulence, constipation, liver ailments including jaundice, and even dysentery. Externally the split peeled leaf is applied to burns, rashes and grazes. On sensitive skins this may cause irritation – so test first on the inside of the wrist. Interestingly, the fibres also contain insect-repelling substances. Crushed and pounded leaves tied at one end into a bundle are still used today as a swatter for flies, midges and mosquitoes, especially over the horses' backs and over cattle, and also over kitchen counter tops. Big round river stones are closely guarded as the 'pounding tool' and kept for that purpose by every family.

The sweet sap, which flows easily from the cut stem, is drunk as a much-loved refreshing juice, or fermented into a 'pulque' with added yeast. The swollen base of the leaves and the young and tender flowering stem is peeled and roasted as a delicious vegetable served with vinegar and mint.

Root extracts with the basal leaves are used in the manufacture of soap, and the coarse sisal fibres are woven into mats, ropes, thick twine and string. Leaf waste concentrate, after processing, is not thrown away as it surprisingly contains sources of hectogenin, which is a precursor for steroid drugs.

Caution

Pure agave juice can be bought at health shops, but be aware of the intensely sweetened agave syrup or nectar that is sold commercially, and which is chemically processed from fructose. Its processing method involves genetically modified enzymes, caustic soda and a list of chemicals that most certainly do not build health. Agave syrup or nectar is not made from the plant itself, but rather from a commercial product that is not diabetic friendly and not beneficial in any way to your body. Read the labels carefully, be alert and avoid these highly processed 'health fads'!

Health Note

Agave is rich in vitamins A, B and E, potassium, phosphorus, magnesium and amino acids.

Leek

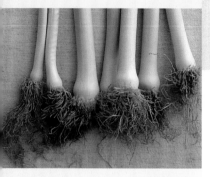

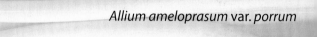

Allium ameloprasum var. *porrum*

Grandmother's Leek Soup

Serves 6–8

6 large leeks, well washed, roots removed, sliced thinly, white parts mainly but include at least 2 cups of the tender green parts

2 cups celery, chopped finely, leaves included

2 cups grated carrots

2 cups grated turnips

2–3 cups finely shredded kale or cabbage, especially the outer leaves

1 cup barley

1 cup split peas

1 cup brown lentils (soak barley, peas and lentils in hot water while preparing the rest of the ingredients)

½ cup olive oil

sea salt and black pepper to taste

juice of 1–2 lemons and a little grated lemon zest

about ¾ cup good homemade chutney, if you have it

2 tablespoons honey

2 litres strong homemade chicken stock, or use boiling water

Fry the leeks in the olive oil until lightly browned. Add all the vegetables and stir-fry briskly, adding a little more oil if needed. Then add the barley, split peas, lentils and lemon juice. Add the chicken stock or boiling water. Stir well and simmer, with the lid on. Stir frequently, adding more stock or water if necessary. When the barley is tender, season with salt and pepper, and if not tasty enough, add the chutney, more lemon juice and the honey. If anyone had a really bad cold, my grandmother added about a teaspoon of cayenne pepper as well. Serve hot in big bowls with crusty bread.

The wild leek, *Allium ameloprasum*, is indigenous to Asia, Europe and parts of North Africa. It is an ancient, respected, cherished and much-loved plant that has an ancient and extraordinary history. It was the Romans who took the leek to Britain, around AD 600. When the Welsh went into battle against the Saxons in AD 640, the soldiers, well fed with leeks for strength and courage, made the leek their emblem and were the victors of the great battle, and that is how the leek became the national emblem of Wales.

In the Middle Ages the monks used the leek as a medicine to treat coughs, colds, 'flu and chest ailments, to improve the voice, for sore throats and laryngitis, and the leek made into a syrup became a traditional winter medicine all over Europe and Britain.

Growing Leeks

Today leeks are as valuable a winter crop as they were in those ancient days – more as a food than as a medicine. As they have a long life and can be eaten small, young and tender as well as thick, mature and huge, it is so worthwhile growing them we should make it part of our winter garden annually. Sow the seeds in mid- to late summer to give the pencil thin seedlings time to fill out. They begin as tiny blades and when they are big enough to handle, they can be planted out in a well-dug, deeply and richly composted trench in full sun, spaced 30 cm apart. They love the cold weather and take heavy frost and even light snow. Water the trench thoroughly and deeply twice a week and you'll be rewarded with such a feast you'll become as addicted as we are!

Using Leeks

I have created so great an array of leek dishes I never tire of them, and they provide the same health benefits as garlic and onions: they help to lower the cholesterol levels, boost the immune system, fight cancer, chronic and degenerative diseases, fight coughs, colds, 'flu, sore throats, bronchitis, pneumonia, chronic coughs, laryngitis, and help to clear toxins from the liver, the pancreas and the kidneys.

The French went on to develop the still popular vichyssoise, a cold soup made of leeks and potatoes, and braised leeks with a mustard sauce are served still today in posh restaurants all over the world as a side dish accompanying poultry. Leeks became the traditional soup flavouring with turnips, carrots and celery, and the monks in Europe and England served this nourishing and warming soup to the poor, which formed the cornerstone for soup kitchens the world over. During the First and Second World War years, leeks were grown in every cottage garden with kale, cabbages, potatoes, turnips and carrots, and on this excellent diet many people survived. My grandmother made a leek soup for us as children and we never tired of it. Today, as I make it for my grandchildren, I go back to being 6 or 7 years old again and I can smell the leeks browning in the big soup pot ready for the rest of the ingredients, and I can hear my grandmother's voice urging speed as we grated the carrots. It seems like yesterday and it tastes the same. Try this wonderful soup; it will sustain you through the winter (see recipe alongside).

Health Note

Leeks are rich in vitamins A, C, K, B6, folic acid, iron, manganese and dietary fibre.

Onion

Allium cepa

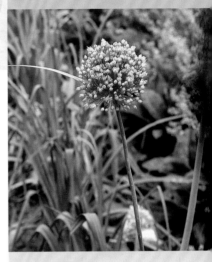

There are some 700 varieties of onions and they are cultivated all over the world, differing in colour, size, shape and even flavour. The history of the onion family is fascinating. Its earliest recordings go back to over 3000 BC and it is thought to have originated in Central Asia, possibly from Iran, spreading to Pakistan and as far as southern Russia. Recordings show that in the 6th century the onion was a valuable medicine in India, Greece and Italy.

There are two main types of onions – the large globe multi-layered type, the popular storage onion that can be successfully grown in cold climates and stored in the long dark winter months, and the smaller bunching onions like spring onions, Welsh onions (*Allium fistulosum*) and also shallots, scallions and pearl pickling onions. Then there are the ever-popular chives (*Allium schoenoprasum*), garlic (*Allium sativum*) and the garlic chive (*Allium tuberosum*) – all have the delicious and characteristic taste like no other, which is loved and enjoyed worldwide!

Growing Onions

Sow onion seed in trays and when the seedlings are big enough to handle, plant them out, about 10–12 cm apart, in full sun in deeply dug, richly composted soil. The bed needs to be kept moist and weeded until the tiny grass-like plants grow sizeable and sturdy. Once established, water the bed well twice weekly, once weekly in the cold months, and remember the more you pick of the bunching onions the more they grow. To start spring onions off buy a packet from the greengrocer, split them up and plant them 30–40 cm apart. Be very sure to keep them well watered, and even shaded, if you plant them out in hot weather.

All parts of the clump-forming spring onions, chives and garlic chives can be eaten – the slender bulbs, the hollow leaves and the flowers. For the big globe onions, which are often biennial, let them 'ripen' in the bed and before they send up a flowering stalk step on the leaves and bend them over. In this way they dry out quickly and can be lifted and hung tied in bunches in a cool, dark shed.

Using Onions

I cannot cook any savoury dish without them! The most versatile of vegetables, we need to be aware of the valuable nutritional and medicinal benefits within them. In addition to their legendary ability to act as a natural antibiotic, clinical studies have shown that garlic and onions lower high blood cholesterol, prevent clot formation, and significantly lower blood sugar levels. Eating fresh garlic and onions will help to cleanse the liver, tone the kidneys, treat asthma, relax muscle spasms, especially in the bronchi, and they even have the ability to arrest tumour growth. It has been found that liberally eating garlic, onions, leeks, chives and spring onions boosts the health thus breaking the disease patterns of many major illnesses, like cancers, atherosclerosis, even diabetes, that are so prevalent today.

Health Note

Onions are rich in vitamins C, B1, B6 and K, folic acid, organic sulphur, phosphorus and calcium. They also have a high pectin content and contain flavonoids and volatile oils.

Onion Salad in Mustard Sauce

This is one of my favourite onion dishes and in a well-sealed container it keeps beautifully in the fridge. Serve it with cold meats, cold chicken or cheese.

Peel and quarter 1 kg small onions. Cook in salted water until tender, usually about 20 minutes. Strain and cool.

In a heavy bottomed pot, whisk together:

3 eggs
1 tablespoon cornflour
125 ml brown grape vinegar
2 teaspoons salt
½ cup brown sugar
2–3 teaspoons mustard powder
250 ml full cream milk

Whisk vigorously until creamy, then, while whisking, heat the pot on medium heat until it thickens. Immediately remove from the stove and pour over the cooled onions. Stir in gently until every piece of onion is well covered. Cool in the fridge. Just before serving sprinkle with freshly chopped parsley.

Garlic

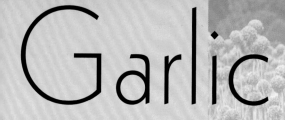

Allium sativum

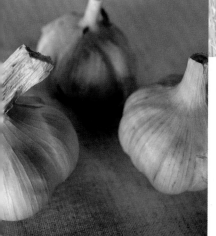

Garlic Health Toast

Serves 1

Many years ago an old doctor told me this is the best way to eat garlic in order to get its full benefit.

Grow your own organic garlic. When it is fully developed, before the thin green leaves start to dry off, pull it up and wash it carefully. Cut the top of the bulb off and with a rolling pin roll and squeeze out the soft flesh, discarding the papery shells around it, and spread onto hot lightly buttered toast. Squeeze over this plenty of fresh lemon juice, dust with a touch of cayenne pepper and a sprinkling of fresh parsley and eat it slowly, chewing well. Wash it down with a cup of mint tea!

Hint

In the garden folklore garlic enjoys high status: planted around roses it is believed to give the rose a deeper perfume (I've never been convinced of this, as the garlic is so pungent!) and it also keeps moles away, they say, and it chases flies, ticks and fleas!

Garlic was found in the tomb of Tutankhamen (who died *c.* 1340 BC) but its recorded history dates back to Babylonian times, 3000 years BC. Its earliest beginnings, it is thought, originate in Asia and Sanskrit documents record garlic remedies 5 000 years ago. The ancient Romans, Greeks and Egyptians also recorded its medicinal uses and it was used in ancient Chinese medicine in AD 500. Since ancient times, garlic was considered to be a protective good luck charm if carried in a pocket or tied in a little bag around the neck; it is believed even to ward off vampires! Throughout history, myth and legend, garlic is woven unforgettably, its ancient uses largely verified today by medical research. Garlic has to be one of the most pungent, powerful smelling of all plants – its pervasive and typical all-engulfing smell is caused by its rich sulphur compounds and therefore its therapeutic value is of the highest value.

Growing Garlic

Garlic bulbs encased in papery husks consist of a number of 'bulblets' known as 'garlic cloves'. It is these that are planted, as garlic does not produce seed. In spring, split the garlic bulb and plant each individual clove, pointed side up, 2–3 cm deep and 15 cm apart in well-dug, richly composted, moist soil in full sun. I find in the hot dry area where I live that a light mulch of leaves helps to maintain the moisture of the soil so that no hard crust forms and the little pointed tips can grow unhampered. Do not let the area dry out in the first weeks. Thereafter a good twice weekly watering, or more in very hot weather, ensures a good crop. Reap when the top growth dies down and dries, losing its greenness, usually by late summer (in a very hot year, even midsummer). Hang in bunches to dry under cover – an open shed far away from the house is ideal! They do need to be kept cool and aired.

Using Garlic

One could say garlic is an indispensable culinary herb with an almost unbelievable medicinal value. It protects against heart disease, atherosclerosis and high cholesterol, it helps to lower high blood pressure, strengthens the heart and improves circulation. It strengthens the immune system and has a long history as a superb treatment for bacterial and viral infections. It contains a compound known as allicin which fights colds, 'flu, bronchitis, asthma, stomach viruses, candida yeast and even diabetes and tuberculosis, and it is a protection against some cancers. New research has shown that garlic not only protects the colon from cancer-forming toxic chemicals, but also stops the growth of the cancer cells once they start to develop.

Ideally a clove of garlic should be eaten daily with plenty of fresh chopped parsley and freshly squeezed lemon juice to help deodorise the smell! But for those who cannot stomach the taste and the aftertaste of garlic, tablets and capsules are available from the chemist.

In 1609 in a book called *The Englishman's doctor* Sir John Harrington wrote:

> *Garlic then have power to save from death,*
> *Bear with it though it maketh unsavoury breath.*
> *And scorn not garlic like some that think,*
> *It only maketh men wink, drink and STINK!*

Health Note

An important medicinal plant, garlic is rich in vitamins B6 and C, phosphorus, calcium, iron, copper, potassium, manganese and selenium.

Amaranth

Amaranthus caudatus · Amaranthus hypochondriacus

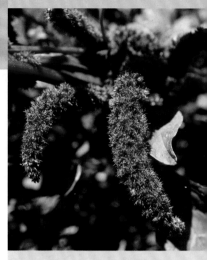

This is one of the most exceptional foods in the world! An ancient, respected and revered medicine, the name *Amaranthus* comes from the Greek word *Amaranton*, which means 'unfading' and it *is* unfading in its vigorousness, its survival mode of growing no matter where – even in the crack of a hot city pavement – its robust prolific flowering and showering of millions of nourishing seeds, and its all summer long luscious leaf growth no matter the drought, the heat, the neglect. Amaranth is a cosmopolitan weed, the leaves used as a beloved *morogo* in South Africa and as a spinach throughout the world, and the seed as a nourishing grain that has been used as a porridge and to make bread since the Stone Age. This genus consists of over 50 annuals. All are used as food and it is found worldwide, and it is loved and cherished everywhere.

Growing Amaranth

It can be found as a tough annual everywhere – along the roadsides, in disturbed ground, in fields and in cities – and once you have it, you'll always have it. At one time I had a collection of amaranth, from tiny, juicy, succulent ankle-high plants to the giant 2–3 m tall one with great sprays of magenta flowers and stems that turned shocking pink in the autumn. I've never been without seedlings since, and they can be transplanted into well-dug, lightly composted moist soil in full sun, or in light shade, when they are quite tiny. I space them 50 cm apart and pick them early on. The more you pick the more they grow!

Using Amaranth

An ancient medicine for blood building, warriors ate amaranth for strength and nursing mothers ate amaranth for breast milk production and to make the baby flourish. Today's research finds amaranth important for treating anaemia and chronic fatigue, and for chronic and intermittent diarrhoea. I am always intrigued that those ancient medicinal uses were so spot-on – modern research verifies them!

Amaranth tea is an excellent remedy for heavy menstrual bleeding, and for excessive vaginal discharge, coughs and colds, and for ulcers in the mouth and stomach the astringent tea soothes and heals. To make the tea, take ¼ cup amaranth leaves, pour over it 1 cup of boiling water, stand 5 minutes, strain and sip slowly sitting down. Take 2–3 cups daily and use the cooled tea as a gargle or as a lotion for burning, scratchy, itching skin. The mist spray of cooled tea is excellent for reducing oiliness, for refreshing and cleansing the skin and for adding to the rinsing water after shampooing the hair to reduce oiliness, dandruff and itchy scalp. Spritz it over sunburn and problem oily skins and use the cooled tea as a wash and a lotion over acne spots.

For the dog's itchy skin, boil up a large pot of fresh amaranth leaves in enough water to cover for 20 minutes. Cool and strain. Add to the dog's bath water after washing him. Add fresh leaves, boiled for 10 minutes in a little water, to the dog's food, and amaranth tea, well strained, to the dog's drinking water. This will soothe itchiness, rashes, insect bites and stop the endless scratching.

Health Note

Amaranth is a low GI food. It is a source of protein, the amino acids lysine and methionine, vitamins B2, B3, B5, B6, C and E, folic acid, iron, copper, calcium, manganese, magnesium, zinc and phytosterols.

Amaranth Spinach Dish

Serves 4

2 onions, finely chopped
olive oil
6 cups fresh amaranth leaves
2 cups water
1 teaspoon salt
juice of 1 lemon

Stir-fry the onions in a little olive oil. Add the fresh amaranth leaves and briefly stir-fry. Add the water and salt. Finally, add the lemon juice and serve hot as a vegetable dish with fish, poultry or meat. You will never tire of it, and just feel the energy it imparts!

Hint

To collect the nourishing seed, spread a large sheet or two of newspaper out on the ground. Shake the ripened flower sprays over it and collect the tiny grey seeds for using like poppy seeds in breads, porridge, cakes, muesli and stir-fries. It tastes nutty and delicious!

Cashew Nut

Anacardium occidentale

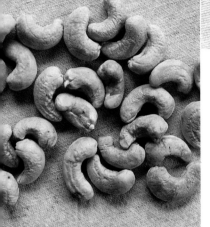

A beautiful and intriguing evergreen tree that grows about 10 m in height, the cashew nut is indigenous to northern Brazil and the West Indies. It was the Portuguese explorers who took it to India, Malaysia and Mozambique, where it is now cultivated as an important commercial crop. What is so fascinating about this huge tree is its fruit. There is a fleshy, elongated 'apple' that is actually the stalk, and the hard-shelled nut develops at first inside the fleshy fruit and is approximately 10 cm long and 5 cm wide. It ripens from a light green colour to bright red or golden yellow, and the nut then protrudes outside below the mature fruit. The swollen stem is tasty and juicy when fully ripe and is usually eaten raw or sliced and sweetened with sugar. The nut is contained in a hard shell in which an acrid, skin-irritating oil is present. The nuts must be roasted in order to render the oil less caustic. The smoke or steam that is produced during the roasting process is also irritating to the eyes and to the skin, so great care must be taken. Once heated, the nuts are harmless and can be easily and safely removed from their shells.

Growing Cashew Nuts

Growers in Mozambique have sent small trees to botanical gardens as curiosities, and although the cashew needs a tropical climate, growers agree it thrives in warm sea air. I have been brought a cashew tree which found the dry hot mountain air an unequal battle and I sadly lost it, in spite of careful nurturing.

Using Cashew Nuts

If we knew of the enormous journey cashew nuts go on to arrive quite inexpensively in our markets and shops we should be gratefully impressed, as the crop is frequently erratic and difficult to reap, and the distances are enormous and much manpower is needed to process the nuts and get them freed from their caustic shells. Next time you pop a rich and creamy cashew nut into your mouth, think a little about the small miracle of the cashew!

In Brazil the fermented 'cashew apple' produces a potent and much-loved wine, also a precious vinegar called *anacard*, and a raw nut butter that has been eaten for centuries. The nuts are highly nutritious eaten unsalted and through the centuries have been used raw to treat emaciation, lack of energy and vitality, also for children who fail to thrive, for teeth and gum ailments and for the elderly. A nourishing drink is made by pounding the raw nuts in milk or water until a thick 'gruel' or soup is made and ½ a cup is taken 3 times a day to treat the above ailments. The fruit stalk is made into jam and candied fruit slices, fruit juices and relishes.

No wonder those ancient Portuguese explorers were so excited about this amazing tree!

Health Note

Cashew nuts are rich in iron, phosphorus and calcium particularly, as well as vitamins A, D, E and K. The fruit stalk is rich in vitamin C.

Cashew Cakes

Makes 12

These cakes are particularly delicious served as a dessert with vanilla ice-cream.

2 cups sifted cake flour
1 cup chopped cashew nuts, raw and unsalted
2 eggs, well beaten in ½ cup of milk
4 tablespoons soft butter
2 teaspoons baking powder
a pinch of salt
3–4 tablespoons honey, warmed over hot water until runny

Add the baking powder and salt to the flour and stir well. Rub in the butter with the fingertips until the mixture resembles fine breadcrumbs. Add the rest of the ingredients and mix to a slack dough. Place small cupcake paper cases on a baking tray and fill each one with a tablespoon of dough – enough to almost fill the little paper case. Place in a warm oven, preheated to 180 ºC, and watch them carefully – they will start to turn light golden brown after 10 minutes. Test to see if they are done by pressing lightly. Serve warm with a dusting of icing sugar.

Pineapple

Ananas comosus

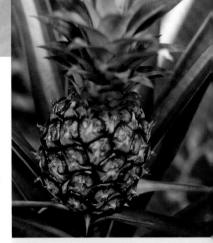

We once again have South America to thank for this fabulous tropical fruit that looks so like a green pine cone that this is where it got its name! Christopher Columbus was the first to bring the pineapple back to Europe, but it was found to be difficult to grow in the cold winters of Europe. 'Hot houses' were constructed to create the warmth it needed – some say these were the first hot houses – so great was the desire for this exotic and fascinating fruit. In the 17th and 18th centuries the pineapple became the symbol of hospitality, and carvings of pineapples often topped the gate pillars of country houses and inns. By the end of the 16th century, Spanish and Portuguese explorers took it further to the warmer tropical areas of the South Pacific and North Africa. The United States of America had by this time established pineapple fields in their warm areas and today they are amongst the biggest producers of one of the world's favourite fruits, with Mexico, Brazil, the Philippine Islands, China and Thailand being the other main producers. South Africa too established good fields and we can proudly compete in the world market.

Growing Pineapples

Propagation is from the crowns – the tuft of leaves above the fruit – and many a child has cultivated a pineapple on the kitchen windowsill, and although a slow beginning, it is fascinating to watch it in a large compost-filled pot. If the conditions are right, it sends down roots and when sturdy it can be planted out in full sun in a frost-free garden in a large hole filled with compost. It is a drought-resistant plant so do not be tempted to over-water and water from below, not into the tuft of leaves. A new fruit will gradually form in the centre of the tuft of spiky leaves within a mass of tiny flowers, one fruit per plant, which, when ripe, can be carefully cut away from its base or axis. The fruit is actually formed from the central core of the plant within the fleshy flowers, which form the outer skin or rind! It is nothing short of intriguing! The leaves, sharp pointed and spiny, must be handled with care and gloves are advised when cutting away the ripened fruits. The pineapple fields nearer the sea are often considered to yield the best and the sweetest fruits, it is claimed, but it is worth trying in dry, frost-free areas just for the interest alone.

Using Pineapples

Rich in the precious bromelain, which is a superb digestive aid, and containing a group of sulphur protein digestive enzymes, which reduce inflammatory conditions, the pineapple is considered to be a protective fruit for the digestive system, and clinical trials are ongoing. To maximise the benefits of bromelain, it is best to have a half a glass of freshly liquidised pineapple juice, or put the fresh slices through a juice extractor with carrots, and sip it slowly between meals. Doctors recommend fresh pineapple and pineapple juice for treating carpal tunnel syndrome, to reduce and clear mucus in pneumonia and severe bronchitis, to treat acute sinusitis, arthritis, throat infections, gout, swollen joints and also to help to restore the body post operatively and after injury.

Serve it frequently in salads and fresh fruit desserts – eaten with other fruits and salads it lessens the sharp sensation on the tongue.

Health Note

Pineapple is rich in vitamins A, C and B6, beta-carotene, calcium, iron and phosphorus, and it contains bromelian, an excellent digestive aid. It also contains sulphur, protein and digestive enzymes, which reduce inflammatory conditions.

Pineapple Grill

For a quick and utterly delicious dessert, it is so delectable it could be served as a party piece.

In a glass ovenproof baking dish, lay slices of fresh pineapple. Drizzle with maple syrup and a little grinding of allspice berries (pimento) or nutmeg and place under the grill. Just as it starts to brown, remove it and serve it hot with plain Greek yoghurt. You'll be surprised by the compliments.

Hint

Dry slices of pineapple in a low oven or in a dryer. It is perfect for school lunches and children love it!

Custard Apple
Cherimoya

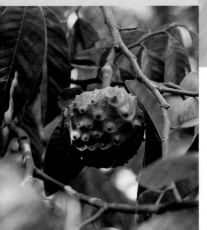

We have a lot to thank Peru for. Many of our delicious tropical and subtropical fruits originate from there and the extraordinary and utterly delicious custard apple is one of their treasures. This fabulous fruit thrives high in the Colombian and Peruvian Andes at altitudes up to 1 200 m above sea level, but it is equally at home in the hot and humid areas of Ecuador. There is no other way to describe it – its sweet, delectable flesh is as soft and as digestible as custard and it has been, for centuries, enjoyed fresh, ripe and scooped out of the sturdy shell – nothing fancy, just that. Commercial plantings are valuable in many areas of India, Java, Ecuador, Malaysia, Jamaica, Peru and even Thailand, for processing the custard apple into juices, ice-cream and jellies. It has never lost its popularity and it has been loved and enjoyed for centuries. Many home gardens are shaded by a tree or two and the fruit is left to ripen on the tree, or, for commercial use, picked just a couple of days before it is fully ripe so as not to soften too much on the journey. The thick, leathery and strong skin protects the soft pulp with its large black seeds, but watch for the birds as their sharp beaks pierce it with no problem!

Growing Custard Apples

The tree is a small, neat grower with large leathery leaves and tubular creamy flowers which turn into larger than fist-sized fruits, 12–15 cm in diameter, which are clearly marked with 'scales' that start off pale green and ripen to dark brown. The tree thrives in full sun in a large, deeply dug, compost-filled hole that can be flooded with water once or even twice a week. The trees bear fruit when they are quite young and a newly planted one a mere 3 years old gave me an unexpected surprise by producing two enormous fruits – so heavy and so perfect that they weighed the branches down. What a feast they provided and as the first cold days of winter tinged its leaves with yellow, the unnoticed summer bounty detached itself from the branch to lie waiting on the path – two huge ripe and perfect custard apples!

Using Custard Apples

The ripe flesh is used still today as a skin softening scrub to clear pimples, oiliness and blackheads, and the skins, once the flesh has been spooned out, are a much-loved skin treatment rubbed over cracked heels, dry calluses on the feet, and for healing rashes, scratches and grazes. Through the decades a tea made of the leaves boiled in water was used as a wash for sore, scraped feet, cracked heels and for corns and rough patches of skin. Cloths soaked in the tea were bound round the feet, often with the leaves, over the rough, sore places, the cloth holding them in place, and then the required 15 minutes of sitting still and letting the leaf infusion do its soothing calming work, resulted in a release from pain and dryness that rivals the best beauty treatments today! The mashed ripe flesh is also a much-loved face mask, the custard consistency a superb skin cleanser and softener, the Malaysians will tell you.

A cooling drink made with mashed fruit, plain yoghurt and cinnamon is a favourite refresher, and if this is frozen it makes a delicious type of ice-cream. The fruit is very sweet so no sugar needs to be added.

Health Note

Custard apples are rich in vitamins, particularly vitamins A, C and D, and also potassium, magnesium and phosphorus.

Custard Apple Yoghurt

Serves 2

This makes a party dish that has guests clamouring for more!

Mix 1 cup of plain Bulgarian yoghurt with 1 cup of mashed fresh custard apple. Sprinkle with cinnamon and chopped almonds or cashew nuts. Serve in pretty bowls as a deliciously light dessert. Sweeten with a touch of honey if liked.

Hint

There are several different species of custard apple – the *Annona* genus – and all have the same delicious custard-like flesh. The fruit ripens at the very end of the autumn, so in early winter greengrocers will have trays of the fragrant, delicious custard apples or cherimoyas for sale. Look out for them – it is a taste experience that is unforgettable.

Celery

Apium graveolens

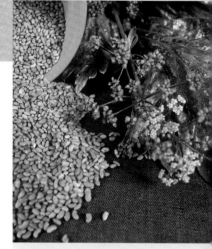

Celery, that easy to grow biennial, has to be one of the world's favourite health foods! Modern celery, as we know it today, actually comes from the ancient wild celery indigenous to the Mediterranean area, Europe and Britain, where it has been much respected and much used since the 9th century when it was widely taken as a medicine – especially the seeds, but also the stalks and leaves – and cherished as a flavouring in soups and stews, a tradition, it is thought, started by the Romans that has been continued through the centuries to this day! I cannot even think of making soup without celery!

During the 16th century the use of celery as a flavouring and food and as a medicine expanded enormously. Salt was a rare and expensive commodity and celery was cultivated, the stems blanched much as we know it today, making it a valuable vegetable that lessened the need for salt. It was then taken to clear the system of toxins and excess fluid, and to soothe arthritic and rheumatic aches and pains. Over 3 000 years ago the ancient Egyptians ate celery to build strong bones, strong muscles and fleetness of foot. In the 5th century BC the ancient Chinese were eating celery and making teas of celery to slow the ageing process, to treat serious illnesses and to flush toxins from the body! Today the Chinese eat a celery salad daily as a tonic and a cleanser and to lower blood pressure and as an anti-cancer treatment. I never cease to be astonished that those ancient uses are verified today by our modern research!

Growing Celery

Sow seeds in trays throughout the year, except in the coldest months. Plant out when big enough to handle into bags to establish the tiny plants before planting out into the garden. Choose a well-composted, deeply dug bed in full sun and space the plants 30 cm apart and fill the hole with water as you lower the plant into it. Do not disturb the roots too much as you peel away the bag in which it is growing. I plant new batches frequently – every 2 to 4 months – and treat it as an annual, except for allowing a row to set seed which I reap for salts and flavoured sauces, and for teas. Do not use the celery seed you buy for sowing for medicinal teas, or for flavouring – reap your own organically grown seed.

To blanch the stems, wrap in a collar of folded newspaper with just the tips of the leaves protruding and pile up the soil around it. This lengthens and whitens the stems. Keep replacing the old newspaper collars with new higher collars as the plant grows taller and taller. Soup celery is unblanched – the leaves on shorter stems are sold in bundles in the greengrocer.

Using Celery

Seeds, leaves and stems lower blood pressure and are a superb diuretic, cleansing both kidneys and bladder and are valuable in treating cystitis. Celery literally clears toxins and is valuable for treating arthritis, gout and rheumatism, as it dissolves and flushes out the urates that cause the stiffness and pain, and it clears acidity from the whole body. It is a well-known anti-convulsant and anti-cancer treatment and tones the vascular system. To make celery seed tea, pour 1 cup of boiling water over 1 teaspoon of organically grown celery seeds. Stand 5 minutes, sip slowly and chew the seeds well. *Do not take during pregnancy or if you have a kidney disorder.*

Health Note

Rich in potassium, sodium, calcium, folic acid, vitamins C, K, B1, B2, B3 and B6, celery is so a valuable health food it should be eaten often.

Celery Health Salad

Serves 1

Chop up 2 celery stalks and leaves, add a little chopped cucumber, ½ cup grated carrots and ½ cup chopped pineapple. Squeeze lemon juice as a dressing and be amazed at how quickly this cleansing salad flushes out the toxins, and migraine sufferers find this salad reduces migraine attacks.

Hint

Celeriac is a close relative to celery that has a swollen root and short stems, and is a popular vegetable in Europe. Its root is grated into soups and sauces and salads, and it can be grown the same way as celery but without blanching the stems. Look out for it in autumn and winter in your local greengrocer. It is an exquisitely tasty addition to a hearty winter soup.

Waterblommetjie
Cape pondweed
Aponogeton distachyos

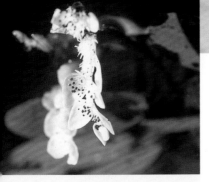

Traditional Cape Waterblommetjie Bredie

Serves 6–8

I learned to make this traditional recipe when I was 22 years old, taught to me by a Cape farmer's wife and I make it every season and love it still as much as I did then!

1 kg fresh waterblommetjies (or 2 tins waterblommetjies)
1–2 kg mutton loin chops, fat removed, or leg trimmed of fat
¾ cup runny honey
3 large onions, chopped
2–3 tablespoons sunflower cooking oil
3–4 cups water
1 cup white wine
4 large potatoes, peeled and cubed
4 carrots, peeled and thinly sliced
juice of 1 lemon
1 cup celery stalks, thinly sliced
1–2 cups sorrel (Cape sorrel, Oxalis pes caprae, is used traditionally, but I use garden sorrel, Rumex acetosa)
sea salt and black pepper to taste

Soak the fresh waterblommetjies in water to remove any grit that may have lodged between the petals and scales of the flower. In a heavy bottomed pot fry the onions to a golden brown. Paint the lamb with the honey and brown with the onions, turning frequently. Add all the other ingredients, except the wine, and simmer with the lid on, stirring gently every now and then. Add a little more water if needed and simmer until the meat is tender. Add the wine last and cook a few more minutes. Serve piping hot on a bed of rice.

This beautiful and fascinating water plant with its exquisite white fragrant butterfly flower is a sight in spring across the shallow dams in the Cape. It is only found in the Western Cape and the flowers and the rhizomes have been part of the diet of the Khoi and the San people for over 1 000 years! Today, thanks to enterprising Boland farmers, fresh and tinned waterblommetjies are available to other provinces and all over the world as well. The plants have adapted well to other countries and are grown in ponds in botanical gardens all over the world as a botanical rarity. Flat oval leaves float on the surface of the water and in spring the small forked white flowers with their double row of 'petals' or bracts held above the water in two separate parts look like a mass of white butterflies scattered over the pond.

Growing Waterblommetjies

Many years ago I was given a plastic pot with a few small rhizomes of the first waterblommetjie I was to grow in the central small pond in the Herbal Centre gardens. Unimpressed with the tangled, somewhat slimy mass of roots and flat leaves, I filled a big new plastic pot with rich compost and replanted the root mass in it, gently sinking it, very, very slowly, into the water. A few flat fairly large pebbles placed on top of the pot kept the roots anchored. Left to grow amongst the water lilies, I confess to not watching it diligently, so imagine my delight when in midwinter in the dry cold of a North West winter a mass of white flowers sparkled in the winter sunshine, delicate, intricate, tiny black stamens enticing the bees. The first waterblommetjies set my heart racing, and from that day I have never been without them.

Each year we pot up new plants – they set seed easily – and tiny new plants, leaves as thin as a match, can be lifted out of the water easily to find a new home in another large compost-filled plastic pot. The tuberous rootstock settles into the mud quickly. Propagation can also be easily done by slicing the large mother rootstock where there is a visible 'eye'. Fill the pots with compost – they need to be at least 40 cm deep – and gently submerge them into a large water-filled tub. Left to stand a few days in the tub of water to settle, it can then be slowly lowered into the pond, the roots held in place by a few pebbles placed here and there. Each year or two we replace the old compost with fresh compost and divide up the roots and rhizomes and replant. Surprisingly tolerant, it needs full sun and at least 60 cm of water in which to flourish.

Using Waterblommetjies

Crushed waterblommetjie stems soothe rashes, cuts and grazes, sunburn, chafed skin and light burns. For mosquito bites, stings and itchy areas, the juicy stems remain a valuable treatment and the leaves, washed and well rinsed, make a comforting poultice over sprains, bruises and strains, held in place with a crêpe bandage. Some of the old recordings of the Cape remedies showed the use of the fresh leaves – warmed first – placed over rheumatic swollen joints. Crushed flower petals can be applied to a pimple or over acne and the crushed waterblommetjie stems make an excellent gel to ease rashes, grazes, burns and hot itchiness.

Traditional dishes abound and the famous waterblommetjie bredie still tops the list (see recipe). Add the flowers to stir-fries with celery, onions, green peppers and mushrooms for a sustaining and delicious lunch dish, dressed with a little olive oil and lots of freshly squeezed lemon juice.

Health Note

The flowers are a source of vitamins C, A, D, E and some B-vitamins, folic acid, calcium, potassium, magnesium, copper, phosphorus. The rhizomes contain starch.

Peanut

Arachis hypogaea

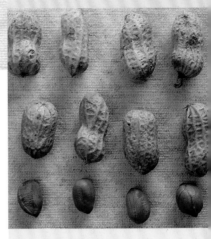

A popular crop worldwide, the peanut that we know today is a cultigen from the wild legume that originated in South America on the southern slopes of the Andes, from Argentina to Bolivia and possibly in Peru as well. It became a staple food and spread from South America to Mexico around 3 500 years ago. The underground nuts could be taken for long distances in their shells without spoiling and, thanks to the Spanish explorers, this valuable food source quickly spread to Africa, where it became known as the 'goober nut'. It soon became entrenched in the cuisine and culture of the African people, and once the slave trade began, it was the African people who introduced it to North America and Europe.

In the 1800s George Washington Carver urged American farmers to plant peanuts as a valuable food source in the cotton fields, after the Civil War ended. He developed 300 ways in which to use peanuts, and was the first American to make peanut oil! Dr John Kellogg – well known for his Kellogg's cornflakes – mashed up peanuts for the now well-loved peanut butter as a protein substitute for his patients who had dental problems and could not chew meat sufficiently well. And from this early beginning the peanut butter we know today was established!

Growing Peanuts

A leguminous annual crop, its above-ground growth is succulent and spreads 50 cm in height and about 1 m in width. Some varieties are low growing. It needs well-dug, compost-rich, sandy soil and full sun. The yellow flowers are self-pollinating. After pollination the stems grow quickly, pushing the tiny pods into the sandy soil – often known as a 'groundnut' – and there they grow underground in a pale 'shell' that protects the soft and oily seeds, the actual nuts. It is quite an amazing crop and it is grown worldwide in all subtropical areas and harvested by hand and piled in heaps or 'stacks' to dry out. In the vast commercial fields it is dug out by mechanical harvesters. The demand for organically grown peanuts is rising, due to the dangerous fumigants that are injected into the soil, as it is a heavy feeding crop and there is often not enough land to practise crop rotation.

Using Peanuts

Buying peanuts still in their shells ensures a fresher nut and ideally crushing your own nuts is healthier eating. Buy peanut oil in small quantities, as it easily goes rancid, and keep it in the fridge.

Rich in healthy monounsaturated fats, the peanut is a protector of the cardiovascular system and it lowers the 'bad' blood cholesterol and maintains the 'good' cholesterol.

Peanuts and peanut oil are included in many commercial products – mayonnaises, salad dressings, sauces, sweets and biscuits, curries, soups, margarines, spreads and tinned sardines, and in baked goods of all descriptions, and even in cosmetics! Great care must be taken for those allergic to peanuts to read the labels with extreme care – the oil is often called arachis oil or groundnut oil.

Health Note

Peanuts are rich in monounsaturated fats, proteins, vitamins B1, B3 and E, folic acid, magnesium, phosphorus and manganese. But salted, roasted peanuts are not a healthy snack! Rather eat them raw, freshly shelled.

Caution

Peanuts with mould on them are extremely dangerous to eat – buy fresh peanuts and keep them in the fridge. Eating rancid or mould-infected peanuts can introduce carcinogenic aflatoxins into the body. Peanuts can cause the mucus membranes to swell and this can lead to anaphylactic shock.

Peanuts are one of the most seriously allergenic foods in the world – a danger food of epic proportions for those who are allergic to it. Commercial products containing the oil as well as the nuts *must be clearly marked on the packaging*. Extreme care needs to be taken at all times by those who are allergic to peanuts. Ask at a restaurant if you are in any doubt, as a rush to the nearest hospital is traumatic.

A final word of caution: avoid eating too many roasted peanuts, and peanuts for children should be carefully monitored. They can become very oily within the stomach and react with other foods and cause vomiting.

Burdock

Arctium lappa

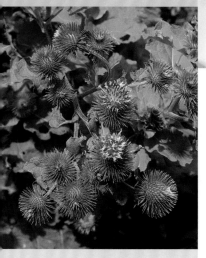

This huge and fascinating robust biannual originates in China and Japan and in the early centuries was introduced into Europe and beyond as a food and as a medicine. It has been part of history and it has been a cherished and precious herb for centuries, and I count myself lucky to have it growing so abundantly in the Herbal Centre gardens. The Chinese have considered it to be a valuable medicinal herb and included it in stir-fries, in drinks and in soups – usually the thinly sliced or grated root – as a daily health booster. In Japan it was considered to be an elixir for energy, for recovery from severe illness and for prevention of illness, and as far back as the 10th century it was made into teas, soups and pickles – the taproot and the young tender leaves and stems – and forms to this day an important part of the pharmacopoeia and medical history of Japan.

Growing Burdock

A robust survivor plant, propagation is from seed that forms in its rounded thistle-like flowers with crowns of magenta 'petals'. It seeds itself all over the garden and its branched flowering head grows to a lofty 1,5 m in height. The seeds are encased in burrs that attach themselves to everything and so spread easily. Sow the seeds in individual pots so that they can be transplanted easily while still small; they have a long taproot that does not like to be disturbed. Start off the little seedling in a deep, moist, compost-filled hole and water it well – literally soak it with water. Do not let the little seedling dry out, keep it moist until it is well established. Thereafter give it a good weekly soaking. It thrives in full sun and has adapted to the heat of the African sun and sparse rainfall amazingly well. In the first year it forms a rosette of huge leaves and often spreads 1 m in diameter – so always space burdock at least 1½–2 m apart. In its second year it will send up the flowering spike. Harvest the long taproot before the flowering spike appears and use the leaves for medicinal teas. With its huge rhubarb-like leaves on velvety silvery white stems and the flowering head, it is simply spectacular in the garden!

Using Burdock

An amazing detoxifier, burdock root particularly has been found to assist in removing and eliminating heavy metals from the body and it helps to clear the lungs. Once grown near the coal mines and industrial areas thick with pollution, dust and fumes, a tea made of burdock leaves, stems and roots was given to the workers daily to clear out the toxins from the body. It has strong cleansing, antiseptic and detoxifying properties as well as anti-tumour action. Burdock also contains an ingredient called arctiin, which is a smooth muscle relaxant, so it is helpful for gout, kidney stones, fevers, muscular aches and pains and swollen arthritic joints, and is excellent in alleviating the symptoms of mumps and measles.

The young and tender leaves, eaten as a spinach and served with lemon juice, soothe psoriasis, eczemas and acne. Make a tea of the leaves – ¼ cup fresh leaf and stalk to 1 cup boiling water, stand 5 minutes, strain and sip slowly, 1 cup a day. The cooled tea can be used as a lotion for psoriasis and eczema and a warmed leaf over a boil or abscess will quickly bring it to a head. The tea is excellent for coughs, colds and 'flu (it has mild antibiotic properties) and for rheumatism, arthritis and stomach disorders it is immediately soothing. Take 2–3 cups daily during times of acute infection, or one cup a day for all other ailments.

Health Note

Burdock contains carbohydrates, vitamins A and E, folic acid, potassium, magnesium, lignans and arctiin, a smooth muscle relaxant.

Pickled Burdock Stems

This is delicious served with cheeses and cold meats.

2 litres of grape vinegar
2 tablespoons coriander seed
2 tablespoons celery seed
2 tablespoons fresh thyme
1 cup of honey

Boil everything together for 10 minutes in a stainless steel pot with a well-fitting lid. Meanwhile chop 6 cups of burdock stems into 1 cm long pieces and simmer in enough water to cover them for 20 minutes. Drain and pack into screw-top jars. Pour over the vinegar pickle mixture, enough to completely cover the stems. Seal the lids tightly, label and store in a cool, dark cupboard.

Hint

Try boiling the young buds and eat them like artichokes served with salt, a little butter and lemon juice, just the way the Chinese do to lower blood sugar levels.

Horseradish

Armoracia rusticana

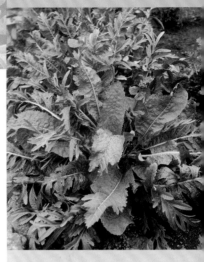

For many centuries the pungent, powerful and extraordinary root of horseradish was grown as a medicine, long before its culinary values were even thought about! Indigenous to Europe and Western Asia, horseradish leaves and roots were used by the Egyptians around 1500 BC, by the ancient Greeks and Romans for toothache, for rubs into painful arthritic joints, for backache and even for phlegm and deep, moist coughs as an expectorant. By 1300 horseradish had spread further and further as a medicine and in the Scandinavian countries and Britain it became a valuable cough medicine and was also used for scurvy and tuberculosis, and as it was easily grown from pieces of the amazingly strong root, it was soon used as trade. By around the 1590s the Germans found that the crushed root mixed with vinegar made a tasty condiment for preserving meat and fish, and by the early 1600s it had spread to France as a condiment and became known as *Moutarde des Allemands* – German mustard! So by the 1640s the culinary use of horseradish was well established in Europe and England, and it was even grown at inns where it was mixed with other herbs as a bitter and pungent and reviving ale for weary travellers!

By the 18th century horseradish was included in the *Materia Medica* of the London Pharmacopoeia as *Rusticanus*, officially recorded as a valuable medicine for the treatment of pain, rheumatism and scurvy, as an anti-scorbutic for improving the digestion, as an expectorant in respiratory ailments and as an emetic. Horseradish poultices applied to areas of gout, sciatica and neuralgias became popular and before long horseradish was introduced to America, where whole farms were started by the 1850s. Today horseradish is so popular in America that the Horseradish Information Council states that 'each year approximately 24 million pounds of horseradish roots are ground and processed into 6 million gallons of sauce, sufficient to season enough sandwiches to circle the world 12 times'!

Growing Horseradish

Propagation is by root pieces and at the end of the summer the clump is lifted, large roots removed for processing and the smaller roots are replanted in deeply dug, richly composted moist soil – I have never been without horseradish since my early plantings over 40 years ago, just by replanting the little roots each year – and a tuft of deeply serrated leaves as well as simple leaves emerges with the warmth of spring. As a companion plant under fruit trees it helps to prevent mildew and fungus development, and it acts as a tonic to the soil – so it is a valuable plant to have in the garden.

Using Horseradish

Medicinally it has been found that horseradish has antiseptic, antibiotic, diuretic and expectorant properties and that it is excellent for chest ailments, for the circulation and that a syrup made from grated fresh horseradish will soothe and ease persistent coughs, colds, 'flu and fevers. A poultice stimulates the blood flow to the area and is thus excellent for arthritis, gout, aching muscles, sprains, stiff joints and aching feet.

The tender leaves – just a little as the peppery taste is strong – can be finely chopped and added to salads and stir-fries, and the roots, freshly grated and mixed with vinegar, make the popular horseradish sauce which should be eaten sparingly as it is so powerfully strong!

Health Note

Horseradish is a source of vitamins C, D and E, copper, sulphur, iron, calcium, magnesium and phosphorus.

Horseradish Sauce

My favourite way of eating horseradish is this simple recipe my grandmother taught me. It is delicious with beef, cheese, grilled fish and spread on a ham sandwich!

Finely grate 3 cups of fresh, well-scrubbed, carefully peeled horseradish roots. Combine 1½ cups of brown grape vinegar and ½ cup of boiling water into which 1 cup of honey has been dissolved. Then add the grated horseradish root and mix well. Spoon into sterilised jars with a well-fitting screw-top lid and seal. Be sure all the horseradish is submerged. Add a little extra vinegar if necessary. Allow to mature for 2 weeks before eating.

Caution

Always be aware of the tremendously strong effect that horseradish has. Its properties can be too strong and too pungent for sensitive skins – so use with care and caution. Inhaling the unbelievably strong fumes when working with horseradish will have the eyes watering far worse than slicing onions, and the throat can be irritated. And overeating horseradish can cause irritation of the stomach lining – *so be careful*!

Jackfruit
Kathal

Artocarpus heterophyllus

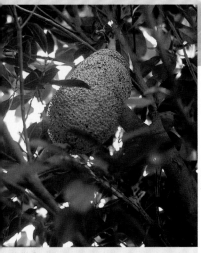

Jackfruit Salad

Our best way of eating jackfruit is in a fruit salad of papaya, mango and granadilla. With cream or vanilla ice-cream it is literally food for the gods – no wonder it was used in ceremonies in ancient days.

Hint

When cutting open a jackfruit, oil the hands and the knife, as its milky sap is sticky. Cut the fruit in half, and with oiled fingers pull out the pockets or 'arils' of divinely scented and delicious flesh which surround the seeds. The Javanese turn the arils inside out deftly and cleverly and in this way are able to remove the seeds with ease!

I write here of jackfruit because I grow it and because I am astonished by this beautiful evergreen tree with its massive fruit, which my grandchildren call the dinosaur's fruit! The jackfruit originated in the rainforests and mountains of tropical India and Malaysia from where it spread into Indo-China, Singapore, parts of tropical Africa and the West Indies and particularly into Java. When Christopher Columbus sailed past Trinidad on his third journey to the New World, he recorded his fascination with the jackfruit trees – so huge, so imposing, so thickly growing alongside great palms, writing that he thought he was close to the Garden of Eden, which was at that time thought to be in Eastern Asia.

It has been revered through the centuries as a thanksgiving to the gods for its food value, its prolific bearing of giant fruits, and for its medicinal value. In Central Java it is the most important fruit of the region where a spicy curry-like dish, known as *gudeg* is cooked in an earthenware pot on a slow fire, sweetened with palm sugar and nutmeg. In the Javanese *Rijstafel* banquet, an ancient ritual, *gudeg* may include chicken or bean curd or hard-boiled eggs. It is part of the ceremony and everyone eats this dish.

Growing Jackfruit

Jackfruit needs a tropical to subtropical climate and it is a relatively fast growing tree that offers so much. Our gratitude goes to Nelspruit Tropical Fruit Research gardens for bringing us our first jackfruits. We tasted the massive ripe fruit for the first time with them and subsequently grew small trees from the large, almost square, brown seeds freshly planted in compost-filled bags. The tree needs full sun and a really deep, richly composted hole, flooded with water at least once a week, and the leaves splashed and sprayed with water whenever you can – remember it is a rainforest tree. We set a pipe into the hole at an angle to allow the hose to be inserted and water to reach the roots.

We constantly look out for the sheathed, pointed, pale green flowers, which enclose the rough-skinned fruit, to emerge, and we watch eagerly as the fruit, oval and pale green, daily swells. The real trick is to know when to pick it – as it lightens in colour and a scent of exotic fruitiness is present. Male and female flowers are borne on the same tree: the male flowers are smaller and grouped together while the female flowers grow directly on the bigger branches. The fruit has as many as 100–500 seeds in pockets of soft pulp, known as arils, within the more dry and fibrous fruit which reaches around 40 cm in length.

Using Jackfruit

Store the soft arils in the fridge until ready to serve – exotic and utterly delicious, they have a taste that is between a granadilla, a mango and a litchi. The harder, drier flesh surrounding the pockets is thinly sliced with an oiled knife and fried as chips. The seeds can be boiled or roasted and eaten like chestnuts. The Malaysians eat the male flowers boiled as a vegetable and served with oil in salads or in curries.

Given as a medicine to boost energy levels and to ward off 'flu and colds, jackfruit is taken as a tonic, and for children it is particularly valuable. It is said the Javanese, who eat if often, have strong bones and teeth and glossy, beautiful long hair because of their devotion to this fascinating fruit.

Health Note

Jackfruit is rich in vitamins A and C, beta-carotene, iron, potassium, zinc, manganese, calcium, phosphorus, magnesium and dietary fibre.

Rooibos Tea

Aspalathus linearis

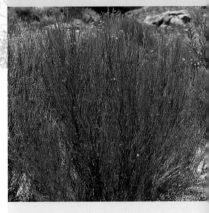

Rooibos is an amazing plant unique to the arid Cederberg mountains in the Western Cape, an extraordinary medicinal plant of such unusual status that new properties are being constantly discovered. The 'tea' was first recorded by Swedish botanist Carl Thunberg in 1772. He was intrigued by the 'Hottentot's tea' as he called it, introduced to him by the Khoi who used it as a health-building beverage, and who developed a traditional manner of harvesting the branches with axes and processing them by beating the branches with wooden beaters or truncheons. Piled into heaps, the branches were left to 'prove' or to 'ferment' in the hot summer sun. Once that period was over, the narrow small leaves, shaken off their branches, were spread in the sun to dry, turning from light green to a rich red, hence the name 'rooibos'. The dry 'tea' was then swept up and sieved through grass mats. This pile of now fragrant and pleasant tasting needle-like leaves would last until next summer as the Khoi now returned to pastures. The branches were used for mulching and for firewood, the ash being returned to the sandy soil. Nothing went to waste. The Khoi worked so diligently with nature that every part of the precious rooibos was utilised. Carl Thunberg took the rooibos tea back to Europe where it was received with much interest. The first marketing of rooibos was done by a tea merchant, Benjamin Ginsberg, who bought the dried and fermented tea from the Khoi people. Today South Africa's own wild tea is an important commercial crop and has become an international favourite!

Growing Rooibos

It *only* grows in the Cederberg; it has been trialled all over South Africa in every condition under the sun, but nowhere else does it seem to thrive or grow, even for a short while. The exact conditions – one could call it a microclimate – it requires are: deep, acid, sandy soil, cold and wet winters, hot summers with almost no rain, and a specific rainfall of no more than 350 mm per year.

In 1985, the Rooibos Tea Board brought me six rooibos plants thinking that perhaps my dry mountainside, newly established herb gardens had the right sort of well-drained soil and hot and dry summers that the rooibos needs. I followed the directions diligently and the officials came fortnightly to check on my little rooibos babies. I studied and experimented with rooibos, I drank the tea, I created cosmetics and medicines, all under the watchful eye of the officials, and so started a life-long admiration for this precious plant. But one by one my brave little plants died off no matter *what* we did, the last one managing to survive just short of a year. I went into mourning! It was an unforgettable experience, but we realised rooibos is unique to only one area in the world. Luckily we can all have the benefit of rooibos tea bought from the supermarket!

Using Rooibos

Japanese medical researchers discovered rooibos contains antioxidants that are thought to retard ageing. Other research on rooibos has found it to improve the digestion, to relax muscle spasms, to assist in colic in infants, and to relieve allergic reactions, particularly in babies but in the aged as well. The tea is taken without milk or sugar to relieve allergic symptoms, milk allergies, skin conditions such as eczema and psoriasis, to ease digestive spasms, for over-indulgence, diarrhoea and to flush the kidneys and bladder, particularly for cystitis, kidney stones, and slow or burning urine.

Health Note

Rooibos is a good source of vitamins and minerals, especially. It is low in tannin and is caffeine free, and has high levels of antioxidants and flavonoids.

How to brew the perfect cup of rooibos tea

The purists say 1 teaspoon of loose rooibos leaves in a cup, pour over this boiling water, stir and let it stand a minute or two or three, depending on the strength you like it. Strain and serve with a slice of lemon and a touch of honey – this is the way I like it best. Some prefer a little low fat milk and a tiny teaspoon of brown caramel sugar. Or 'stew' it in an enamel tea pot on the back of the stove all day, the way the 'Kaapse boere' did, to make it *so* strong you could run around the farm barefoot all day without getting breathless, my old neighbour of 86 once told me!

An excellent source of vitamins and minerals, rooibos is a health tea each one of us should be taking. I have it with a sprig of lavender (*Lavandula intermedia* 'Margaret Roberts', so named by the nursery trade) to help me wind down at the end of a rushed and frantically busy day.

Rooibos Iced Tea

Try this wonderful iced tea as a summer refresher. For those who like their tea unsweetened, leave out the honey.

Take 3–4 teaspoons loose rooibos tea leaves, and pour over this 2 litres of boiling water. Add 3 or 4 lemongrass stalks. Stand to cool until it is the strength you like. Strain. Add a little honey to taste, a slice or two of fresh lemon and the juice of 2 lemons. Serve chilled with ice.

Asparagus

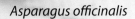
Asparagus officinalis

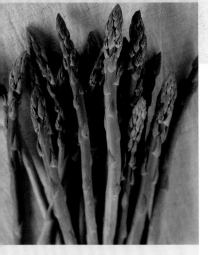

Asparagus Soup

Serves 4–6

This is the best detoxifying soup I know!

enough fresh asparagus spears, chopped up into small 1 cm pieces, to serve 4–6 people (about 3 bunches that contain 20 stems each)
2 large onions, chopped
2 green peppers, finely chopped
4 cups chopped celery

Simmer the vegetables in about 1½ litres of water (enough water to cover everything). Simmer gently for about 30 minutes or until the vegetables are tender. Whirl in the liquidiser and add Himalayan rock salt or crushed coarse non-iodated sea salt and a grinding of black pepper if liked. Serve hot.

Asparagus originates in the Mediterranean area, Europe, parts of Asia, North Africa and, surprisingly, some species even in South Africa! There are around 100 species of asparagus, but only about 20 are edible.

Asparagus has been cultivated for over 2 000 years as a vegetable but even more importantly as a medicinal herb, specifically for its extraordinary diuretic qualities. Most of the asparagus species are used medicinally for their asparagin content, which is a strong diuretic that gives urine its characteristically strong odour within half an hour of eating it, and cleanses the body amazingly. The ancient Greeks and Romans harvested spring asparagus spears from the wild, and in 200 BC precise growing instructions recorded by Cato indicate cultivation on a large scale. Louis XIV in France introduced it to the courts of Europe as a gourmet food, and its medicinal powers became legendary.

Growing Asparagus

Asparagus crowns are sometimes available from nurseries – keep an eye out for them. This is the quickest way to start off. I have imported seed through the years from reliable sources in Europe, but found it extremely slow and erratic to germinate. Far easier is starting with crowns. Space them 75 cm apart in rows of compost-rich soil that has been deeply dug, in full sun, and water well twice a week, three times a week in late winter and early spring. Bonemeal added twice yearly with extra compost gives sturdy root development. Replace the crowns every 8 to 10 years. Cut the spears off below the soil surface with a sharp knife in spring. Plant tomatoes, beans, cabbages, carrots and parsley alongside the asparagus to encourage growth. Asparagus is well worth growing for its amazing health boosting properties.

Using Asparagus

This is the most superb restorative herb that cleanses the kidneys (flushing out toxins), the liver and the bowels, and acts as a tonic to the whole system. When preparing fresh asparagus, save the water in which they were boiled as it is a superb treatment for cystitis, kidney ailments, rheumatism, gout and oedema from heart problems. It is probably one of the most extraordinary detoxifiers known to mankind – no wonder it has been so popular throughout the centuries.

Eating asparagus to treat arthritis and rheumatism has been done for centuries, and it remains a popular treatment today. Do remember if you have severe gout, limit asparagus to twice weekly as it contains a fairly small amount of purines, which may aggravate the gout.

This ancient health food is still one of nature's best diuretic detoxifiers, and in this day and age vital to include in our diets. To cook fresh asparagus, simmer the well-washed spears until tender in enough water to cover them. Serve the asparagus spears with a squeeze of fresh lemon juice and a grind of black pepper and the tiniest sprinkle of sea salt. If you are serving them hot, a dot of butter on the tips of the spears makes it melt in the mouth.

Health Note

Asparagus is an excellent source of vitamins A, C, B1, B2, B3, B6 and K, folic acid, potassium, phosphorus and iron.

Oats

Avena sativa

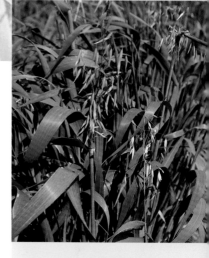

A familiar and comforting breakfast food, oats is one of the most treasured ancient grains that has never lost its popularity. Our grandmothers gave us a bowl of oats porridge at the end of an over-excited day when we are tearful and overwrought, or had a cold or 'flu coming on. Today medical research finds oats to have calming, restorative properties for both physical and mental exhaustion and a host of debilitating ailments. It stands today as an enormously important health food as it has through the centuries.

The oats we know today is actually a hybrid between the ancient grasses recorded archaeologically around 1000 BC in Europe. Cultivation began around 500 BC and the ancient Greeks and Romans grew it extensively for their horses, and as a nourishing gruel, and as a valuable medicine. Later it became a commercial crop in Britain, particularly in Scotland, in the Scandinavian countries and in Germany. Used as a staple food for centuries, oats as a commercial crop thrived easily, and spread further and further into distant lands.

Growing Oats

Sow oats as an annual crop in well-dug, well-composted moist soil in rows in full sun. It can be sown at any time of the year but best is in autumn for a winter crop. Excellent as a fodder crop for cattle and horses, it is a quick grower and germinates easily. Rake over the area once the seeds have been scattered and water in gently and thoroughly. A sprinkler set over the area will give it a good start. Every 2 or 3 days repeat the watering so that the soil does not dry out. Water well twice weekly in hot weather, less in the winter months. Allow the grain to ripen fully before reaping. The grain can be threshed and the straw kept for teas (see recipe below). The husks are removed in the milling process and the oats are rolled.

Using Oats

Cut green for cattle feed and horses, and allow to ripen to a golden colour for *oat straw tea* for osteoporosis. Chop the stems of the oats into small pieces, ¼–½ a cup, pour over this 1 cup of boiling water and stand 5 minutes, strain and sip slowly. A cup or two a day is soothing, comforting and a valuable bone-building and digestive tea. It is also taken as a restorative tonic for stress, depression and panic attacks, degenerative diseases like multiple sclerosis, recurring colds and 'flu, thyroid deficiency and lack of energy, and for menopause symptoms, as oat straw assists in oestrogen deficiency. Medical studies found that oats has beneficial effects on blood sugar levels, and type 2 diabetics saw significant changes when oats was included in the daily diet. Oats and oat bran contain polyunsaturated fatty acids that help to lower 'bad' cholesterol, and oats porridge, oats muffins, breads and oat straw tea should be included in the diet daily. You can also eat oat sprouts. Pull up the little newly emerged seedlings, rinse well and add to soups, stir-fries and stews. Rich in vitamins and minerals and tender and delicious, you can also sprout the long, pointed seeds in a sprouter or on wet cotton wool.

Oat flakes softened in hot water are a superb beauty aid for problem skins. Used as a gentle scrub oats are the perfect cleanser, toner and oil remover and cooled oat straw tea used as a lotion will soothe sunburn, windburn, eczemas and psoriasis.

Health Note

Oats has the highest protein content of all cereals; it is rich in vitamins B1, B2, D and E and has high levels of beta-carotene. Oats is an excellent source of minerals, specially magnesium and calcium, and dietary fibre. It is this dietary fibre that is rich in beta-glucan which helps to bind cholesterol and remove it from the body via the bowel.

Oats Health Breakfast

For an energy building, health building breakfast, this is my favourite. Once you've had this fully guaranteed breakfast you'll not want that coffee and a doughnut midmorning!

1 cup of large flake oats, simmered in 2½ cups of water with ½ teaspoon salt until tender. Stir frequently. Spoon into a bowl. Stir in a teaspoon or two of honey and add plain Bulgarian yoghurt or skim milk. Add 2 tablespoons of mixed sunflower seeds, flaxseed, almonds, sesame seeds and pumpkin seeds that have been ground in a seed grinder. (I make at least a cup full at a time and store it in a sealed glass bottle in the fridge.) Add a sliced banana or a grated apple or a peach or a slice of papaya or even 5 prunes if you are constipated.

Hint

Do not buy instant oats as it has been partially cooked and stabilised, losing some of its valuable nutritional content in the process. Choose rather the large flake, non-instant kind that needs longer cooking.

Star Fruit
Carambola

Averrhoa carambola

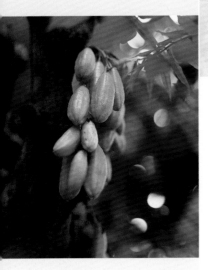

Star Fruit Dip

Our favourite way of eating star fruit is by making a satisfying dip served with rye bread.

1 carton cream cheese
1 tablespoon crushed coriander seed
2 tablespoons finely chopped celery leaves and stalks
about 1 tablespoon of fresh lemon juice
black pepper and sea salt to taste
a teaspoon of paprika OR 2 finely chopped fresh paprika peppers OR 1 very finely chopped fresh chilli, depending on how hot you want it

Mix everything together. Slice two or three star fruit and serve with the cream cheese dip and fresh buttered rye bread. Delicious!

Hint

The fruit, specifically along the ribs, is high in oxalic acid which makes it an excellent cleaning material for copper and brass, and it has been used for centuries to clean brass goblets and candlesticks in churches, and places of worship and ceremony in its lands of origin.

I have grown star fruit for several years in the hot Herbal Centre gardens and never cease to be intrigued by it! It is a fragile and fairly small tree away from its exotic beginnings in Southeast Asia and Malaysia and particularly Sri Lanka and there, and in other tropical countries, it can reach between 7 and 10 metres in height and its branches become bowed with the weight of the fruit! The five-ribbed fruit has a thin translucent skin, ripens to a golden yellow and the sliced fruit, exotically ripe and juicy, is the perfect star shape with tiny seeds and sweet and succulent yet crisp flesh.

It is a treasured fruit in its native lands and its history goes back centuries. It was an early trade commodity, as half ripe fruits nestled in grass packaging could travel far. Travellers took tiny trees, established in coconut shells filled with rich, moist soil with them and bartered the fruits, and commercial cultivation in tropical areas soon began. Visiting ships took the half-ripe fruits on board, as well as fresh leaves for teas. Today cultivation in tropical countries such as Brazil, Malaysia, Hawaii and the West Indies, even in the Seychelles, is big business as the world remains intrigued by this star-shaped fruit!

Growing Star Fruit

It does not take frost, so always plant it in a sheltered position. Propagation is by seed or by grafting onto rootstock of the more easily grown acid cultivar, and several nurseries offer established little trees for sale. Start the little tree off in a deeply dug, compost-filled hole in full sun. It can take afternoon shade and it needs a deep, twice weekly watering. It loves having its leaves sprayed with a light fine spray of water. Remember it comes from the tropics, so it enjoys the frequent tropical storms or short showers of rain! The fruits take a long time to ripen on the tree and we pick our best in the still warm autumn. For the gardener the star fruit offers intriguing specimen plantings and constant interest as the fruits develop.

Using Star Fruit

In Malaysia it has been used for centuries to treat coughs, colds, 'flu and bronchitis as well as for ear infections. Ripe fruit minced and mixed with honey is an ancient cough mixture. A poultice of warmed thinly sliced ripe fruit is an ancient treatment for boils and suppurating or slow-healing wounds.

Star fruit is treasured and enjoyed by the Malaysians, who serve it for breakfast almost daily, freshly sliced, dribbled with a little honey, covered in plain yoghurt and thickly sprinkled with sesame seeds. Or try slices dipped in a honey and ginger sauce and served with fresh cream, sprinkled with flaked almonds as a dessert as it is served in South America, or sliced and marinated in fresh grape juice with coconut flakes and served with grilled fish as it is done in the West Indies.

The ripe fruit, used as a beauty treatment for oily problem skin, has a refining effect on enlarged pores. Its acidic content tones and tightens the skin, and mashed into grape-seed, sesame or olive oil it is a popular skin treatment for sunburned skin and dry skin.

A very effective cleanser is made in the Seychelles for toning and tightening the skin on both the neck and the face by mashing ripe star fruit with soft thin coconut flakes – even the men use it. Spread onto the face and neck and left for 10 minutes, it cleans, softens and smoothes the skin very effectively.

Health Note

Star fruit contains vitamins C, A and B (particularly thiamine, niacin and riboflavin), carotenoids, iron, phosphorus, calcium and potassium.

Brazil Nut

Bertholletia excelsa

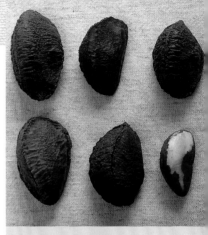

This huge and beautiful evergreen tree that originates in the forests of the Amazon valley in Brazil and in the forests of Peru, Colombia, Bolivia and Venezuela, reaches a height of over 40 metres and produces masses of woody capsules filled with the divine nuts the world has come to know and love. For centuries the precious nuts have been a source of food, income and trade for the local people who have treasured the wild harvest, and through the years have established plantations so that literally tons of harvested nuts go worldwide. The indigenous tribes make a variety of nourishing dishes and nut-milks from the nuts, and the rich oil, which is used to keep the skin smooth and supple, is highly valued.

Growing Brazil Nuts

These are real rainforest trees needing the moisture and humidity of that rich environment. Botanical gardens in tropical areas and on some islands have been able to grow Brazil nut trees to an extent, but as the nuts take around 15 months to ripen they need special heat and moisture to reach maturity. It is a slow and exacting growth – it takes 15–30 years before it produces fruit in any significant quantity – but that tree will live 500–800 years with a trunk of almost 2 m in diameter! I never cease to be amazed that so luscious and relatively inexpensive a crop of such richness is available to the man in the street. Think for a moment of the distance that nut has travelled and from where it has come across the seas to become a treat fit for a king!

Each big wooden pod houses about 20 creamy rich and smooth seeds within it, and with an expert swipe of a sharp axe the nut gatherers will split it open to reveal the undamaged smooth seeds in hard shells within. It is an art taught by the father to his son through generations. The harvesters carry shields as they work in the forest to protect themselves from the ripe falling pods. The weight of the pods, some up to 3½ kg, falling from the height of the huge tree – several stories high – impacts the seed in the moist fertile soil below so that it can grow into a tree alongside its parent tree. No wonder shields are necessary! These forests of Brazil nut trees are known as *catanales* in Brazil, and *manchales* in Peru, and the fallen nuts are collected carefully. Local factories shell the hard outer covering of the nut. Some are left on and the nut is dried before packing and selling.

Using Brazil Nuts

One of the most ancient of remedies is to take one crushed and pounded nut mixed with ½ a cup of warm water for stomach aches. Brazil nuts are one of the richest and most stable sources of selenium and eating two Brazil nuts twice weekly, loaded with health-giving polyunsaturated fats and selenium, will help to lower the risk of heart disease and cancer and will also provide the rare trace mineral chromium – one could call it a *tonic nut*! Brazil nuts are also rich in oxalates, and two or three nuts a week are all the body needs in most cases. *Those with a tendency to kidney stones should avoid them.*

The husk of the Brazil nut is burned as a mosquito and insect repellent around campfires and in forest homes. The carved husk is a valuable container and has become a favourite trinket box for tourists. Brazil nut oil is used for cooking, for lamps, for skin care and hair care and for rich, soothing healing creams and moisturising soaps. This precious oil is worth its weight in gold and in the last century it has become a sought-after ingredient for the cosmetic industry worldwide.

Health Note

Brazil nuts are rich in selenium, chromium, polyunsaturated fats, vitamins A, C, D and E, phosphorus and magnesium.

Brazil Nut Milk

This is a favourite Brazilian recipe, for energy and vitality.

Grate 10 shelled Brazil nuts on the fine side of the grater. Add 2 cups of hot (not boiling water). Stand 10 minutes, then liquidise. Spoon 2 tablespoons over mashed fruit salad or into plain Bulgarian yoghurt. Keep the rest in the fridge for the next day.

Hint

½ cup finely chopped Brazil nuts well mixed with ½ cup mashed ripe strawberries makes one of the most effective face masks loved by models. Use as a gentle scrub and leave on as a mask for 10 minutes.

Beetroot

Beta vulgaris

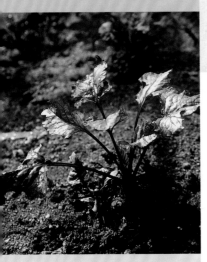

Beetroot Booster

Makes 1 glass

This is the most valuable drink I know. In a juice extractor push through 3 scrubbed and quartered medium-sized beetroots with all their roots, stems and leaves. Add 2 sticks celery with their leaves, 2 peeled apples (I use Golden Delicious), 3 large sprigs fresh parsley and 1 cup watercress when in season. Catch the precious juice and sip slowly.

Old-fashioned Beetroot Salad

In a covered pot, simmer 10–12 beetroots, unpeeled but well scrubbed, in enough water to cover them until tender. Drain and cool. Peel by rubbing the outer skin off. Slice thinly and layer into glass screw-top jars. Pour over this: 3 cups of grape vinegar simmered with 2 cups of water and 1 cup dark caramel sugar for 15 minutes. Pour over the sliced beetroot and seal. Store in the fridge. Serve with cold meats and salads.

Cultivated and cherished for thousands of years, this important food and medicinal plant originally came from the Mediterranean and North African coastal areas and has been part of the diet in many cultures as far as history takes us. The first to actually cultivate the beetroot is thought to be the Germans; the Italians reaped only the leaves and used the roots and stems to treat jaundice and other liver ailments. The Germans further developed the swollen root, which they ate with vinegar. So the beetroot as we know it today, is grown primarily for its rich and succulent below ground 'root' and began its history in the late 15th century in Germany. The improved variety was later recorded in France and Italy and today it is grown commercially in many parts of the world and it is available virtually all year round.

Growing Beetroot

Prepare a well-composted, deeply dug bed in full sun and mark rows spaced 30 cm apart with the end of a rake. Thinly sprinkle seed into the small furrow and then rake over carefully to cover the seed. Set a gentle sprinkler over the area to wet the soil thoroughly and evenly. Scatter leaves over the area to shade the little seeds and never let the soil dry out. Once the rows of seeds have germinated, thin out so that the little plants have space to grow, and replant the pulled-out seedlings in bare areas. They will transplant easily while they are still small. Keep them well watered. Pull up the beetroot plants when the 'bulb' starts to thicken and cook them whole – leaves and all – or cut the leaves for salads and spinach and grate raw beetroot with apple as a summer salad – it is packed with health-giving minerals and vitamins.

Using Beetroot

Never underestimate the power of this easy to grow and quite amazing plant! Both the leaves (to a larger extent) and the root contain an abundance of minerals and vitamins (see Health Note). And then there is the importance of their rich deep red colour – betacyanin is a powerful anti-cancer agent, and the combination of betacyanin along with the beetroot's high fibre content makes it particularly beneficial for treating the colon and preventing colon cancer and stomach cancer.

Through the centuries beetroot has been used with excellent results in the treatment of jaundice and diverticulitis, clearing pockets of acidity, as it is an excellent liver and blood and intestinal cleanser. It clears the blood of toxins, eliminates kidney stones, clears the kidneys and gall bladder and literally puts a glow back into the general health of the body. Raw beetroot grated with apple in equal quantities and served with lemon juice and fresh chopped parsley is a valuable health salad served daily that you will never tire of.

The beautiful natural red 'dye' from unsalted water in which beetroot has been cooked can be used to colour ice-cream, milk puddings, jellies, cake icing and more and was once used as a paint on cloth.

Health Note

Beetroot is a rich source of iron, calcium, magnesium, phosphorus, potassium, manganese, folic acid, vitamins A, C and B6, beta-carotene and dietary fibre.

Annatto
Lipstick Tree

Bixa orellana

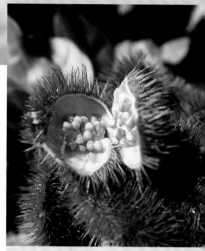

Indigenous to tropical America and the Caribbean Islands and introduced in the 17th century by the Spanish to the East and West Indies, the Philippines, Hawaii, Jamaica and the Seychelles, the annatto tree is now extensively cultivated as a safe and natural orange-red dye for foods and cosmetics – especially lipstick and rouge and even eye shadow – and also as a spice for flavouring. Annatto seeds are slightly peppery and are used to flavour many dishes across the world, and they give a rich colour to cheeses, meats, dried sausages and many Chinese delicacies, *and* the tree is considered to be lucky!

Growing Annatto

The annatto tree is a large, shrubby, colourful tree that can reach 3–4 m in tropical areas. It is sensitive to cold, the leaves are deciduous, large and heart-shaped, and the clusters of pink many-stamened, wild rose-type of flowers turn into furry pointed pods that are filled with masses of seeds. If they are crushed when still soft, they will give a bright orange-red juice much loved by young girls who carefully spread it on their lips as a natural lipstick, hence its Hawaiian name of 'lipstick tree'.

Propagation is from fresh seed sown in bags to mature. Dig a large hole in full sun, fill with compost and water and sink the small tree into it (now about 60 cm tall – the plant grows rapidly). Make sure all the roots are well covered with compost – be careful not to bend the taproot – and make a sturdy dam around it. Once a week flood the dam with water – it will thrive, offering much fascination and beauty. After about 18 months the first flowers will appear.

Using Annatto

The entire plant has been used as a medicine for centuries, particularly by the Native Americans. The young shoots made into a tea are taken for dysentery, fevers, hepatitis and skin ailments. In Brazil it is taken as a purgative, a diuretic and for heartburn, and in Mexico it is also taken for headaches, epilepsy, inflammatory ailments, malaria, throat and stomach ailments and as an aphrodisiac and a wash for skin ailments. It has also been taken for cancer, diabetes, kidney ailments and stones, and its high antioxidant properties have been listed in worldwide pharmacopoeias, *and* annatto is also found to be an insect repellent!

There is very little food value in annatto, but by its very colour it is becoming an important part of many dishes throughout the world, and some specialist delicatessens sell annatto oil (see recipe alongside) and annatto and chilli pastes which are becoming gourmet foods.

Loved by the Jamaicans, crushed annatto seeds are added to fish dishes, oils and meats with ease, and the Mexicans and Chinese add it to curries and chilli pastes.

The bright red colour is a precious pigment called bixia, which is used extensively to colour the waxy red rind of many cheeses, and as a colouring agent for smoked fish. The cosmetic industry is making full use of the beautiful natural colour and soon natural lipsticks will become available. Paint, varnish and lacquers also use bixa.

Health Note

Due to the recent trend to avoid unnatural colourants and flavourants in foods, some manufacturers have started to replace chemicals like tartrazine with annatto. The artificial yellow-orange tartrazine has been found to cause allergic reactions in certain people, and annatto does not have any adverse effects.

Annatto Tea

Pour 1 cup of boiling water over a thumb length young sprig, buds and flowers included. Add 6–10 seeds, crushed lightly. Stand 5 minutes, strain and sip slowly (can be sweetened with a touch of honey).

Annatto Oil

Warm whole or crushed seeds in sunflower oil – one tablespoon seeds to 2 cups of oil – in a double boiler and simmer for at least 30 minutes. A vibrant and beautiful oil will emerge. Once strained, this oil can be used in sauces, dressings, for stir-frying and for rice dishes.

Hint

Let the pods mature on the tree before reaping. They can be dried out in the shade. The inner small seeds are the spice, and they need to be stored in screw-top glass jars.

Mustard

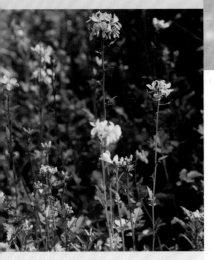

Brassica juncea

Mustard belongs to the great *Brassica* genus of which there are around 30 species of annual and biennial plants (including the cabbages) that originate in Europe and Asia. Gathered in the wild this great genus has provided food, flavourings and green herbs from the beginnings of time, and mustard was used as a condiment and a green vegetable even before 400 BC! It was the Chinese who used it first as a medicine in AD 659 and it is thought that it got its name from the Romans who mixed ground and powdered mustard seed with grape juice as one of the first flavourants known, and the word 'mustard' comes from 'mustum', which is grape must, and 'ardens', which means burning. The original trade with mustard began as seeds and the trade routes can be traced historically as the different seeds – black mustard (*Brassica nigra*), white mustard (*Sinapis alba*) and brown mustard (*Brassica juncea*) – found their way into different cultures. The seeds of white mustard – which are of a golden colour, larger than the black or brown mustard, and with a milder flavour – form the base of the popular 'American mustard' and blended with the seeds of the black mustard make the favourite English mustard, but are not used in French mustards!

Growing Mustard

I have grown mustard seed on wet cotton wool as a child. My Scottish grandmother encouraged us to garden from an early age and her childhood favourite was growing mustard and cress. So it became a part of our lives. We reaped the tiny seedlings already rich in their hot and biting components, neatly snipped off with kitchen scissors, and sprinkled onto baked potatoes with butter or onto hard-boiled egg and mayonnaise sandwiches. And to this day I still relish the taste as I encourage my own grandchildren to grow these precious golden seeds on wet cotton wool for an instant crop.

Other than on cotton wool, mustard sown year round is a quick and rewarding annual crop. It thrives in deeply dug, richly composted soil in full sun, scattered where it is to grow. In the midsummer heat it bolts very quickly, so I prefer spring and autumn sowing, and add mustard greens, grown in a protected area, to my winter salads.

Using Mustard

Our grandmothers used finely ground mustard powder in the bath, in bandages around a sprained ankle, for arthritic joints and over boils and bruises, and ate the green leaves and stems for respiratory infections, chilblains, coughs, joint pains and neuralgia. The green fresh leaves have the same antibiotic properties, stimulant and warming and pain relieving, that the seeds have, as well as being a digestive, an expectorant, a diuretic and an excellent circulatory herb. For painful feet mustard is a long respected treatment. Mustard is also strongly preservative and discourages moulds and bacteria.

Leaves, flowers and green seedpods are all delicious, particularly in stir-fries and salads. Use the seeds whole in vinegars, relishes and pickles.

Health Note

Mustard is low in calories and rich in antioxidants, vitamins B1, B2, B6, C and E, calcium, folic acid, manganese, copper, phosphorus, potassium, magnesium and iron, as well as glucosinolates, which are particularly important for women going through menopause due to their ability to protect against osteoporosis, breast cancer and heart disease.

Caution

Mustard mixed with water can be extremely irritant to the skin and mucous membranes, and I do not advise using mustard powder compresses without medical or professional assistance. Huge red weals are often experienced on tender, sensitive skin.

Honey Mustard

Making your own mustard is a most satisfying experience, especially when you reap your own seeds. This also makes an excellent 'marinade' for meat and fish.

Soak 2 cups of mustard seeds in cold water for 30 minutes. Strain through a fine sieve. Add 1 cup of honey and ¾ cup of dark grape vinegar and briskly stir in to coat each seed. (I prefer thick raw honey. Mix the honey and vinegar well before adding to the seed by whisking it together.) Spoon into sterilised screw-top jars and label.

Hint

Mustard is a natural emulsifier, so when added to homemade mayonnaise a mere teaspoon of mustard powder smoothes and emulsifies it to a deliciously creamy consistency. The secret is to mix the mustard powder with *cold* water and let it stand for 10 to 15 minutes. The enzyme that causes the glucoside to react brings the amazing taste of mustard to the fore, but that same enzyme is killed by adding hot water or vinegar. But once it has been mixed with the cold water and allowed to stand for 10–15 minutes, vinegar can be added and it will not change the taste.

Rape

Oilseed Rape ■ Rutabaga ■ Swede

Brassica napus

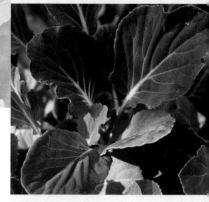

The origin of this extraordinary plant is shrouded in mystery. It is thought that its ancient beginnings in medieval gardens were because cabbages and turnips were grown in close proximity to each other and, both belonging to the huge *Brassica* genus, it was an easy cross-pollination! The root part became known as the 'swede' and was thought to have developed in Bohemia in the 17th century, and was documented by a Swiss botanist in 1620. By 1664 it was documented growing in England and it became a staple vegetable in the cold countries of Northern Europe and a valuable food during World War II. It became hugely popular, as it is so easy to grow, yielding masses of delicious leaves for soups, stews and stir-fries, particularly through the long winters – it even thrives under the snow – and a nutritious turnip-like root, which is so long lasting and so versatile in its uses that traditional dishes are woven around it. It even became the traditional dish known as 'neeps', served as an accompaniment to Scotland's famous haggis!

Growing Rape

Sow seed where it is to grow in well-dug, well-composted, moist soil in full sun. Thinly sprinkled into rows and raked over, it needs to be kept moist in its first months of growing. It is a cold weather crop, so sow the seeds in early autumn for winter reaping. Pick the young leaves fresh for salads and pull up the little seedlings, sown in trenches, when they are only a few centimetres in height to add to salads and stir-fries.

For the 'swede', grow as you would turnips (see page 87) but reap before the tall flowering head emerges.

Using Rape

A long-treasured fodder crop, rape is grown everywhere and what is interesting is that the leaves of rape contain three times more calcium than phosphorus, which is a beneficial ratio for treating osteoporosis (high phosphorus consumption has been linked to osteoporosis as it reduces calcium absorption). As part of the cabbage family, rape exhibits the same anti-cancer properties and as well as its high chlorophyll content, rape also has lutein, beta-carotene and a valuable health-building component known as zeaxanthin.

The young leaves, stripped off their strong white stalk and midrib and finely chopped, form a substantial 'spinach' dish and served with butter, salt, black pepper and lemon juice is much enjoyed through the bitterly cold winters. The flowers, brilliantly yellow, with buds, and the very young and tender seeds, are made into pickles with onions and mustard seeds, which are served with traditional fish and meat dishes. Or try eating the flowers fresh, sprinkled over hot soups or added to salads, stir-fries and fritters.

The swede is delicious finely grated into soups, stews and stir-fries, or boiled, quartered and served with a cheesy sauce, or grated into a fritter dough and fried and served with a thick hot vegetable soup as they do in Sweden.

Health Note

All parts of the plant, particularly the root, are rich in vitamins, vitamin C particularly, and a host of minerals. Vitamins B6, B1 and B2 and vitamin E are high, as are manganese, copper, iron and calcium.

Quick and Easy Ways with Swede/Rape

Add boiled mashed swedes to your favourite pancake batter, pan fry, and then top with mushrooms in white sauce. This is a party dish and much enjoyed all over the world.

Chopped fresh rape leaves steamed with chopped apples and raisins that have been pre-soaked in warm water, are a valuable immune-boosting dish. Served with balsamic vinegar and chopped walnuts, it is a much-loved dish in the Scandinavian countries.

A Note on Rapeseed Oil

Rapeseed oil, also known as canola oil, is a valuable salad and cooking oil and great fields of canola are grown for the food industry as its main use is for margarine, mayonnaises and spreads. Its incredible popularity in a relatively short time is due to its high levels of omega-3 oils, much higher than those found in sunflower and safflower oils. During processing, a toxic component known as erucic acid is removed and canola oil is perfectly safe. But we still have to be alert to the fact that canola has had bad publicity under the broad heading of 'genetically modified', which puts fear into the hearts of many. I have been careful over the last several years to find only organically grown rapeseed, and the canola oil used in the 'Margaret Roberts Garlic & Canola Insect Spray' sold countrywide is **not** from genetically modified seed.

Broccoli

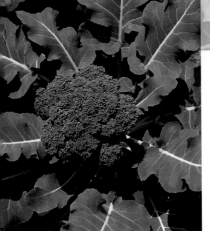

Broccoli Salad

Serves 4–6

This is my favourite broccoli dish and one salad I never get tired of!

about 6 cups of broccoli florets, their
*   stems peeled and pared and trimmed*
juice of 2 lemons
½ cup plain Bulgarian yoghurt
½ cup good homemade mayonnaise
sea salt and black pepper to taste
chopped spring onions
½ cup sesame seeds

Steam the broccoli pieces until bright green and only just tender. Remove from the heat and quickly rinse under cold water. Drain and combine all the other ingredients except the spring onions and sesame seeds and pour over the still warm broccoli. Toss and spoon into a pretty salad bowl, sprinkle with the spring onions and sesame seeds.

Hint

Broccoli has to be the most upfront health food of all, but *only* if it is organically grown and unsprayed!

A member of the huge cruciferous family, along with cabbage, kale and cauliflower, broccoli stands out as a healing food that developed from the wild cabbage native to Europe and the Mediterranean area. For over 2 000 years broccoli has been planted as a food, it was improved upon by the Romans and was well known in Italy by the 16th century. It gradually spread throughout the world, popularised by Italian immigrants, but it only became a vegetable of note in the new world in the 1920s. In 1923 the D'Arrigo brothers planted trial fields of broccoli in California and in 1929 the brothers started the first radio programme advertising broccoli and also placed stories of broccoli and its virtues in the press, and after that the broccoli industry took off and spread all over America.

Growing Broccoli

In very hot areas plant broccoli only as a winter crop. Broccoli is a short-lived annual and propagation is from seed. Sow seeds in boxes to mature to about 10 cm in height before planting out in full sun in deeply dug, richly composted, moist soil. Space them about 50 cm apart and plant out extras to leave to go to seed, as broccoli seed becomes the most incredible sprouts so filled with nourishment and medicinal value that whole organic fields should be devoted to growing broccoli sprouts.

During the cooler months and even deep into winter, start several batches of seeds so that you can have continuous batches of broccoli coming along. In the very hot summers broccoli does not thrive and is often riddled with aphids, scale and black fly. Heavy spraying programmes are the only way commercial farmers can get a return on their investment. *So do not eat chemically sprayed broccoli* – it breaks down health instead of building it up. Rather grow broccoli sprouts in summer.

Using Broccoli

Broccoli appears to be a superb cancer protector and fighter. It has rapidly become a four star vegetable, thanks to President Reagan's bowel cancer scare, where the White House chefs devised an eating plan to fight the cancer with large amounts of organically grown broccoli, fresh carrots and broccoli and alfalfa sprouts daily. It has been advised that ½ a cup of broccoli lightly steamed a day can protect against several cancers, particularly breast cancer, colon and lung cancer, but also cancer of the oesophagus, pharynx, larynx, stomach and prostate. Broccoli and other dark green vegetables, like cabbages and spinach, help to fight irradiation as well, and as our daily exposure to irradiation in cell phones and computers increases we should be aware of broccoli's ability to protect. Smokers should also seriously include broccoli in the diet at least 3 times a week to protect the lungs. Interestingly, researchers at the Johns Hopkins School of Medicine in Maryland have found broccoli sprouts contain 30–50 times the amount of protective chemicals that mature broccoli plants contain.

Low in calories and high in nutrients (see Health Note), broccoli is also a rich source of lutein, which shows anti-cancer effects and also helps to prevent the development of age-related ailments such as macular degeneration in the eyes. We should add broccoli to the daily diet for obesity, toxaemia, high blood pressure, constipation and kidney ailments.

Health Note

Broccoli is an excellent source of vitamins C, A, K, B6 and E, folic acid, magnesium, calcium, potassium and phosphorus.

Cauliflower

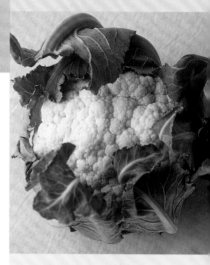

Brassica oleracea var. *botrytis*

The much-loved cauliflower originates in the eastern Mediterranean region and Asia Minor, and has been a cherished food for centuries. Records show it has been widely known and eaten since the 6th century BC, and was grown in Turkey and Egypt around 400 BC, and from there it spread to Italy and the rest of the world, arriving in England only around 1586 where it became known as 'Cyprus colewart' and was considered to be a great delicacy. Later, due to the hypertrophied inflorescence – the creamy head – it became known as coleflower and from there it became known as cauliflower. It became so popular that cultivation in France, northern Europe and England began in earnest and before long its health benefits were recognised and seeds and plants of the whole cruciferous family, the cauliflower being the favourite, became available to the man in the street, and small gardens and allotments began to spring up all over the countryside. The monks at the local monasteries tended cauliflower, kale and cabbage gardens and learned to pickle their produce in vinegar to treat the sick during the winter months.

Growing Cauliflower

Cauliflower is mainly a winter annual, although in perfect conditions it can be grown virtually all year round. It really is a superb vegetable to grow and I have never ceased to be enthralled by its beauty, and the ease with which it grows. It is the grand star of the vegetable garden and thrives in the winter sun like a row of creamy posies! Start the easy to grow seeds in trays in autumn and prick out when they are big enough to handle. Plant them in well-dug, richly composted, moist soil in full sun 75 cm apart. They will take frost, cold winds and even rain.

One of the most spectacular show gardens I ever created was for a spring flower show and I planted curved grey stone terraces of lines of cauliflowers, Savoy, drumhead and red cabbage varieties, ornamental kale in both pink and cream, and the taller growing kale. Kohlrabi and broccoli featured in profusion, and it was so beautiful everyone who saw it was inspired. All the path edges were planted with thick bands of the exquisite (and edible) ornamental kales, their pink and white hearts giving colour to the fascinating shades of grey and green of the other members of the *Brassica* genus. It was simply quite breathtaking!

Using Cauliflower

The monks used cauliflower soup cooked with onions and celery to treat coughs, colds, bronchitis and pneumonia. The entire cabbage family is now proving to be an immune system booster as well as an excellent treatment in cancer prevention. All the cruciferous vegetables such as kale, broccoli, cabbage and Brussels sprouts, contain compounds that appear to increase the action of the enzymes which eliminate and disable carcinogens.

Rich in vitamins, minerals and fibre, the cauliflower is an excellent vegetarian choice and is at its best served steamed with lemon juice and black pepper, picked straight from the garden. Small cauliflower florets, uncooked, are delicious in salads and their leaves can be finely shredded and added to soups and stir-fries.

Health Note

Cauliflower is a good source of vitamins C, B3 and B5, folic acid, potassium, iron and fibre.

Cauliflower Pickle

This precious little recipe is similar to the one the monks made to treat winter colds.

Cut a fresh cauliflower into florets, pack into a wide-mouthed jar. Boil 3 cups of grape vinegar with 1 tablespoon each of caraway seeds, dill seeds and coriander seeds, and 4 tablespoons of raw honey, for 10 minutes. Pour over the cauliflower until fully covered. Seal well and store for 1 month, if you can wait that long, before eating. Serve with cheese and crusty bread.

Cauliflower Cheese

A rich white cheesy sauce poured over a perfect head of steamed-until-tender cauliflower, sprinkled with grated cheese and melted under the grill, is today as popular as it was in Victorian times – known as 'the dish of hospitality' that everyone loved!

Cabbage

Brassica oleracea var. *capitata*

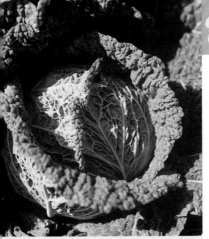

The cabbage as we know it today is indigenous to Asia and was brought into Europe around 600 BC by the roving Celtic people, and from those ancient early beginnings its value as a food crop quickly spread into Russia, Poland, China and Japan who remain some of the leading producers today. A cold weather crop, the cabbage adapts easily and soon became one of the most valuable of food crops, and it was probably one of the most important medicinal plants as well, taken as a remedy for many ailments. It is not known which forms of the cabbage family were used in those ancient times, but early recordings show kale, mustard, radishes and cabbages in various forms, and even flowering rape! Cabbage is without doubt the King of the cruciferous vegetables, and it is not surprising that it is grown everywhere and in all its varieties.

Growing Cabbage

Remember, cabbages grown in the hot months will need an extensive spraying programme. Grow cabbages in the cold winter months *organically* as this is a valuable health food but only if it is grown without the use of dangerous chemicals.

Sow seed in trays and plant out in well-dug, richly composted, moist soil in full sun. Space them 75 cm apart, as the head grows large. Watch for aphid attack and spray with a strong jet of water to clear the aphids or spray with a natural spray made from khakibos or soap water. Cabbages thrive with companion plants – beetroot, celery, chamomile, chives, dill, onions, pennyroyal, rosemary, sage, southernwood and thyme – which will keep it insect-free.

Using Cabbage

The outer dark green leaves are packed with the goodness of vitamins and minerals (see Health Note) and all the Brassicas have extraordinary natural antibiotic properties. The whole cabbage family contains cancer-fighting phytochemicals, more than any other group of vegetables. Cabbage and other members of the family lower the rate of cancer, particularly colon, lung, breast and prostate cancers, and the medical studies are ongoing. The cabbage also contains substances known as glucosinolates, which increase the antioxidants within the body and improve the body's ability to detoxify and to eliminate harmful pollution and chemical substances that increase the risk of illness. There is also research being done on a valuable amino acid known as glutamine, which has the ability to regenerate the cells lining the digestive tract, and fresh cabbage juice is being included in treatments for peptic and duodenal ulcers. Cabbage in the diet has also been shown to assist in the breakdown of harmful hormones through the liver's detoxification process.

From medieval times onwards, cabbage leaves were warmed in hot water and used as a poultice over slow-to-heal wounds, swollen, sprained ankles, for stiff, sore shoulders, knees and backs, and for engorged breasts in new mothers. It became a true panacea and was widely used. Even today, some maternity hospitals ask the young mothers to bring a cabbage on admittance!

Warmed fresh cabbage leaves soaked in hot water and bound over tired aching feet, and wrapped in a towel were a soothing poultice used by the Crusaders after a heavy day. The Roman gladiators used warmed cabbage leaves as a poultice too!

Freshly picked cabbage leaves, organically grown, and finely shredded, steamed for only a few minutes and then served with freshly ground black pepper and a squeeze of lemon juice, should be on everyone's plate at least three times a week. Cabbage salad is a world favourite salad, and sauerkraut has been part of German, Polish and Russian diets for centuries and is the reason, it is thought, why those nations remain so healthy despite the snow-bound winters.

Cabbage Stir-Fry

Serves 4–6

Quick and easy to prepare and any vegetables in season can be added to it.

1 small cabbage, finely shredded, green outer leaves included
3 onions, thinly sliced
juice of 1 lemon and a little lemon zest
about ¾ cup finely chopped parsley
2 teaspoons freshly grated ginger root
2 tablespoons olive oil
sea salt and freshly ground black pepper
thinly sliced celery, green peppers, mushrooms, can also be added

In a hot wok fry first the onions in the olive oil and brown lightly. Then add all the other ingredients and about 1 cup of water. Stir-fry until tender. Serve hot with steamed rice.

Health Note

Cabbage contains folic acid, calcium, magnesium, phosphorus, beta-carotene, boron, potassium, vitamins C, E and K and even some iodine.

The following members of the great cabbage family are valuable healing foods in their own right and we should not only be growing these but we should be eating some of them daily!

Brussels Sprouts

Brassica oleracea var. *gemmifera*

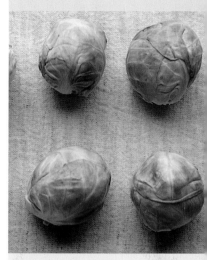

A much-loved biennial grown in Southern Europe and possibly brought into Belgium by the Romans, the first mention of Brussels sprouts was in 1500 near the town of Brussels, hence its name, from where it spread literally everywhere in Europe. Thomas Jefferson introduced it to North America in 1812 and it became so popular a vegetable that to this day it is traditionally served with the Christmas turkey in the Northern Hemisphere!

Attractive in the vegetable garden, this useful biennial grows tall with a mass of leaves on long stems, and the miniature 'cabbages' form along the stems. Sow seeds as you would sow cabbage seeds (see page 84).

An excellent source of folic acid, vitamins C, K and B6 and numerous cancer-fighting chemicals as well as being rich in beta-carotene, potassium and lots of fibre, they are well known for reducing the appetite, promoting bowel regularity and preventing colon cancer. They are included in health-building diets all over the world, steamed and served only with lemon juice and if you are not on a slimming diet, Brussels sprouts in a creamy cheese sauce are fit for a King!

Kale

Brassica oleracea var. *acephala*

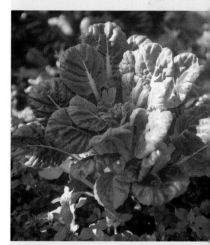

A lso known as collard greens, bore cole or boerkool, this easy-to-grow winter crop is literally a kind of cabbage that does not make a head. Bundles of luscious leaves are available all through the winter, some with curlier leaves than others, at the greengrocers and are waiting, begging to be made into a really delicious soup. I am always thrilled when I see the first kales in the market, as my own rows are nowhere near picking.

It is so worth growing your own as they grow readily and quickly from seed (plant them out the way cabbages are planted). Rich, well-dug compost-filled beds in the sun will ensure a great crop of leaves all winter and well into spring.

Rich in calcium, potassium, phosphorus, magnesium, vitamins, especially vitamins A, C and B6, as well as all the cancer-fighting compounds and iron, kale is power packed with goodness. It makes a delicious steamed vegetable, thinly shredded and served with a little butter, salt and black pepper – perfect with a rich, meaty stew!

Kohlrabi

Brassica oleracea var. *gongylodes*

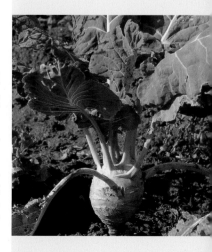

A nother member of the marvellous cabbage family is this rather unusual spacecraft-shaped cabbage–turnip cross! Like kale, which has been cultivated in Europe for over 2 000 years, kohlrabi has been around since before the first century – Pliny the Elder called it a 'Pompeian cabbage' – and it is the swollen turnip-like stem that is eaten!

Kohlrabi is easy to grow, just like its close cousin the turnip! (See 'Growing' instructions under Turnip on page 87.)

Rich in vitamins and minerals, it can be steamed and served with a tasty cheese sauce or grated into soups, stews and stir-fries. Pull them up when they are smaller than a cricket ball and try peeling them and eating them raw in salads with lemon juice. Served this way, it is crisp and refreshing and full of goodness that fights colds and 'flu. The leaves are edible too and are delicious shredded into soups and stir-fries.

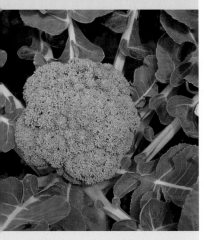

Calabrese

Brassica oleracea var. *italica*

Then, still in this superb family of *Brassicas*, is the sprouting broccoli, the Romanesco broccoli and the purple Cape broccoli – almost like heads of colourful cauliflowers, some lime green with a pointed top, some so incredibly purple they look as though they've been dipped in dyes, and some like great heads of pale broccoli! Most of these beautiful cauliflower-style vegetables come from around the Mediterranean area – Crete, Italy, Belgium, Cyprus and France – and the heads and the tender leaves surrounding the heads are used in mouth-watering traditional dishes. Records go back to around the end of the 16th century and they have never lost their popularity!

To grow Calabrese, follow the 'Growing' instructions given under Broccoli on page 82.

Feast on them, as they are loaded with vitamins and minerals and quickly steamed or added to soups, stir-fries and casseroles, they'll provide a health-packed winter feast. Their best accompaniment is a squeeze of fresh lemon juice.

Chinese Cabbage

Brassica rapa var. *pekinensis*

Also known as celery cabbage or Chinese leaf, this huge and luscious wide-ribbed, pale-leafed cabbage originates in southern China and it has a history that goes back thousands of years. There are several delicious Chinese cabbage varieties – one has mustard-flavoured leaves and is known as Chinese mustard cabbage, another one has a mass of succulent flowering stalks known as Chinese flowering cabbage (*Brassica rapa* var. *parachinensis*), and then there is the crisp, leafy rosette known as pak choi or bok choi (*Brassica rapa* var. *chinensis*), also a Chinese white cabbage, and all are rich in vitamins and minerals, especially iron, calcium and potassium.

A large variety of easy-to-grow Chinese vegetables can be bought in seed packets as, over the last few decades, the world is becoming aware of the value of growing these important vegetables and adding them to our daily diets to build health. Sow the seeds in trays first and when big enough to handle plant out in richly composted, well-dug moist soil in rows spaced 30 cm apart. They are all delicious at any time during their prolific growth and they look beautiful in the garden and do well in big pots at the kitchen door too.

Medicinally Chinese cabbage has been used through the centuries to fight colds and 'flu, bronchitis, pneumonia and kidney and bladder infections. Chinese cabbage leaves softened in hot water makes an excellent poultice over a sprained ankle or to draw out a suppurating sore or to bring an abscess or boil to a head, a simple yet effective treatment that has been used for centuries!

All are delicious in stir-fries and soups, salads and stews, and as a winter vegetable they are simply charming and very decorative to grow in the garden. In China the leaves are finely shredded with onions, mustard greens, radishes and ginger, to make a deliciously hot and tasty soup. Thinly shredded Chinese cabbage in vinegar and thick molasses, rich moist brown sugar or honey, has been an ancient pickled relish that is eaten every day in winter to keep the circulation going.

I use Chinese cabbage to make a quick, light, refreshing and warming soup that will take away the aches and pains of an exhausting day (see recipe alongside). It is my basic recipe and I add whatever vegetables I have available. This is a detoxifying soup to treat 'flu and coughs and revive exhaustion, so don't be tempted to add stock cubes, spices or other flavourings.

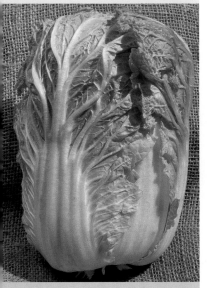

Chinese Cabbage Soup

Serves 6

This is a basic recipe; you can add any vegetables to suit yourself.

In a heavy bottomed pot fry 3 finely chopped onions, 3 cloves of garlic, finely chopped, and 1–3 red chillies without their seeds in a little olive oil. Stir-fry until they start to lightly brown. Now add 3 cups thinly shredded Chinese cabbage and 1½–2 litres homemade chicken stock or water, 2 cups thinly sliced celery, 2–3 cups other Chinese greens or mustard leaves or pak choi leaves, and simmer for 15 minutes. Add sea salt and black pepper to taste and the juice of 2 lemons and about 3 tablespoons of honey. Simmer for another 5 minutes and then add, just before serving, about ¾ cup finely chopped parsley.

Turnip

Brassica rapa

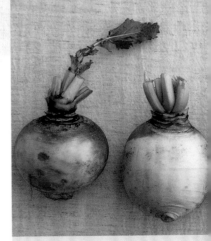

The turnip is one of the oldest root crops and was cultivated over 4 000 years ago in Asia. The wild turnip, it is thought, originated in Europe and Theophrastus described it in early writings around 400 BC. The Greeks and the Romans grew fields of turnips and they were the first to discover and plant new varieties. Trade of turnips and turnip seeds became brisk between Italy and Greece in the Middle Ages, and turnip cultivation spread quickly. The early European settlers introduced turnips to America and 'turnip greens' became a valuable part of the winter diet. Later on with the slave trade between Africa and America, turnip greens were utilised in the spinach dishes that formed part of the traditional African cuisine. The turnip leaves became a valuable asset as the leaves supply many times the nutritional content of the turnip root! Gradually the turnip spread across the world. Travellers bartered turnip seeds for other items and carried the turnip further and further away. The monks – those first healers or medicine men – in their cloister gardens reserved space for this easy-to-grow annual plant, turning the root part into a medicinal 'wine' for coughs, colds, bronchitis, excess phlegm and even for the aches and pains of old age, and the leaves into a valuable tonic for the ailing aged.

Growing Turnips

My fascination with turnips began as a child with my father and his grand passion, his compost making. He specially made compost for the root vegetables like carrots, beetroot, radishes, parsnips and turnips! In those years seeds were quite difficult to find, and we gathered a lot of our own – so I know all about turnip seed. We often tagged a really luscious plant and the seed was carefully collected in a separate packet.

Like those medieval gardeners who quickly learned underground vegetables like the carrot, potato and turnip really thrive in richly composted, deeply dug trenches that can be flooded with water weekly, we learned that turnips love trenches. At the Herbal Centre we choose to grow turnips as a cool weather crop, sowing the seed in April and thereafter a fresh batch each month until July. We're still reaping both the roots and the leaves in September, but the heat, often over 34 °C, quickly dries them out. In cooler parts of the country turnips will survive later into the summer months. Long, slow and deep twice weekly watering will ensure tender, flavour-filled and juicy turnips that are delicious finely grated into a salad or a stir-fry!

Using Turnips

Quite a fabulous food, the turnip is almost a forgotten vegetable relegated to the soup pot! But pause a moment and consider its extraordinary values. It is invariably thought of as a root vegetable, and its exceptionally valuable leafy tops are cut away and thrown out, but for the soup pot the turnip itself *and* its leaves were a valuable ingredient. The turnip became so popular in the early centuries and was included in many dishes because it was considered a 'plant of warmth', and eating turnips could help to withstand the long cold nights of the intensely long, cold Northern Hemisphere winters!

Health Note

Turnips are rich in fibre, copper, calcium, manganese, potassium, magnesium, folic acid, the B vitamins, especially B6, as well as vitamins E and C. Interestingly, the leaves contain all these minerals and vitamins but in a far greater abundance than in the actual root vegetable itself!

Quick and Easy Ways with Turnip

Mashed turnips are a delicious vegetable side dish. Peel, dice and cook the turnips until tender and mash. Add to an equal amount of mashed potato, and serve with a sprinkling of grated nutmeg and butter.

Often a row of turnips that has been sown too thickly will produce a rich source of tender leaves with small unformed roots, and these are a terrific bonus – quickly steamed and served with crisp fried onions, lots of freshly squeezed lemon juice and salt and black pepper.

Lightly stir-fried and sautéed in butter, the tender green leaves cooked with sweet potatoes and cubes of tofu is a favourite dish in Italy that has stood the test of time.

Caution

The leaves of the turnip contain oxalates, so those who have a history of kidney stones should avoid eating turnips and their leaves more than twice a week.

Pigeon Pea
Cajan Pea

Cajanus cajan

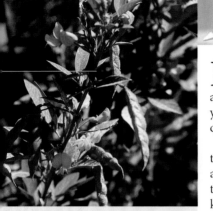

I am intrigued by this little tree! It is a small upright perennial shrub, a legume that is grown in plantations in its native India, which shows a great variety of cultivars. Some have a dark almost russet-coloured pea, some are pale and some are greyish and some speckled. Even its bright yellow flowers, pea-shaped and honey-fragrant, are in some varieties marked with red and some are quite pale.

Thousands of years ago it was cultivated in India and from there it spread as a valuable dried food trade – the pea pods fetching an excellent price – into Egypt, East Africa and on into the Caribbean area, and from Malaysia with the slave trade into distant lands. The Malay name for pea is *kacung* and the name 'cajan' comes from its botanical Latin name, *Cajanus cajan*, and this is why it is commonly known as cajan pea, and also pigeon pea for it is much loved by pigeons and chickens and was grown as feed in the Barbados Islands.

Growing Pigeon Pea

Undemanding and a quick grower, it is both drought tolerant and grows easily in any soil. In many areas it survives with rainfall only and begins bearing the flowers and pods in clusters along its leafy branches while still quite young, and within 6 months it bears heavily.

Seeds quickly germinate sown in full sun, spaced 2 m apart in a richly composted hole. (I plant 2 or 3 seeds and keep the strongest plant once it reaches about 30 cm in height.) Be sure to keep the area moist every day until the little plant is well established. Thereafter water once or twice weekly.

Sown in early spring, by late summer in the heat its pods are abundant and in frost-free areas it is a strong perennial little tree that stands up to heavy winds and neglect surprisingly well. In areas where there is light frost, protect the little tree with plant fleece.

Using Pigeon Peas

History records its use as a medicine in the early centuries. A pulp of cooked mashed pigeon peas and leaves was used as a wound dressing over infected wounds, and a hot poultice held in place with banana leaves bound over a boil or an abscess or over a suppurating sore, and applied three or even four times daily, is still used today in many countries. Crushed, pounded leaves are used over insect bites, scratches and grazes, or the leaves are cooked and made into a paste and then applied warm to the area and bound in place, freshly applied every day until the area heals. This has long been a traditional first aid in many countries.

Rich in protein, vitamins, amino acids and minerals, both green and dried pigeon peas are packed with energy-giving goodness and form the base of many dishes that are sustaining and beneficial for the poorest of people – a staple food that has been treasured and respected and cherished for thousands of years. Cooked into nourishing stews and soups, and the dried peas stored in clay jars for long journeys and as trade, the pigeon pea has become almost a legend in its history, and dried cakes and meal made from pigeon pea today form the base of many dishes in many cultures.

Health Note

Pigeon pea is high in vitamins A, B, C, D and E, and minerals like magnesium, potassium, calcium, phosphorus and iron are also abundant.

Green Pigeon Pea Mash

This is my favourite way of eating pigeon peas.

2 cups hulled green pigeon peas
2 cups fresh green pigeon pea leaves
juice of a lemon
sea salt and pepper to taste
2 onions, finely chopped
2 sweet potatoes, peeled and grated
   (enough for 2 cups)
1 green pepper, finely chopped
a little olive oil for frying

Brown the chopped onions in the olive oil. Add the green pepper and stir-fry. Now add all the other ingredients and stir-fry well. Add a little water and turn the pot down to a gentle simmer. Check that it does not burn and add a little more water when needed. Serve as a vegetable with poached eggs or with chicken or on its own – it is nourishing, filling and delicious!

Hint

A companion plant of note, pigeon pea becomes a catch crop for black aphids, taking away the infestation from other crops grown near it. Its light shade in very hot areas ensures abundant crops of green peppers, spring onions, garlic, chives, buckwheat and even lettuces in the summer heat. A light spray of any of the insect-repelling herbs 3 days in a row will clear the aphids and the little tree will produce an abundance of edible pods and leaves as if nothing ever bothers it!

Tea

Camellia sinensis

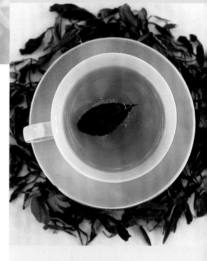

It is China we have to thank for the popular and fascinating tea plant! Indigenous to Northern China, Thailand, Cambodia and Laos, where it grows in glossy wild abundance, it is part of myth and legend that goes back almost 5 000 years! Around 2737 BC 'tea' was discovered by accident when an aged Chinese Emperor on a journey through his Empire stopped to rest with his entourage under an evergreen hedge one afternoon. Being old and frail, his pages always made the Emperor a cup of hot water and some food to settle him for the evening. On this day, while they prepared his tent and his food, 3 or 4 leaves from the hedge under which they sheltered on the windy afternoon, blew into the pot of boiling water on the fire. The food and the hot water seemed to revive the Emperor so quickly that he wanted to continue the journey, much to the servants' surprise! On the return journey, the servants collected a whole box of the leaves to take with them and that is how tea was discovered! From that time on tea consumption spread throughout Chinese culture – it became a ritual and it remains so to this day.

European explorers began the tea trade, the Portuguese explorers took it to Lisbon and the Dutch ships took it from there to France, Holland and Germany. These tea trade routes spread further and further until finally it reached Britain around 1652 where it quickly became the most popular drink, replacing English ale! Tea mania began and it swept across the New World. The colonists took tea to North America and the great tea trades began in Boston, New York and Philadelphia. Tea was then heavily taxed and it was smuggled into the colonies, setting the stage for the American Revolution. The Boston Tea Party made history and by the 1800s, after the Revolution ended, America traded directly with China. Its popularity never waned and today around 2,5 million tons of tea are produced yearly!

Growing Tea

Specific conditions are needed and the acidity of the soil, the moisture of the air, the temperature of the days and the nights, all need to be considered. Perhaps it was the sea breezes in 'Ceylon' that made the 'Ceylon tea' so popular, or the soft mists over China, or the cool valleys of America that established viable plantations, and trial plantings in full sun with sufficient watering and the correct soil type are the only way to begin.

Using Tea

Both green and black tea are rich in riboflavin and polyphenols, particularly the first picked green tea (tea leaves before they have been rolled or fermented). The polyphenols in green tea are flavonoids which increase antioxidant activity, and green tea has been found to have excellent cancer-fighting activity, specifically cancer of the intestinal tract, digestive tract, breast and prostate. Tests have shown that green tea polyphenols can inhibit the growth of cancer cells by blocking the formation and activation of cancer-causing compounds like the nitrosamines and other carcinogens.

Black tea is rolled and fermented to increase its flavour and is more processed than Oolong tea (which is only partially oxidised), and black tea contains far more caffeine than green tea or Oolong tea. Brewing black tea in a warmed teapot, in only a little boiling water, releases the tannins and caffeine, and the twisted and fermented leaves become softened and expanded, producing the flavour-filled black tea. During processing, the leaves are allowed to oxidise, and it is during this time that the enzymes convert the polyphenols into substances that are much less potent than those in the less flavour-filled green tea.

It is all in the processing that the teas differ and, interestingly, studies are now indicating that excessive consumption of black tea may actually increase the risk of certain cancers.

Health Note

Both green and black tea contain calcium, magnesium, zinc, iron, fluoride, and vitamins C, D and K.

Green Iced Tea

This remains my favourite.
Steep ½ cup dried unprocessed green tea leaves in 1 litre of boiling water. Stand until cool and strain. Add the juice of 2–3 organically grown lemons, a little grated lemon zest and honey to sweeten if liked. Serve chilled in a tall glass.

Caution

Black tea contains high levels of both caffeine and oxalates and should be avoided by those who are predisposed to the formation of kidney stones.

Green tea can interfere with the blood thinner Warfarin, so it is always advisable to discuss every food or drink you take with your doctor first.

Chilli Pepper

Capsicum frutescens

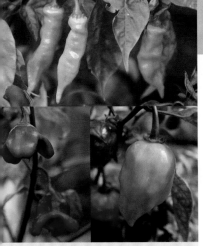

There is surely no other food in the world that inspires so great a passion as the chilli does! The incredible diversity in this group of easy-to-grow plants, its colours, shapes, forms and intensities and its flavours ranging in such amazing variety, put the chilli in a class of its own. And it has an equally amazing history. Discoveries at archaeological sites in Mexico show that as far back as 7000 BC chillies were part of life. The Aztecs and the Mayans actually named the varieties – names that are still used today – and although their cultural records and their historical recordings were destroyed by European invaders, the chilli and its names are still found in their carvings and burial sites. During the 15th century, Christopher Columbus, seeking India's pepper, *Piper nigrum*, found the peppery chillies on his voyages and so began the trade as he introduced the chilli to Europe, and from there it spread into Africa and Asia.

Growing Chillies

So easy to grow, it is worth growing your own. Finding your favourite chilli is a matter of taste, and seed merchants offer a wide range of so many different varieties you'll be spoilt for choice. Here are a few varieties to try: Anaheim (mild to hot), Ancho (mild to hot; delicious dried), Cayenne (everyone's favourite, long red and fiery hot!), Habanero (orangey yellow, it is the hottest of all – *beware*!), Helmet chilli (mild, red helmet-shape, seeds are fiery), Hungarian Wax (a long yellow chilli, mild to hot), Jalapeño (dark green, ripening to dark red and very fiery), ornamental chillies like the Black Pearl and Fireworks (start off tiny and yellow, ripens to fiery red), Serrano (very hot, dries well) and Tabasco (bright orange and very fiery).

Sow seed in early spring in a protected area in full sun in a deeply dug, richly composted furrow or bed that can be flooded with water twice weekly in the heat of summer. Small chilli plants transplant easily: plant them in moist soil and keep them wet and cool until they recover. Most chilli bushes reach 40–80 cm in height, so plant them 80 cm to 1 m apart. Chillies need winter protection and pruning in late winter to tidy them up. They take a while to recover, which is why many chilli lovers prefer to start each spring with new plants, especially if you want to pick constantly!

Using Chillies

Hot and spicy, chillies are a mainstay of Mexican, West Indian and Indian cuisines. Chillies actually can easily become addictive: the compound responsible for both the pleasure and the pain in chillies is capsaicin. It is an intensely powerful compound that, if a fraction of a tiny drop touches the nerve endings in the tongue, it triggers pain messages that are transmitted to the brain. The burning sensation signals the brain to release endorphins, which are natural painkillers that create a feeling of well-being. Each mouthful creates a dramatic response – heat, sweating, pain and discomfort – and this continues to trigger the endorphins! The overall effect is a sensation of such pleasure – once the 'fire' within is calmed – that chilli lovers literally crave it!

Caution

Chilli burns are well documented, especially when working with intensely hot chillies. The skin and mucous membranes around the eyes, the nose and the lips are all affected. *Wear gloves and never touch your face while picking or preparing chillies.*

Chilli Pickle

2 kg of chillies (a combination is very attractive)

4 litres cold water

3 cups coarse sea salt (not table salt)

Wash the chillies well, trim the stalks and pierce with a toothpick all over. Seeds remain inside. In a big, non-chipped enamel or stainless steel basin, submerge the chillies in the water and sprinkle in the salt. Cover with a weighted plate to keep the chillies under water and leave for 24 hours. Refrigerate if it is very hot weather. Next day, drain the chillies well and rinse twice in fresh water.

Prepare the pickling liquid

In a large stainless steel pot, combine the following ingredients:

12 cups white grape vinegar • 2 cups water • 1 cup coarse salt • 1 cup coriander seed • ½ cup mustard seed • ½ cup fennel seed • ½ cup star anise • ½ cup black peppercorns • ½ cup cumin seed • 5 cups brown sugar

Simmer for 5 minutes. Now gently drop the drained chillies into the liquid. Time this carefully. Let the chillies boil for only 3 minutes after the pot has begun to boil again. Take off the stove and with a slotted spoon fill prepared sterilised glass jars with the chillies. Ladle spoons full of the liquid over them to completely cover the chillies. Make sure you fill the jars to the brim. Seal and label. Leave to stand 2 weeks before opening.

The following two capsicums need to have a space of their own in the garden, as no summer is complete without them.

Bell Pepper

Capsicum annuum

Indigenous to South and Central America, these green, red and yellow sweet peppers have been used for at least 7 000 years! Portuguese and Spanish explorers spread this valuable food throughout the world from its early beginnings. This was relatively easy as they adapt so well to different climates and to different cuisines.

Bell peppers are an annual crop and are easily grown from seed. See Growing instructions under Chilli Pepper on page 90.

One of the most nutrient-rich foods available, the bell pepper has to be one of the best health foods we know: rich in vitamins C, K, B6, beta-carotene and folic acid and a source of phytochemicals with outstanding antioxidant activity. Red bell peppers are even higher than the green sweet peppers in their nutrient value and they also contain lycopene, which offers protection against heart disease and cancer. They also have the effect of protecting the eyes against the formation of cataracts. So eating bell peppers daily could lessen the need for cataract surgery. For high cholesterol levels, to reduce the risk of heart attacks and for irregular heartbeat, bell peppers in the diet are high on the list and their vitamin C and capsaicin content helps to prevent blood clot formation.

Thinly sliced into salads, stir-fries, stews and soups, this is one vegetable that is so versatile you will never tire of it.

Paprika

Capsicum annuum

Commonly known as Hungarian pepper, paprika was probably a Turkish variety brought into Hungary around the 16th century where it acclimatised when the Turks conquered Hungary and allowed some Belgian farmers to settle there. The Belgians were the first to plant the mild and delicious paprika. Soon the Hungarians included it in their diets and in time it became so popular it was known as 'the spice of Hungary'.

To grow paprika, follow the instructions under Chilli Pepper on page 90.
High in vitamin C, A and E, paprika is taken to boost the immune system to resist the winter colds and 'flu. Hungarian children sprinkle paprika over their bedtime milk because it eases a sore throat and soothes a cough. No medicine shelf in Hungary, Czechoslovakia or Russia is without a bottle of paprika where it is used today as it has been for centuries to clear wounds, scratches and grazes by sprinkling it into the washing water. To stimulate and treat a sluggish bladder and kidneys, to ward off 'flu and colds and as an anti-cancer food – it is high in valuable minerals and beta-carotene – paprika is used in many dishes. Grow your own paprika and slice the mild, crisp pods into salads and stir-fries.

Hint

Make your own paprika powder by grinding the fully dried paprika pods, seeds and all, into a fine powder and bottle in glass bottles with a screw top. Or you can pickle the ripe paprika pods – follow the recipe for Chilli Pickle on page 90 but replace the chillies with paprika.

Health Note

Chillies and sweet peppers are rich in vitamins C, A & E, B6, K, beta-carotene, folic acid, lycopene, amino acids and capsaicin (the active ingredient in chillies, which is responsible for the heat factor).

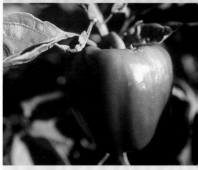

Bell pepper

Baked Bell Peppers

A dish I serve often, it is so quick and easy it can become a party dish.

In a roasting pan lay out rows of bell peppers that have been cut in half and de-seeded. Choose red and yellow bell peppers. Fill each half with a layer of breadcrumbs that have been lightly browned in olive oil and sprinkled with chopped parsley. Then a layer of cherry tomatoes cut in half and thickly packed in like little rows of bright scales. Sprinkle with more fried breadcrumbs, grind a good black pepper and sea salt over everything and finally cover with finely grated Parmesan cheese. Put under the grill and melt. Remove when the cheese bubbles and serve hot as an entrée or as a side dish with roast beef or chicken. It is melt-in-your-mouth delicious!

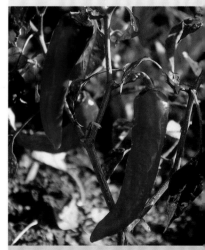

Paprika

Papaya
Pawpaw ▪ Pepino

Carica papaya

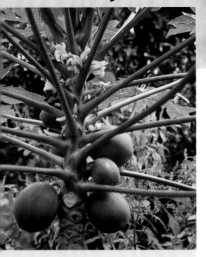

One of nature's most effective natural laxatives and an extraordinary aid to the digestion, the much enjoyed papaya or pawpaw is an easy-to-grow fruit that originates in the warm and tropical areas of Central America. It closely resembles the babaco, which is native to the Andes Mountains of South America. It is thought that the Spanish and Portuguese explorers took the papaya seeds into the West and East Indies and later into Europe, but even before the arrival of the Europeans it was already being cultivated well beyond its native lands. The trade routes mapped its journey and its Carib name was 'ababai' which gradually became 'papaya' as it spread, and by the 1800s it was being widely cultivated in all tropical and even subtropical areas. Interestingly, Hawaii and South Africa are today among the main exporters of this delicious and much-loved fruit.

The babaco (*Carica pentagona*) comes from Ecuador and is similar to the papaya and although it is not found in the wild, botanists agree it could be a hybrid of the mountain papaya (*Carica candamarcensis*), grown in New Zealand and in Europe as far north as the Channel Islands, and although similar to the much-loved papaya it is a softer and more tender fruit, normally seedless and liquidised to make a refreshing commercial drink. The babaco is more acidic than the papaya and so tender it is not often for sale in the marketplaces when ripe.

Growing Papayas

A tall, usually unbranched, tree with a soft stem and a bunch of huge, hand-shaped leaves on long stalks forming a crown, the flowers are borne on male and female trees tight against the stem. Fragrant, creamy and luscious, they scent the night air with a lily-like fragrance loved by moths. Both male and female trees are necessary for the fruiting, but one male tree is sufficient for 10 or 15 or even 20 female trees.

Full sun and a huge, deep, compost-filled hole that can be flooded with water twice weekly, is needed for an abundant crop, and even in areas where the winters are mild it will need a little protection. Grown against a north-facing wall is often protection enough, and a barrow load of compost around its roots in autumn will protect it well. Let the fruit ripen to its golden beauty on the tree for the maximum goodness – if you can protect it from the birds and monkeys!

Using Papayas

Rich in antioxidant nutrients, the precious carotenes, the papaya is superb as an anti-cancer food. It is a natural laxative, a fabulous digestive, anti-parasitic, and soothes, eases and disperses intestinal gas, bloatedness, flatulence, tummy rumblings, colic, heartburn, hiccoughs and intense discomfort in the bowel, and cleanses, clears and detoxifies generally. Ancient medicinal treatments urged the eating of a few of the ripe seeds within the fruit for inflamed joints, rheumatism and arthritis, and the wrapping of a warmed softened leaf over an aching elbow or shoulder or knee. The papain in the fruit, and to an extent the leaf, meant it could ease aches and pains in the body and generally soothe burns, scratches and grazes.

The inside of the skin makes a superb beauty aid, used as a mask over inflamed problem oily skins. In fact, papaya is a fabulous skin treatment for sunburn, very dry flaky skin and for scalp problems. Even the milk from the stems and leaves will clear away warts and crusty dry callouses.

Green papaya – matured to almost fully ripe – makes delicious chutneys, relishes and pickles, and is part of the colourful and delicious diet of the West Indies.

Health Note

Papaya has masses of vitamin C, E and A, beta-carotene, magnesium, calcium, dietary fibre, and it contains papain, a very necessary enzyme that helps digest proteins! It is a seriously valuable health food!

Papaya Salad

Try mixing cubed papaya in a green salad with avocado, cold chicken and cucumber. You'll think you're dining out in Hawaii!

Note

There is some confusion around the name 'pawpaw' which arises from Asimina triloba, a type of custard apple, native to southeast United States. In some parts of the world this is called 'pawpaw'. In South Africa, pawpaw is the common name for the Carica papaya.

Hint

The papain in papaya skins makes an excellent meat tenderiser. You need the skin of green (raw) papaya . Peel the skin and add 1 teaspoon of salt to a cup of papaya skin and grind down to a paste. Use one tablespoon of this paste per kilogram of meat. Tenderising time may take from 30 minutes to 2 hours depending on the type of meat, age and cut.

Safflower
False Saffron

Carthamus tinctorius

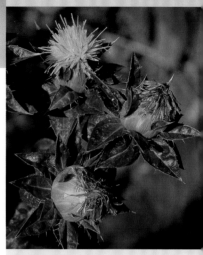

A slightly prickly annual herb, the safflower is an ancient crop much treasured for its large white seeds that are so rich in oils, and also for its thistle-like flowers that were much sought after as one of the first of the world's cloth dyes. The dried florets of the flower head contain a reddish-orange pigment called carthamine – hence its Latin name. The safflower belongs to the thistle family and the orange thistle heads have become a substitute for the precious saffron stamens! The name *Carthamus* comes from the Arabic word *quortom* or the Hebrew word *qarthami*, which means 'to paint', referring to its bright orange pigment used as a colouring agent in food, cloth, feathers, body paint and the robes of the monks. The flowers yield a yellow dye in water, and a brilliant fiery red in alcohol. Through the ancient days there was so great a demand for it and for the dyeing of the Buddhists' traditional golden robes that it became a valuable annual crop, and foods prepared for celebrations and festivals and religious ceremonies were coloured by safflower. Real saffron (*Crocus sativus*), the world's most expensive spice, grown only in the Middle East and parts of Europe, has become so expensive that safflower is used extensively in its place. Although safflower does not have the flavour of saffron, it imparts the same rich colour to food.

Growing Safflower

A hardy annual, sow safflower in spring in well-dug, richly composted soil in full sun and keep moist (we cover with raked leaves to keep the soil from drying out – check it every day) and water gently until the seeds come up. Thereafter water alternate days until the little seedlings become stronger. They grow fast and the flower heads in spiny bracts form quickly. The whole plant branches into several flowers, reaching 75 cm or even 1 m in height in favourable conditions.

Using Safflower

The flowers and the seeds are the parts used and the seed crop with its valuable oil extracted is grown in America, India, Mexico, Spain and even Australia, harvested mechanically for salad oils, margarines and cooking oil and is one of the cholesterol-reducing oils that is quickly gaining importance. Safflower oil has a higher proportion of polyunsaturated fatty acids than any other cooking oil that is commercially available today.

A tea of the flowering heads (see recipe alongside) can be taken for any of these ailments: to lower high blood cholesterol; to improve the circulation and to stimulate the heart; to stimulate the uterus (so it is not safe to take if you are pregnant); to relieve pain; reduce inflammatory conditions such as arthritis, painful joints and fevers; to ease the symptoms of menopause and ease menstrual problems, premenstrual tension and heavy bleeding. Externally, flowers softened in hot water can be applied to bruises, sprains, an aching back and neck and shoulder pains, and bound in place with a crêpe bandage or kept in place with a hot-water bottle lying on a pillow. For wounds, scratches and grazes a lotion made by boiling 1 cup of flowers and leafy tops in 1 litre of water for 10 minutes, then cooled, strained and used as a wash is a soothing and comforting treatment used for centuries.

The edible deliciously chewable seed is a snack enjoyed all over the world, much like a hulled sunflower seed. A few seeds, crushed and mixed into fresh milk will coagulate it, so it is often used in cheese making along with its yellow stamens to give a rich colour to cheese.

Health Note

Safflower oil is high in polyunsaturated fatty acids and is starting to gain importance as a cholesterol-lowering oil, and as a delicious cooking oil.

Safflower Flower Tea

I am fascinated by the medicinal value that safflower is so respected for. To make a tea of the flowering heads, take ½ cup of fresh flowering tips, pour over this 1 cup of boiling water, let it stand 5 minutes, then strain and sip slowly. It can be used for a multitude of ailments – see main text.

Safflower Skin Rub

This skin rub makes an excellent dressing for scratches, bites and grazes.
Add 1 tablespoon of safflower oil to 1 cup of good aqueous cream with 2 teaspoons of vitamin E oil. Store in a screw-top jar and apply frequently to the area.

Hint

To reap the flower petals, wait for the whole flower to dry. Pull off the tuft of petals and spread the tiny petals out on paper in the shade. It will take 2 days to dry. Store in a labelled screw-top glass jar and use as you would use saffron.

Pecan Nut

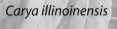

Carya illinoinensis

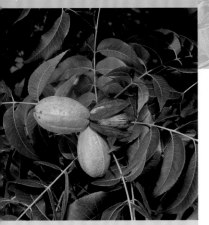

This large, beautiful and stately tree is native to North America around the Mississippi River valley area and parts of Mexico. It is now cultivated commercially in many countries. There are several types of 'hickory nuts' that have played a large part in the diet and the history of the Native Americans (American Indians). They used the wood of mature trees for bows and arrows, for structuring their dwellings, for furniture and utensils. Prehistoric archaeological sites offered an enormous amount of evidence, the fossil remains along the river banks clearly showed the pecan nut was a treasured food, and that it was indigenous to the area. The first historical reference to this popular nut was by the Spanish explorer Cabeza de Vaca who survived a shipwreck and was washed ashore on Galveston Island around 1540. The Indians shared their store of autumn gathered nuts, which they ground into a sustaining milky drink, with him. The same milky drink could be fermented into a powerfully intoxicating drink for ceremonies and feast days, known as 'pawcohiccora' and it is thought this is where the word 'hickory' was derived from.

By the 1700s French explorers of the New World discovered the pecan nut when they visited Natchez and the surrounding areas, which later would become New Orleans. It is thought that the French were the first to create the much enjoyed pecan pie! Today there are literally hundreds of varieties of pecans and from its beginnings in America, it is now grown in Brazil, Peru, South Africa, Australia and China – but America still produces over 80% of the world's crop.

Growing Pecans

They are easy to grow, but do not take heavy prolonged frost. The secret to success is to plant them in full sun, in a large, deep (1 m × 1 m × 1 m), compost-filled hole into which a plastic pipe is inserted at an angle in order to get the hosepipe into it to allow the water to reach the roots. A deep watering once a week is all it requires, and a barrow load of compost in late winter and in midsummer will ensure abundant nuts. The nuts ripen and fall from the lofty branches when their outer green, tough cases split to reveal the thin, shiny brown shell of the nut.

Using Pecan Nuts

The Native Americans camped in the pecan forests at the end of summer to gather the valuable nuts for winter and restock their medicine chests. As they gathered the nuts, they ate them to boost their immune systems. Eating pecan nuts before winter helps to protect against 'flu and colds, and crushed pecan nuts assist with the healing of wounds. Pecan nuts are rich in arginine, a valuable amino acid that plays an important role in strengthening the immune system, healing of wounds and clearing suppuration, secretion of natural insulin and growth hormones, and detoxifying the liver and kidneys. It also exerts a relaxing effect on the walls of the blood vessels and so helps to improve the blood circulation generally. Research also found that eating a mere 4 pecan nuts a day helps to lower 'bad' or LDL cholesterol! Abundant in monounsaturated fatty acids and vitamin E, the best way of eating pecans is freshly shelled as, like all nuts, they can go rancid. Keep the nuts in the refrigerator to prolong their shelf life.

Health Note

Pecan nuts are a good source of vitamin E, the B-vitamins, calcium, iron, magnesium, phosphorus, manganese, zinc and copper. They also contain the amino acid arginine and monounsaturated fatty acids.

French Pecan Pie

For fun make this as a showstopper!

Basic Sweet Pastry

1½ cups flour
½ teaspoon salt
1 tablespoon sugar
120 g butter cut into small pieces
2 egg yolks well beaten with
  2 tablespoons iced water

Mix flour, salt and sugar. Rub in butter until the mixture resembles fine breadcrumbs. Stir in the egg mixture. Add a little more water if necessary to make a dough that can be easily rolled out on a floured board. Pat into a 22 cm flan tin and trim to shape.

Filling

About 1½ cups pecan nuts
3 eggs
1 cup dark soft sugar
2 tablespoons golden syrup
Grated rind and juice of 1 lemon
2 tablespoons butter melted
1 teaspoon vanilla essence

Preheat oven to 175 °C. Pick out ½ a cup of pecan halves and set aside. Chop the rest coarsely. Beat the eggs and sugar together. Add in the golden syrup, lemon rind, juice, then the melted butter and the vanilla essence, and finally the chopped pecans. Pour into the pastry case and set in the half cup of pecan nuts in a circle or in a pattern. Bake on a baking sheet on the middle shelf of the oven for about 40 minutes or until the filling is set. Cool on a wire rack and serve warm with whipped cream.

White Sapote

Casimiroa edulis

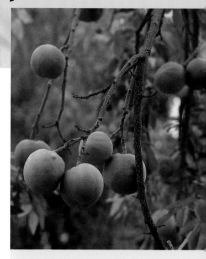

This is an extraordinary tree! Its fruits take a long time to ripen and in midwinter the birds go wild as its large apple-sized green fruits start to soften and ripen, and when it is pale yellow its deliciousness is a combination of soft succulent white flesh and sweetness, something like a pear, that has you searching for more.

Native to Mexico and Central America where it is known as the Mexican apple or *matasano*, it is rare and very precious in other parts of the world. It is a beautiful, fast-growing tree that reaches 15–17 m in height with evergreen trifoliate leaves the size of your hand. Masses of small buds form during spring and summer and the round green fruits vary in size as they grow. At any one time there will be golf ball-sized hard green fruits on the same branch as huge apple-sized ripening fruits, which can be picked hard and green to ripen indoors before the birds and monkeys get them. The tree is tough, resilient, drought, cold and heat tolerant, and produces this luscious and productive crop year after year. The fruits ripen in the coldest months when little else does but it cannot take heavy frost.

The black sapote (*Diospyros digyna*) has a darker flesh and skin and is not related to the white sapote. It is also a subtropical tree and grows into a vigorous, large tree.

Growing Sapote

Choose a site in full sun and dig a deep hole. This becomes a big tree so give it space. Fill the hole with rich old compost and set a wide pipe into the hole at an angle in order to get the hose into it to water the roots. Stake the tree while it is young and water deeply once a week. All it will require is a barrow load of compost in spring and another in autumn but the rewards are astonishing! Baskets of fruit can be picked all through the late summer and winter and will ripen when placed on layers of newspaper on the kitchen shelves. New trees are easily grown from the large seeds or pips pushed into moist, compost-filled bags.

Using Sapote

There are usually 6 large seeds almost the size of the first joint of the thumb in each fruit. Some seeds are smaller than others, and in Mexico the seeds are dried and ground to make a powder. One teaspoon of this powder in warm water is taken as a sedative and a calming medicine. A natural sleep potion that has been used by the Mexicans for centuries is made by taking 2 teaspoons fresh seeds, finely chopped, in 1 cup of boiling water, stand 10 minutes and take an hour before bedtime.

In addition to its high vitamin and mineral content (see Health Note), the sapote with its high fructose content is considered to be beneficial to health and is planted around villages, farms and homesteads all over Mexico. Many trees are planted along the roadsides and a few commercial sapote orchards have been experimented with.

The sweet creamy flesh of a ripe sapote lends itself to ice-creams, fruit salads and creamy desserts.

As the sapote is generally not well known and the large unripe fruits can only be transported at that stage, like the pear, it needs to be eaten quickly as soon as it is ripe, as it has a short shelf life once it becomes soft. This is possibly the reason why it is relatively unknown.

Health Note

White sapote contains vitamin C and some B-vitamins, calcium, phosphorus, a little iron, potassium and magnesium and several amino acids.

Warm Sapote Dessert

Serves 4

This is quick, easy and simply divine. Whisk 3 eggs in 2 cups of milk. Add ½ cup of sugar and 2 tablespoons of corn flour and mix well, whisking over medium heat until it thickens. Stir in a teaspoon of vanilla extract and pour over thinly sliced sapotes in individual glass bowls. Add a dollop of whipped cream and a sprinkling of chopped pecan nuts, and eat while it is still warm. Delicious!

Hint

In some areas the sapote ripens in late summer. The large, green fruits that fall can be swept up and dumped onto the compost heap where they seed easily. Transplant the sturdy seedlings into bags and keep them protected until they strengthen.

Chestnut

Castanea sativa

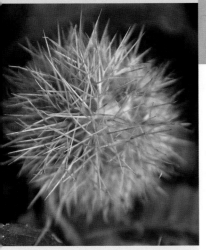

One of the oldest known nuts, indigenous to Europe and Asia, chestnuts are part of history, folklore, myth and magic, and they have been loved and cherished since ancient times. No tree has ever been as useful as the chestnut and there are hundreds of varieties in the *Castanea* genus whose nuts have been relied upon through the centuries as food and medicine for both people and animals. The American chestnut, *Castanea dentata*, the Chinese chestnut, *Castanea mollisima* and the Japanese chestnut, *Castanea crenata,* all have their place in history, and during famine and wars it is the chestnut that has saved millions of lives. Stately, spreading and beautiful, the chestnut tree's bounty has been so valuable through the ages that it was cultivated as far back as Roman times. Avenues of trees were planted in the towns and today, wherever the winters are cold all over the world, chestnuts are cultivated, with France, Italy and Spain the main producers.

Growing Chestnuts

Huge and spreading and slow growing, the chestnut needs full sun and an extra large compost-filled hole. It thrives in the colder areas of the country and will reach 30 m! Deciduous and fascinating, the catkins are produced with the first spring leaves and the prickly outer burrs are green at first and then, as the shiny brown nuts grow inside them, turn light brown to split open in autumn revealing the treasure within.

Using Chestnuts

Once considered a staple food, the nuts were eagerly gathered and cooked in boiling water or roasted over hot coals. Chestnut flour was once a favourite porridge or gruel and formed a thickener in soups and stews, and chestnut tea made of the leaves was taken for coughs and colds and used in gargles and mixtures made by the monks. Chestnut soup or gruel as it was then known, made with parsley, celery, turnips, parsnips, cabbage, potatoes and onions, all peeled and finely grated or chopped or mashed, was the diet for the soldiers during the winters and was made by the monks from their cloister gardens to feed the poor and the sick, and it had such incredible energy-giving, immune system-boosting qualities that it literally became legendary.

As it was usually wild harvested, each country made traditional dishes with chestnuts and my Scottish grandmother made us the most marvellous chestnut puddings and sweets that I have never forgotten. Chestnuts were planted around Cape Town's suburbs and in the first rains in the winter she would take us to places she knew when she first came to South Africa to gather the fallen chestnuts which littered the roadside round Constantia and Bishop's Court. From these gatherings we made *marron glacé* and sugared chestnuts and chestnut spread for scones. Chestnuts had been so much a part of her Scottish childhood she made the journey from Gordon's Bay yearly to collect 'her memories'.

Health Note

Chestnuts are rich in vitamins B1, B2, B6, folic acid and vitamin C (the only nut that contains a good quantity of vitamin C) as well as manganese, magnesium and copper. Just eating 3 boiled chestnuts will supply enough vitamin C for a day!

Chestnut Syrup

In France, *marron glacé* – chestnuts boiled in a syrup – became one of their national dishes and if you've ever tasted it you'll never forget it! This is my grandmother's recipe.

Boil a pot full of chestnuts until tender. Peel away the thick skins and slice into pieces. Simmer 1 cup brown sugar in 1½ cups water with 1 cinnamon stick and a grating of nutmeg for 15 minutes. Stir frequently. Add the chestnut pieces (usually about 3 cups). Simmer another 10 minutes, stirring frequently. Pour into bottles and seal. Serve a spoonful with homemade ice-cream or on hot oatmeal porridge with a spoonful of whipped cream.

Chestnut Leaf Tea

Take this soothing tea for coughs and a cold.

Take 2 fresh chestnut leaves, enough for ¼ cup, and pour over this 1 cup of boiling water. Stand 5 minutes, stir and bruise the leaves. Strain. Sweeten with honey, add a slice of ginger if liked, and sip slowly.

Carob
Locust Tree

Ceratonia siliqua

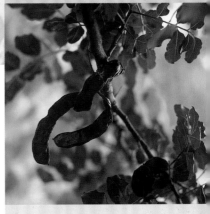

A huge and beautiful evergreen tree that originates in the Mediterranean area, the carob is legendary. It has been used as a food since biblical times. An ancient, cherished and nurtured tree whose rich dark ripe pods, which the tree prolifically bears, are thought to be the 'locusts' that sustained John the Baptist during the time he lived in the wilderness. Valued for thousands of years, the pods have a natural chocolate taste and are a source of exceptional nutrients for both humans and animals, and the seeds were used as trade or barter. In the early centuries, due to the uniform weight of those seeds within the pods, they were used to weigh both diamonds and gold – the *carat* that jewellers use still today as a measurement.

In the Middle East the carob pod is a much loved snack food. The pod is ground and soaked in water and allowed to ferment for 2 to 4 days. The strained liquid is boiled with sugar to make a syrup called 'dibs', and almonds and dates and pieces of fruit, like apples and pears, either fresh or dried, are dipped into the syrup which coats them enticingly in chocolaty deliciousness. Wire racks of 'dibs' sweets can be seen drying in the sun in many villages.

Growing Carob

The tree grows easily and fairly quickly from the seeds and as it grows needs a stake to keep it upright. I trim off the lower branches as it develops into a strong, small tree. It makes an exceptional evergreen shade tree, and some nurseries offer beautifully pruned lollipop trees on thick straight stems, sturdily planted in large plant bags that need merely to be slit and lowered into a large compost- and water-filled hole. A thick plastic pipe, a metre long, set at an angle, which makes an excellent 'watering pipe', can be 'planted' at the same time. This is a means of getting precious water to the roots, especially in times of intense heat and drought, and the eight carob trees in the Herbal Centre gardens bear testimony to this life-saving practice.

Carob trees are undemanding and thrive with a deep weekly waterering, flooding the large 'dam' securely built around their trunks. A barrow load of compost twice yearly ensures masses of flowers and pods, and so my trees bear pods while quite young.

Using Carob

Carob flour or powder contains pectin, which has been taken through the centuries for digestive problems – 1 tablespoon in 225 ml of warm water taken 3 times a day in acute conditions, once or twice in non-acute conditions. Interestingly, carob also contains a high percentage of protein, and added to the formula assists babies who are unable to keep any food in their little stomachs.

Carob flour can be made by grinding the pods finely, excluding the seeds. This, used in baking, replaces cocoa and chocolate, and because it is so sweet it also reduces the need for sugar. Buy ready ground carob flour from health shops to use for baking and milkshakes. The finely ground carob seed powder or gum is used in both pharmaceutical and cosmetic products as well as in foods as a natural thickener, called tragasol, in sauces, salad creams, ice-creams and processed cheeses.

Boil up the crushed seed-free pods with enough water to make a molasses-like consistency, which can then be poured into moulds to make the increasingly popular natural chocolate confectionery. Carob easily replaces chocolate and has no caffeine, less fat and as cocoa beans are high in oxalic acid, it is safer to use carob. Oxalic acid locks in calcium making it unavailable to the body, and carob has a natural sweetener in it, so no sugar needs to be added.

Health Note

Carob is an excellent, well-balanced food, rich in vitamins and minerals, especially vitamins A and B-complex, calcium and phosphorus, and also contains good quantities of iron, copper and magnesium.

Carob Squares

Makes 12 small squares

1–2 cups dark soft sugar (depending on how sweet you like it)
¾ cup ground carob pod
⅔ of a cup of full cream milk
¼ cup of butter
2 teaspoons vanilla essence
½–¾ cup chopped pecan nuts or almonds

Simmer the first 4 ingredients together in a heavy bottomed pot, stirring all the time. Keep stirring – this is the secret – until it reaches 110 °C (225 °F) or the hardball stage. It literally needs to cook through thoroughly so it will set. Remove from the stove, cool 5 minutes, then add the vanilla essence and, if liked, the pecan nuts or almonds. Pour into a well-buttered dish, spread carefully and allow to cool. Cut into squares with a knife dipped first into very hot water. Pack into a tin lined with greaseproof paper. What a treat!

Hint

Here is how to use your own carob pods. The pods need to be dry and brown and brittle. Give them a bash with a stone on a flat stone to open the pod so that you can remove the hard 'carat' seeds. Then push the pieces through a seed or coffee grinder. It needs to be finely powdered or it will taste gritty. Now use the chocolate-like powder as you would cacao with hot milk as a night cap or make it into carob squares (see recipe).

Garland Chrysanthemum

Chrysanthemum coronarium

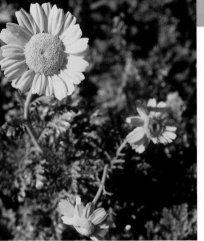

The spectacular yellow daisy-like flowers of the chop-suey greens is so fascinating in the garden and comes up year after year, that it has crept into my heart by its sheer persistence! Many years ago I was given a matchbox of seeds by a Chinese visitor to the Herbal Centre gardens who urged us to plant it as it is so valuable a part of Chinese cooking – she called it *shungiku* – and she said it was used in health-building soups and stir-fries for a variety of ailments and was considered to be an excellent tonic and anti-ager! From then on – almost 20 years – I have grown it every winter and have loved its spring flowering display!

Its taste is strongly pungent – the young leaves are used extensively in Chinese cooking and it is indigenous to the Mediterranean region and Southern Europe where, in the early centuries, the buds were pickled and eaten with meats to ease the digestion. Garland chrysanthemum was taken to Japan and China around the 11th century where it became popular as an ingredient in soups and stir-fries. All parts of the plant have the distinctive chrysanthemum smell and taste. The Chinese were the first to cultivate *Chrysanthemum morifolium* and *Chrysanthemum indicum* in 500 BC. The Mikado adopted the chrysanthemum as his personal emblem in AD 797, and the cultivation of chrysanthemums by the Japanese began in earnest by AD 900, amongst them several edible ones which were all considered to be valuable for the digestion and for blood cleansing.

Interestingly, tansy, feverfew and costmary are all part of the chrysanthemum family, but it is the pretty garland chrysanthemum that remains the favourite in Japanese and Chinese cooking, and many recipes include it. If you ask for the popular chop suey dish in a Chinese restaurant, it will usually contain garland chrysanthemum.

Growing Garland Chrysanthemum

Sow the seeds in autumn for an abundant spring display. Seedlings transplant easily and flourish in well-dug, richly composted soil in full sun and thrive with a deep watering once or twice a week.

Small and succulent plants – a mere posy of finger length leaves – long before the flowers establish, is the part used and loved. These little plants can be transplanted while still tiny into well-dug, well-composted soil in full sun – space 50 cm apart, or a mere 20–30 cm if you intend to reap them young and tender.

Somehow ours are never all reaped at once, so we get these bright, almost hip height, brilliantly yellow daisies in happy abundance and the display in our kitchen gardens is charming. Some flowers are bright yellow, some are creamy yellow with a darker centre, and some are tipped with light butter yellow. We use the petals in salads and stir-fries, and mixed with the petals from our rows of calendulas, we make the spring salads in the restaurant quite spectacular and very tasty!

Using Garland Chrysanthemum

Chinese and Japanese recipes often include young leaves, sometimes young buds and petals, and although the taste is distinctive, it is a much enjoyed health-building ingredient in many dishes, and well worth experimenting with as it is so easy to grow. Look out for self-sown seedlings in early winter and add them to soups and stews.

Health Note

The leaves contain vitamins A, C and a little D, and phosphorus, copper, potassium and some iron.

Chop Suey Greens Stir-Fry

In a wok or pan heat a little sunflower cooking oil. Add 1 medium onion, finely chopped, and stir-fry briskly, then add 1 cup finely chopped green peppers, 1 cup finely chopped mushrooms and 1 tablespoon grated ginger. Keep stir-frying until the onions start to brown and the mushrooms soften.

Now add 1 cup chop suey greens, lightly chopped, and stir in well, ½ cup chopped parsley and ½ cup finely chopped celery stalks and leaves. Briskly stir-fry, adding a little more oil if needed.

Add the juice of 1 lemon and a little grated zest, 2 tablespoons soy sauce, salt and black pepper to taste and ½ cup of spring onions, thinly chopped, and finally add 1 tablespoon of honey dissolved in ½ cup of hot water. Stir well.

Serve hot on a bed of brown rice. To vary the stir-fry, add 2 cups of cooked cubed chicken breasts or thinly sliced lean beef and stir-fry well.

Chickpea
Garbanzo Bean

Cicer arietinum

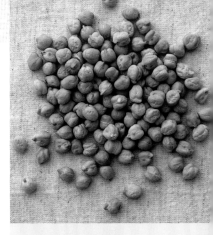

An ancient cultivated crop, the chickpea was revered, cherished and respected for it is as perfect a food as one can get. Known in ancient Greece, India and Egypt, the chickpea has been around forever, but its exact origins are a mystery as archaeologists debate the actual area. At the time of the Pharaohs the chickpea grew wild in Turkey and Egypt, and the dried peas were stored in clay vessels in the tombs of the Pharaohs. From Egypt it spread to Palestine and Mesopotamia, and the traders took it with them to North Africa and east into India.

The mystery deepens as merchants and explorers took the chickpea, an essential survival food for the long journeys, further and further afield, and in ancient burial sites in Asia and in parts of the Mediterranean, pouches and clay pots of chickpeas have been unearthed, as well as ancient food vessels filled with chickpeas still in their pods – presumed to be the seeds for the afterlife.

There is no doubt as to its vital importance and through the centuries chickpea flour, unripe pods and the tips of the branches, and coarsely ground ripe chickpeas made into the much-loved North African couscous, all formed part of a sustaining diet.

Growing Chickpeas

Easy and undemanding, growing your own chickpeas is a lot of fun. Dig a bed in full sun and add generous amounts of compost, water it well and press in the chickpeas, which have been soaked in warm water for at least 2 hours before planting, 50 cm apart in moist and friable soil. Do not let the seeds dry out until the little shoots reach 10–12 cm. Thereafter water well two or three times a week. A bushy and prolific annual, little round pods develop with a point at one end, following the white pea flowers, each holding one or sometimes two chickpeas which ripen slowly.

Dig in the bush once the chickpeas have been harvested. It makes an excellent green manure addition to the soil. I find slashing it up first the easiest way to digging it back into the soil where it quickly breaks down.

Using Chickpeas

One of the best sources of vegetable protein, this is one of the most important foods for treating malnutrition. Children in India suffering from the protein deficiency disease kwashiorkor were treated with chickpea flour and the results proved the chickpea treatment far superior to even milk. A diet of roasted chickpeas and skim milk resulted in more weight gain and the children grew taller than the other groups who were treated with milk and other supplements. Interestingly, the chickpea provides nearly double the amount of iron that is found in most legumes.

Benefits are huge with chickpeas in the diet: they help to lower high cholesterol, assist kidney function flushing toxins from the body, and they literally cleanse the whole digestive system and ease constipation. The chickpea contains a group of compounds called protease inhibitors. These compounds have been found to inhibit cancer cells. In the digestive tract the chickpea molecules are indestructible and these inhibit the protease enzymes and the oncogenes, which can promote cancer cells. So it is certainly worth including chickpeas in the diet, even if it is only twice a week.

Add chickpeas to soups, stews or just have a bowl of freshly cooked chickpeas very lightly salted as a snack. Green chickpeas are delicious boiled in their tender pods and served with butter and lemon juice.

Health Note

In addition to protein, chickpeas are high in calcium, zinc, manganese, magnesium, potassium, phosphorus, vitamins C, A, B1, B2, B6, folic acid, beta-carotene and absorbable iron.

Chickpea Salad

Serves 6–8
This is my favourite way of serving chickpeas.
Soak 4 cups of chickpeas overnight. Next morning boil up in fresh water; simmer gently keeping the pot covered. I usually find 2–2½ hours makes them soft and tender. Drain and cool.
Pour over a **mint sauce dressing**:
½ cup brown grape vinegar
½ cup hot water
½–1 cup finely chopped fresh mint
½ cup honey
Pour into a large screw-top glass bottle and shake well. Serve with cold meats, salads, pizzas, etc.

Hint

Dried chickpeas last well in sealed containers in the fridge. Every week, from this store, boil up 2 cups chickpeas that have been soaked overnight. Cook until tender and drain. Stir in a touch of butter and salt, cool and spoon into a bowl as a delicious quick snack for the children – they love it!

Chicory

Cichorium intybus

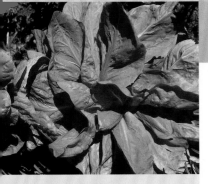

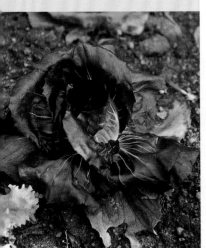

When we think of chicory we think of bitterness! Grown for its roots, mainly as a coffee substitute, this pretty blue-flowered biennial or perennial has been cultivated commercially since the 18th century. It originates in Europe and Asia and there are many cultivated chicories which are all varieties of the same original species, *Cichorium intybus*. Some varieties are grown for their roots (*Cichorium intybus* var. *sativum*), some are grown for their blanched leaves, the best known being witloof (*Cichorium intybus* var. *foliosum*), and some for their bitter salad leafy ingredients known as endive (a separate species, *Cichorium endiva*).

Belgian endive was first discovered purely by accident in the mid 19th century when some chicory roots left forgotten in a dark cellar produced white and tender leaves. The Brussels Botanical Gardens then experimented, and by the 1880s the technique for producing white, tender and mild flavoured 'chicons' was established in Flanders, situated in western Belgium along the North Sea.

Chicory is much loved in its native Mediterranean region and has been used by the ancient Greeks and Romans mainly as a medicine. Today Belgian endive and witloof chicory are grown all over the world as a sought after delicacy. In Europe chicory's cultivation increased substantially when it was discovered that the roots could be roasted and ground into a pleasant tasting and healthy coffee substitute.

Growing Chicory

I grow chicory mainly for its exquisite sprays of starry blue flowers which are edible, and for its blanched 'chicons'. I grow it as a biennial and sow seed in trays individually in autumn for planting out as they get stronger. Dig a deep, thickly composted bed in full sun and water well, then plant out the sturdy little plants in rows spaced 30 cm apart. As they grow tie the leaves together with sisal string, wrapping the whole plant in a tube of thick brown paper and mound up the soil all around it. I also do this with the endives and the beautiful red chicories commonly known as 'radicchio'. The hearts remain tender and crisp and not nearly as bitter as the unblanched leaves. Served with white wine vinegar as a salad, the Italian varieties of radicchio are now a gourmet delight and are grown worldwide.

Using Chicory

The wild chicory, *Cichorium intybus*, is still used today all over the world as a medicine the way it was in the early centuries. The bitter compounds in chicory are considered to be health-building digestives and laxatives that have both tonic and diuretic action, and eating chicory for dinner is believed to purify the blood and ease insomnia. The red Treviso and Verona chicories as well as the beautiful Castel Franco variegated chicory are now grown worldwide and Italians buy them constantly wherever they are, due to their superb tonic effects.

Because the roots, roasted and ground, do not have the same stimulating effects as coffee, many people enjoy chicory as a healthy coffee substitute. So this ancient herb has never lost its place as a precious medicine throughout the centuries.

Add the chopped blanched leaves to soups, stews, or sauté the leaves in butter and stew with lemon juice, honey and mustard, covering the pan and simmering gently until tender.

Health Note

Chicory is rich in vitamins, especially vitamin A and C, carotenes and folic acid, as well as inulin, which is a 'sugar' that is safe for diabetics.

Belgian Chicory and Pears

Serves 6

My favourite way of serving chicory is as a starter.

Break up 2 or 3 'chicons' into little 'boats' – the leaf lends itself to holding a delicious filling. Slice 2 pears into thin wedges and arrange in the 'boats'. Chop ½ a cup of fresh walnuts and crumble about ½ a cup of strong blue cheese (the Belgians love Gorgonzola), sprinkle these over the pears and finally add a splash of raspberry vinegar. Serve chilled on pretty small individual dishes.

Cinnamon

Cinnamomum verum

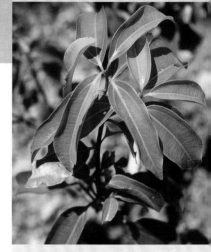

A precious and much-loved evergreen tree that, in its native Sri Lanka, southwest India and parts of Asia, sometimes grows up to 8 metres in height, cinnamon is one of the oldest spices known and in the early centuries was so treasured it was considered to be even more valuable than gold. In Chinese medicine it is recorded in their ancient writings, as being valuable for treating many ailments that today have been verified by modern research. Used in embalming in ancient Egypt, as well as a beverage and flavouring and a medicine, it has never lost its popularity, and through the centuries, featured in religious ceremonies. Quills of cinnamon were burned in churches and on shrines, and incense made of cinnamon still features today in ceremonies throughout the world.

There are several species of cinnamon, but Ceylon cinnamon (*Cinnamomum verum*) and the Chinese cinnamon or cassia (*Cinnamomum aromaticum*), a coarser thicker variety, are the most popular and feature in the spice trade all over the world. The greatest demand for cinnamon was during the Middle Ages and cinnamon was used in many dishes, some surviving to this day, like Christmas mince pies. It became so popular that it actually launched sea explorations by the Dutch and the Portuguese during the late Middle Ages!

Growing Cinnamon

In its tropical native environment it grows to an attractive tree – its typical glossy leaves with the three veins are still used medicinally so it flourishes unchecked along roadsides, in plantations and, in the Seychelles, in fertile valleys. It needs heat, humidity and deep, moist, compost-rich soil and it survives astonishingly well in my hot mountainside gardens and forms attractive prolific bushes with clusters of small creamy buds. Fresh leaves give wonderful flavours to teas and cool drinks, but we have yet to strip the bark, which is scraped to remove the outer bark, every 2 years. The curled 'quills' we buy is the inner bark that dries and rolls up tightly to form that familiar and fragrant bundle.

Using Cinnamon

Not only is it utterly delicious as a ground spice in puddings, cakes and biscuits, chutneys and sauces, and even in curries, but we are only beginning to learn of the amazing healing powers stored in cinnamon. A recent and compelling discovery is cinnamon's extraordinary effect on blood glucose levels, on cholesterol and on blood triglycerides. Cinnamon has insulin-enhancing properties, which for diabetics, including type 2 diabetes, is good news. It is a known antibacterial and its rich and gloriously fragrant essential oil – applied in almond oil as a carrier oil and massaged into the area – is used to treat bacterial and fungal infections, including the yeast fungi of candida. Cinnamon tea has even been found to be effective in fighting *E. coli* bacteria.

Used for many centuries to treat insomnia – just ½ a teaspoon of ground cinnamon in a cup of warmed milk with less than a teaspoon of honey – is soothing, calming and quietening for old and young alike, and can be taken for arthritis, diarrhoea, heart ailments, menstrual problems, peptic ulcers and muscle spasms, and also as a circulatory stimulant, for flatulence and for travel sickness. Cinnamon oil was a favourite rub and massage oil in Europe around 1850, made by warming crushed cinnamon sticks – not the powdered cinnamon – in vegetable oil for 6 hours. Once strained and bottled it could be warmed when needed over hot water and used gently as a comforting treatment for aching backs and sprains and strains.

Health Note

Cinnamon is a natural antibiotic, a natural antiseptic, a diuretic and an excellent digestive, and for coughs and colds and 'flu a mere ½ a teaspoon at a time in warm milk, usually 1–6 grams a day, will bring relief. If you are a diabetic, speak to your doctor about including cinnamon in your diet.

Cinnamon Bark Tea

Pancakes with cinnamon are now considered to be a health booster and combined with cinnamon tea it is a force to be reckoned with.

1 cup of boiling water
½ teaspoon cinnamon powder or
  2 teaspoons crushed cinnamon bark
1 teaspoon grated ginger
1 tablespoon fresh lemon juice
honey to taste

Mix and sip slowly.

Cinnamon Leaf Refresher

Serves 4

Cinnamon leaf tea is a delicious, revitalising drink, and cooled with fresh fruit juice added, becomes a favourite with children.

Pour 2 cups of boiling water over 2 fresh cinnamon leaves. Leave to stand until cool and strain. Add 2 cups of freshly squeezed pineapple juice or litchi juice, or a mixture, and add lots of ice. Pour into glasses and enjoy.

Melon

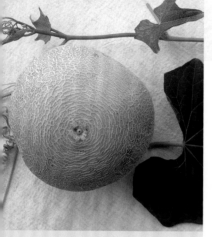

Know Your Melons

Watermelon (*Citrullis lanatus*) – the biggest of all fruits – has shocking pink flesh, thick green or mottled skin and a thick rind. The lime green mottled variety is called 'Charleston Grey'. The baby watermelon or 'Sugar Baby' is pale lime green, often with markings. Slightly bigger than your head, the flesh is like a watermelon's pink, succulent sweetness but denser. The following melons are all varieties of *Cucumis melo*:

Spanspek or **Netted Melon** is a golden-fleshed, richly sweet and flavour-filled melon with a beige-orange skin often with a net-like marking. The stronger it smells the riper it is.

Honeydew Melon is smooth and scented with pale, almost white skin with a touch of green. The flesh is crisp and pale green.

Cantaloupe is similar to spanspek, but with a denser, smoother skin and sectional lines or grooves. The flesh is orange and fragrant, dripping in sweetness.

Casaba Melon has ribbed yellow skin and creamy flesh, and can sometimes be found in greengrocers.

Sprinkled with a little powdered ginger and a dusting of crunchy brown sugar, melons are a summer favourite and the beautiful varieties offered in the greengrocers go on for months.

In my mind the word 'melon' conjures up hot summers and cool, sticky, sweet, crisp flesh of summer picnics and the Christmas holidays! From the great, shocking-pink watermelons, the juice dripping off your chin, to crisp green honeydew melons, to the headily fragrant spanspeks, melons are a feast!

The first melons came from Africa, and also from the Middle East down to Afghanistan. The honeydew melon is thought to have originated in Persia, and was so prized by the Egyptians that it appears in their hieroglyphics dating back to 2400 BC! Melons were in cultivation by the Romans and from there were introduced to Europe, but only became popular around the 15th century. Meanwhile in China the real domestication of the melon began and ancient Chinese writings indicate it was used as a medicine for flushing the kidneys in the early centuries and to this day it remains a valuable food and medicine in China. Christopher Columbus took the seeds to America and it made its American debut in the warmth of California, which remains one of the biggest producers of melons today. It is thought that the melon became a means of barter and trade and some historians have mapped out a seed route of the melon's journey from the top of Africa on into the world. Today, the cantaloupe, the honeydew and the watermelon are produced by not only America but in vast abundance by China, Spain, Turkey and India, and by South Africa as an annual summer crop.

Growing Melons

It is a quick annual vine that creeps along the ground and needs full sun and sandy well-drained soil – remember its sub-Saharan beginnings – and if the summer rainfall is reliable, it does well in dry land. But in the early summer heat I found furrow planting suits the melons better as their roots could go down to get moisture from the flooded furrows for weeks on end.

Using Melons

Melon seeds were found in the tombs of the pharaohs, so valuable was this precious fruit, and ancient documents show the seeds being crushed and utilised as a poultice over wounds bound in place with the skin of the melon. Tests done on the honeydew and spanspek reveal they are helpful in maintaining blood pressure levels and they flush the kidneys and bladder, as they are an excellent diuretic. For cleansing problem skins, face masks or 'masques' made of mashed melons have remained a popular choice all over the world. Eating melons helps to clear skin problems in teenagers – particularly the watermelon, as it is rich in vitamin C and has a slightly astringent skin. So applied mashed to the face it will act as a soothing skin-tightening mask, which is good for acne, rashes, oily skin and pimples. With their excellent cleansing and rehydrating properties we should enjoy them while the season lasts!

Definitely a cooling food, melons are best served chilled as a delicious hot afternoon treat. Eat them on their own for maximum benefit as they digest so quickly. Serve with chopped mint, iced and sliced into bite-sized pieces – seeds removed – and taste summer!

Health Note

With their high levels of vitamin B and C and beta-carotene, melons are an antioxidant powerhouse and an exceptional health food. They also have a high calcium, magnesium, potassium and phosphorus content, especially the spanspeks!

Lemon

Citrus limon

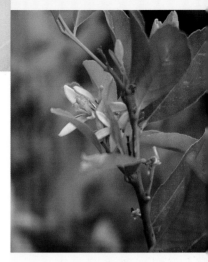

I am mad about lemons! I grow several varieties and I love each one for what it puts up with – heat, drought, searing winds, hail storms and endless picking. No garden should be without a lemon and it is so valuable a food and a medicine that it has to have its own place in these pages. The lemon is thought to have originated in Asia, possibly India and China, and it belongs to the great Rutaceae family. The *Citrus* genus contains many evergreen perennial shrubs or small trees that flourish in mild climates.

The lemon grows in mild climates and it has been cultivated for around 4 000 years. The *citron*, as it was then known, was taken to the Middle East between 400 and 600 BC. Later, Arab traders took the fruits to Eastern Africa and the first lemons, limes, oranges and shaddocks arrived there between 100 and 700 AD. Christopher Columbus took them to the New World, and by the 16th century the lemon became quite well known. After the 1890s, physicians found that the dreaded scurvy – a vitamin C deficiency – could be cured by eating citrus fruits, especially lemons and drinking the juice, so the demand increased substantially, and wherever the climate was suitable citrus trees were planted.

Growing Lemons

The Cape rough skin lemon does better than the other lemons in a colder climate. It will need winter frost cover and a north-facing protected area in full sun. The Eureka lemon thrives in a frost-free area and is a heavy bearer of smooth-skinned lemons. The Meyer lemon is the only real lemon I know that thrives in a huge pot and it needs a frost-free winter, but can survive wheeled onto a protected veranda in full sun if it is covered at night. Caffea or makrut lime, *Citrus hystrix*, is grown mainly for its extraordinary double leaves used in cooking, and also does well in a large pot, but its fruit is inedible, the zest is the best part and it is fascinating to grow. All the different limes grow best in frost-free areas and they are all valuable for drinks, for flavouring and for juicing.

All the varieties of lemons need full sun, a huge, deep, compost-filled hole, adequate and thorough and slow weekly watering and a barrow of compost twice a year. For the rest, they need no attention except the picking of the winter bounty of fruit that is simply stunning!

Using Lemons

I literally cannot cook without lemons and have found it so valuable for coughs, colds and 'flu that wherever I have lived I have always grown lemon trees. Lemons contain the phytochemical limonene, which is currently being tested in clinical trials to dissolve gallstones. Limonene is found in the white pith of the lemon and it has also been found to have promising anti-cancer properties. Lemon juice helps to detoxify us, to clear a spotty oily skin, to brighten our hair, rejuvenate our scalps, to lighten our freckles and to tone our skin and close our pores and cleanse away the cares of the day. Add lemon slices and fresh leaves to the bath or squeeze out the juice from a freshly picked lemon into the bath water and use the skins as a nail and cuticle strengthener and cleanser! Take the hollow skin of half a lemon, spoon in some coarse sea salt and add a little hot water. Spread some aqueous cream thickly over your cracked heels and, sitting on the edge of the bath, work the moist salt and lemon peel deeply into the heel in your cupped hand. This is the most softening and soothing treatment you can give your heels. Do it often and keep squeezed-out lemon halves for your elbows too!

Homemade lemon curd, lemon syrup, lemon marmalade, lemon ice-cream, lemon sponge cakes, lemon marinades and lemon desserts are nothing short of divine, and no one ever tires of them. Lemon is the most valuable tree in your garden!

Health Note

Lemons are rich in vitamins A, C, B6, potassium, folic acid, calcium, magnesium and phosphorus.

Lemon Cough Mixture

My grandmother's cough recipe is equal quantities fresh lemon juice, honey and finely chopped sage leaves. Mix and pour into a little jar – each one has their own. Take a teaspoon at a time, frequently, for a cough and sore throat.

Lemonade

Sit back on a hot afternoon and sip your own lemonade.

Squeeze 6 lemons, add 1 litre of iced water, about ¾ cup of sugar (taste as you go) and mix well. Pour into a tall glass, add crushed ice and sip slowly, looking at your lemon tree!

Hints

Mix lemon juice and mustard and spread over meat or poultry as a pre-grilling marinade.

Mix chopped fresh mint into freshly squeezed lemon juice, mixed with a little honey, as a mint sauce over pasta or baked potatoes or over a salad.

Just squeeze the juice of a fresh lemon over fish or meat or chicken and taste the magic of it – it really has to be the most versatile fruit on earth.

Grapefruit

Citrus paradisi

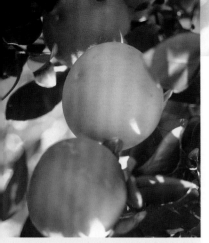

Grilled Grapefruit

This is the most delicious way of eating grapefruit – include a little of the pith as well.

Cut a grapefruit in half, sprinkle with cinnamon and a little soft caramel sugar or maple syrup, add a dash of nutmeg, freshly grated, and place under the grill for 2 minutes.

Grapefruit, Avocado and Sweet Pepper Salad

Cut segments out of fresh grapefruit with a sharp knife and add to avocado, sweet peppers, salad leaves and fresh coriander. Pour over a dressing made with 2 tablespoons each honey and olive oil, 1 teaspoon mustard powder, 2 teaspoons crushed coriander seed and a grinding of black pepper.

Caution

Always discuss any medical condition with your doctor – some doctors will advise against including grapefruit in the diet. In particular, grapefruit and grapefruit juice have the potential to interact with many medicines. For a list of medicines that are affected by grapefruit, see http://en.wikipedia.org/wiki/List_of_drugs_affected_by_grapefruit.

Although the oranges and lemons have been around for many centuries, the grapefruit was first noticed in the 1700s on the Barbados Islands and West Indies where it was thought to have been a natural crossbreeding between the abundant pomelo or shaddock and the oranges that grew there. It was only around 1823 that even a mention of the grapefruit was first recorded and, known locally as the 'forbidden fruit' in 1830, it was officially named *Citrus paradisi*. From then on it was gradually introduced to Florida in the United States, from the Bahamas, and only by 1885 were the first commercial consignments shipped to New York and Philadelphia and introduced as a health food. The rest, as they say, is history! Production increased, trees were trialled in many tropical and subtropical regions of the world, and Argentina, Cyprus, Israel, South Africa, Cuba and Mexico became the biggest growers. The Ruby grapefruit became the favourite. Astonishingly, it was discovered only in 1970 on the property of a Mr R. Ruby in Texas! Every year more and more varieties emerge, but the high health value remains – the grapefruit is a really remarkable fruit.

Growing Grapefruit

In the hot, frost-free summer rainfall areas of South Africa the grapefruit thrives and it is a rewarding small tree to grow – it demands nothing except a few barrows of compost every autumn and spring and a long, deep and thorough weekly watering. It always looks good and it has masses of headily fragrant blossoms in spring that fill the air with so a nostalgic and incredible a scent that it literally envelopes one. The heavily laden branches bow down with fruit that can remain on the tree for a long time – the longer it remains on the tree the sweeter it becomes, the locals say.

Using Grapefruit

Grapefruit is a valuable source of lycopene, which is an antioxidant that is also found in tomatoes, and which fights macular degeneration, heart disease and cancer. In addition, it contains glucarates, which are compounds that help to prevent breast cancer by helping the body to get rid of excess oestrogen. Grapefruit pectin has been extensively researched and results show it has a valuable cholesterol-lowering action and it has been shown to normalise the percentage of red blood cells per volume of blood (known as hematocrit levels), which are normally 40–54% for men and 37–47% for women. Lower hematocrit levels usually indicate anaemia, and high hematocrit levels reflect severe dehydration or an increased number of red cells with an increased risk of heart disease. Naringin, a flavonoid in grapefruit, has been shown to promote the elimination of old red blood cells. So doctors recommend eating ½ to 1 grapefruit for breakfast daily. It really is an amazing thought that a mere ½ a grapefruit in the daily diet, while they are in season, can make so huge a difference!

Grapefruit marmalade is becoming the designer breakfast jam and it is particularly delicious served with cream cheese on toast. It is a commercially viable product and easily made. Follow the recipe for Orange Marmalade on page 105, but replace the oranges with 6 large grapefruit and leave out the lemon juice and zest.

Health Note

Eating fresh grapefruit for breakfast or drinking grapefruit juice will provide good amounts of vitamins A, B & C, folic acid, beta-carotene, potassium, lycopene (an antioxidant) and flavonoids.

Orange

Citrus sinensis

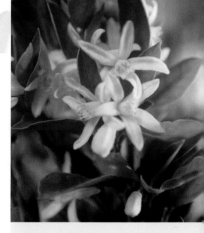

Of the many varieties of citrus fruit the orange is surely the king – one of mankind's favourite fruits that originated in China where it has been in cultivation for thousands of years! The first known reference to the orange was found in China around 500 BC in a text known as 'The Five Classics'. During the 15th century the first sweet oranges were brought into Europe by the explorers and early traders, and their bright presence caused much excitement! By the 16th century the Spanish explorers brought the oranges and tiny trees to Florida, in the United States, and later Spanish missionaries brought the orange trees to California where they thrived. In Europe 'orangeries' or special conservatories that could over-winter this precious crop were built with glass to keep the trees warm and to this day the orange remains a treasured and valuable crop in many countries. The biggest producers of oranges in the world today are China, Brazil, Spain, Mexico, Israel and South Africa, all the warm frost-protected areas of the world, and many varieties have developed from those original Chinese oranges. The word 'orange' comes from the Arabic *narandj*, which comes from the Sanskrit *nagarunga* meaning 'fruit favoured by the elephants' and it is thought that the first oranges were also found in India and Indo-China where the elephants ate them in the wild. It was during the expansion of the Arab domination in the Mediterranean region that the sweet orange became a heritage there and where it flourishes today and cultivars of those original sweet oranges are numerous. We are familiar with favourites like Navel and Valencia and grow them to perfection in South Africa.

Growing Oranges

All it requires is a huge, deep, compost-filled hole in full sun and a long, slow watering weekly in very hot weather and every two weeks in winter when its glorious ripe oranges are at their peak. Pruning is kept to a minimum and we give two full barrow loads of compost to every tree twice a year and every now and then a small bucket of Epsom salts. This is an old-fashioned way of looking after our citrus trees and they have always been so beautifully healthy we continue with this method.

We are dedicated to organic growing in the Herbal Centre gardens, and so watch carefully for any signs of thrips or knobbly leaves, which we remove at once and burn. But through the almost three decades of growing citrus here against the hot northern slopes of the Magaliesberg mountain range, we have remained free of any problems.

Using Oranges

The health benefits of the orange are legendary. A glass of freshly squeezed orange juice from your own organically grown oranges is one of the most enjoyable of drinks. No bottled orange juice, no carbonated orange juice, no preserved orange juice for us – only freshly squeezed from our own trees. In this way, as well as eating fresh oranges, you can get the valuable health benefits known by the ancient Chinese doctors. Rich in vitamins and minerals (see Health Note), oranges protect the lens of the eye, the adrenal glands and the connective tissue of the body. Its stimulating, cleansing and digestive qualities – it even acts as an internal antiseptic – make the fresh, organic orange a valuable health builder that fights cancer and viral infections. And don't forget the important flavonoid hesperidin which is found in the white pith under the skin. Hesperidin has been found to lower high blood pressure and high cholesterol. Chinese doctors have used the white pith for centuries to treat many ailments, as well as the finely scraped orange zest, which is rich in oil glands, for various ailments, including toning of the reproductive organs, treating bladder and kidney ailments and boosting the immune system. The flowers contain the exquisite essential oil called neroli oil. The September orange blossom scents the whole valley and we make our own orange flower water and orange blossom oils in heady concentration all through spring.

Health Note

Oranges are rich in vitamins C, B1, B2, B6 and folic acid, and are a wonderful food to boost the immune system. They also contain carotenes, potassium and calcium.

Grandmother's Orange Marmalade

The winter making of our much-loved orange marmalade, made the way my grandmother did, is a ritual we love. Serve with hot buttered toast for breakfast or spread onto sausages before grilling for an unforgettable treat!

10 oranges quartered, then finely sliced – remove all pips
3 kg sugar
juice of 2 lemons
about 2 teaspoons finely grated lemon zest
about 3 litres of water

Tie the lemon pips and any orange pips in a piece of muslin. Simmer the orange slices, the lemon juice and the muslin tied pips in the water in a big heavy bottomed pot for about 1½ hours. Meanwhile warm the sugar in the oven while the oranges cook. Remove the bag of pips. Now add the warm sugar to the oranges and water and bring to the boil. Stir well. Boil rapidly for about 20 minutes or until setting point has been reached (105 °C). Test by dropping a few drops onto a cold saucer (keep the saucer in the fridge) – it should set immediately. Stand 10 minutes with the lid on. Bottle into sterilised jars with good screw-top lids. My grandmother always covered the surface of the marmalade with a neatly cut circle of greaseproof paper which fitted perfectly into the bottle mouth. Label and date.

Coconut

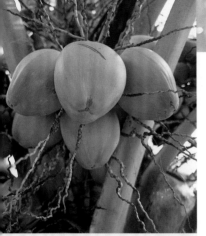

Cocos nucifera

The coconut is one of the world's most incredible trees. It is that exotic looking palm on Africa's beaches, but it originates in Southeast Asia. King of all the plants in tropical areas, it is a primary and vitally important crop as all parts of it are used. In Sanskrit it is known as *kalpa vriksha*, which means 'the tree that provides all that is necessary to survive'. Probably the oldest of all food plants, the coconut palm is thought to have originated somewhere in the Malayan Archipelago, but was dispersed by the sea. The huge coconuts have been known to survive for years floating in the sea, securely sealed in their fibrous cushioned outer shell before being washed up on other shores far, far away, there to take root and to grow. Used for over 4 000 years as a remedy for skin diseases in Ayurvedic medicine, it remains one of the most cherished and respected plants in the world today.

Growing Coconuts

If you are living on the tropical coastline of Africa or Latin America, or in the Philippines, India or Indonesia and the Pacific Islands, you have a chance. Otherwise we need to buy the oil from the chemist or the coconuts from the greengrocer.

Using Coconuts

A rich, clear, pleasant-tasting oil is extracted from the endosperm, which is the white, fleshy part of the fruit. Coconut oil consists of saturated fatty acids, known as lauric acid and myristic acid, but these are medium-chain triglicerides – unlike the long-chain triglicerides found in animal fats – so there are no health risks in adding coconut oil to the diet. Coconut oil is excellent for frying, baking and grilling; only a little is needed *and* it has an extra long shelf life.

Both desiccated coconut, which is used in baking, and coconut milk are obtained from the flesh of the endosperm. Palm sugar is a sugary sweet sap tapped from the flowering stalks and it is used to make palm wine and palm vinegar. The soft top of the stem is the sought-after gourmet ingredient 'palm heart'. The young flower buds, about the size of a golf ball, are cooked and eaten as a succulent vegetable, known as 'palm cabbage', and are made into pickles and stews to give energy and vitality, and to soothe the aches and pains of old age.

The roots are made into a tea to treat dysentery, colic and diarrhoea, and the softened and finely scraped bark from the palm stem is made into a poultice, warmed in hot water, for earache and toothache. The ash from burned bark is used to clean the teeth, to wash out the mouth, as an antiseptic and to treat skin diseases. The flowers are made into a tea to treat bladder infections, diabetes, leprosy and kidney stones. A tea made from the young buds is used to cool a fever and as a diuretic. The stringy fibres inside the bark made into a tea are taken for a sore throat and inflamed tonsils, to bring down a fever, and to expel tapeworm. Added to this tea, the watery juice or milky liquid is also used as a diuretic and to treat tapeworm and to soothe a sore throat. The sap from the trunk is an excellent and mild laxative.

The trunk provides excellent wood and is topped with a cluster of 20–30 long palm leaves which are used for thatching. The fruit is also a source of coir, a rough fibrous lining between the outer shell and the hard inner fruit shell. Coir has been used for centuries to fill mattresses and cushions, to make mats and sacks from, and is still valuable today for lining hanging baskets in which to grow flowers.

Health Note

The fleshy endosperm, rich in oils, contains calcium, zinc, selenium, phosphorus, magnesium, potassium, iron and copper, and the oil contains immune-boosting medium-chain fatty acids.

Coconut Tart

My grandmother made this tart for Christmas every year.

500 g short-crust pastry, bought or homemade
¾ cup apricot jam (homemade, if possible)
½ cup brown sugar
½ cup butter, softened
2 large eggs
½ teaspoon salt
1 teaspoon vanilla extract
½ teaspoon allspice (pimento)
2 cups desiccated coconut (I store mine in the fridge)
1 teaspoon finely grated lemon zest

Line 2 pie dishes with the short-crust pastry. Spread the apricot jam over the base of each. Beat the brown sugar and butter until creamy. Whisk the eggs with the salt until pale yellow. Gradually and slowly, beating constantly, add the whisked egg mixture to the creamy butter and sugar mixture. Add the vanilla extract and allspice. Whisk well. Add the desiccated coconut and mix in thoroughly. Lastly add the lemon zest and mix well. Divide the mixture between the 2 pie dishes, and evenly spread it over the jam. Bake at 200 °C for 30 minutes or until it is firm and turning a light brown. Cool before cutting into wedges.

Coffee

Coffea arabica

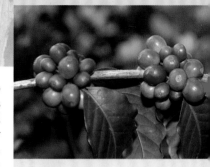

Coffee is thought to have originated in Ethiopia where it grows wild in the forests. An ancient Arab story tells of a priest named Mullah, who was troubled by constantly falling asleep during his prayers. Upset by his apparent lack of devotion, he begged Allah for help. The next day he happened to meet a shepherd whose goats foraged in the fields and forests, and the shepherd told him how the animals played and ran about all night after they had eaten the ripe berries of a particular tree. The shepherd gave the priest some of the berries – for he too ate the berries and cooked the seeds in water in order to stay awake to watch his goats! The priest prepared a brew and drank it prior to his prayer time. He remained awake all night, and that is why it is believed coffee came from Abyssinia, or Ethiopia, as it is known today!

Whatever its true origins, its energising effect soon became widely known and it spread through Egypt, the Sudan and Turkey, reaching the Mediterranean region in the 16th century. With speed the coffee legend gathered force and was introduced into Europe. The Dutch, realising its potential for cultivation in their colonies, introduced the coffee bean plant to the Americas. Mexico, Brazil and Colombia grew it in vast areas and different varieties started to develop. Today South America produces 80% of the world's coffee.

Growing Coffee

The attractive little coffee tree thrives in a tropical, frost-free, hot climate in moist, shady, compost-rich soil. Give it a twice weekly deep watering and spray the leaves regularly.

Using Coffee

Coffee beans need to be prepared with care, as they cannot be used until they have been roasted to 200 °C. During roasting, they will dry up and shrivel, as the sugars and cellulose become caramelised. Freshly roasted, sealed and kept in airtight tins, will keep the beans at their best. Grinding your own coffee as you are about to drink it retains the incredible flavour and aroma.

Several recent studies have suggested that coffee may be a beneficial drink, but note this is *not* instant coffee but freshly ground, filtered coffee. Researchers have found that coffee could reduce the risk of diabetes, cirrhosis of the liver and heart disease (but this does not include the milk and the sugar!). It has been found that coffee, pure and unadulterated, contains high levels of antioxidants, which help to slow down cell damage, as well as chlorogenic acid, which may decrease the risk of cardiovascular disease. New research also shows that coffee may reduce the risk of cancer of the mouth, larynx and oesophagus, the prostate gland in men, and endometrial cancer in women. Coffee is thought to enhance exercise as the caffeine in it signals the muscles to draw energy from the body's fat reserves, which makes more energy available and lessens the discomfort of intensive exercise. Scientists at the University of California also found that a group of over-65-year-olds who drank a cup of coffee at least 5 times a week, significantly reduced their memory loss, and similar results were seen in Alzheimer patients.

This interesting list of the benefits of coffee drinking is thought to be largely as a result of the high concentration of antioxidants found in it. The research continues but the evidence suggests that those without specific conditions and who enjoy a cup or two of coffee per day need not be afraid of negative health effects. Our own research finds organically grown, decaffeinated coffee made with milk and sweetened with stevia or a little caramel sugar, is refreshing and mood lifting but we remain cautious and vigilant and urge discretion. If you are overstressed, tense and anxious, rather choose a cup of lavender or rose-scented geranium or melissa or chamomile tea – it is soothing, safe and comforting and it will instantly calm and relax you.

Health Note

Coffee contains high levels of caffeine, a stimulant that excites the nervous centres of the brain and stimulates activity. Too much caffeine is not good for you! Caffeine is addictive and even a little can cause varying degrees of indigestion, lack of attention, irritability, insomnia, agitation, quick tempers, the shakes and palpitations! If you absolutely have to have the occasional cup of coffee, it must be filtered. And although it does contain a little potassium, some B-vitamins and antioxidants, eating the little ripe fruits is far more healthy than drinking a cup of coffee, which will contain between 100 and 150 g of caffeine!

Decaffeinated coffee is considered to be a 'healthier' choice by some. There are two methods of removing the caffeine from the coffee beans. The first is by soaking the freshly picked berries for many hours in hot water, and then drawing off the water, which now contains all the caffeine. Then by rinsing the berries twice, before drying and roasting them in the normal way, all the caffeine is safely removed. The second method involves using a solvent to remove the caffeine from the freshly picked berries, and this raises serious health concerns because of the harsh chemicals that are used in the process. Look out for decaffeinated coffee that is labelled 'naturally decaffeinated' or 'Swiss Water Processed', to make sure it contains no harmful chemicals.

Taro

Madumbi

Colocasia esculenta

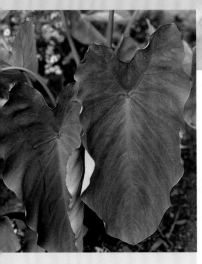

Roasted Madumbi

Wash and peel at least 3 madumbis per person and cut in half or in thirds, depending on the size. As you work keep squeezing lemon juice over them. In a bowl pour in a little sunflower or olive oil mixed into a little sunflower oil. Sprinkle each piece of madumbi with salt and turn in the oil. Place into a baking tray and tuck in wedges of onions (at least 1 medium-sized onion for each person) between the madumbis. Drizzle a little of the oil over everything and roast in a hot oven at 190°C turning every now and then until golden brown. Serve with roast chicken and vegetables.

Taro Leaf Stir-Fry

Serves 4

This is a popular street food in Malaysia.

Roll up several taro leaves and slice thinly (enough for 2 cups). Brown 2 large onions in a little olive oil. Add 2 cups of sliced tomatoes and stir-fry until soft. Now add the taro leaves with 1 tablespoon of honey, 2 teaspoons crushed coriander seed, and salt, pepper and lemon juice to taste. Stir-fry until soft and tender and serve on rice.

An exotic and fascinating plant, the taro looks rather like a giant elephant's ear, but has dull grey-green leaves and a smaller growth and sometimes has purple leaves or purple stems or purple veins on the dull green leaves. **Caution: the elephant's ear (*Alocasia macrorrhiza*) is poisonous – do *not* confuse the two plants.** Thought to be of Polynesian and Indian origin, this extraordinary plant has been cultivated in Asia and the Spice Islands for over 10 000 years! It is a valuable food source, its rich tubers thriving in marshy furrows and wetlands and in exotic and tropical places where it is a staple food and was grown in China since the Han Dynasty. Often grown in furrows alongside the rice paddies in Asia, it was part of a thriving trade between Egypt, the Middle East and the Mediterranean region for centuries. The Spanish and Portuguese explorers took the tubers on their ships as a valuable food – it is long lasting when well stored in moist grass. They spread the taro into Africa as trade and also introduced it to the New World. It is an ancient food that has never lost its popularity and various cultivars have been established in different countries.

Growing Taro

Wherever there is a moist furrow it will thrive. I keep a watchful eye out for the neat piles or boxes of madumbis from KwaZulu-Natal, appearing in local greengrocers at the end of the summer, and often buy them not only for roasting but to plant. They need deeply dug, richly composted soil where a slow hosepipe can be easily lead to irrigate the furrow twice a week in hot weather and once a week in winter. Taro cannot take frost so the area needs to be tropical and hot – KwaZulu-Natal's hot and steamy coastline is ideal. Moisture is essential and the huge leaves love being sprayed. We dig up the tubers in autumn when they are palm-sized and return the smaller ones for replanting.

Using Taro

The tough, huge leaves have been used as dressings over wounds, scratches, grazes and burns for centuries. Peeled and pounded tubers spread onto the leaves have made a comforting poultice over bruises, sprains, arthritic joints, swellings and aching feet. For backache, hot pounded peeled tubers wrapped in the leaves, which have been immersed in hot water, to this day make a pain-reducing poultice over the back, and bound in place with sisal strings or thin ropes the hot leaves literally encase the whole body. Resting is essential and the patient lies on a bed of taro leaves in the shade for two days, and the poultice is replaced twice a day.

The whole tuber or corm, well scrubbed, can be roasted like a roast potato with salt and oil and lemon juice, otherwise it literally turns black. Cut into cubes and drenched with lemon juice to stop them from discolouring, the tubers can also be steamed or boiled, the starchy water discarded once they are tender, and then mashed with either salt or sugar and fried, or even baked, into a 'cake'. The Hawaiians cook thin slices with tomatoes and onions, and in Egypt taro features in a beef stew with garlic, beetroot and fresh coriander leaves. In China a popular snack called *woo kok* is made from taro flour dough, which encases minced meat and when deep-fried is deliciously feather light. The Chinese also use taro flour to thicken soups. Fresh taro leaves, neatly rolled up, can be bought in Asian shops for spinach or for wrapping foods which are cooked in the coals or in the oven in sealed pots. You have only to read about these fascinating far away places to get inspired with this simple, easy-to-grow staple food.

Health Note

Taro is rich in vitamin C and some B-vitamins, iron, phosphorus, potassium, calcium and magnesium.

Melokhia

Corchorus olitorus

Jew's Mallow ■ Jute

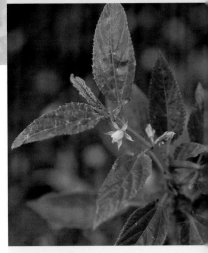

This is an extraordinary plant that I came across growing in a community garden in the Hoedspruit area, that offers so much and with the potential of becoming so popular a survival food that we all need to take notice! Grown as an annual or short-lived perennial, it thrives in full sun in literally any soil, needs little or no attention and it offers so much I am both astonished and excited. It grows 1–2 m high into a multi-branched bush with a spread of over a metre, offering pointed, thumb-length-sized leaves which are cooked as spinach or served fresh in salads, and edible small yellow flowers that develop into seed-filled pods just less than a thumb length in size. But even more fascinating is its journey from its native India as a fibre crop. It is also known as 'tassa jute' or 'nalta jute' and branches tied together make excellent brooms. So this plant is probably one of the first brooms used by mankind! Melokhia is an ancient food and can be found growing in tropical and even subtropical regions of the world where, since the early centuries, it has served as a valuable pot herb, a medicine and as a strong and durable fibre.

Growing Melokhia

The seeds germinate easily and from the few pods I gathered in Hoedspruit instant germination caused great excitement. We planted 6 or 7 in compost-filled bags. Plant the little plants once they reach 15 cm in height in full sun in well-dug, moist soil to which rich compost has been added. Planted in rows spaced 2 m apart it grows quickly from those small seedlings, but needs to be watered well for a few weeks to establish it. Thereafter a weekly watering is enough. Mulched with raked leaves and grass cuttings to keep the soil moist, friable and soft, the little seedlings thrive. It quickly forms a much-branched little bush and the young and tender leaves can be picked daily for salads, stir-fries, soups and spinach dishes.

Using Melokhia

Melokhia leaves, flowers and stems have been used as a medicine in India and China for centuries for building stamina and endurance, as a poultice for sprains, strains, broken bones, and for childbirth, for the elderly and for children who fail to thrive. A poultice of fresh leaves over wounds, tied in place with melokhia jute string, is today as important a medicine as it was centuries ago.

Even more exciting is its potential as a fibre crop, a substitute for sisal or hemp, and as building material melokhia branches give strength and long life to structures – perhaps in our modern-day search for natural and organic building materials, melokhia could become a giant in the not too distant future!

Made into soups, stews and eaten with porridge, melokhia leaves have become more and more valuable as an easy-to-grow, inexpensive pot herb, and in many countries have become a sustainable survival food. Eaten young and fresh, the leaves are delicious served with a little olive oil, lemon juice, and a grinding of black pepper with dried coriander seeds, and in markets from China to Israel, Turkey to Egypt to Malawi, packets of melokhia leaves are for sale and enjoyed by everyone! In parts of Israel it is a spinach dish served with olive oil and salt or made into fritters, and cultivated plants thrive where not much else does.

Health Note

The fresh leaves are rich in health-building vitamins, vitamins A, C and E particularly, and in minerals, particularly iron, magnesium, calcium and potassium.

Molokhyia

Egypt's national dish, known as *molokhyia*, is a thick soup made from rich beef stock, fried garlic and onions, fresh coriander leaves and fresh green melokhia leaves, all cooked together, with rice, lemon juice, a little finely grated lemon rind, sea salt and sometimes a little hot chilli. The Egyptians grow melokhia abundantly for this delicious and sustaining dish.

Melokhia Relish

The Malawians eat this relish with stiff mealie meal porridge.

Fry 2 large, finely chopped onions in a little olive oil until golden. Add 3 cups fresh melokhia leaves and stir well. Season with the juice of 1 lemon, salt, 2 teaspoons crushed coriander seed and 1 finely chopped chilli (just a little at a time, it should not be too fiery hot – taste as you go!). Now add 1 cup thinly sliced green peppers, 2 cups grated sweet potato and about 2 cups of water. Stir and simmer until the vegetables are tender. Serve hot.

Coriander
Cilantro ▪ Danya
Coriandrum sativum

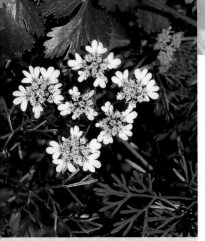

Although this precious plant falls under the heading 'herb' or 'spice' and I have written of it extensively in my other books, I feel it needs to find a prominent place within these pages as it has become so valuable a 'health food' and, like parsley, its tender young and succulent leaves as well as its exquisite flowers and seeds find an ever-widening circle of benefits and enjoyment in so many dishes. An ancient annual herb of antiquity, native to the Mediterranean area and parts of Asia, Southern Europe and the Middle East, it was cultivated extensively in ancient Greece and Egypt and the Roman Empire. Over 7 000 years ago it was recorded as a meat preservative and a medicine. India and China used coriander as a much-respected medicine thousands of years ago and coriander trade was a valuable asset between many countries. The spice trade route became so vibrant and so exciting that spices like ginger, cinnamon, cardamom, coriander and cumin were bartered for cloth and jewels as well as food staples like salt and honey. Much myth and magic surrounds the trade routes and many wondrous stories are locked into the very fragrance of these precious seeds.

Growing Coriander

I grow great swathes of coriander all through the year, except in the coldest months of June and July. An easy-to-grow and rewarding annual, it needs well-dug soil that has been richly composted and raked level, in full sun – but in the heat of midsummer it thrives in afternoon shade. Scatter the seeds over the surface and then rake them over thoroughly. Set a soft sprinkler over them to moisten them thoroughly and in the next two weeks do not let the soil dry out. The tiny seedlings grow quickly but need to be watered gently and frequently. The first pickings of young leaves, known as danya or dhania, are much loved in Indian cookery and sell quickly daily at the market stalls.

Using Coriander

Use the fresh leaves and flowers in teas, medicines and as flavouring. The green seeds are delicious in curries, stir-fries and pounded into sauces. The essential oil in the seed makes it a valuable digestive, and it has been used through the centuries as a treatment for diabetes – it is referred to as an anti-diabetic plant. Traditionally used as an anti-inflammatory and an anti-microbial, modern medical research confirms many of these ancient treatments. Even more interesting is that coriander has proved to be one of the best treatments for removing heavy metals from the body, including the effect of amalgam from the fillings in the teeth.

A few seeds chewed or made into a tea will ease flatulence, colic, bloating, griping and belching. Sip a tea made from the leaves and flowers for nervous tension, anxiety, temper tantrums, bad moods, irritability, and to lower cholesterol and clear infections. A poultice of warmed fresh coriander leaves was used as a pain-relieving treatment for swollen, painful joints. To make coriander tea using the seeds, add 1 teaspoon of seeds, lightly crushed, to 1 cup of boiling water, stir well, steep for 5 minutes and sip slowly. Using the leaves and flowers: Pour 1 cup of boiling water over ¼ cup fresh leaves and flowers and stand 5 minutes. Strain and sip slowly.

Recent research shows that coriander is valuable as an anti-tumourigenic in treating certain cancers due to the important phytochemical concentration found in its leaves and seeds, and its thinning action on the blood lipids reduces the risk of a stroke or heart attack.

Health Note

Coriander is rich calcium, phosphorus and magnesium and together with its vitamin A & C content, it is a valuable addition to the diet.

Cucumber

Cucumis sativus

The cucumber is an ancient plant that originates in India and Southeast Asia and has been in cultivation for over 3 000 years, and was well known and much enjoyed by the ancient Romans and Greeks. Used for over 10 000 years as both medicine and food, ancient explorers took it to Egypt and China around 200 BC, and it was finally introduced to the New World by Columbus around 1494. Its journey from ancient Asia and India to where the cucumber is today, is nothing short of astonishing. During the 17th century greenhouse cultivation began in earnest and cucumbers were taken to the Americas. It is thought that the Spaniards were the first to pickle them. This much-loved, treasured and nurtured vegetable – a simple and easy-to-grow summer annual – is still around today, still in commercial cultivation and although improved upon and many varieties have been developed from those ancient beginnings, it is still a cucumber and it is still going strong!

Growing Cucumbers

In my childhood garden we grew cucumbers along the fence where they could trail and climb. Seed was sown every spring in a deeply dug, richly composted furrow that could be flooded with water below the fence at least twice a week. The strong little seedlings, spaced 50 cm apart, had to have collars of stiff cardboard tucked in around them to protect them from cutworms. Today 2 litre plastic cool drink bottles can be sliced into 10 or 12 cm high rings which will last longer than the cardboard rings did. But cardboard is biodegradable and the plastic rings are not, so save the rings for next year and keep recycling!

Help the vines to start their climb onto the fence and keep an eye on the flowers – their bright yellow petals lure those voracious rose beetles who can devour a single flower in an hour or two. Strips of tinfoil hung over and near the flowers, moving in the breeze, frighten them and the birds away. I use little coverings over the tender new fruits as they form, made from soft white 'plant fleece' – a lightweight fabric that allows light in but keeps birds, beetles, frost and sunburn off. Buy it from your local nursery and cut out small pockets roughly tacked with needle and thread, roomy enough for the fruit to grow to full size within its protection, and tied or clipped loosely over the fruit.

Plant garlic chives in a row alongside the cucumbers and you'll reap a healthy and abundant crop.

Using Cucumbers

The cucumber is an excellent source of silica, which is a valuable trace mineral that builds and strengthens the connective tissue within the body. It acts literally like an intercellular 'cement' for muscles, tendons, cartilage, brain cells and bone! The cucumber is an excellent diuretic and laxative and it dissolves uric acid that builds up in the joints, the kidneys and the bladder, preventing the formation of stones and stiffness. It also helps to regulate the blood pressure and eases the digestion, and it flushes out toxins and acid build-up within the body. No wonder it is so treasured! A cucumber sandwich is one of the world's favourite snacks, so include it, and cucumber salads, often in the diet.

As a skin treatment cucumber was probably the first cosmetic and is still used today to treat sunburn and as a scrub – use it grated – to clear impurities, remove oiliness and to deeply cleanse the skin. For puffy eyes, for itchy dermatitis, for rashes, even light burns, apply thin cucumber slices and relax for 15 minutes. Cucumbers contain both ascorbic and caffeic acid, which release and prevent water retention and this is why cucumber is so popular as a topical skin treatment.

Health Note

Cucumbers are rich in silica, magnesium, potassium, folic acid, beta-carotene, and vitamins A and C.

Bread and Butter Pickle

This is a favourite old-fashioned and still much-loved recipe.

Wash and slice 4-6 cucumbers very thinly. Place on a clean tea towel and pat dry. Layer into wide-mouthed preserving jars with mustard seeds and coriander seeds sprinkled between the layers, about ½ cup of each. Tuck in fresh dill or fennel leaves around the sides. Boil up 2 cups of white grape vinegar with 1 cup of white sugar and 1 cup of water for 10 minutes. Cool for 10 minutes, then pour over the cucumber slices to the top of the jars and seal well. Eat after 2 weeks with bread and butter.

Cucumber and Aqueous Cream Scrub

This is invaluable for problem skins and oily acne.

Mix 1 cup of coarsely grated cucumber, unpeeled but well-scrubbed, with 1 cup of good aqueous cream and 1 tablespoon of apple cider vinegar. Use as a face mask, a scrub or a cleanser. Use daily and keep the excess in the fridge, it lasts 3–4 days.

Pumpkin & Squash

Cucurbita species

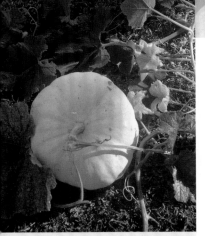

Pumpkin Soup

Serves 6–8

I reap the big flat boerpampoen with its stalk dry and the first frosts glistening white on its shiny skin and make my usual mashed pumpkin soup on a bitterly cold winter morning.

4 large onions finely chopped

4 cups celery leaves and stalks, finely chopped

2 cups flat-leaf parsley, finely chopped

1 medium-sized pumpkin, peeled and chopped (save the seeds for roasting and for planting next season)

1 cup good homemade peach chutney

1 tablespoon cinnamon

1 cup soft brown sugar

sea salt and freshly ground black pepper to taste

2 litres good chicken stock

½ cup sunflower cooking oil

Fry the onions to light brown, then add all the other ingredients and simmer gently for 1 hour. Mash when tender and serve hot with crusty bread.

Pumpkins and summer squashes, gourds, butternuts, pattipans, courgettes and hubbards and big flat 'boerpampoen' are so much a part of our everyday lives that we have come to think of them as commonplace, yet seldom do we ever think of their early beginnings which go back in time to over 5000 BC! The Incas were amongst the first to cultivate the vines of the pumpkin and the squash. The vine tips boiled in water and the flowers were as important as the fruits and so were the seeds, which were valuable as a survival food roasted in the coals and carried in a small 'purse' on the belt by travellers and explorers as a life-sustaining 'food'. Today we know how rich in vitamins and minerals pumpkin seeds are but those ancient Incas already knew this and small pots of pumpkin seeds have been found in burial chambers and tombs as a precious sustenance for the afterlife. The first squash and pumpkin plants were cultivated for their seeds, as those early wild fruits from long trailing vines were somewhat bitter and dry, not as fleshy and succulent as we know them today, but as cross-pollination is a simple and easy matter, soon many new varieties of pumpkin and squash came to the fore.

Growing Pumpkins

Soft, deep, well-dug, richly composted soil in full sun is needed for a good summer crop. Plant 8–10 seeds in a circle, equally spaced and about 25–30 cm apart, with a 'dam' surrounding them, which is raked in place to hold the water in dry, hot areas. Water well and cover the circle lightly with grass and leaves to keep the moisture in. Plant in spring when all fear of frost is passed. Inspect the plantings regularly for mildew and insect damage. Plant garlic chives near them – this will help against mildew – and mealies and runner beans. All are summer annuals and all are beneficial to each other.

Using Pumpkins

The pumpkin was possibly one of the first medicines used by mankind, and ancient herbals document its role in medicine from the 15th century onwards. The flesh, roasted in the coals, was applied as a hot poultice to arthritic joints, aching backs, boils and suppurating wounds. It was used to treat worms in both humans and animals, and ½ cup each of pumpkin seeds (the hard outer skin removed) and finely chopped onions, liquidised with soya milk to bind it, and a teaspoon or two of honey mixed in, was an ancient remedy for clearing parasitic worms from the body.

Pumpkin seeds are rich in protein, amino acids, minerals and fibre and stand strong and steady in treating lack of energy and low fertility. They are particularly rich in zinc, which is a valuable mineral for protecting against free radical damage and for protecting the liver. Remember, white spots on the nails tell you clearly you are zinc deficient, so top up on pumpkin seeds!

A nourishing baby food and a favourite vegetable worldwide, pumpkin soup, roasted pumpkin slices, stuffed marrows, pumpkin pies and pumpkin fritters have remained family favourites, comfort food and part of tradition and family gatherings and homecomings.

Health Note

Pumpkin is rich in vitamins and minerals, particularly beta-carotene, vitamins A, B, C and E, iron, calcium, magnesium, phosphorus, potassium, manganese, copper and dietary fibre. Pumpkin seeds are an excellent source of zinc, and also provide calcium, iron, phosphorus, magnesium, copper, manganese, omega-3 and 6 fats, protein and amino acids.

Turmeric

Curcuma longa

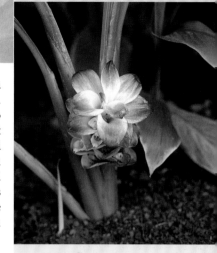

Turmeric is truly a plant that is worth its weight in gold. Believed once to be indigenous to India and Southern Asia, its beginnings are lost in the mists of time and wild turmeric is unknown. In Southern Asia it has been used as a protective charm and as an ancient medicine, and Marco Polo recorded it being used as a food, its thick rhizomes much treasured in China in 1280. The bright yellow dye – a pigment known as curcumen – within the rhizomes was used for ceremonial and religious robes – think of the bright saffron coloured robes of the Buddhist monks. The Chinese in the 7th century had already developed delicious dishes with turmeric and to this day grow several varieties of turmeric. There are around 40 species of perennial rhizomatous plants belonging to this genus, found seasonally in the tropical forests of Asia. *Curcuma aromatica* and *Curcuma zedoaria* are amongst them and are sometimes available as fresh or dried rhizomes from markets in China and in India.

Growing Turmeric

I have found this to be easy and so rewarding I constantly search for new tubers. Propagation is by rhizomes in late winter to early spring. Plant in semi-shade in moist, compost-rich, deeply dug soil in a tropical or subtropical climate with no winter frosts or prolonged cold. Watering 3 times a week is essential.

Huge, often 50 cm long, leaves emerge and in midsummer exquisite flower-tiered bracts, pale or deep pink with yellow and with stamens between the bracts, emerge – way down at ground level deep within the thick stalks of the leaves, hidden and rare. In winter the entire plant dies down, so cover it with a protective thick mulch, and in the warmth of the spring the big luscious leaves emerge.

Using Turmeric

The volatile oil within the tubers has been found to have an excellent anti-inflammatory effect, even greater than that of hydrocortisone. Extracts from the rhizomes have been found to significantly reduce allergic reactions on the skin, and inflammatory arthritis in the sub-acute stage. Its bactericidal and anti-allergenic properties have been proven in clinical testing and through the centuries the powdered rhizome mixed with other oils, or thin slices of the tuber have been used as a treatment for external sores and wounds on animals as well as humans. The rhizomes ground to a paste not only cleanses and disinfects the skin without drying out the natural oils, but will soothe and heal skin ulcers, acne and skin problems quickly and effectively. Turmeric tea is a valuable ingredient in Ayurvedic medicine for treating respiratory ailments. It is also found to be effective in treating uterine tumours, digestive ailments, circulatory disorders, liver ailments, jaundice and menstrual problems, as an anti-inflammatory, for asthma and eczema and to reduce the risk of strokes and heart disease, and even for diabetes. New research verifies the many ancient uses – we should be including this fascinating plant in our diets far more than we do.

A traditional Indian face cleansing oil is made with almond oil to which a few drops of turmeric oil (bought from Indian specialist shops) is added – it gives the skin a golden glow. Lentil flour mixed with a few drops of turmeric oil is the centuries old 'paste' that is thought to give that perfect skin so admired of Indian women.

Buy powdered turmeric to use in pickles, curry powders, chutneys, mustards and relishes. Use it as a substitute for saffron in rice dishes and to colour pumpkin soups.

Health Note

Turmeric is rich in rare oils, beta-carotene, enzymes, phosphorus, copper and magnesium.

Turmeric Tea

Brush your teeth well after drinking it and don't splash it on your clothes – turmeric stains!

Add 1 scant teaspoon turmeric powder (the fresher you can get it the better) to 1 cup of boiling water, stand 5 minutes, stir slowly and carefully. Sip slowly.

Homemade Curry Powder

Make your own mixtures for spicy curries and enjoy one of nature's most fascinating plants.

Mix together:

2 tablespoons turmeric powder
1 tablespoon ground coriander
1 tablespoon ground cumin
2 teaspoons ground ginger (even nicer is 1 tablespoon freshly finely grated ginger)
2 teaspoons cayenne pepper
½–1 tablespoon mustard powder

Mix gently and carefully and store in a screw-top glass jar. Use a little at a time in fish, poultry and meat dishes or add very little to pickles and relishes.

Quince

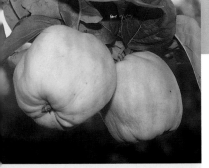

Cydonia oblonga

The quince has got to be one of the most extraordinary and fascinating trees anyone could ever grow. Its history is spellbinding and the traditional recipes from Israel to Turkey, Portugal to Greece, Morocco to Romania, take us through so exotic a journey its very beginnings are lost in antiquity. All my life, I have grown quinces and to this day I sell quince trees in my little nursery and urge gardeners to experience this historic fruit, as I never tire of exploring its many uses.

Originating in the Caucasus where they still grow wild today, the quince spread to southeast Europe and the Levant long before the apple. Easily cultivated rootstock and small trees became a rapid trade and a 'confection of quinces' cooked with honey became so popular that the quince is thought to be the first 'sweetmeat'. Known in Palestine around 1000 BC, 'quince gardens' became the sign of great wealth. The 'apples' mentioned in the 'Song of Solomon' it is thought, were actually quinces. Turkey remains to this day the place where the quince is most treasured and, like the Moroccans, the Turks use the quince in both sweet and savoury dishes.

Quince Leather

In a dryer, quince leather can be made within a couple of hours. Rolled up into little tubes, the children clamour for more.

Thinly slice and chop 8–10 large well-washed quinces, skin and all. In a large stainless steel pot add 4 cups of water and simmer with 2 cups of soft brown caramel sugar and ½–1 cup of chopped fresh stevia leaves. (Stevia is 300 times sweeter than sugar, so start gradually!) Stir frequently and add a little more water when necessary. Once the quince is tender, switch off the stove and leave the pot covered to cool.

With a blender whisk the cooked quinces to a smooth paste. Spread thinly onto an oiled tray and place in the sun or on the solid rack of the dryer. Keep the excess in the fridge to use as each batch dries. Store the dried quince leather in an airtight glass jar.

Growing Quinces

Today there are new varieties of the old-fashioned smaller hedgerow quinces that I grew up with. A multi-stemmed, spreading, small, deciduous tree, the quince will live to a great age, demands nothing except a barrow load of compost twice a year and a long, slow and deep weekly or twice weekly watering. Very occasionally a quick light pruning or tidying up of the many branches can be done, but usually it is so adaptable and undemanding it requires no attention.

It needs full sun to ripen the golden fruits and mulches and retaining dams ensure large and firm fruits that ripen in late summer. Do not wait for the hard granular flesh to ripen to softness – the quince remains hard but the skin becomes bright yellow and then it is ready for picking.

Using Quinces

Fresh grated quince, cooked in water until tender, has been an ancient treatment for stomach ailments, diarrhoea and dysentery. In many countries cooked quince pulp spread onto hot rocks to dry and carefully stored for the winter, was part of the traditional medicine chest and was taken mixed with hot water for digestive problems, to clear kidney and bladder ailments, and even for coughs – cooked up in honey.

Quince skins and cores of the fruit – which is rich in pectin – boiled up with a few leaves make an extraordinary hair rinse that, once strained and added to the rinsing water after shampooing, will make the hair soft and shiny. This brew is also used to comb into the tails and manes of the beautiful Arab horses to encourage hair growth and sheen! Massaged into the scalp, the lotion was used to treat scalp problems, dandruff and falling hair during the 17th and 18th centuries, and is still used in rural Europe today. This lotion was also used as a wash for rashes, grazes and scratches.

Used in centuries past by the 'ladies of the court' quince paste was one of the first beauty treatments recorded. As a cleanser the paste was mixed with crushed fresh rose petals and used as a gentle scrub. Boil up quince slices in enough water to cover and add 10 cloves. Simmer until tender. Remove the cloves and blend until smooth. This makes an excellent face mask and cleanser for oily problem skin, its astringency helps to refine large pores, to cleanse, tone and refine the skin and to clear away spots and rashes.

Quince Cleanser

I found this recipe in an ancient herbal and tried it and was so surprised to feel the softness of my skin afterwards.

Boil 2–3 quinces, thinly sliced and chopped, in just enough water to cover. Simmer until soft (around 30 minutes). Push through a sieve. Add 1 cup of finely chopped fresh rose petals (that have not been sprayed with any chemicals). Spread onto the face after washing in warm water. Massage gently into the skin. Relax for 10 minutes to allow the quince paste to penetrate. Wash off with warm water and pat dry.

Health Note

Quince is a very good source of vitamin C and dietary fibre, and also contains some beta-carotene, potassium, phosphorus, calcium, iron, copper and magnesium.

Cardoon

Cynara cardunculus

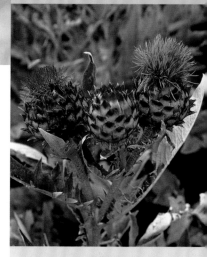

The cardoon is thought to probably be the wild relative of the globe artichoke, and there is some confusion regarding the actual origin of the cardoon. Some botanists believe both vegetables came from *Cynara cardunculus* var. *sylvestris*, which grows in Southern Europe and parts of North Africa still today. Some taxonomists believe the globe artichoke and the cardoon are two distinct species and if you grow them both side by side as I do, you'll see they are definitely related, but quite different, and both of them are enduringly fascinating!

The cardoon has huge, deeply lobed leaves in the palest silvery grey with a thick and succulent midrib. The flowers appear on beautiful branched candelabra-shaped flowering stalks and the buds are smaller than the globe artichoke and not quite as tasty, but if eaten no larger than golf ball size are deliciously delicate and intricate, revealing a succulent little heart. The flowers, if left to open on their great-branched candelabra stems, are breathtakingly beautiful topped with a shock of brilliant purple stamens, which send the bees and butterflies dizzy with delight! They dry beautifully too, maintaining that brilliant purple colour.

But the real surprise is the midrib of the leaf! This is the part that is eaten and its popularity goes back thousands of years. The ancient Romans and the Greeks used the cardoon usually as a plant going into its second year. The leaf base and stalks were reaped and sliced and boiled in broths, stews and thick vegetable soups with carrots and pumpkins and their vine tips. Eaten raw or blanched, succulent and flavour filled, the cardoon is a stunning addition to salads and stir-fries.

Growing Cardoon

Treat the cardoon as an annual. Plant small plants out at least 1 m apart in deeply dug, richly composted soil in full sun and make a 'dam' around each one, which you can flood with water twice a week. When it is about 50 cm high, tie the big leaves together at the top and circle with tube cardboard packaging material so that it is open on top and only the tips of the tied-up bunch of leaves are visible. This is the blanching process, and the leaves that mature and new ones that form inside the tube of cardboard are pale, tender, succulent and without a trace of bitterness. I draw the soil up on the base of the cardboard to keep the sunlight out. Hessian around the cardboard helps it not to disintegrate. Don't use plastic as it becomes too hot inside. Flood the dam twice weekly and inspect the plants every now and then to see if they are 'breathing' by removing the cardboard tube and checking for mildew. When the stems are thick and juicy, slice the whole plant off at the root and wash carefully, then slice it thinly and boil until tender. Or, you can leave it to grow untied, its huge and beautiful leaves in the sun! Then you would need to cook the midrib twice, to get rid of the bitterness. Throw away the first cooking water, then repeat.

Using Cardoon

Like its close cousin the artichoke, the cardoon is a superb medicinal plant – it has diuretic and purgative action, it clears acidity from the body, rebuilds and repairs the liver and the kidneys and flushes out toxins, and lowers high cholesterol. As a diuretic the cardoon has an ancient history, cleansing and clearing the blood of impurities, and the cooled water in which the blanched stems were cooked was used to wash to face to clear acne and pimples and oiliness. The cardoon is good for diabetics too and, like the artichoke, acts as a tonic to the whole system.

Health Note

Cardoon is rich in vitamins A, B, C, iron, potassium, magnesium and phosphorus.

Cardoon in Cheese Sauce

Boil up 4 cups of thinly sliced cardoon stems and young leaves (best is blanched – otherwise select younger leaves and cut away the leaf, saving the midrib only). Boil until tender. Drain, rinse thoroughly under the running hot water tap. Spoon into a baking dish and cover while you make the sauce.

Fry 2 chopped onions in a little olive oil until brown. Add to the cardoon slices. Whisk 4 eggs into 1½ litres of milk with 2 tablespoons of cornflour. Add 1 teaspoon of mustard powder, sea salt and black pepper to taste. Add 1 cup of grated cheddar cheese and ½ cup chopped parsley and pour over the cardoon slices and onions. Bake at 180° for about 30 minutes or until set. Serve hot with a green salad.

Boiled Cardoon Buds

Pick 2–3 buds, no bigger than a golf ball, per person. Simmer in enough water to cover for 40 minutes or until tender enough to insert a fork through the base. Drain. Slice in quarters and dot with butter. Season with lemon juice, salt and pepper and serve hot.

Globe Artichoke

Cynara scolymus

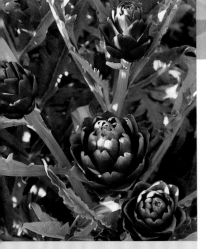

The globe artichoke is a strikingly beautiful, short-lived perennial with huge, deeply lobed, grey-green leaves and spectacular scaled, purple thistle flowers on thick-branched stems. The young and tender unopened buds are the edible part and are enjoyed all over the world as a gourmet food.

Native to the central and western Mediterranean region, the artichoke grew wild along the sea cliffs and roadsides over 3 000 years ago. Used both as a food and a medicine, it was introduced into Egypt over 2 000 years ago and really only gained popularity when Catherine de Medici of Florence introduced it to France in 1533. From there it spread to England and by the 18th century it was taken to America. In those ancient times the stems and buds were taken as a medicine, also the water in which they were boiled, and the tender heart eaten for anaemia, rheumatism and dropsy, and ancient writings and paintings featured the 'Al-Kharshuf', its original Arabic name, frequently.

Growing Globe Artichokes

Propagation is by seed or by side shoots that form after the flowering branches have matured. Plant in full sun 1½–2 m apart in deeply dug, well-composted soil in spring. The plant will only flower in its second year and the young and tender buds are at their best in early spring. Water deeply twice a week and dig in extra compost twice yearly in winter and after flowering in midsummer. Sow seeds reaped from mature heads every autumn.

Using Globe Artichokes

Those ancient healers were right – eating artichokes is excellent for rheumatism, over-acidity, for liver ailments, regenerating and repairing the liver, obesity, kidney ailments, glandular disorders, anaemia, diarrhoea and even for halitosis, and it helps to lower high cholesterol.

Low in calories the globe artichoke is beneficial to diabetics, particularly when it is very fresh, as it contains inulin, a polysaccharide, which improves blood sugar control. The whole plant contains cynarin, which is predominant in the leaves, and which improves the functioning of the cells lining the arteries. Current medical research is showing that artichoke extracts can boost the immune system. Just including boiled globe artichokes in the diet will promote the flow of bile to the gall bladder and to and from the liver, and so is excellent in keeping the liver healthy, actually acting like a tonic.

Even the seed is considered to be hugely beneficial if crushed and taken as a tea. Add 1–2 teaspoons artichoke seeds (reaped from your own organically grown plants) to 1 cup boiling water. Stand for 5 minutes, crush the seeds with a spoon, then strain and sip slowly. Add a squeeze of lemon juice for extra benefits for all the above ailments and as a tonic. To make a tea of the leaves, pour 1 cup boiling water over ¼ cup fresh chopped leaves, stand 5 minutes, then strain and sip slowly. Sprouting the artichoke seed is well worth it. Soak the seeds in water overnight. Line a dish with wet cotton wool, sprinkle the seeds over it and cover with a layer of more wet cotton wool. Keep moist and check daily. As soon as the seeds sprout, remove the top layer of cotton wool. Keep the seeds moist and use in salads after 2 days.

Health Note

The bases of the fleshy scales on the buds as well as the tender heart are rich in vitamin A and C and the B-vitamins, especially biotin, niacin and folic acid, and are also excellent sources of iron, phosphorus, potassium, magnesium and manganese.

How to Eat an Artichoke

Boil the freshly picked buds in enough water to cover them, until tender. Test by pulling out one of the leafy scales. If it comes out smoothly it is ready. Drain and serve with a little dipping sauce of lemon juice and salt mashed into a little soft butter. Dip the base of each 'leaf' or scale into it and pull away the fleshy base between the teeth, discard the tough part and work your way down to the heart. Should there be any fibres that are the start of the flower, known as the 'choke', these are inedible. So lift them out with a knife tip and discard. The soft, exquisitely flavoured 'heart' – the base of the flower – is the true gourmet prize. In France I ate it spread onto a savoury biscuit with fresh lemon juice and a touch of coarse salt, the way Catherine de Medici did, and I surely knew why this fascinating plant has been loved and cherished for so many centuries.

Artichoke Dip

This is an Italian recipe similar to the Romans' way of eating artichokes. Mix 1 tablespoon good olive oil with 1 tablespoon balsamic vinegar and season with a grinding of coarse sea salt and black pepper. Dip the base of each leaf scale into it.

Tree Tomato
Tamarillo

Cyphomandra betacea

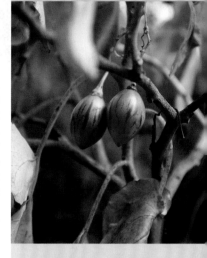

A productive, slender little tree, the tree tomato is a great favourite with gardeners in subtropical and tropical areas all over the world. It belongs to the great Solanaceae family – its close cousins are the tomato, potato, brinjal and chillies – and it is a much-loved and treasured little tree everywhere. Its exact origins are uncertain, but it is believed to have originated in the Andes Mountains in Peru, also in Chile, Ecuador and Bolivia, but it has been grown so extensively in Brazil, Colombia and Argentina for so many centuries that the arguments remain. The name 'tamarillo' is fairly recent. The tree was introduced into Spain in the 19th century and spread quickly into France, Germany and England, where it was grown in hot houses. From Southern Europe its trade routes clearly defined its spread to the top of Africa. From Egypt it went to Jamaica and from Jamaica to Madeira and from Madeira to the Cape of Good Hope, and on into India to Sri Lanka, Hong Kong and to Australia! In 1891 it arrived from India into New Zealand and today New Zealand is the largest grower of tree tomatoes and they coined the name 'tamarillo' in 1967! Tamarillo seemed far more a romantic name and has been accepted worldwide – even in the lands of its origin!

Growing the Tree Tomato

A small shrub or neat small tree that grows between 2–5 m tall, small clusters of white, richly scented flowers at the branch tips are borne in spring and the fruits, egg-shaped and bright red or yellow or almost maroon in some varieties, ripen in clusters. Tough skinned, sometimes with longitudinal dark, uneven purple stripes, the ripe fruit has a sweet pulp, rich in seeds.

We start off new trees in our nursery by squeezing out the pulp, which is thick with seeds, onto a double layer of kitchen paper towel. Labelled and dated it will await a seed box filled with moist compost into which the whole paper towel with its seeds will be patted down, well watered and covered with a thin layer of finely sieved compost. Keep the seed tray moist at all times in a shady area away from draughts. Within about 2 weeks, tiny seedlings will pop through. Once they are big enough to handle, prick them out and carefully plant into compost-filled bags. Now let them strengthen and grow, staking the plants to ensure a tall, neat stem. Move them gradually out into the sunlight to harden off before planting them out.

It thrives in full sun in a large compost-filled hole, and a long, slow weekly watering, less in winter, will ensure frequent fruit. Easily damaged by strong winds, hail and heavy rain and by the cold, the little tree has a shallow root system so plant it in a sheltered place and cover it with plant fleece if the winter is cold. Young trees are very frost tender, so keep them well protected in their first 2 years. Be diligent about pruning off old wood every winter as new fruit is borne only on new wood and the tree can become leggy and untidy.

Using the Tree Tomato

It has a long history as a medicinal plant. Taken for centuries to boost the immune system, a syrup of the soft inner seeds and juice, as well as the thick mesocarp, finely chopped – enough for 1 cup (the thin outer skin is peeled away with a potato peeler) – then simmered in a double boiler with ½ a cup honey with a teaspoonful powdered cloves for 15 minutes, is an ancient treatment for colds, coughs, bronchitis, congestion and 'flu symptoms. In Brazil a teaspoon of cayenne pepper is added and a teaspoon of the mixture is given at a time – at least 6 or 8 times during the day – followed by a cup of hot lemon tea.

The fresh fruit pulp is delicious scooped out with a teaspoon or squeezed into the mouth like the children love to do. It can be used like a tomato, sliced and grilled with sausages or made into a sauce with onions and green peppers or made into a chutney or jam. Mixed with fresh tomatoes it makes a delicious salsa.

Health Note
Tree tomato is rich in vitamins C, A, B6 and E, beta-carotene, phosphorus and potassium.

Tree Tomato Chutney

1 kg ripe peeled tree tomatoes, thinly sliced
1 kg ripe tomatoes, peeled and chopped
6 medium-sized onions, roughly chopped
1 cup seedless raisins or sultanas
2 cups celery, finely chopped
2 cups soft caramel brown sugar
2 teaspoons salt
1 teaspoon ground cloves
2 teaspoons powdered turmeric
550 ml dark grape vinegar
2 tablespoons coriander seeds

Simmer all the ingredients together, stirring often, at a low heat. Simmer until thick – be sure it does not burn – it usually cooks about 1–1½ hours. Spoon into sterilised bottles. Seal when cold and store in a cool, dark pantry or cupboard. Give it 3 weeks to mature before opening. Once open store in the fridge.

Hint

In New Zealand, a favourite way of serving tamarillo is to cut off the tips of ripe tree tomatoes and squeezing the juicy, sweet pulp over individual bowls of rich vanilla ice-cream. Sprinkle with a few chopped pecan nuts and enjoy!

Carrot

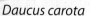

Daucus carota

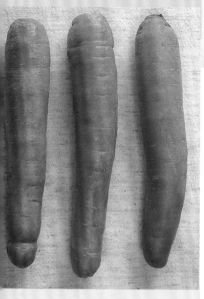

In ancient times a small, tough pale-fleshed wild carrot flourished in Afghanistan. Carrot seeds were found in ancient Bronze Age archaeological sites which dated back 2000 to 3000 years BC. In the early centuries, carrots spread into Europe and the Mediterranean area and Central Asia, cultivated from that original wild carrot. Better and better forms were gradually grown from seeds collected, and then by the 12th century in Spain the literature includes descriptions of a red juicy sweet carrot and also a bright yellow juicy sweet carrot, and it was then eaten cooked with vinegar and salt. By the 13th and 14th centuries it became a popular food, and in Holland the feathery, pretty leaves were used as hair decorations by the ladies of fashion! Flemish refugees, arriving in England during the reign of Elizabeth I, started up the growing of bright orange juicy carrots in the fields of Surrey and Kent, and from then on up to this day the carrot remains one of the world's most loved vegetables.

In the 1980s I brought back wild carrot seed from England which I sowed in a meadow, amongst blue flax, red field poppies, royal blue cornflowers, white ox-eye daisies and wheat. It was one of the most breathtaking spectacular things I have ever done. The exquisite white lace flower heads still come up every now and then after a season of good rain. Interestingly, when I pulled up the maturing plant, the 'carrot' was pale, thin and not very tasty. So I salute those carrot growers of the early centuries for their diligence in persisting in the search for the flavour-filled vegetable that we enjoy today.

Growing Carrots

Easily grown from seed, it does well virtually all year round, except midwinter, in richly composted, deeply dug trenches in full sun. Seeds thinly scattered over a bed or in the trench, covered lightly with soil, kept moist and shaded by a light layer of leaves or coarse hay, will quickly germinate. Flood the trench with water twice weekly as the carrots mature, and pulling up individual carrots for the evening meal is a 'chore' that the children love. Nothing tastes quite so delicious as a freshly pulled baby carrot! Remember, the minute it is pulled out of the ground the sugars begin to turn to starch!

Using Carrots

Raw, freshly grated carrots is a delicious health food that we should be eating daily! Rich in vitamins and minerals (see Health Note), carrots are a valuable treatment for toxaemia, high blood pressure, constipation, asthma, obesity, acne and skin ailments, bladder and kidney ailments, sinusitis, catarrh, painful menstruation, and eating carrots keeps the skin healthy and glowing.

For those whose immune system is compromised, eating carrots and drinking carrot juice daily is vital, and incidentally will increase your ability to smell. A deficiency in vitamin A dries up the mucous membranes and skin, and the thyroid and pituitary gland can also be affected. Add carrots to soups, stews, salads and stir-fries. Drinking carrot juice from 2 fresh carrots daily will soothe peptic ulcers and prevent infections of the throat, the tonsils, eyes, lungs and the sinuses. And for nursing mothers, carrot juice enhances the quality of the breast milk. Best of all, carrots in the diet will literally kill viruses and bacteria.

Health Note

Carrots are rich in vitamins, including vitamin A, B6, C and E, beta-carotene, as well as traces of vitamin G and K. It contains the minerals calcium, phosphorus, magnesium, potassium, selenium and zinc.

Carrot Salad

Serves 4

Finely grate 6 large carrots. Add the juice of a freshly squeezed orange, half a cup of finely chopped fresh parsley, a cup of finely chopped celery and ½ a cup of sesame seed. Sprinkle with a little freshly grated nutmeg.

Hints

For an energy boost, add 2 fresh carrots, 2 fresh beetroots, 1 cup parsley and 2 stalks celery to your juice extractor. Catch the precious juice and sip slowly.

Eat a raw, well-washed carrot every day as a snack, chewing it really well. Do this while driving or studying and feel the quick energy and alertness just that simple action will give you!

Air Potato
Potato Yam

Dioscorea bulbifera

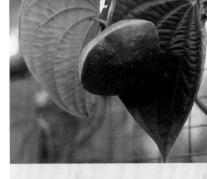

This is an extraordinary plant and a fascinating one to grow! Indigenous to tropical Asia and parts of West Africa, and possibly India, this strange vine has been around for centuries, and cultivated as a food crop and a medicine for almost as long. Both the 'air potatoes' and the huge underground tubers are eaten and used as an ancient medicine. And what makes it so valuable is that the air potatoes can be stored for a long time. Today, from those ancient beginnings, it is grown commercially in parts of India, Africa, Indonesia, Japan, and even in Australia. In Indonesia and India even today it is still used as trade and as a medicine. The Chinese potato yam, *Dioscorea batatas*, is a similar plant but with smaller 'air potatoes' and a lobed leaf.

Once considered to be a peasant food, it is now reaching a popularity that will encourage gardeners to grow it. This prolific perennial creeper twines engagingly through its restraining wire enclosures, climbing to great heights, and offering a great number of tiny 'potatoes' at its huge leaf nodes. The giant, heart-shaped leaves, frost tender and soft, arise all along the thick twining stems that in midwinter dry off and turn brown, awaiting the spring growth of fresh new tendrils from its huge underground 'bulb' or storage tuber. It is so astonishing to see a new plant arising from the actual potato, which can be stored for months, and equally astonishing is to see the flowers, soft drooping short tender stalks covered in tiny creamy bud-like flowers, dangling in the breeze on the new early summer vines.

Growing the Air Potato

Although its great tuber is perennial, the vine needs hot, tropical or subtropical regions to really thrive. In both our great plant conservatory and in our huge caged granadilla and grape areas in the kitchen gardens it thrives, remaining undisturbed in a deep, compost-enriched bed. It seeks sun in which to produce its potatoes, but also does well in light, bright shade.

Start off with an air potato that has a growing shoot. Place it in a shallow, compost-filled hole that has been deeply dug and thoroughly moistened. Nestle the air potato into the hole and leave the top of the air potato and its growing shoot out. Do not over-water it at this stage as it can rot, but keep an eye on it – water when the soil dries out. Train the vine up over a fence or a frame or a lattice. It literally grows 'a mile a minute' once it establishes and at least once a week you'll need to very gently guide the succulent and tender tips – they very easily escape and do their own thing!

By midsummer, tiny bulblets form at the leaf stalk that can grow into palm-sized potatoes. These can be picked at any time, and mature potatoes picked and stored through the winter on a kitchen shelf will sprout new vines. Established vines each spring need a barrow of compost and a deep dam around them flooded with water weekly.

Using the Air Potato

Warmed 'potatoes' cooked wrapped in banana leaves in the hot coals, are used still today the way they were used centuries ago as a dressing over boils, suppurating wounds and abscesses. Thin raw slices were used to soothe burns, grazes and rashes, eczemas and itchy inflamed areas. Ancient Chinese documents reveal that eating a mash of boiled or steamed air potato was taken as a tonic to treat bedwetting, nerve pain, diarrhoea and 'irritable bowel syndrome' as we know it today.

Peeled and thinly sliced and boiled in water for 3 minutes, then drained and boiled up again in fresh water until tender, the air potato can be fried, added to soups, stews, stir-fries, fritters, desserts, and even made into jams and jellies. It is enjoyed both savoury and sweet in Japan and Indonesia. Air potato baked with a little oil and salt and served with lemon juice and butter, is given to children who do not thrive and as a soup to invalids and convalescents, with onions, garlic and thinly shredded cabbage. The air potato is peeled, parboiled and then grated into the soup.

Energy-Giving Air Potato Soup

Serves 6–8

2 onions, finely chopped
2 cups celery, finely chopped
3 cups peeled, parboiled and coarsely grated air potato
2 cloves garlic, finely minced
4 cups thinly shredded Savoy or drumhead organic cabbage, specially the dark green outer leaves
1 teaspoon cayenne pepper
2–3 teaspoons sea salt (taste first)
2 tablespoons olive oil
2 tablespoons sunflower oil
3 tablespoons fresh chopped parsley
juice of 1 lemon
2 teaspoons lemon zest
1½–2 litres chicken stock

Lightly brown the onions in the oils. Add the grated parboiled air potato with the garlic and stir-fry until it lightly browns. Add the cabbage and celery and stir-fry briskly. Finally add all the other ingredients (save the parsley for serving) and simmer 30 minutes or until tender. Serve hot sprinkled with fresh parsley.

Health Note

The air potato is rich in vitamin C and the B-vitamins, magnesium, potassium, iron and phosphorus.

Persimmon

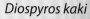

Diospyros kaki

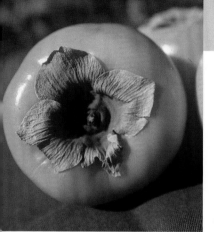

Persimmon Purée

Serves 4

This is one of the most delicious ways of eating persimmon.

You need 6 ripe persimmons. Peel of the tough outer skin of the ripe persimmons and mash the pulp or push it through a sieve. Add 4 tablespoons of thick, plain Bulgarian yoghurt (or thick fresh cream to make it really rich and delicious) and a sprinkling of cinnamon powder. Spoon into individual glass dessert bowls. Sprinkle with chopped almonds and serve chilled.

- - - - - - - - - - - - - - - - - - - -

Health Note

Rich in beta-carotene, vitamins A & C and in iron and a host of minerals, especially potassium, if eaten fresh, one a day, the persimmon will boost the immune system for the winter ahead.

Now a rare tree, the once popular persimmon has sadly all but disappeared from our gardens! Not so long ago most gardens had one – a beautiful spreading, slow-growing deciduous tree that hung heavy in late summer with soft and scented orange fruits that looked like a tomato. With the large calyx cut away gently with a sharp knife a teaspoon was needed to scoop out the fragrant flesh – the riper the better! Today it is known as Sharon fruit and its soft flesh with no 'keeping' or 'travelling' benefits, has been out-bred with crisper, harder fruits that can reach the shops bright, ripe and saleable from faraway places such as Israel!

Interestingly, the persimmon is indigenous to China, Japan and Korea, and has been in cultivation for many centuries, and they remain the biggest producers of persimmon today. It was introduced to America in 1856 by Commodore Perry, a ship's captain who found it so delicious he took the seeds back to America, and from there it spread to the rest of the world. The Americans were the first to make persimmon ice-cream. From the early centuries the Chinese dried persimmons – flattened and pressed into flat rounds – and these became a sweet trade, fetching good prices. Used in Chinese medicine from the early centuries for several ailments, the high sugar content of the ripened fruits, dried for the winter months and made into luscious thick syrups for coughs, colds and respiratory ailments, made the persimmon a much sought after item and the trade routes record its advance into the New World.

Growing Persimmons

I mourn the absence of these spreading and beautiful trees, but as many cultivars are becoming available, and as the world searches for food trees, we may be lucky enough to find a persimmon tree in our local nursery one fine day. They do take a certain amount of frost, and Israel is proving that it can take the heat. I have grown persimmon trees in the Herbal Centre gardens and they bear erratically, even enclosed in cages to keep the monkeys and the squirrels away. The fruits we have picked are richly sweet when fully ripe. We keep trying as they are very slow growing.

They need a deep, compost-filled hole in full sun with a twice yearly barrow load of compost – one in late winter and one in midsummer – for the ripening fruit. By late autumn the leaves turn reddish and fall, often leaving a fruit or two on the bare branches. The rich carpet of leaves is excellent for the compost heap and slow-ripening fruits picked for transport can be ripened to their full potential by placing them in a cardboard box with a good fitting lid with a ripening banana. The banana gives off ethylene gas, which helps to ripen the persimmon.

Using Persimmons

Recipes have been developed through the ages in Japan and China which include both fresh and dried persimmons in a variety of dishes. Long ropes of dark dried persimmons can be found in Chinese markets and have been part of the Chinese New Year celebrations each February since ancient times. Interestingly, dried persimmons are so rich in sugar it can be scraped off the fruits and can be compacted into moulds. These ornamental 'tablets' of sugar are part of the wedding ceremonies in China and are served at Chinese banquets with tea as the first course.

Used in desserts, jams and ice-creams and dried, the persimmon is an extraordinary fruit that we don't fully appreciate. As a child we grew a persimmon tree in our Pretoria garden, and it bore the soft and delicious fruits abundantly. My grandmother made a delicious jam from them – rather like a lemon curd – and added lemon pulp and juice to make it set. Try drying slices of persimmon (see page 23) for energy and for the exceptional fruit sugars – no wonder it was known as the Chinese date!

Warmed persimmon cut in half and applied to a boil, will quickly bring it to a head, and slices over grazes, rashes, infected scrapes and cuts will soothingly heal it. Chinese medicinal texts list persimmom as panacea – a golden fruit of preciousness.

Enset

Ensete ventricosum

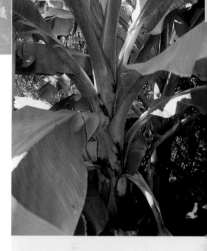

This extraordinary plant is nothing short of miraculous! It is certainly one of the most valuable plants in Africa for creating food security. Indigenous to Southern and East Africa, it looks so like a banana plant people are often confused when they see it. It is a huge, single-stemmed plant with massive, flapping leaves that actually form a stem in sheaths. As it grows older, leaves peel back and die off and are then used as firewood, thatching and processed into ropes and ties. In Ethiopia it is a staple food that has been in cultivation for over 5 000 years.

In the Herbal Centre gardens we grow a spectacular variety that has a dark red midrib to each of the massive leaves, and every visitor mistakes it for a banana tree. The long, conspicuous, massive, dark red flowers in thick purple bracts are each around 75 cm to 1 m in length. A visiting Ethiopian university student told us that the juicy flower bracts, when young and tender, are fried crisp and eaten where he grew up in southern Ethiopia. The flowers give way to leathery fruit resembling a bunch of small bananas, but instead of the sweet and delicious banana within the tough skin, a mass of hard, black, tightly packed pea-sized seeds form. Propagation is not from the seed, but from the offsets or sucker shoots that form around the huge underground stem, the base from which the large and succulent leaves arise. Travellers often take the seeds with them, as they are considered to bring good luck to the owner!

Growing Enset

Rich, compost-laden, moist, deeply dug soil is what this beautiful plant thrives in, although its wild habitat is along streams and in the moist and hushed rain-spattered forests and along tree-lined ravines and wherever there is moisture and deep soil. I grow them in full sun against the hot harsh northern slopes of the great Magaliesberg mountain range, and in semi-shade in the rich soil of the herb garden, and they thrive – I am sure because they are tough survivor plants, and every visitor is enthralled by their beauty.

Using Enset

Dig out the entire root or corm of a mature 'tree'. The corm is actually the underground stem, which is made up of the leaf bases. Replant the side shoots to ensure continuation of the crop, then do as the Ethiopians do: Chop up the leaf bases, wrap them in the great leaves and store for 20 days in a cool moist pit, lined with leaves so no soil comes in contact with it. It will ferment and the resultant 'kocho', a starchy porridge-like mass, is spread flat onto green leaves, baked on the hot coals covered with more leaves. 'Kocho bread' is part of the Ethiopian diet. Interestingly, the starchy enset can remain enclosed in the leaves in the pits for a long time and it does not deteriorate.

Finely chopped and crushed, the corm can be made into porridge or pancakes or, when young, corms are dug up, carefully washed and cut and fried over the fire. They taste rather like potatoes and are called *amicho*.

Hot mashed corms are used as a poultice to bring a boil to a head or to cleanse a suppurating wound. The leaves are also used as wound dressing and as a cool, smooth and comfortable sleeping mat for those with fever, with burns, and with grazes, scratches and wounds. Sap from the succulent leaf bases is used as a 'wash' or lotion over rashes and stings, which are then covered with a poultice of warmed leaves to quickly bring relief.

- -

Health Note

Enset is rich in starch, calcium, magnesium, phosphorus and vitamins A, C, D and E.

Enset 'Potatoes'

Boil young corms that are cut into wedges until tender. Drain and fry lightly in a pan with a little olive oil and butter, browning and turning both sides. Serve with lemon juice, black pepper and sea salt.

Hint

Strangely fibrous and tasteless, enset corms need to be almost roasted to get them to become like the beloved Ethiopian staple. We dug up one and it was huge – 75 cm wide and 50 cm thick – and dripping with clear sap housed in fibrous 'cells'!

Loquat

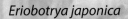

Eriobotrya japonica

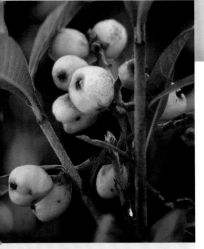

One of the most beautiful spreading trees with huge, glossy, dark green leaves, the loquat is a feature in many a garden. Originally from China and cultivated since ancient times as both a food and a medicine, the loquat has a place in history in both China and Japan. Imported from Japan at the end of the 18th century to France, it was grown then for its beautiful leaves as a tree of stature in the gardens of the palaces, and later as a street tree. Most fascinating of all is that the tree flowers in late summer and fruits earlier than most trees, often in winter! The ancient Chinese used the fruit in syrups and drinks for coughs and colds, and the candied fruit was sold to travellers as an energy food. The sweetly scented flowers on their velvety stems and the leathery leaves have been used through the centuries as a decoration during celebrations and festivities, and placed around altars and shrines.

Growing Loquats

The tree needs a huge, compost-filled hole in full sun and with a large pipe set into the hole at angle so that a hosepipe can be set into it to get the roots well watered. I remember my parents watering the big loquat every week in this manner and in our suburban garden it set luscious fruit every year thanks to the diligent watering and the barrow loads of compost dug in around it every six months. The fruits need to ripen on the trees to encourage the sugars within them to fully mature, but because they bruise easily they are only sold at local markets. Note that in South Africa the loquat tree is no longer available at nurseries as it has been included in the alien invader list.

Using Loquat

The creamy white sprays of flowers, heady with perfume, make fascinating flower arrangements, and floated in a shallow glass bowl with candles made our Saturday night family dinners very special. Drying carefully chosen small loquat branches, by standing the branches in a mixture of 1 part glycerine and 2 parts hot water, was once a popular practice amongst flower arrangers, especially for the church flowers. The leaves would gradually turn flexible and soft, and a light, coppery tan colour. These long-lived branches became a focal point in the big flower arrangements and could be used over and over with whatever flower was in season.

Included in China's medical texts as treatment for building strength and vitality, it was given as a food to their warriors. Made into a liqueur dispensed by the priests and monks in the early centuries, the loquat was considered to be an excellent after-dinner digestive. Candied loquats are still today given to children as a cough treatment, and loquats cooked in syrup and spread onto a biscuit with cream cheese and grated ginger is often eaten as a cough and cold treatment – and it tastes delicious!

Trim and cut ripe loquats into small pieces. Refrigerate and add to plain Bulgarian yoghurt, with a dribble of honey, as a refreshing energy boost on a hot afternoon.

Health Note

The fruit is rich in fruit sugars, digestive enzymes, vitamin A, some vitamin C, folic acid, beta-carotene, calcium, iron and some phosphorus and selenium.

Loquat Sauce

Serves 6

This is delicious served hot or cold with mutton, beef or pork.

3 Granny Smith apples, peeled, cored and chopped

3 cups of stoned, sliced loquats (topped and tailed – meaning the little stem is cut off, as well as the opposite end where the flower remains)

½ cup honey

½ cup water

½ cup thick caramel brown sugar

6 cloves

1 teaspoon grated nutmeg

1 dessertspoon crushed coriander seeds

1 tablespoon apple cider vinegar

Simmer everything together in a heavy bottomed pot on low heat, stirring frequently until tender (about 10–15 minutes). Add the apple cider vinegar and mix well. Spoon into sterilised jars. Keep refrigerated.

Rocket

Arugula ■ Rucola ■ Roquette

Eruca sativa • Eruca vesicaria

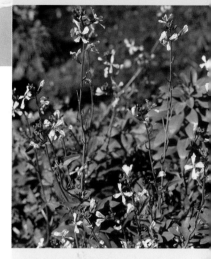

The flavour of this easy-to-grow and abundant annual is powerful to say the least! The Italians say it 'fills your mouth with flavour' and they eat it with gusto – especially with mozzarella cheese and crisply fried bacon on Italian bread dipped in olive oil. Native to the Mediterranean area, it has been a much-loved salad ingredient for centuries, but to the rest of the world it has only in the last few years become a popular ingredient and taste.

A new rocket variety has emerged as a favourite fairly recently. Known as Wild Rocket (*Dipsotaxis tenuifolia*), this is a smaller, more refined plant, an untidy perennial, which we find in our gardens needs really to be treated as an annual for continuous leaves. With thinner and smaller leaves and small bright yellow flowers and possibly a more peppery, more pungent flavour, it is definitely less prone to bolt in the long hot summers. Seeds are available from seed merchants now, and our plantings have proved to be exciting. Originating in the Mediterranean areas, Franchi Seeds of Italy sent us this true wild rocket, which thrives in the over 30 °C heat of our mountainside gardens, and it reseeds itself where the soil is soft, moist and friable. The seed is easily collected from the fine pods and we have found cutting back the plant when it starts to go to seed is often very successful as new growth, tender and filled with flavour, reappears, but don't count on it, as suddenly it becomes stringy and dries off.

Growing Rocket

A quick annual with a mass of succulent leaves, flowers and long sprays of the valuable seeds, rocket seed is sown in full sun in deeply dug, well-composted soil in a shallow furrow that can be flooded with a gentle trickle of water twice a week. It will quickly germinate and the little seedlings must not ever dry out in the early days. Seedlings can be transplanted 50 cm apart when they are big enough to handle, into moist, composted beds.

Using Rocket

Rocket was used in the early centuries as a treatment for digestive disorders and circulatory disorders and the steamed hot leaves as a compress over bruises, sprains and aching muscles. A cough syrup, made of the leaves and seeds with honey, remains valuable today. The uses of rocket have been almost forgotten today, but in some rural areas the grandmother of the house will still be applying hot rocket leaves to a sprain. The early Romans used green rocket seedpods, pounded with honey and lemon juice, for coughs and bronchitis and the church cloister gardens grew enough for the monks to dispense over the winter to keep the villagers free from chest ailments. Today that rocket seed mixture is still made and kept in the medicine cupboard of many Mediterranean households.

The abundant seeds are sometimes pressed for oil the way rapeseed is, and rocket oil was once a profitable trade. The oil was not only used for cooking but for medicinal purposes as well. Known as Jamba oil, it is still sold in the street markets in India, Iran, Pakistan as well as Israel and parts of Turkey today.

Leaves can be picked from the early stages onwards for salads – the younger and more tender they are the more delicious the salad becomes. The flowers, small pale creamy and four-petalled like little propellers, are edible and are added to salads and soups and stir-fries, and so are the young and tender seedpods. Sprouted rocket seeds are delicious served with grills or sprinkled over pasta as the Italians do.

Interestingly, crushed flower petals were used as a cosmetic herb to treat skin blemishes – the flower pounded to a soft pulp was spread over the blemish and left to dry there. Mixed with olive oil and used as a scrub, rocket flowers and crushed green seeds remain to this day, one of the best beauty treatments to refine and moisturise the skin in the Italian countryside. Squeeze rocket stems over itchy insect bites or crush the fresh leaves and rub them onto the area to relieve the itch and redness the way the ancient field workers did under the heat of the Mediterranean sun.

Italian Misticanza Salad

For our salads we find the best rockets should be sown in early autumn for winter growth in our frost-free gardens, then the succulent flavour-filled salads are a treat. This salad is a mixture of young salad greens and can vary with what we have in the garden. It can include:

chervil (another cool weather plant)
young dandelion leaves
our abundant winter butter lettuces and oak leaf lettuces
rocket leaves and flowers
*young new baby spinach leaves (**not** Swiss chard leaves)*
dill or fennel leaves, finely chopped
flat-leaf Italian parsley, finely chopped
endives – just a little if we have them

Tossed together with olive oil, black pepper, a squeeze of lemon juice and a sprinkling of toasted sesame seeds, and served in individual small shallow bowls with olives or walnuts or even small squares of mozzarella cheese, this salad never fails to have visitors ask for the recipe!

Health Note

Rocket leaves are rich in vitamins A and C, folic acid, calcium and iron.

Buckwheat

Fagopyrum esculentum

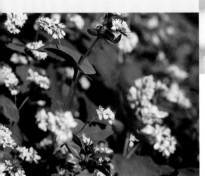

An ancient, much revered food, buckwheat was brought into Europe from its native Asia by the Crusaders who named it 'Saracen corn', and it has remained one of the world's most important grains for centuries. One of the most valuable medicines during the Middle Ages, records going back to the early 14th century detail its versatility in treating many ailments, and vast buckwheat fields were established all over Europe and Asia during the summers for this quick-and-easy-to-grow grain, which could be easily stored for the long snowbound winters. Buckwheat seed trade was profitable and it spread easily because of its ease of growing and its abundant seed production. All parts of the plant are edible and form part of many traditional dishes in many countries.

One of its most enduring uses was, and still is, as a rich and rewarding green manure crop, dug back into poor soil to revitalise it. Early records show it was often used to revitalise depleted soils near the villages, its seeds reaped and the remaining plant ploughed back into the soil with chicken and goat manure. One could say buckwheat became one of the first plant fertilisers, and in many countries this remains so today.

Growing Buckwheat

Easy to grow and quickly maturing, we have found it to be a reliable and prolific crop that can be sown all through the year except in the coldest months. Prepare beds by digging deeply and adding compost – the more the better. Rake the area level and scatter the seed. Rake the seed in and set a sprinkler over the area to keep the soil moist. You will get almost 100% germination, but water it daily to ensure the little heart-shaped seeds do not dry out. Buckwheat also makes a nutritious and delicious sprout and can be grown in compost-filled seed trays in light shade for quick pickings for salads and stir-fries.

In the vegetable garden buckwheat rows are valuable next to mealies and globe artichokes, each enhancing the other's growth. Buckwheat stimulates the growth of any plants near it, even in the poorest of soils. It loosens heavy clay soils and so is excellent for root crops like carrots, turnips and potatoes. But don't plant it next to winter wheat as they retard each other's growth.

Using Buckwheat

Buckwheat leaves, flowers and seeds are packed with vitamins, minerals, amino acids, and easily and accessible protein that act as a tonic to the whole body. Its earliest recordings found buckwheat to be important for controlling bleeding, dilating the blood vessels and lowering blood pressure. By eating the leaves and the flowers fresh in the daily salad, winter chilblains and circulation were vastly improved and it became known as 'the winter tonic'.

Today's research finds buckwheat strengthens the walls of the veins and so is a valuable treatment for varicose veins, spontaneous bruising, poor circulation, haemorrhages of the retina, reducing capillary permeability, and for lowering high blood pressure quite drastically. By eating the green leaves and flowers, and by adding buckwheat flour to the diet, or eating buckwheat groats (the hulled grains) as porridge and steamed groats as a rice dish at least twice a week, great changes can be recorded.

The Chinese and Japanese have included buckwheat in their cooking for over 1 000 years, and it remains a favourite ingredient in many dishes. Added to stir-fries with mushrooms, the leaves and the cooked groats have become exciting and delicious dishes and are worth experimenting with. Big tubs of buckwheat greens stand outside in the sun near many eateries in China and in America, and even today are known as grano saraceno, or trigo saraceno, and it is a valuable food included in the diets of many cultures for radiation damage. We need to sit up and take notice!

Health Note

Buckwheat is a good source of vitamins B, A and E, magnesium, manganese, copper, iron, phosphorus, potassium, zinc, selenium and amino acids.

Buckwheat Pancakes

Serves 4–6

Try these quick and easy pancakes with both savoury and sweet fillings.

1 cup buckwheat flour (bought from a health shop)
½ cup cake flour or Nutty Wheat flour
2 teaspoons baking powder
pinch salt
1 egg whisked into 1 cup of milk or soya milk

Mix all the dry ingredients and then add in the milk and egg mixture. Mix to a slack dough. Should it be too stiff, add a little water and whisk thoroughly. In a pan heat a little olive oil, enough to spread all over the pan, then pour in about ¼–½ cup of pancake batter and tip to cover the bottom of the pan. Keep it on medium heat and wait until it bubbles. Flip it over to cook on the other side. Serve with a filling of fresh sliced fruits – strawberries, berries and nectarines – or stewed apples and rhubarb or salad ingredients like avocado and tomato and butter lettuce, savoury mince or chicken and tomatoes with soy sauce like the Chinese do. The combinations are endless and delicious!

Caution

In some people with sensitive skins buckwheat may cause light-sensitive dermatitis if it is consumed daily. In those who are allergic to nuts or other proteins, it may irritate the mucous membranes of the mouth and throat – an allergic reaction due to its high protein content. Usually the leaves and flowers are safely eaten, but the grain and the flour may be an allergenic in some sensitive people.

Feijoa
Pineapple Guava

Feijoa sellowiana

This fascinating and beautiful shrub originated in Brazil, Uruguay, Paraguay and Argentina, where it remains a much-loved ingredient in jams, ice-creams, crystallised and dried fruit, juices, jellies and fruit cups. It is an unusual shrub that is a monotypic genus, which means it is the sole representative of its genus. It was 'discovered' around 1819 by a German explorer named Sellow who found it growing abundantly in Brazil and named it after a San Sebastian botanist, Don de Silva Feijoa. The 'pineapple guava' as it became known, was introduced to Europe around 1890 by a French horticulturist, Édouard André, and from there it went to the tropical and semi-tropical gardens of Australia, New Zealand and California around 1900.

Very little research has been done on this exotic fruit, but in its native countries it is a firm favourite and hedges, avenues and orchards of feijoa make it a valuable market fruit, as each 'tree' or shrub produces an abundance of both fruits, small, green and guava-like with a rich and delicious scent and flavour, and the luscious pink sweetly edible, juicy flowers.

Growing Feijoa

I am simply thrilled with feijoa! Not only is it a most versatile garden focal point, but it is so easy and undemanding to grow and it is a charming feature plant wherever it grows. Try it in a really big compost-filled pot in full sun – it can be clipped and pruned topiary style. Try it espaliered along a north-facing wall, tied onto firm trellises in deep, compost-filled holes. Try it clipped into a neat evergreen hedge, or try it in rows along the drive, free and unrestrained, or train it over arches – it will be fascinating in all seasons! The grey-green leaves are the perfect foil for the small clusters of fragrant pink flowers and unrestrained it can become almost tree-like.

Planted in a huge, compost-filled hole, it adapts to virtually any soil but flourishes in warm, protected frost-free areas in full sun. It thrives with lots of compost and a twice weekly deep watering. Give it a barrow load of compost every winter to ensure abundant spring flowers.

Hang a tin with molasses and water in the tree to attract the fruit flies, which love the pineapple guavas and under-plant with tansy to deter the fruit flies.

Using Feijoa

Feijoa tea is taken for certain thyroid conditions as it contains iodine, and the same brew is used in its native lands to treat dysentery, diarrhoea and stomach cramps. Add ¼ cup of flowers or fruit, or both, to 1 cup of boiling water, stand 5 minutes, then strain and sip slowly. A lotion for sunburned, windburned skin is made by boiling 1 cup of flowers in 1 litre of water for 10 minutes. Once cooled and strained it can be splashed on, dabbed on or sprayed onto the area. When the fruits and flowers are not in season, a brew or 'tea' can be made of the leafy tips of the branches. In Argentina this warm brew is added to the bath to soothe the children's scratches and grazes.

In Paraguay fresh crushed flowers or a lotion of leaves in boiling water, is used as a wash over rashes, mild burns, insect bites, stings and itchy inflamed areas, or slices of the fresh fruit are used as a soothing poultice.

Eating freshly sliced chilled feijoas with coconut flakes has to be one of the most delicious tastes imaginable. The Spanish serve this delectable dish set in jelly and with a dollop of fresh cream! They call it 'Food for the Gods' and it is often served at feasts and celebrations.

Health Note

Feijoa provides vitamin C, some B-vitamins, folic acid, calcium, iron, magnesium, potassium, manganese and iodine.

Pineapple Guava Stir-Fry

Serves 4–6

This pineapple guava stir-fry on pancakes is a dish no one can ever get enough of!

3 cups sliced pineapple guava fruits (check for insect damage)
3 tablespoons butter
1 cup cream
1 cup coconut flakes (not desiccated coconut)
a pinch of ground cinnamon
¾ cup chopped macadamia nuts
1 tablespoon toasted sesame seeds (shake over a hot plate in a pan for a minute to toast them)

Melt the butter in a heavy bottomed pot. Add the pineapple guava pieces and, using a wooden spoon, stir well. Add the cream, coconut flakes and cinnamon and stir-fry for 2 minutes. Now add the macadamia nuts and stir well to coat everything. Spoon onto hot pancakes and sprinkle with the sesame seeds. Serve warm.

Hint

Add the fresh flowers to fruit juice, especially granadilla juice served in tall glasses with ice, for a party treat.

Fig

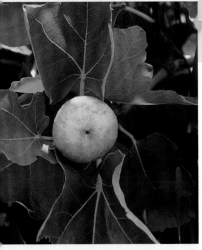

Ficus carica

Summer Fig Lunch Dish

Serves 6

Our family favourite is this delicious summer salad. We grow black figs as well, which look spectacular in this dish.

Arrange 20 ripe figs, halved, 20 thin slices Parma ham and slices of mozzarella cheese on a platter. Serve with freshly baked bread.

Syrup of Figs

This is my grandmother's recipe. Thinly slice and chop 10 figs and place in a double boiler over gentle heat with 1 cup of honey. Warm over gentle heat, stirring frequently for 30 minutes. Strain, bottle and label. Take 1 dessertspoon daily.

Hint

Place a fig twig without leaves in your flour bin – it keeps weevils out of grains!

The fig has to be one of the most loved and the most precious plants ever known to mankind, and is one of the most ancient of all cultivated food crops. It was a major crop in ancient Greece. Pliny the Elder (AD 23–79) described then around 29 cultivars including Kadota, which we still grow today. The fig's origins are lost in the mists of time, but it is thought to be indigenous to Syria, western Asia and the eastern Mediterranean, and ancient archaeological evidence in many Old World countries shows it has been a valuable part of the diet in Egypt, Mesopotamia and Italy, and drawings of the fig were found in the Gizeh pyramid and in ancient Babylon. The Phoenician trade caravans spread it into China and India and it became, through the centuries, one of the most valuable of medicines.

Figs have been cultivated from around 4 000 years before Christ, and present-day cultivation, particularly in Turkey, Spain and Italy, is extensive and the biggest part of the fig production is dried figs. The original wild figs, which grow in an enormous area from the Canary Islands through the Mediterranean area to eastern Iran, are still tended and cultivated and traded today. Fresh figs, sold in markets, are still a favoured item, and for many small farmers figs are still their most profitable income. There are at least 700 varieties today which have evolved out of the single species *Ficus carica* and from the subspecies *Ficus carica sativa* which is commonly known as the domestic fig.

Growing Figs

I urge every homeowner to find a space for a fig tree or two. Not only is it a fascinating tree in its all-year-round beauty, but it is so easy and undemanding to grow and the rewards are so great. Choose a spot in full sun and dig a really huge hole. Fill with old compost and set a large pipe into the hole at an angle in order to get the hosepipe into it to enable water to reach the roots. It needs a twice weekly watering – in fact it would love to have its feet in a furrow. We lead a rainwater tank's overflow into the fig trees after a summer of good rain, and the crop was so abundant, we turned to fig jam making almost daily after Christmas! A barrow or two or three of compost in late winter ensures good fruiting, and make a huge dam around it to flood it with a slowly trickling hose twice weekly in summer, once every 10 days in winter.

Using Figs

The health boosting tonic properties in figs are legendary. The fig has a high fruit sugar content and it is a natural laxative – it will literally move sluggish bowels if 4 fresh or dried figs are eaten first thing in the morning. (Soak the dried figs overnight and eat next morning accompanied by a cup of herb tea.) Figs are restorative, increase energy, vitality and well-being. Figs in the diet help to clear toxins and to build bones – remember their high calcium content. They are one of the highest plant sources of calcium and they are excellent for children.

Made into syrups with a little honey for coughs and colds, the fig has been part of the home medicine chest for centuries. When I was a child, 'syrup of figs' could be bought from every chemist, made then only with honey and figs – no preservatives, colourants or stabilisers! And when we did not have our own supply, my grandmother made her own syrup of figs (see recipe alongside).

Health Note

Figs are abundant in vitamins, especially vitamins A and C, beta-carotene, and a mass of minerals, in particular calcium, potassium and phosphorus.

Fennel

Florence Fennel

Foeniculum dulce

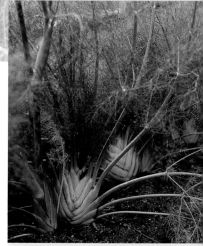

Fennel is a popular, easy-to-grow perennial herb that can reach up to 1,5 m with a froth of fine leaves. This is *Foeniculum vulgare*, but here I want to bring Florence fennel to your attention.

This is the annual fennel, grown particularly in the cooler weather, widely known and loved in ancient Greece and Rome, that has a luscious swollen, above ground stem that features in many delicious recipes dating back to the early centuries. In fact, fennel is mentioned in a papyrus botanical collection that goes back to 1500 BC! Fennel is also described by Pliny the Elder as so valuable a medicinal plant that he urged everyone to grow it near their homes!

It has a long history of use as a valuable medicine, particularly in its native Mediterranean area. Traditionally used as a digestive, it came to Europe in the Middle Ages as a medicine of such great value that fennel seeds became a prized commodity that spread into India, China and North Africa by the 15th century. Small leather pouches of fennel seed were often used to barter, and the remains of these 'fennel trade relics' have been found in tombs and churches in distant lands. If was considered to be so valuable that the seeds were precious enough to take with one into the afterlife!

Growing Fennel

The more perennial fennel, *Foeniculum vulgare*, is tough and weather resistant and grows easily, often becoming a wayside weed. But the Florence fennel, *Foeniculum dulce*, is the real treasure, a winter annual in very hot areas. Grow it first from seed, then transplant into richly composted, deeply dug soil in full sun, spaced 50 cm apart. The leaves as well as the bulbous swollen root stem can be eaten, as well as the flowers and seeds. Reap Florence fennel as soon as the bulbous stem is about the size of a tennis ball.

Using Fennel

All the fennels have a fresh, delicious slightly anise taste that is perfect with fish, pasta, cheese, poultry and salads. The seeds produce an aromatic antispasmodic essential oil that contains anethole, which is used as a flavouring, a digestive and a natural treatment for spastic colon and other digestive ailments. Refreshing and cleansing, all parts can be used, and fennel leaf tea, made by pouring 1 cup of boiling water over ¼ cup fresh leaves and stems and even flowers and seeds, leave to stand 5 minutes, then strain and sip slowly, is an excellent tea for flushing out toxins, it acts as a natural diuretic and it is fondly known as 'the slimmer's herb'. It reduces the effects of over-indulgence in both food and alcohol and it is excellent for constipation, heartburn, colic and respiratory ailments. Just chewing fennel seeds will ease heartburn and indigestion so effectively you'll want to carry a little pouch of seeds everywhere with you the way the ancient Romans and Greeks once did!

As fennel contains phytoestrogens, it makes it a valuable remedy for menopause and female ailments and new research finds fennel beneficial in treating excessive facial hairiness in women. Experiments are ongoing and are finding fennel exerts an anti-testosterone effect in certain cases. Fennel is also high in anti-cancer coumarin compounds and anethole oil, which also shows it is a competent anti-inflammatory.

The most valuable way of eating Florence fennel is by shaving the succulent and flavour-filled 'bulb' into a salad or stir-fry. Add the leaves and the finely sliced bulb to coarse salt and use as a scrub in the bath, tied in a facecloth, soak it well and then with soap use it as a scrub particularly over the feet and legs to clear toxins, cleanse and refresh.

Health Note

Fennel is rich in vitamins C, A and D, potassium, magnesium, manganese, phosphorus and folic acid. It is also a good source of iron, calcium and dietary fibre.

Fennel Slimming Salad

Serves 4

Sustaining and refreshing, this is a meal for a slimmer, with a perfect balance of nutrients!

2 cups fennel root, thinly shredded
1 avocado, peeled and cubed
1 cup chopped green pepper
1 cup chopped celery
2 cups cubed pineapple
1–2 cups cooked and cooled butter beans
½ cup chopped parsley
2 teaspoons fennel seeds

In a glass bowl, mix all the ingredients together, leaving the avocado until last so as not to bruise it. Place the avocado slices on top of the salad and dress by squeezing over the juice of a lemon and, if liked, a drizzle of olive oil, a grinding of black pepper and a sprinkling of sea salt. Serve chilled.

Hint

Mix 2 cups chopped fennel leaves into 2 cups Epsom salts and store in a screw-top jar. 1 cup of this added to the bath makes an excellent skin toner and cleanser.

Kumquat
Fortunella

Fortunella margarita

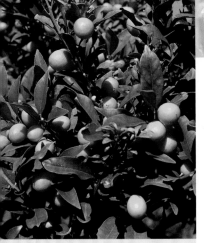

Pixie's Kumquat Marmalade

I use the fruits in this much-loved marmalade recipe given to me by an old and dear friend.

Slice kumquats thinly, to every heaped cup of the sliced fruit add 3 cups of cold water and leave overnight. Next morning, boil until tender, about 2 hours – the water will be gluey and thick.

Leave and stand covered overnight. Next morning weigh the whole mass and add 1 kg of sugar to every 1 kg of pulp. In a heavy bottomed pot and on low heat boil it gently, stirring often so that it does not burn – usually about 2 hours – and watch it carefully. Test a drop or two on a cold saucer to see if it sets. Fill sterilised bottles and seal well. Label and store in a cool cupboard. Delicious served on toast with strong cheddar cheese!

Hint

Thinly slice 12 kumquats and push into a bottle of brandy. Add 1 cup of warmed honey to the bottle and shake well. Keep in a dark cupboard and shake every now and then. At the first sign of a cold take a spoonful or two of this excellent mixture.

P art of the great citrus family but not a true citrus, the kumquat belongs to the genus *Fortunella*, and as such are a rare and precious fruit, indigenous to China. Ancient, loved and respected, this little miniature orange is part of history, legend and myth. I am mad about kumquats. I love their mass of sweetly scented flowers, their long bearing capacity of basket upon basket of glowing little sour fruits, and their undemanding presence in my gardens.

The history of the kumquat is fascinating. Grown in the Emperor's gardens and preserved in honey, the kumquat became an item of trade. Their sweet golden rind pared from the intensely sour fruit, was cooked in honey and taken as a treatment for coughs and colds. Small kumquat trees in beautiful Chinese pots where taken by the emperors on their visits to their subjects as a symbol of friendship and good fortune. As the little tree is slow growing, yet bears fruit at a young age, there was space for it in the tiniest of gardens or in the sun in the front of a house.

The flowers, infused in sugar water or honey water, were given to children who could not sleep or who were restless and noisy. The leaves, evergreen and leathery, were threaded and hung over the doorways and over windows to repel flying insects, and trade was brisk and consistent. The tree of Good Fortune or 'Fortunella' became so loved that it formed part of tradition, ceremony and celebration.

Growing Kumquats

They need full sun and a large, deep, compost-filled hole. They are grafted onto the Cape rough skin lemon root stock, so always be on the look out for a long thorny branch emerging from its almost ground level graft and prune it carefully away. Space 2–3 m apart, for although it is neat, small growing and dense, it does need air around it and it will grow into a perfectly shaped little tree that is laden with its exquisite little bright fruits for at least 4 months of the year.

I never prune them as they form so perfectly and they thrive with a long slow weekly watering in hot weather, less in winter. A barrow load of compost in spring and in late summer will ensure an overwhelming crop of fruits.

They do well in big pots but feeding once a month and watering more often is essential. For a small garden they are simply stunning and will give years of evergreen pleasure.

Using Kumquats

The ancient Chinese healers used the fruit as a treatment for many illnesses, including skin conditions and kidney and bladder ailments. Introduced into Europe in 1846, it became a much-loved preserve and a brandied sugary sweetmeat was served at banquets. In the cold winters of Europe and America it is still a valuable cough and cold medication with honey (and often brandy). Within its rind are the precious essential oils, and a soothing massage oil for aching feet is made by warming 1 cup of rind with 1 cup of almond oil in a double boiler for 40 minutes. Strain and bottle in a dark glass bottle to protect the essential oils.

A charming way of using kumquats is to prick holes all over a ripe kumquat and to insert cloves into it, tightly packed together. Dry it in the sun, hanging by a ribbon that has been pinned into it. Once dry, place a few drops of oil of cloves on the clove-studded kumquat and hang a little cluster of these dried kumquats in the bathroom, or toilet, or the kitchen cupboards, to keep the air fresh smelling. It makes a beautiful gift too, and one that lasts many years.

Health Note

Kumquat is a good source of vitamins C and A, calcium, iron, magnesium, phosphorus, potassium and dietary fibre.

Strawberry

Fragaria ananassa

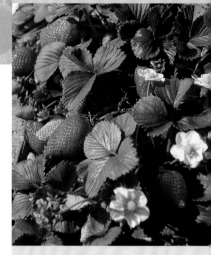

Indigenous to Europe and to many parts of the world, the wild strawberry was a much-loved fruit that was brought into the limelight by a happy accident around 1714. A French engineer working in Peru and Chile noticed the strawberries growing wild there was bigger and juicier than the ones he knew and grew in France, and took some plants home to grow when his job was completed. The plants struggled to adapt in France and a natural crossbreeding occurred between his own European strawberries and some from North America he was already growing, and the new plants from Peru and Chile. The result was a large, sweet, intensely flavoured and very juicy hybrid-strawberry that became the foundation of the strawberries we enjoy today!

Once a luxury food of the rich, it was only in the 19th century when the railways were constructed that the strawberry could reach the faraway places and many varieties have subsequently been established from those original species: the Chilean strawberry (*Fragaria chiloensis)*, the American strawberry (*Fragaria virginiana*) and the European wild strawberry (*Fragaria vesca*).

Interestingly, it was only by the 13th century that the wild strawberries began to be grown in cottage gardens and the monks grew enough in their cloister gardens to make medicinal remedies, and in medieval times the strawberry, in syrups or mashed with honey, became a treatment for many ailments. The monks even made a strawberry wine for the winter months – which was thought to be a cure for almost anything! For headaches and for backaches strawberry compresses became so popular that they were preserved in vinegar for easy application.

Growing Strawberries

Choose a sunny site with deeply dug, richly composted soil. Plant out the runners or established small plants 30 cm apart in moist, friable soil and keep them well watered until they root well. Tough and weather resistant, low growing and easy to manage, a twice weekly watering will ensure strong mother stock and the best time to start new runners is in the autumn, but plants can be set out at any time of the year.

Mulching in late winter with straw is invaluable so as to keep the berries off the soil and avoid insect damage. Cover the area with strong woven bird nets to ensure the ripening fruits are safe or you will have no crop! Not even scarecrows scare the birds, but black strings tautly stretched crisscross over beds about 40 cm high will protect the ripening fruits to a large extent.

In the late winter the first strawberries can be protected by plant fleece, a thin fabric that can be placed over the beds supported by wire hoops. This creates a warm 'hot house' effect and protects the fruit, and you'll be picking in late winter!

Using Strawberries

I learned to make strawberry jam from our own strawberries at the age of seven, and from that day to this I crave my own strawberry jam. It was many years later that I learned about their high levels of flavonoids, which protect against cancer, inflammation, heart disease, arthritis, asthma, and are gaining prominence as a potent anti-aging food. With their antiviral, antibacterial and anti-cancer activity, we should all be growing strawberries and fill every available space with pots and hanging baskets. Pick these succulent beauties to add to your muesli, or add them to homemade ice-creams, jellies and smoothies.

Mashed, fresh strawberries, spread evenly over the face for 10 minutes while you relax in the bath, make an excellent face mask, and mixed with rolled oats, they make a superb cleanser for spotty skin.

Strawberry Smoothie for Get-up-and-go

Serves 1

6–8 large ripe strawberries freshly picked
¾ cup plain Bulgarian yoghurt
1 peeled and sliced apple
1 teaspoon honey
1 tablespoon freshly ground almonds
1 tablespoon freshly ground flaxseed
1 tablespoon freshly ground sesame seed
½ teaspoon cinnamon
½ a banana

Whirl everything together in a liquidiser. Serve in a glass with a spoon and taste summer!

Health Note

Strawberries are a fabulous source of vitamins C, K B1, B5, B6, folic acid, beta-carotene, biotin, potassium, iodine and manganese.

Soya Bean

Glycine max

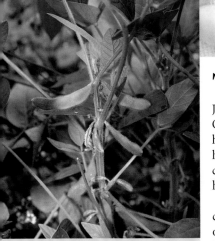

The soya bean is one of the most ancient annual crops. Indigenous to China, it has been grown for over 13 000 years as a staple, treasured food crop. It was part of the ancient trades between China, Japan, Korea, Taiwan and Malaysia and spread slowly into Asia and eventually into the New World. Originally used in Chinese medicine to treat fevers, respiratory ailments and circulatory disorders, it has its roots firmly in ancient Chinese traditional medicines and writings. For thousands of years it has been known as the 'meat of the earth'. In 2800 BC Emperor Shen Nung of China recorded it as his country's most important food crop. Legend and history are woven around soya and few other plants have ever matched its noble status.

The first soya beans reached Europe only by the 18th century and the United States by the early 19th century where it was grown mainly as cattle feed. A useful and versatile crop, prized for its valuable oils and proteins, therapeutic properties and exceptionally high nutritional value, the soya bean became, and has remained, one of the world's most sought after commodities, not only as a health food but also for its industrial applications where it is used in the manufacture of soaps, linoleums, paints, inks, even synthetic fibres and adhesives.

Growing Soya

Sown directly in spring into moist, richly composted, deeply dug soil in full sun, the small hairy pods develop quickly. The soya bush grows about 40–50 cm in height and ideally needs to be spaced 40 cm apart. Watering needs to be consistent in its early development and a furrow is the ideal way to allow the soil to be kept evenly moist. Thereafter once the plants have established well, a slow watering twice a week is usually sufficient.

Using Soya

Soya beans contain over 35% protein, 20% fixed oil, 22 health-building amino acids and lecithin, making it not only the perfect vegetarian food but also a valuable benefit for both the circulatory system and the nervous system. With its polyunsaturated acids, isoflavones and a host of exceptional properties, soya beans are also excellent for treating menopause symptoms, mimicking oestrogen in the body; acting as a general tonic, toning muscles and stimulating the liver and the kidneys; and helping to reverse the toxic effects of overmedication and wrong eating. For diabetics soya is superb. It contains phytoestrogen, which medical research suggests could help to prevent breast cancer and ovarian cancers – interestingly, Chinese women remain the healthiest after menopause. Soya milk is often recommended as an alternative to cows' milk and is enjoyed by many suffering from milk lactose intolerances and high cholesterol. Soya has an alkaline effect on the body, regulates the bowels, is good for treating high cholesterol and can help to dissolve gallstones and repair the arteries. The Chinese eat a bowl of soya bean soup daily as a health builder.

You can eat soya sprouts and green soya 'peas', or use the mashed cooked beans as a facial scrub over problem, oily skins, or use it as a cleansing mask – it acts as a gentle exfoliator removing oily build-up, softening blackheads and for teenage acne and spots, soya mash is an excellent beauty treatment.

Fresh green pods can be reaped and the beans, called edamame, cooked like green peas. Sprouting soya and eating those young and tender sprouts in a salad with lemon juice is a superb health food, or add the sprouts to stir-fries and spring rolls.

Soya flour is used in baked goods, pancakes and sweets, cakes and desserts and a bowl of cooked cooled mature soya beans served with lemon juice and a sprinkle of herbs and salt is an excellent snack replacing peanuts. When cooking dried soya beans, soak them overnight in warm water and cook them slowly in plain water with no salt or flavourings until tender.

Health Note

Soya is rich in phosphorus, iron, calcium, vitamins B1, B2, B6, C and E, beta-carotene as well as the omega-3 fatty acids.

Caution

Be aware that soya is a common allergen.

Those with thyroid problems should limit their consumption of raw or sprouted soya beans. (Cooking soya beans will inactivate the goitrogenic compounds within the soya bean, so cooked soya beans are safe.)

Women who have had breast tumours should limit their soya intake if these tumours are oestrogen sensitive.

Hint

Soya beans grown in poor, overgrazed, overused soils make an incredible green manure crop, a green fertiliser or 'smoother crop' that in one season, ploughed back into the soil, will literally revitalise and rejuvenate the soil. Green soya plants laid over compost will reactivate it, adding superb vitamins and minerals to the heap.

Niger
Ramtil

Guizotia abyssinica

I have only recently become familiar with a strange and fascinating plant known as 'niger' or 'niger seed'. My first rows sown in spring yielded a metre-high crop of rough textured leaves and small yellow flowers which, like little miniature sunflowers, hold the extraordinary oil-rich seeds. Narrow and black, shiny and quite soft, the seeds of this precious plant, which originated in Ethiopia and East Africa, are fiercely guarded due to their oil content.

Little is known about niger other than it became an early trade with India because it is tolerant of low rainfall, poor soil and neglect and in times of famine the seeds can be stored for long periods without becoming rancid. It has been a cultivated crop in Ethiopia and India for centuries where it is known by the Bengali name of ramtil and where both the seeds and the bright yellow flower petals are fried, often with coriander or cumin or caraway seed, and added to fruits or other seeds to make a relish or chutney. It is thought that 'niger seed cake' – crushed seeds mixed with honey – were traded and sold for religious ceremonies in the early centuries and also sold or traded as a medicine for skin ailments, and crushed and applied to wounds and sores. Ground in hollow stones with smooth river rocks, the elders of the tribe became the medicine makers and the growers of this precious oil-rich seed.

Chickens picking at the rough leaves and at the fallen seeds became succulent and fat with glossy feathers. Today most niger seed is sold as an oil-rich seed for caged birds and can be found in commercial bird seed mixes, but the Ethiopians still grow it, treasure it and use it, as do the Bengalis as a substitute for ghee (see note). Its precious oils are so health-building, niger seed has remained, one could say, a national treasure for Ethiopia.

Growing Niger

I am fascinated by its strong presence in our kitchen gardens. The leaves are rough and tough and survive hot winds, heat, hail storms and last all summer long as a survivor plant. It is an annual and we sow the elongated black seeds in full sun into deeply dug, well-composted soil that is raked into a flat wide 'furrow' so that moisture can be retained within its raised edges. A quickly maturing annual, it starts flowering soon after it gains height and where it has access to good compost and deep watering it reaches 1½ m in height. The small yellow flowers are abundant and are harvested as soon as they have matured and have begun to dry out. Harvesting is often by hand but in India, which has become the major producer, it has become mechanised.

The rough hairy leaves and stems are a valuable addition to the compost heap, adding much-needed silica to the heap and they break down quickly when smothered with grass clippings and raked leaves.

Using Niger

The ripe seeds are the main part of the plant that is used. The oil from those seeds is known as 'noog' in Ethiopia and 'negrillo' in Spanish and is sold as a cooking oil, or ground fried seeds are made into a delicious small sweet cake or sweet, much loved by children. Mixed with honey, fruit like mangoes and dates, or green peppers and brinjals, niger is a delicious ingredient in chutneys or relishes.

After the oil has been extracted, the 'oil cake' is a nutritious and much sought-after cattle feed, so enriching the milk of milk cows that farmers to this day have a bartering system that pleases everyone! I look at the rough textured leaves with much interest and wonder if the leaves could be added to the feeding system for cattle mixed with the oil residue cakes. My farm life for 25 years with a Friesland milk herd never leaves my thoughts!

Health Note

It has been established that niger seed contains linoleic and oleic fatty acids as well as vitamins A, B and E, and it has a high mineral content, in particular silica, calcium and potassium.

Niger Seed Dressing

Look out for niger seed oil – specialist Indian delicatessen shops sell it. It is clear, nutty and delicious and can be mixed with olive oil or other oils as a salad dressing with fresh lemon juice. Or try the following mouth-watering condiment:

1 tablespoon niger seeds, crushed or minced
1 cup homemade peach or apricot jam
½ tablespoon crushed coriander seeds
1 cup chopped fresh green coriander leaves
½ cup lemon juice
honey to taste

Mix everything together and serve with hard-boiled eggs or cold meats or on baked potatoes or pasta or add to curries. The taste is tantalising!

A Note on Vegetable Ghee

The vegetable ghee, known as vanaspati, could contain niger seed and much discussion rages around it. As it is a largely unsaturated vegetable fat product, made from oil-producing seeds, it has the advantage of containing less cholesterol than ghee, which is based on butter. Vanaspati is eaten where religion forbids the consumption of any animal products. As niger seed has a low rancidity it is thought that vanaspati could incorporate this delicious nutty-flavoured oil.

Sunflower

Helianthus annuus

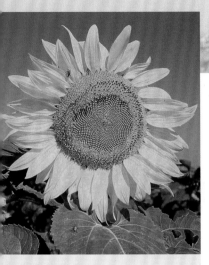

Sunflower Energy Sweets

For cyclists, hikers and joggers, this is a power-packed energy booster and is equally loved as a school lunch box treat or as a snack at anytime. It is an excellent and healthy substitute for a chocolate bar!

1 cup sunflower seeds
¾ cup sesame seeds
¾ cup flaxseed (linseed)
2 teaspoons cinnamon powder
1 tablespoon carob powder
desiccated coconut (or coconut flakes)

Grind the seeds together in a seed grinder. Mix in the cinnamon and the carob powder, then mix in enough runny honey to bind it all together into a stiff dough (about ½ to ¾ of a cup of honey, but start with a little and add more as needed). Pinch off pieces and roll into balls between fingers that have been smeared with a little sunflower oil. Now roll the little ball in fresh desiccated coconut or in coconut flakes and store on greaseproof paper in an airtight container in the fridge.

Hint

A bowl of hulled pumpkin seeds, sunflower seeds and almonds and pecan nuts is the perfect snack food for children and teenagers as this combination literally bursts with vitamins and minerals.

A robust, spectacular and much-loved food plant, the sunflower in all its glory is indigenous to North and South America. In cultivation for over 5 000 years by the Native Americans who have used all parts of the plant for so many centuries, its history is long, fascinating and exciting. It is a giant, not only in its actual height and size, but also in the rich diversity in its oils, its seeds, its flower buds, its dried stalks as a fuel and in its pollution cleansing properties. The sunflower is a symbol of hope, of light, of nourishment. It is the state flower of Kansas and Russia's national flower! One of the biggest flowers in the world, it has been adopted by many countries and today it is a valuable oil crop in South Africa, Spain, France, China, Peru, Russia, Argentina and in several states of the USA. Its history is incredible: the seeds sold as food were spread first by the Spanish explorers who took it to Europe, and its great presence extended quickly into adjoining countries. It was received as a spectacular gift from the New World and European countries went wild with excitement! Never had there been so astonishing and huge a flower and the Greeks named it 'Helios', the Greek word for sun, and 'Anthos' the Greek word for flower, and so its Latin name *Helianthus* was born. Trade in sunflower seeds was brisk and trade routes throughout Europe and beyond flourished by the 16th century.

Growing Sunflowers

An easy-to-grow annual crop, seed sown in spring brings a quick harvest and new crops can be sown well into summer, as it matures quickly. Sow the seeds in full sun in well-dug soil to which rich compost has been added. Plant in a row in a furrow so that water can be run in from one end once or twice weekly. It grows astonishingly quickly and needs watering more frequently in the very hot summers. In heavy winds a stake is sometimes needed to support the massive heavy head as it ripens and bird-scares with flapping streamers or shiny CD disks or scarecrows are needed to chase the ever-watchful flocks who relish the seeds! Leave the plants to dry before reaping.

Using Sunflowers

In the 16th century Russia grew it as a valuable oil crop and oil-rich cultivars were gradually introduced, trialled and recorded. Sunflower seed oil, mild, bland and rich in vitamin E and polyunsaturated fats, became one of the world's favourite oils and remains so to this day. The oil helps to lower cholesterol levels and is a favourite and inexpensive cooking oil all over the world, and is used externally as an excellent massage oil for aching muscles, dry cracked skin and for rheumatic swellings and pain. Interestingly, sunflower oil supplies more vitamin E than any other oil. The seeds have been taken medicinally for centuries to treat bronchial infections, tuberculosis and to treat malaria. The entire plant has been used for centuries – the leaves and petals included.

As the plant matures into its main huge head, along the stem secondary buds that may ripen into small flowers, form. It is those young and tender buds, when about the size of a golf ball, that make a delicious vegetable dish boiled until tender and served with a rich cheese sauce and lemon juice.

Sprouted seeds are a superb health food, rich in anti-cancer, anti-inflammatory and anti-allergenic properties as well as vitamins and minerals (see Health Note). It is worth growing your own sunflowers to reap organic seed for sprouts to add to salads as a superb energy booster.

Health Note

Sunflower seeds are high in vitamins E, B1, B5 and B6, folic acid, calcium, copper, zinc, iron, phosphorus, potassium, sodium, and mono- and polyunsaturated fats. The seeds are also an excellent source of protein and dietary fibre.

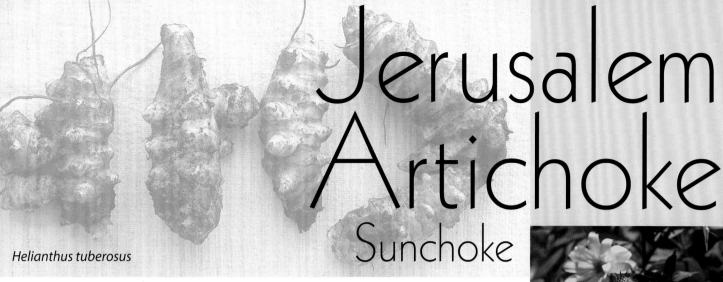

Jerusalem Artichoke
Sunchoke

Helianthus tuberosus

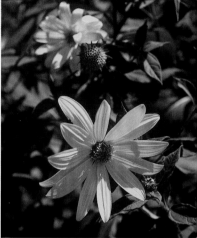

The Jerusalem artichoke is a root or tuber, and no relation whatsoever to the globe artichoke and the cardoon. It produces a tall and vigorous 2-metre-high branched annual flowering spike – the flowers are small and dazzling 'sunflowers' – and below the ground the treasure trove of juicy edible rhizomes or tubers, often enough to fill a bucket if the soil has been rich and the rains good.

Indigenous to North America, it grew wild along the eastern coastline, from the Great Lakes in Canada down to Georgia. It spread with ease as a delectable trade, a strange and remarkable delicacy cultivated by the Native Americans living along the coast. They called the tubers 'sun roots' and introduced it first of all to the pilgrims. Around the early part of the 1600s a French explorer, Samuel de Champlain, first tasted the Jerusalem artichoke in a gruel or soup made by the Native Americans, and so enjoyed it that he took the tubers back to France and from there it quickly spread through Europe.

The artichoke reached England by 1617 and Germany by 1632, and by then it was called 'Jerusalem artichoke' officially for this reason: The English had acquired their first consignment of tubers from the town 'Ter Neuzen' in the Netherlands, and Jerusalem sounded similar and easier to say. Others believe the Italians gave the plant the name 'girasole', literally meaning 'turning to the sun', and so perhaps it was this name that got corrupted to 'Jerusalem'. Either way, the actual plant has nothing whatsoever to do with Jerusalem as we know it today!

Growing Jerusalem Artichokes

Tuck the tubers into deeply dug, richly composted soil that is moist and loamy, loose and friable. Space them 40 cm apart as each tuber will produce several 'babies' which will mature to its own size. Water deeply twice a week in hot weather. The 2 metre tall, branched flowering stem with its bright array of small 'sunflowers' makes a spectacular show – so plant the artichokes at the back of the vegetable garden.

Dig up the tubers once the flowering head dies down at the end of the summer. Leave them in the ground to keep them fresh until needed otherwise they quickly shrivel and dry out.

Using Jerusalem Artichokes

The Native Americans used the boiled tuber as a dressing as hot as could be tolerated over a ripe boil or abscess, or over a suppurating wound or as a comforting treatment over sprains, strains, bruises and arthritic joints. Fresh, raw artichoke is an ancient remedy for clearing blocked noses and catarrh, and for opening blocked ears. Chew a small piece or two thoroughly. For diabetics the artichoke is a much-loved plant as it produces levulose sugars (a type of fructose) which diabetics can eat.

It can be added to soups, stews, grated fresh into salads, dipped in batter once parboiled and then fried, or served boiled with a white cheese sauce as the French do, as a lunch dish. Note that eating artichokes too quickly and in too great an abundance causes flatulence! So always eat caraway seeds and fresh mint with artichokes and sip a cup of strong mint tea after eating them.

Health Note

The Jerusalem artichoke is rich in carbohydrates and potassium, with some calcium, phosphorus, magnesium, chlorine, sulphur and a small amount of iron, as well as vitamin C and a little vitamin E.

Jerusalem Artichoke Soup

Serves 6–8

sunflower oil
4 medium onions, finely chopped
8 cups of well-scrubbed, chopped fresh Jerusalem artichokes tubers
6 medium-sized potatoes, peeled and chopped
2 litres of good, rich chicken stock
sea salt and black pepper to taste
2 teaspoons caraway seeds
1 tablespoon crushed coriander seed
½ cup parsley

In a heavy bottomed pot in a little sunflower oil, brown the onions lightly, then add all the other ingredients except the parsley. Simmer gently, stirring often until the vegetables are tender (usually 1 hour). Whirl in a liquidiser and serve in bowls sprinkled with parsley.

Hint

Buy tubers, when you see them, from the greengrocer and plant them to start this fascinating crop.

Rosella

Roselle ▪ African Mallow ▪ Jamaica Sorrel

Hibiscus sabdariffa

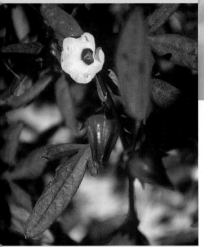

'Karkade' – Rosella Drink

In a heavy bottomed pot pour 2 litres of boiling water over 2 cups of rosella calyxes, either fresh or dried. Add 1 stick of cinnamon and 1 tablespoon of cloves. Simmer with the lid on very gently for 45 minutes. Top up the water as it boils away.

Now strain out the spices and the calyxes and discard. Return the beautifully coloured rosella to the pot. Add 2 cups of sugar, stir well and simmer for a further 15 minutes. Stand aside to cool.

Dilute the syrup with iced water to taste (usually ¼–½ glass of rosella syrup), fill up the glass with iced water and ice and a slice of fresh lemon. Sip it slowly, thinking of 'the ladies of the court'!

Health Note

Rich in vitamins, especially vitamin C, and several amino acids, and high in potassium, iron, calcium, riboflavin, rosella makes an excellent health drink (see recipe above).

This is a most beautifully inspiring plant, a colourful annual that fascinates everyone who seeds it. It grows to between 1 and 2 metres in height and its typically *Hibiscus* flowers are pale yellow, in a succulent and predominant dark red calyx. The sour, dark red leaves are prized as a type of spinach and in its native countries it is a treasured plant diligently planted every spring.

Indigenous to India, Malaysia and North Africa, rosella is grown in all subtropical regions of the world with passion. An extraordinary trade has always been woven around rosella and the ancient Arabic word *karkade* names a delicious sour drink that has been served to royalty in several countries through the centuries. It has been known as 'the drink of the ladies of the court'.

The first records of its health-giving properties go back to Java in 1687 where the leaves were sold as a food – a type of spinach – and the calyxes as as a medicinal tea. As a trade it fetched high prices and it spread with speed onto the ships of the explorers who made a tea of the brilliant red calyxes for treating the sailors' scurvy, sore throats, colds, 'flu and chest ailments.

It reached Mexico and then Australia during the 17th century. There was an interesting interlude in 1895 when the Australians shared seed with the Californian Agricultural Experimental Farms hoping to promote a 'rosella jelly industry' as rosella is similar in taste and in medicinal properties to the cranberry and is so much more prolific and easier to grow than the cranberry, which only grows in certain moist areas in the Californian bogs. This never took off, but the dream remains, and my own experiments with rosella jellies, jams, syrups, teas and cool drinks as well as chewy sweets have been profitable enough to inspire extra plantings.

Growing Rosella

I started growing rosella in the mid 1970s from seed I had been able to buy from German farmers in the Muden area in KwaZulu-Natal. A Portuguese visitor later brought me new seeds, calling it 'vinagreira'. I grew the rosella from Muden in one area and the rosella from Portugal in another, both partnering mealies, chillies and cassavas, as the West Indians do. It thrived and I had enough calyxes to sell and I sold this strange red tea for winter coughs and colds to a steady stream of visitors. My plantings in full sun thrived in their compost-rich soil, no insect damage, no aphids and no mildew. Under-planted with creeping oregano, we kept having bumper crops with only a weekly watering.

I start off the rosella plants in the hot house in August in bags for planting out in full sun and in richly composted soil in September's heat when all chances of frost are gone. It thrives with a twice weekly watering in hot weather. By the summer's end the calyxes are swollen and we reap the whole plant, we peel off the calyx by hand, save the marble-sized seed capsule and toss the stems onto the compost heap.

Using Rosella

Rosella tea is a superb remedy for sore throats, tonsillitis, 'flu, coughs, colds, bronchitis, tuberculosis and chronic chest ailments, taken daily or even twice daily in acute stages. Pour 1 cup of boiling water over ¼ cup of fresh or dried calyxes, stand 5 minutes, stir well, sweeten with a touch of honey and sip slowly.

A lotion can be made of the fibre-rich stems by boiling 4–6 cups of chopped stems and leaves in 2 litres of water for 20 minutes with the lid on. Cool, strain and use as a wash for rashes, insect bites, stings and for sunburn. Keep the excess in the fridge in a spritz spray bottle. Use the lotion or the cooled tea for treating acne, oily problem skin and for oily hair and dandruff. Use the cooled tea as a hair rinse after shampooing the hair.

Food industries across the world are using the brilliant red of rosella as a substitute for tartrazine and other coal tar dyes.

Barley

Hordeum distichon

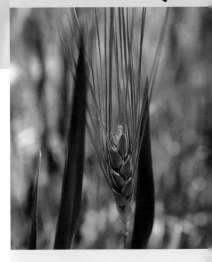

This ancient precious grain, grown in the winter months, has been cultivated all over the world since prehistoric times. In the 1st century AD, Dioscorides urged the consumption of barley gruel and barley water for sore throats, stomach ailments and to build health and warmth into the body.

Indigenous to Europe and the Mediterranean area, Roman gladiators ate barley for strength and endurance, and barley remains an important grain and, even though it was gradually supplanted by wheat during the Middle Ages, it is still today one of the most trusted and respected foods known to mankind. Its medicinal qualities are legendary, and today it is extensively marketed as 'green barley' products in every health shop.

Growing Barley

Sow in rows or scatter over deeply dug, richly composted soil in full sun during early autumn. Keep it moist and covered by a thin protective layer of dried leaves, as the birds love it, and this light mulch helps to retain the moisture too – do not let the area ever dry out – and the tiny vivid green little spears will soon push through.

Once the little barley sprouts reach 3–5 cm in height they can be pulled up and the whole little plant eaten – they are delicious in stir-fries. Or soak organic barley seed in warm water for at least 6 hours, drain and spread over a thick layer of wet cotton wool that has been placed in a large flat glass dish or on a tray, and allow the little seeds to sprout there. Keep the cotton wool wet at all times and set up trays a week apart for a continuous supply of succulent health-boosting sprouts.

Using Barley

Barley is one of the most superb natural cholesterol treatments we can take daily in the form of barley water – it literally sops up cholesterol. The bland and soothing barley water (see recipe alongside) soothes and heals stomach ulcers, digestive problems, cleanses and repairs and strengthens the liver, treats diarrhoea, helps to prevent hair loss by nourishing the hair and the nails, and even prevents tooth decay – it strengthens the gums. For asthmatics, barley should actually be part of the daily diet as it contains hordenine, which relieves bronchial spasms and releases tension in the lungs – this is worth talking to your doctor about. Barley is also one of the ancient treatments for releasing kidney stones. The monks during the Middle Ages gave barley water to those suffering from bowel and bladder ailments. Today irritable bowel syndrome responds beautifully to barley water.

Use the warmed strained grains as the most soothing and cleansing scrub on oily problem skin. This was an ancient treatment used to restore a healthy glow to the skin.

Our grandmothers used pearled barley in soups, stews and a jug of chilled barley water was always in the fridge to refresh with a good squeeze of fresh lemon juice and a slice or two of lemon at the end of a busy day. Generally the less processed the barley the better. Look out for wholegrain barley, barley flakes, barley grits and cracked barley in health shops.

Grow your own green barley in trays of rich compost, and make this barley health drink often: when the little sprouts reach around 10 cm in height, cut 2 handfuls and push through a spiral juicer, along with 1 peeled apple, 2 well-washed beetroots and 2 carrots, 2 celery sticks with leaves, 2 thick slices of peeled pineapple and 1 cup of fresh parsley sprigs. Drink it immediately – it is like a turbo boost!

Health Note

Barley is rich in the B-vitamins, especially vitamin B3 and folic acid, as well as vitamins C and K, and full of minerals – potassium, phosphorous, magnesium, zinc, manganese and calcium.

Barley Water

Simmer 1 cup of pearled barley, or better still organically grown unpearled barley if you can get it. Pour over this 2 litres water and simmer gently with the lid half on until tender – about 1 hour. Keep topping up the water. Cool. Strain through a colander, catching the water in a bowl. Pour the barley water into a glass jug and cover it. Store in the fridge. Save the soft grains and serve warm as a 'rice' with a little salt, black pepper and fresh lemon juice. Drink a glass of barley water daily, even 2 glasses, for high cholesterol, and eat the cooked barley grains once or twice a week.

Hint

Grow barley in the garden and once it turns golden, cut and twist it into small bundles tied into a net. Sink this into a pond, weighted with a stone, to keep the water clean and clear.

Sweet Potato

Ipomoea batatas

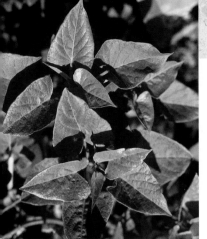

Easy Ways with Sweet Potato

Serve them well scrubbed if they are organically grown or lightly peeled, and steamed with a squeeze of lemon juice and a sprinkling of freshly grated nutmeg and a dab of butter – a simple, quick and easy dish that goes equally well with chicken, fish or meats.

Any leftovers can be mixed into fritters with finely chopped onions, green peppers and parsley and a beaten egg, which make a delicious lunchbox treat. You'll find you'll never tire of having sweet potatoes on the menu.

Health Note

The leaves and tubers are rich in vitamins A, B, C and E, folic acid, carotenes, phosphorus, copper, potassium, manganese, enzymes and unique proteins.

The sweet potato has proved through the centuries to be a true superfood! A perennial vine with a mass of tuberous roots that form along the nodes of the vine, the sweet potato is indigenous to parts of South America and it has an extraordinary and ancient and colourful history. Sweet potato relics dating back 10 000 years were discovered in Peruvian caves – making the sweet potato one of mankind's most ancient foods. A treasured food in prehistoric times, sweet potatoes became a hugely valuable crop and the ancient Colombians, Guatemalans and Peruvians were possibly the first growers of the sweet potato around 4500 BC.

Christopher Columbus, after his first voyage to the New World, returned to Spain with sweet potatoes and the first crop began on Spanish soil. Soon they were exported to England and King Henry VIII enjoyed them in sweet potato pies! Soon France showed interest in sweet potatoes and the first were planted in the gardens of Louis XV and by the 16th century Africa, southern Asia, India and Indonesia were all caught up in the sweet potato trade introduced by the Portuguese explorers.

Even more fascinating is that it has never ever lost its popularity nor been lost or neglected by any country, and today the greatest producers of sweet potatoes worldwide are China, Japan, Vietnam, India, Indonesia and Uganda! Not even its native lands can compete! In South Africa alone it is one of our main crops and sweet potatoes are available almost all year round as a staple food.

Growing Sweet Potatoes

Rewarding, easy and infinitely satisfying to grow, sweet potatoes thrive in deeply dug, richly composted soil in full sun. Planted in trenches spaced 75 cm to 1 m apart and lightly covered with soil and compost, run a hose gently down the trench twice a week in hot weather. The vines spread easily – train them into the furrow, as new potatoes will form at the nodes. Reaping the crop is done usually from late summer onwards. Dig carefully so as not to pierce or damage the tubers and to see if they are mature enough to dig out. If not, leave them another month or so.

Many cultures eat the sweet potato leaves as a green spinach and here I introduce a variety given to me by a young and dedicated vegetable farmer several years ago. Different to the ordinary sweet potato, this variety is thought to have originated in Mexico and came to Africa via Egypt. It has long and luscious vines with heart-shaped leaves and is grown more for its leaves, which when lightly cooked or steamed quickly make a superb spinach dish served with a dab of butter, a grinding of coarse sea salt and black pepper and a squeeze of lemon juice. A rampant and undemanding grower, the Mexican sweet potato is becoming hugely valuable for communities struggling to survive. It thrives in poor soil, often in adverse conditions, taking intense heat and drought as well as surviving deep into the winter when its leafy vines become dormant. It is then that the succulent yellow sweet potatoes can be dug up and turned into nourishing dishes.

Using Sweet Potatoes

Sweet potatoes are rich in valuable nutrients: their unique proteins have significant antioxidant effects and the high vitamin and mineral content (see Health Note) makes the sweet potato an excellent immune booster. Classified as an 'anti-diabetic' food, research finds the sweet potato actually helps to stabilise blood sugar levels and to improve the response to insulin.

Excellent for the whole digestive tract, for stomach ulcers and for a detox regime, the sweet potato will bind heavy metals and remove them from the body. Nutritionists suggest serving sweet potatoes at least three times a week to take advantage of their unique qualities.

Lettuce

Lactuca sativa

I f you say the word 'salad' anywhere in the world, it usually means lettuce! It is the most important of all salad crops and is grown in most countries across the globe and it has never lost is popularity. A huge and increasingly fascinating diversity of forms is cultivated today and it is thought that all these cultigens have been derived from the original wild lettuce, *Lactuca scariola*, indigenous to the eastern Mediterranean region and western Asia.

Used by the ancient Romans and Greeks as a medicinal plant, Augustus Caesar even had a statue made in honour of lettuce in gratitude for his recovery from a long illness! In Egypt cultivated lettuce goes back to 4500 BC, and in China, where lettuce has been cultivated since the 5th century AD, lettuce represents good luck and lettuce dishes served on birthdays, New Year's Day and special celebrations are traditionally accompanied by delicious sauces and condiments.

Lettuce belongs to the great Compositae family, along with daisies and sunflowers, and to the genus *Lactuca*, and there are four main categories within this genus and all are steadfastly popular:

Iceberg Lettuce: A large-head lettuce, darker leaves on the outside, pale to almost white in the heart. Known as 'crisp-head lettuce' in some countries, this is the basic salad lettuce.

Romaine or Cos Lettuce: A continental favourite with a long, deep-green, crisp head and much enjoyed with bacon and croutons. Traditionally used for the well-known dish, Caesar Salad.

Butterhead: Tender, large, soft leaves that form a loose head. Easy to grow, sweet and buttery, it is served often with chopped hard-boiled eggs and mayonnaise or with diced avocado pear and lemon juice as a summer luncheon in France and Italy and here in our own sunny South Africa as well.

Loose Leaf: Easily raised from seed, new varieties are emerging every season, from 'Lollo Rosso' to 'Oak Leaf' in shades of green and burgundy, to curly-leafed 'Ruby' and pale lime-greens, and frills and serrated edges, the choice is endless. These are the cut-and-come-again varieties – you only pick the outer leaves, leaving the rest to grow on. As an added bonus, they look beautiful for a long time in the garden.

Growing Lettuce

In the heat of summer lettuce needs to be partially shaded. If you live in a very hot area leave the lettuce growing for the winter months as in the heat it bolts easily, leaving it bitter and inedible.

Sow the seeds thinly in autumn in a long, deeply dug, well-composted, moist furrow. Lightly sprinkle with sand or soft soil, just enough to cover them, and then sprinkle a layer of dry leaves or leafy sprigs to shield the tiny seeds from the sun. They must not dry out, so water daily. When they are big enough to handle, carefully prick out the seedlings that grow too closely together and plant out in moist, deeply dug, richly composted soil 30 cm apart. Lettuce thrives with water, so water it twice or even three times a week if the weather is hot.

Using Lettuce

Lettuce soup or gruel, served with onions and celery, has been used by the monks since medieval times to treat anaemia, insomnia, constipation, obesity, catarrh, tuberculosis, gout and circulatory conditions. Modern research verifies these uses and adds that eating lettuce is good for arthritis, urinary tract ailments, rheumatism, acne and problem skin, and nervousness, anxiety and high stress levels.

French chefs include lettuce in potato and pea soups or with leeks and green peppers as a vegetable dish in a white sauce.

Health Note

Lettuce is the slimmer's favourite salad ingredient as it is so low in kilojoules! It has an array of vitamins – A, B, C, E – as well as the minerals phosphorus, potassium, calcium and iron, especially in the darker green leaves.

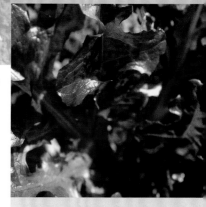

Green Lettuce, Leek and Pea Soup

Serves 6

4 cups leeks, thinly sliced
olive oil
6 cups thinly shredded lettuce leaves, especially all the outer leaves (our favourites are butter lettuce, cos lettuce and the outer leaves of green or red oak leaf lettuce)
2 cups celery, thinly sliced
1 cup finely chopped parsley
4–6 cups young pea pods, chopped with tendrils and tips of the pea vines
freshly squeezed lemon juice
4 cups peeled, coarsely grated sweet potato
sea salt and black pepper to taste
2 litres strong chicken stock

Sear the leeks in enough olive oil to cover the bottom of a heavy stainless steel pot. Stir-fry until they are golden. Add the celery and stir-fry, then the chopped pea pods and the chopped vine tips and tendrils and stir-fry. Lastly add the grated sweet potatoes and stir well. Now add the lettuce, the parsley (keep a little aside for sprinkling on as you serve it), the lemon juice and finally the chicken stock. Taste as you stir and add more lemon juice, salt and pepper. Simmer gently until tender, usually no more than 10–15 minutes. On a very cold day add a little grating of fresh ginger and a sprinkle of cayenne pepper and a spoonful or two of a rich fruit chutney to really warm you up.

Calabash
Bottle Gourd

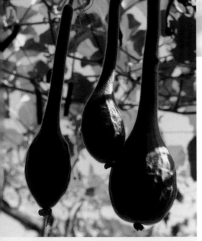

Calabash Stir-Fry

Serves 4

Select a young and tender calabash, soft enough to sink your thumbnail into the skin. Peel and slice it thinly and chop up into squares. Leave the seeds in if they are still soft.

Fry a thinly sliced onion in a little olive oil. Add the calabash squares and stir-fry. Add the juice of one lemon, 2 cups of sliced brown mushrooms, salt and black pepper to taste, and 1 cup of chopped green pepper. Stir-fry until tender. Serve with crusty bread.

Calabash Soup

Serves 4–6

a little olive oil
3 medium onions, finely chopped
3 tender calabashes, peeled and cut into small pieces
3 cups vine tips and young leaves
2 green peppers, finely chopped
6 potatoes, peeled and chopped
2 litres good chicken stock

Stir-fry the onions in the olive oil until brown. Add the rest of the vegetables and lastly the chicken stock. Simmer until tender. Season with the juice of 2 lemons, sea salt and black pepper. Serve hot.

This wonderful annual climber was one of the first crops I grew as a young bride on a distant farm. I was given the seeds by an old Zulu gardener at Pretoria University where I studied Physiotherapy. He told me I would always be rich if I grew calabashes, and I have grown them all my life. And yes, you are rich growing calabashes: rich in food, rich in interest, rich in utensils!

As a plant of Africa and used as trade since the early centuries, the calabash has spread throughout the world where it always has been a loved and cherished crop. Records show it began life well before 5000 BC in Africa from where it is believed it floated across the seas buoyantly and safely sheltering its seeds, and ended across the Atlantic Ocean in South America. There it grew, produced a crop and was carried on to Asia, where today it is a cherished crop.

The gourd or calabash was one of mankind's first utensils – a spoon, a storage vessel, a bowl – and in South America an ancient tradition of tracing and carving out an intricate pattern on its ripening and hardening outer shell or skin, still continues today. It is grown, eaten and used as receptacles throughout China, Malaysia, Burma, the Philippines, Java and Sri Lanka today, and forms part of traditional ceremonies and feasts.

Growing Calabashes

At the first sign of warmth after the winter, prepare a bed in full sun and dig in lots of compost and moisten well. In this way the soil will warm up. Wait until all signs of the frost and cold have gone and spring is well and truly here. Set a fence along the bed where the calabash vines can climb and plant the seeds 30 cm apart, two or three next to each other. Cover with grass and leaves to keep the soil warm and protected. Watch for the little plants to peep through the leaves and keep a close watch for cutworms.

Train up the vines as soon as they are long enough and keep the plants well watered. They will grow prolifically. Keep training the velvety vines as they spread and cover the small fruits gently as they form in fine netting to prevent the birds and the wasps from getting to them. It grows rapidly and attractively with masses of five-petalled white flowers.

Using Calabashes

Rich in nutrients, the calabash is an important part of the diet in many countries. The young tips of the vines and tender young leaves can be steamed like a spinach and are delicious in stir-fries and soups. The young and tender gourd can be eaten steamed and sliced, or fried in batter, or grated into soups.

As the fruit matures it can be sliced and boiled and mashed to make a thick soup with dried beans that have been soaked and cooked until tender. This is the soup that forms a base for many other ingredients and is given to travellers for energy, to young nursing mothers to increase milk flow, and to growing children and the elderly to strengthen the bones.

There are many varieties of gourds and many dishes are traditionally prepared using the young and green fruits. Dried calabashes are a favourite tourist memento and I have sold so many thousands of calabashes to visitors through the years from my farm shop. I often think this must be what the old Zulu meant – trade in calabashes has been on-going for centuries.

I stored water in my biggest giant calabash in the cool shade under the thorn trees, with a ladle made of a smaller calabash with which to 'skep' it out. On a hot summer's day no water ever tasted so cool, so delicious or so refreshing.

Health Note

Calabash is rich in vitamins C, D and E, as well as potassium, and contains moderate amounts of iron and zinc.

Lentil

Lens culinaris

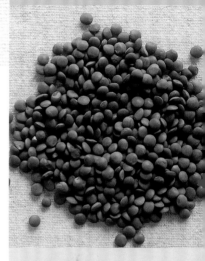

One of the most ancient foods on earth, the lentil is a Biblical food, its very beginnings going back some 6000 BC! It is nothing short of miraculous that so tiny a little 'bean', a pulse, could have been, and still is today, so precious a food that it was found in the pyramids, in the tombs of the Egyptian pharaohs, and it is mentioned in the Old Testament in Genesis in the story of Jacob and Esau, how Esau considered the bowl of lentil soup, 'mes of potage', so tasty, far more valuable than his inheritance!

The lentil is so ancient and so precious a cultigen that it has literally been a part of history. It is thought to have originated as a wild lentil, *Lens orientalis*, in the Near East, Turkey and Afghanistan, as shown by ancient archaeological excavations that date back to 6500 BC, and one at Qalat Jarmo in Iraq that dates back to 6750 BC! Chinese archaeologists found canisters of red lentils in the Han tombs, so by this it is evident that over 2 000 years ago the Chinese ate red lentils. In Bronze Age settlements in Switzerland excavators discovered lentils, indicating how widespread and valuable this food became.

Growing Lentils

Just for fun try to grow some lentils. There are three colours: red lentils, green lentils and the easy-to-sprout and easy-to-grow brown lentils, which are still in their 'skins'. They thrive in well-dug, well-composted soil in full sun. Mark off rows and scatter the little seeds thinly over moist soil and rake in. Often rows of lentils were sown in cooler weather between rows of wheat or barley, both of which take the frost and which protect the lower-growing lentils. But it is also grown as a summer crop.

Little pods form following tiny pea-like pink or white or mauve flowers, and the pods hold one or two 'lens'-shaped seeds, hence its Latin name. The ripe seeds are reaped by hand as the tiny leafed bushes are too tangled and small to reap by mechanical means.

A quick annual, the green leafy bush is a superb compost maker, and rich in nitrogen once the lentil pods have been reaped. The only part used is the ripe seed and to this day it remains a valuable and nutritious and tasty food the world over.

Using Lentils

Often used as a staple food to replace meat, before the 1st century AD lentils were introduced to India where to this day they are made into a deliciously spiced dish known as *dahl*. Lentils are considered to be an excellent heart tonic and body builder and are particularly valuable in cases of low blood pressure, anaemia, emaciation, and for ulcerated stomachs and ulcerated digestive tracts.

Lentils are a superb source of dietary fibre and this is extremely valuable for lowering high cholesterol and managing blood sugar, as their high protein and high fibre content helps to control the rapid rise of blood sugar levels after a meal. Research between 1991 and 1995 showed a significant reduction in breast cancer in the women who ate lentils (or beans) daily or even 2 or 3 times a week, and subsequent trials prove this.

Traditional lentil dishes from many countries offer so huge a variety of tastes, and it is becoming more important to include them in the diet and to encourage the whole family to eat this valuable food. Lentils are an excellent meat substitute and are easily digested as a soup or mash by invalids, the very elderly and babies, and by the most picky of eaters. Lentil soups, stews and casseroles are an excellent standby for energy, vitality and for hypoglycaemia. For anaemia a daily helping of lentils is of such great value we need to sit up and take notice.

Health Note

Lentils are rich in protein, dietary fibre, the B-vitamins, vitamins A and C, calcium, iron, potassium and phosphorus.

Lentil Salad

2 cups brown lentils
1 chopped green pepper
1 cup chopped spring onions
1 cup chopped pineapple
1 cup chopped celery
½ cup chopped parsley
½ cup olive oil
juice of 1 lemon
sea salt and black pepper

Cook the lentils in 1½ litres of rapidly boiling water until tender – do not cook with salt – about 40 minutes. Drain and cool. Add the rest of the ingredients to the cooled lentils. Serve with cold chicken or baked potato.

Lentil Soup

Serves 4–6

a little olive oil
2 large onions, finely chopped
2 cups brown lentils
2 cups chopped celery, leaves included
4 large tomatoes, peeled and finely chopped
4 cups finely shredded cabbage
2 litres chicken stock
juice of 2 lemons

Brown the onions in the olive oil. Add all the other ingredients. Simmer until tender (about 40 minutes). Season with sea salt and black pepper. Serve hot.

Lovage

Levisticum officinale

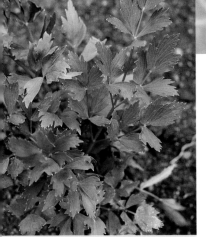

Lovage has to be the most flavour-filled herb known to mankind! It literally bursts with flavour and became so popular among the ancient Greeks and Romans that it was used as a trade. Known as the 'Maggi herb' for its extensive use in flavouring commercial soups, condiments, sauces and chutneys, lovage is still today grown extensively in its native Mediterranean areas to satisfy the demand for this extraordinary herb.

Lovage spread quickly through Europe during the Middle Ages and the monks and priests grew it in their medicinal cloister gardens to treat the sick, and to soothe the travel-worn, aching and battered feet of the weary traveller. Lovage tea, hot and steaming, was a much sought after brew for easing nausea, vomiting and over-imbibing and over-eating, and in rural Europe today lovage seeds, steeped in brandy, is still a much respected folk medicine – a teaspoon or two added to a glass of warm water for the 'morning-after' headache and nausea!

The ancient Romans gathered lovage leaves in the autumn before the plant died down for its winter dormancy, and preserved the leaves in vinegar, a practice that continues to this day. The roots were dug up during the winter to make hearty soups for the travellers coming to the 'ale houses', and the ancient Greeks made lovage gruels or thin soups served with their rich meals to aid digestion.

Growing Lovage

A robust and long-lasting perennial, lovage has adapted to many climates and grows easily in many parts of the world. It thrives in deeply dug, richly composted soil in full sun and it is propagated from seed. It has a long taproot and once it is planted does not like to be disturbed. Plant 50–60 cm apart and water slowly and deeply twice weekly.

Native to southwestern Asia and the Mediterranean areas, it takes as easily to the heat of a long summer as it does to the winter frosts, and it becomes dormant even in a mild winter.

It acts as a tonic to all the plants growing nearby and is particularly invigorating to beans, green sweet peppers and chilli, and it is attractive enough to grow amongst the flowers.

A tall flowering head with yellow umbels appears often in its third year and the seeds form, which are also used to flavour food. New plants are easily propagated from the ripe seed and an essential oil is commercially processed from the seeds, stems and roots in Europe today.

Using Lovage

Medicinally, lovage is a superb digestive herb and it has deodorising, sedative, anticonvulsant and anti-microbial properties. It is a warming, soothing tonic herb for both the respiratory and the digestive systems. It eases colic, treats coughs, makes a gargle for sore throats, clears catarrh, eases bronchitis and removes mucus, soothes urinary tract infections and menstrual cramps, and stimulates the kidneys to flush out toxins. It also clears problem skin, eases rheumatic pains, and is a strong diuretic – and all this from a cup of lovage tea! (Pour 1 cup of boiling water over ¼ cup of fresh lovage leaves, stand 5 minutes and sip slowly.)

Fresh leaves, finely chopped, can be added to sauces, chutneys and condiments, and will give taste to the blandest of soups – just a little, as it is a strong herb – and for stir-fries a sprinkling of freshly chopped leaves with fresh lemon juice will turn it into a feast. The stems can be candied (see recipe) and the roots grated into rich casseroles and meaty stews.

Health Note

Lovage is rich in digestive and volatile oils and natural flavourants.

Lovage Salt

Mix 1 cup of coarse sea salt with 1 cup of finely chopped lovage leaves and thin stems. Pack into a pepper grinder and use as a delicious flavouring over tomatoes, baked potatoes, stir-fries, and more.

Candied Lovage Stems

Fresh trimmed lovage stems can be candied by simmering them in a sugar syrup. Add 2 cups sugar to 1 cup water and simmer for 30 minutes. Then dry on greaseproof paper. Cut into pieces and use as cake decorations with cherries.

Hint

Make a quick lovage sauce for cheeses or cold chicken by adding ½ cup chopped lovage leaves to 1 cup apricot jam warmed in a double boiler with 2 teaspoons cumin seeds crushed with black pepper and sea salt to taste.

Linseed
Flax

Linum usitatissimum

An ancient cultivated crop that goes back into the mists of time, linseed originates around the Mediterranean area and was used for food over 5 000 years ago. It is thought the original wild plants were found in Mesopotamia, and historic documents show it was cultivated as a crop 3000 BC in Babylon, not only as a food but also as a fibre for the first linen cloths.

Hippocrates recorded its medicinal uses in the relief of abdominal pain and also for coughs and mucous treatment. In the 8th century, King Charlemagne of France considered it to be so valuable as a health builder that he ordered his subjects to grow it all around the city so that its energy-giving seeds could be eaten daily. From then on linseed or flaxseed became a valuable food source and a most useful plant for its fibre. The long, tough stems, stone crushed, yield strong strands that did not break in the weaving process. In the 1st century AD Pliny the Elder, the Roman philosopher, wrote: 'What department is there to be found in active life in which flax is not employed and in what production of the earth are there greater marvels to us than this?'

If you think of it, this beautiful, easy-to-grow crop offers really a most bountiful reward – food, medicine and fibre: there is no other plant anywhere like it!

Growing Linseed

A cool weather plant, although in the cooler parts of the country it can be grown all year round, linseed is an exceptionally easy crop to grow and with its sky-blue edible flowers it is a simply charming plant in the garden sown *en masse*.

Scatter the shiny little seeds into well-dug, well-composted, moist soil in full sun in autumn and rake them in. Keep the area moist – do not let it dry out – lightly cover with raked leaves and watch as the little seedlings push out quickly.

Allow the seeds to ripen to a golden colour and to become dry before reaping them. The seeds easily scatter if bunches are threshed on a smooth floor and the light outer casing can be blown away. The seeds need to be stored in glass bottles with a tight screw top. The stems, added to the compost heap, aerate it well, as the strong fibres take time to break down.

Using Linseed

The lignans in flaxseed have been found to show significant anti-cancer activity. A mere 5–10 grams of ground flaxseed every day sprinkled over your breakfast fruit or porridge, will lower the risk of breast cancer by reducing oestrogen, and even shrink breast tumours already present. Use flaxseed baked in muffins, or mix with sesame seed and sunflower seed and grind it all together for not only a super taste but for an energy boost! Ground flaxseed helps to reduce blood cholesterol, reduces prostate cancer and prevents it. For both men and women there is no doubt that flaxseed and flax oil are seriously valuable, and in medical tests worldwide there is a huge amount of exceptionally positive information.

Even a poultice of flaxseed soaked in hot water over an inflamed painful arthritic joint will comfort and soothe it, and have a cup of pleasant-tasting 'linseed tea' for chronic coughs, bladder infections, cystitis, arthritic aches and pains, aching joints, back pains and spasms, and use the crushed seeds as a face pack for problem, spotty, oily skin and acne.

A little precious flaxseed oil mixed with a good olive oil in a salad dressing with lemon juice makes a delicious way of getting the valuable minerals and vitamins and amino acids into the body.

Ground seeds, reaped from your own organically grown linseed, freshly crushed every day in a small seed grinder, sprinkled over breakfast muesli or oats porridge or over a fresh fruit salad – papaya and mango is my favourite – will give you energy and vitality and even ease those aching joints, and reduce the risk and impact of heart disease and cancer! Don't neglect this simple and exceptional food – it is literally nothing short of miraculous!

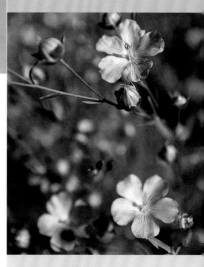

Linseed Tea

Take ¼ cup fresh leaves and flowers and stems, and pour over this 1 cup of boiling water, stand 5 minutes and strain. Then sip slowly.

Breakfast Turbo Boost

King Charlemagne would have loved a modern seed grinder and this would certainly have been his magic potion!

In a seed grinder, grind together:

2 tablespoons flaxseed
1 tablespoon sesame seed
1 tablespoon sunflower seed
2 tablespoons almonds

Sprinkle over a small bowl of plain Bulgarian yoghurt into which a banana has been sliced and to which about half a papino or a slice of papaya or a grated apple has been added. Make this part of your daily breakfast – you'll feel the difference very quickly.

Health Note

Flaxseed is an excellent source of omega-3 fatty acids, alpha-linolenic acid and phytoestrogens, also known as lignans, and is rich in phosphorous, iron, copper, vitamins A, B, D and E, manganese, magnesium and potassium.

Litchi
Lychee

Litchi chinensis

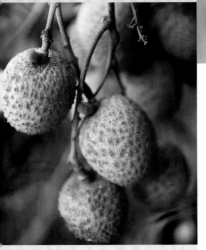

The beautiful litchi tree is one of the most celebrated trees of China. Tall, spreading, voluptuous and evergreen, it can grow up to 25 metres tall. In its native tropical China and parts of Malaysia and Southeast Asia, it is heavily weighted with succulent bunches of pendulous fruit in varying shades of pink and pale pink-brown. Related to another sort of litchi – the rambutan (*Nephelium lappaceum*), which has a thick, hairy shell around each fruit – these two delicious fruits form part of China's traditional food repertoire.

Cultivated in China for thousands of years, during the first century AD it became so popular that a special coach and horses was started so that the delicious litchis of tropical China could be swiftly taken to the Imperial Court. One could say that this was the first courier service! The fruit travelled well just before it was fully ripe and was packed in strong baskets, nestled in its own leaves – great bunches of the fruits, still attached to their stems. Imagine opening so precious a delivery!

Cultivation of litchis from the early centuries began to extend through to Thailand, to Bangladesh and all along Malaysia's warm tropical forest edges to northern India. Now South Africa grows its own good harvest of litchis in the hot areas, but tins of Chinese litchis and rambutans are still imported today.

Growing Litchis

This is a truly tropical tree that grows quickly – both male and female flowers grow on the same tree – and as litchi trees are propagated by grafting, buy your tree from a reputable nursery. They need a frost-free winter and a humid hot summer and around Christmas time they come into full fruit – and what a treat they are!

Plant in a really big, compost-filled hole 1 m wide and 1 m deep, as they are heavy feeders. Set a thick pipe at an angle deep under the roots so that you can set a hosepipe into it to get the water well down to the roots. Twice a year – in winter and in midsummer, June and November – give the tree two barrow loads of rich compost, dig it in well and water thoroughly. Don't forget this, as this heavy feeding ensures an excellent crop.

Using Litchi

The Chinese still preserve litchis today as they did centuries ago by drying them whole in their skins. When the inside rattles as the distorted skin dries, it is peeled and stored – soft, brown and as sweet and as wrinkled as a raisin – for winter stews and stir-fries. Chinese and Thai dishes include litchis, both fresh and dried, with fish and meat and in stuffings, and finely chopped with water chestnuts in stir-fries.

To dry litchis it is worth investing in your own dehydrator. Peeled, sliced litchis placed on the racks dry quickly and remain soft and chewy – a delicious addition to the lunch box!

Preserved in sugar syrup, litchis can be enjoyed all year round and tinned and bottled litchis are sold in Chinese markets all over the world. But the best way to eat them is fresh, and included in fruit salads with mango and granadilla and pineapple.

Keep ripe litchis in the fridge and serve them cold in their skins. There is nothing as refreshing.

Health Note

Litchis are high in vitamin C, phosphorus, calcium, iron, carbohydrates and fruit sugars.

Sweet Lupin

Lupinus albus

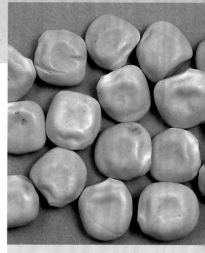

This is quite an extraordinary plant and one so easy to grow I cannot believe we don't grow more of it. It is an ancient, pretty annual that originates in the Mediterranean area – some believe it is of North African origin – and it has been much loved and much cherished since the early Egyptians used it – long before 300 BC it features in their wall paintings.

An Andean variety of lupin was grown in Peru by the Incas around 2000 BC and from these early beginnings more and more varieties with lesser amounts of the bitter alkaloids were cultivated and used as trade and the seeds spread quickly. Today low-alkaloid cultivars are grown for their sweet flavour – the seeds are the part that is used and can also be processed into a flavour-filled cooking oil.

The original lupins (not the colourful hybrids so spectacular in the gardens of Europe but the pale-coloured white or blue lupins) and the seeds carefully boiled to release the alkaloids before consuming, have become a traditional dish in several countries, and in South Africa we are able to buy cooked lupin seeds in salty sour sauces in some Portuguese delicatessens, and sometimes imported from Madeira.

Growing Lupins

The big, thick white seeds are available from farmer's co-ops and are planted in early spring for a summer crop. Choose a site in full sun and dig in as much compost as you can find – around 1 bucket per square metre – as the lupin is a heavy feeder.

Before planting set a spray over the bed to thoroughly soak the soil. Overnight also soak the lupin seed in warm water to hasten its growth. Plant the seeds 40 cm apart, about 3 cm deep. Make a hole with a stick first and drop the seed in and gently cover it. Do not let the bed dry out. Water thoroughly every 2 or 3 days. Mulching around the plants in the midsummer heat is essential to maintain the moisture the lupin needs to flourish.

In some countries the green pods are eaten before they mature and whole plants are chopped off as cattle feed. Best of all, with its high nitrogen content the lupin makes a superb green manure!

Using Lupins

In Europe the lupin is used as a vermifuge for both humans and animals, and has a long history in that respect – cooked seeds are given on an empty stomach first thing in the morning to rid the body of internal parasites. Also the cooked seeds (see recipe alongside) macerated in hot water have been found to be an excellent hypoglycaemic treatment.

Roasted and ground, the cooked lupins make a delicious coffee substitute and have been a much-loved Arabian delicacy known as 'troumis' in Arabic and 'lupini' in Italian.

The protein content in lupins is well established, as well as some vitamins and lecithin, and a substance called inosite phosphoric acid. The seeds yield an excellent edible oil.

Crushed and powdered dried cooked seeds are an ancient cosmetic known as lupin flour used as a beauty mask with water to rejuvenate the skin.

Health Note

Lupins have a high protein content (up to 45%) and provide vitamins B, C and D and some vitamin E. Lupin oil is rich in unsaturated fatty acids, including linoleic acid.

Cooked Lupin Seeds

Serve as a snack with salt and a squeeze of lemon juice the way the Italians love it, or in a dressing of mustard, olive oil and vinegar the way the Portuguese love it.

Soak the lupin seeds in warm water overnight. Rinse well before cooking, then boil up in fresh water for 10 minutes. Drain and again boil up in fresh water and cook until tender – it takes about 1½ hours for the seed to become tender. Drain, rinse in cold water and then stand in fresh cold water until ready to process. Drain. Now add 3 cups cold water with 1 tablespoon of salt to every 1 cup of cooked lupins. Store in this brine in the fridge and change it every 3 days. Keep tasting to see if the seed has no more bitterness – this usually takes 7 or 8 days. Drain and serve with a dressing of your choice.

Caution

Lupins contain bitter alkaloids, so be sure to boil them well before eating. Simmer them in water for 40 minutes, drain and discard the cooking water. Cook again, in fresh water, for another 30–40 minutes and again drain off the water. The lupins can now be eaten as a snack, or added to salads, soups or stews.

Tomato

Lycopersicon esculentum

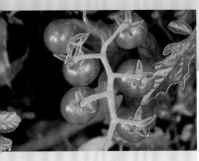

Homemade Tomato Sauce

4 large onions, finely chopped

½ cup olive oil

1½ kg finely chopped organically grown tomatoes (if they are large, peel them by submerging them in boiling water for a few minutes to soften and remove the skins)

6 green peppers, seeds removed and finely chopped

2 tablespoons crushed coriander seed

½–1 tablespoon freshly ground black pepper

4 teaspoons coarse sea salt that has been ground in a pestle and mortar

4 tablespoons soft brown sugar

juice of 1 large lemon

2 teaspoons lemon zest

½–¾ cup finely chopped basil (we use the perennial High Hopes basil as it retains its fabulous flavour)

½–¾ cup finely chopped flat-leaf parsley

4 tablespoons homemade apricot jam

In a large stainless steel pot, brown the onions in the olive oil. Stir-fry until golden brown. Add the chopped tomatoes and green peppers, stir well and reduce the heat. Then add the coriander seed, black pepper, salt and brown sugar. Mix in well, constantly stirring, and simmer on low heat for 15 minutes. (It burns quickly so be sure to keep stirring.) Now add the lemon juice and lemon zest, basil and parsley and finally add the homemade apricot jam. Stir well and spoon into sterilised hot jars or wide-mouthed bottles. You'll never want to eat bought tomato sauce again!

The tomato as we know it today had its early beginnings, like many other plants in the nightshade family, in Central and South America where it was known as the 'apple of Peru'. The first wild tomatoes were similar to the small cherry tomatoes we know and enjoy today, and the first cultivation of this easy-to-grow plant was in Mexico. The Spanish conquistadors, who arrived in Mexico soon after Christopher Columbus discovered the New World, took the seeds back to Spain as they saw how the Mexican Indians grew the bright 'berries' in abundance.

In Europe it was a slow beginning as it was considered to be poisonous – belonging to the deadly Nightshade family – and by the 16th century when it reached Italy, it was first grown as a garden ornament rather than a food. Much mystery and speculation surrounded the tomato. The Latin name *Lycopersicon* given to it, means 'wolf peace' and like a wolf it was considered dangerous! Yet the French named it 'pomme d'amour', the apple of love, and they believed it was an aphrodisiac. The Italians named it 'pomorodoro' as the first species were actually yellow in colour! By the late 19th century the tomato made its way into North America with the first colonists, and started to slowly gain popularity as a summer crop.

New varieties developed, and with new and better means of transport developing, the tomato became a steady favourite. Today the tomato is a top seller and the United States, Spain, Russia, Turkey and China are amongst the biggest producers.

Growing Tomatoes

The most popular of all summer crops and grown in many home gardens all over the world, the tomato needs warmth, full sun and richly composted soil. Start the seeds off in protected trays and plant the seedlings out in deeply dug, compost-filled trenches, in rows spaced 1 m apart when the weather is warm. Water them well two or three times a week until they are established, and stake them or tie them to simple wire supports as they grow. This is a worthwhile and fascinating crop and one that will give so much pleasure, as homegrown, sun-ripened tomatoes have that extra delicious taste.

Using Tomatoes

Tomatoes are rich in lycopene, a powerful and protective antioxidant some believe is even more valuable than beta-carotene. The lycopene found in tomatoes is a red carotene, which has been shown to prevent and lower the risk of cancers of the breast, lungs, skin, colon and prostate gland. It also lowers the risk of heart disease, eye cataracts and macular degeneration of the eyes by neutralising the free radicals before they damage the cells.

The tomato was used in the early centuries as a medicine to cleanse the liver, to build the blood, to fight infections and, interestingly, to clear acidity. Today's research states it is an excellent food, raw and fresh, eaten to help clear the liver of toxins.

Organically home-grown tomatoes have to be one of the most loved treats in the world, and cut in half and grilled and served on toast with quickly fried mushrooms and sprinkled with lots of fresh basil, is one of the most delicious of breakfasts, perfect for a Sunday morning!

Health Note

In addition to lycopene, tomatoes are rich in calcium, magnesium, phosphorus, beta-carotene, vitamin C and folic acid.

Macadamia Nut

Macadamia integrifolia

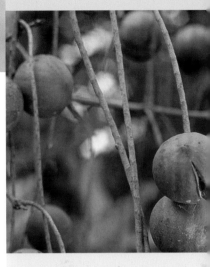

The macadamia tree is a stunning tree – thick, evergreen, sturdy, tough, a dramatic feature of dark-green, toothed, hard, leathery leaves, and the most exquisite pendulous delicate sprays of pale pink or creamy white flowers. These flowers form the fruits, which hang on short stalks from the pendulous flower stalk – 6 or more, even up to 12, round, fleshy, green pods encase the exceptionally hard-shelled nuts. It is pure fascination growing a macadamia – it is endlessly interesting to watch the tiny, tough little tree grow into a giant – the tree can reach 12 metres or even up to 15 metres in its native Australia. A valuable food tree, its history with the Aborigines dates back many centuries. Found in the tropical forests of Queensland and northern New South Wales, the Aborigines so respected and revered this marvellous tree that every winter they would come from far and wide to gather on the slopes of the 'Great Divide' to feast on the nuts of those trees they call 'kindat kindal' in a ceremony of thanksgiving.

The colonisation of Australia by the British began in 1788, and by 1875 the first beginnings of the history of the macadamia were recorded. Two botanists exploring the forest along the Pine River in the Moreton Bay area discovered the trees covered in nuts. Walter Hill, director of the Botanic Gardens in Brisbane, and Ferdinand Müller, a botanist from Melbourne, found no information on the macadamia and so in 1878 they established a new genus *Macadamia* in honour of John Macadam MD in Victoria.

By the 1890s the macadamia was taken to Hawaii and it thrived in the moist, semi-tropical climate there, and today Hawaii is the largest grower of 20 000 acres and exporter of macadamia nuts, with Komatiepoort, South Africa, coming second with over 4 000 acres! Mexico, Costa Rica, Guatemala, Kenya, Brazil and California all grow macadamias today.

Growing Macadamias

Start off with an extra large hole filled with compost with a wide pipe set into the hole at an angle to enable a hose to be inserted in order to get water to the roots. The site must be in full sun and the tree needs a twice weekly watering in summer and once a week in winter. Remember, it will not take frost – it is literally a tropical tree. Give it a barrow of compost twice yearly and the rewards will be huge.

Using Macadamias

High in unsaturated fats, macadamia nuts are considered to be a valuable and beneficial addition to the diet for their cholesterol-lowering action, for their energy-boosting abilities and for their high antioxidant levels. Most nuts have a short shelf life, but the macadamia nut has a long-lasting storage life, especially if it is encased in its hard, thick shell.

Macadamia nut oil is considered to be superior as a cooking or salad oil because of its lower level of polyunsaturated fat. Statistics measure 3% for macadamia oil, 8% for olive oil and 23% for canola oil – to give an idea – and macadamia oil is stable at high temperatures. And, like olive oil, it is very high in natural antioxidants and contains 4,5 times the amount of vitamin E as olive oil does!

Macadamia farmers have devised a clever gadget for cracking the nuts without casualty! No one I know of who has ever tried to crack a macadamia has escaped without a bruised thumb! And it defeats the monkeys – so our macadamia gatherings often entail going far into the bush where the monkeys have abandoned them. Baskets of macadamias intrigue our visitors and our basil pesto with macadamia nuts has become legendary.

Health Note
Macadamias have high levels of unsaturated fat, and are rich in magnesium, copper, iron, phosphorus, vitamins B1, B3 and E, and zinc; the nuts also contain some protein and carbohydrates.

Macadamia and Basil Pesto

This is delicious served over pasta or baked potatoes, or as a spread on bread, or served with cold meats.

1 cup chopped macadamia nuts
½–1 cup finely shaved Parmesan cheese
1 cup fresh basil leaves
½ cup olive oil or, if you can find it, macadamia nut oil
3 tablespoons freshly squeezed lemon juice
1–3 cloves garlic, if liked (we make pesto often without garlic)
1 teaspoon sea salt

First in a food processor pulse the chopped macadamias with the oil, then add all the other ingredients and whirl until smooth and creamy. Add a little water if too thick.

Hint

Store shelled macadamia nuts in the fridge – this maintains their crispness so that they roast easily. Roast them in a shallow pan by stirring over medium heat, sprinkle with a grinding of sea salt and a little freshly grated ginger, and serve while warm.

Acerola
Barbados Cherry
Malpighia glabra

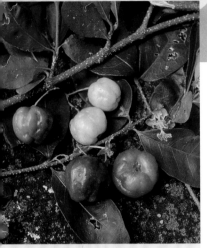

A pretty, dense shrub, the acerola originates in the Caribbean, Barbados Islands, West Indies and parts of America. The tiny five-petalled mass of pink flowers are followed by cherry-sized red fruits, so exceptionally high in vitamin C that it has between 20 and 60 times more vitamin C than an orange! The fresh acidic fruits have been cherished through the centuries as a treatment for coughs and colds, eaten raw (it has three pips inside it that fit together closely) or cooked with honey as a cough mixture, or cooked into jams and jellies and preserves. It was introduced into Reunion Island around 1826 and I saw beautiful specimens growing in the gardens there laden with fruit which the Creoles turn into a zesty and delicious drink.

Growing the Acerola

The dense, spreading shrub can reach up to 3–4 m. The ones growing in the Herbal Centre gardens are 2 m in height after 6 years of growth. So it grows quite slowly and propagation is by seeds and cuttings. It thrives in full sun in a large, deep, compost-filled hole and needs to be flooded with water weekly.

The small pink flowers are edible and are frequently on the shrub, and the fruits start off small, round and green – it is then that the level of vitamin C is at its highest – the fruits then turn orange and finally red, and at this stage vitamin A is at its highest.

Light pruning to shape the shrub can be done in midwinter and compost twice yearly ensures masses of fruit. This is a tropical fruit that will need winter protection in cold areas.

Using the Acerola

Because of its high vitamin C and vitamin A content, the acerola has through the years become important in boosting the immune system, and orchards of acerola shrubs have been planted in Puerto Rico, Hawaii, Jamaica, India, Israel, Australia and Guatemala for both medicine and food. Throat lozenges are excellent for sore throats and acerola syrups for children have been on the market all over the world for decades. At one time acerola tablets and capsules were the only available source of vitamin C and as a young mother on an isolated farm, I was eternally grateful for these soothing capsules for my children's sore throats and coughs and colds. I remember well Natrodale's imported lozenges, so sour *and* soothing for a sore throat.

After the initial excitement and lengthy work on the acerola subsided, financially the natural ascorbic acid the fruit contained gradually became too costly to extract and synthetic ascorbic acid was developed at a fraction of the price. Regrettably, natural ascorbic acid was virtually replaced by synthetic ascorbic acid and those huge orchards of thousands of acerola trees, hectare after hectare of them in Florida, Puerto Rico, Hawaii, Jamaica, Israel, Australia and the Philippines, fell into disuse, and today only a fraction of the harvest is reaped and it is all but impossible to find acerola cherry products around. Sometimes you may be lucky enough to find acerola in apple juice for babies.

Perhaps one day a dedicated farmer might reconsider this precious fruit and plant again an orchard of natural vitamin C – I would be the first to buy his crop!

Health Note

The fresh fruit pulp is one of the richest known sources of vitamin C and also contains good amounts of vitamin A, as well as thiamine, niacin, riboflavin, iron, phosphorus and calcium.

Acerola Syrup for Coughs and Colds

I am intrigued with the growing of my own acerolas and make this cough syrup whenever I get the chance.

1 cup ripe red acerola berries
¼ cup green acerola berries
10 cloves
1 cup raw honey
½ cup grated ginger root

Simmer everything together in a double boiler for 20 minutes, stirring occasionally. Cool 10 minutes, strain, squeezing the pulp through as much as possible. Pour into a glass jar with a screw-top lid. Take 1 teaspoon at a time, holding it in the mouth as long as possible first. Or add 1–2 teaspoons to ½–¾ cup of green tea, stir well and sip slowly.

Hint

In the Caribbean Islands, the pulp from fresh acerola berries is spread to dry in the sun. The dried pulp is chopped finely and mixed with a little honey and a sprinkling of coconut, and rolled into little balls to become a traditional 'sweet' that is much loved by the children.

Apple

Malus pumila

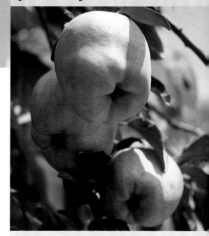

The apple is probably the most loved of all fruits and is internationally known, enjoyed and respected. 'An apple a day keeps the doctor away', our grandmothers drummed into our heads, and if you look at its amazing vitamin and mineral content you can see that this is a health food of great exception.

The apple originated in Asia Minor and Eastern Europe and was one of the first fruits to be cultivated, and archaeologists have found quartered dried apples stored for the winter in many sites all over the world, some dating back to about the 10th century BC. In the 12th century BC Ramses III ordered apple trees to be cultivated in the fertile soils of the Nile Valley and by the 4th century AD the Romans had 37 varieties growing well and producing the precious health-giving fruits.

There are thousands of varieties today and it is one of the most important of all commercial fruits, with China as one of the main producers worldwide. An attractive, small and fascinating tree, the apple grows easily in cool temperate climates and many varieties are available grafted onto dwarf rootstocks, and even a small apple orchard is an enviable possession and a never-ending fascination.

Growing Apples

Apples need cross-pollination, real winter cold, coolish summers and will thrive in a deep, compost-filled hole with a thorough weekly watering, and twice weekly in the hot and humid summer days. Pruning must be judicious, careful, light and gentle, and bonemeal and a little wood ash should be occasionally spread around the trunk.

Using Apples

A ripe apple contains high quantities of juice and 85% of water, which makes it an immediate thirst quencher. It contains pectin which fights irradiation within the body and the freshly pressed juice from ripe apples with this precious pectin, which is a superb digestive, will ease chest infections, coughs, colds and whooping cough, reduce fevers and soothe bladder, kidney, liver and gastro-intestinal infections. It is a natural detoxifier and will modify the whole intestine by recharging and reactivating the good bacteria within it. So peeled, finely grated raw apple that has stood for 5 minutes in order to oxidise – that is by turning a brownish colour – is the best thing one could take for a stomach ailment.

The apple stimulates the intestinal flora, it is a health tonic and a bowel regulator, and it keeps the liver toned and the kidneys flushed. Apples contain malic and tartaric acid, and eating an apple will strengthen the gum tissue, polish the teeth, revive the digestion, soothe headaches, emotional upsets and even skin ailments. In fact, it is both a medicine and a beauty treatment, and grated apple used as a scrub is a superb cleanser and tonic for greasy, spotty skin and acne.

Apples in the daily diet treat obesity, anaemia, insomnia, catarrh and sinus headaches, halitosis, tuberculosis, heart disease, gallstones, asthma, gonorrhoea, nausea, vomiting and even worms! Eating an apple or two a day will help lower cholesterol, ease constipation as well as diarrhoea, and help to protect against computer and cell phone irradiation in our world of technology.

So eating an apple a day will really keep the doctor away – but it needs to be an organic apple and if you're not sure, wash it carefully in a biodegradable chemical-free produce wash.

Health Note

Apples are rich in vitamins A, B, C and K, calcium, magnesium, phosphorus, potassium, pectin and dietary fibre.

Quick and Easy Apple Pie

Serves 6

Make the flaky pastry (or use ready-made pastry)

500 g flour
2 teaspoons cream of tartar
500 g cold butter, grated on the coarse side of the grater
1 teaspoon salt
about 150 ml iced water

Sift the flour with the cream of tartar and the salt. Rub in the butter lightly. Now mix in the iced water, cutting it in with a dinner knife. Turn out on a piece of greaseproof paper, lightly form into a ball and refrigerate for about 1 hour.

Make the filling

Peel, core and thinly slice 8–10 large apples. Cook them in a little water with ½ cup brown caramel sugar, 3 heaped tablespoons of sultanas and 3 heaped tablespoons of currants. Simmer until the apples are tender and the sultanas are swollen and soft. Drain off most of the liquid, leaving only about 1 tablespoon.

Assemble the pie

Roll the pastry dough into a rectangle, fold like an envelope and roll again. Repeat twice. Cut a piece to fit a pie dish and add the fruit. Cover the top of the pie with a circle of pastry and pinch the edges. Prick a few holes in for air to escape, brush with beaten egg and bake at 180 °C for 10 minutes or until golden brown. Sprinkle the top with castor sugar and serve hot with whipped cream.

Mango

Mangifera indica

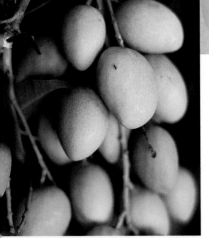

The mango belongs to the same family as the cashew nut – the Anacardiaceae – a group of exotic evergreen and divinely delicious fruiting trees native to the East Indies and Malaysia. Cultivated for over 4 000 years in India, it is one of the world's most loved and cherished tropical fruits, and it seems likely that the Portuguese traders spread it to Africa on to South America, and during the 18th century to the West Indies and America. China, India and Mexico remain the biggest growers of this exotic and much-loved fruit.

The wild mango originated in the hills of India and Burma at the base of the great Himalayas – it is believed – for some of those wild mangoes still grow there today. The fibrous hairiness and strong turpentine taste of those ancient wild fruits bear little resemblance to the luscious beauties we consume so happily today. The real cultivation of the mango began in Moghul India in the 16th century, and this technique is still used today as even the best of the cultivated mangoes will revert back to the fibrous turpentine-tasting fruit of its ancestry.

Growing Mangoes

Mangoes need a site in full sun and a wide, deeply dug hole filled with rich compost. In the orchards each tree is linked to the next by furrows so that a flood of water can seep around each tree, often twice weekly in very hot weather. In many hot areas drip irrigation is used and I still use the pipe, a wide one deeply inserted below the roots at an angle so that the hosepipe can be inserted into it to take water deep into the soil down to the roots. Gentle, long and deep watering will keep the tree prolific and the flowers will form abundantly. Add a barrow load of compost to each tree twice a year.

Using Mangoes

In India the flowers are crushed and used in healing lotions and oils, often rubbed over the area, especially over aching joints and for backache. In certain areas the mango flowers are used in bathing and in hair washing.

Long esteemed as a health booster, it is the high concentration of carotenoids, antioxidants, minerals and vitamins (see Health Note) that make mangoes so valuable. They are also rich in soluble fibre, the sort of fibre that shifts cholesterol build-up – so mangoes in the diet help to prevent cardiovascular disease. Mangoes also help to fight cancer and the University of Hawaii conducted a research in 1997 and found that when mice exposed to cancer-forming substances were given mango extract it stopped normal cells from forming into cancerous cells. Compounds in the mango include water-soluble nutrients and flavonoids which contribute to the mango's anti-cancer effect. Other research has shown that fresh mango and naturally dried mango consumption results in a 60% reduction in the risk of cancer.

Mangoes also contain digestive enzymes similar to the papain found in papayas. These enzymes act as a meat tenderiser and an excellent digestive. The well-known traveller's diarrhoea responds beautifully to mango as it effectively protects against giardia – the organism responsible for many cases of debilitating diarrhoea. Mango actually eliminates it and does as well as the diarrhoea medications! For anaemia, mango's blood-building abilities are well known in India in pregnant women and during menstruation. For muscle cramps, stress and heart palpitations, the high magnesium and potassium content in the mango is highly beneficial. Best of all the mango, the most loved and desired of all tropical fruits, can be enjoyed by those with diabetes as the mango has a low glucose response.

Health Note

Mangoes have significant quantities of vitamins A, B, C, E and K, folic acid, beta-carotene, as well as potassium, magnesium and copper.

Mango Chutney

1,5 kg semi-ripe mangoes, sliced off the pips and chopped into small pieces
sea salt
600 ml dark grape vinegar
500 g soft brown caramel sugar
1 cup finely grated fresh ginger
2 cups sultanas or small seedless raisins
1 cup chopped stoned dates
1 teaspoon cayenne pepper OR a crushed chilli, seeds removed (or more if you like it hot!)
2 teaspoons powdered cinnamon
1 teaspoon powdered cloves

Place the mangoes in a large stainless steel or glass bowl, sprinkle with a little sea salt and add enough cold water to submerge the mango pieces. Cover the bowl and leave it to stand overnight. Next morning, drain and set aside.

In a heavy bottomed stainless steel pot, bring the vinegar and sugar to the boil and add the rest of the ingredients. Mix in the drained mangoes and simmer gently, stirring often, for about 1 hour until it thickens. Keep an eye on the heat so that it does not burn. Spoon into sterilised jars.

Hint

Ripen mangoes in a brown paper with an apple – leave it at room temperature for a couple of days.

Cassava

Manihot esculenta

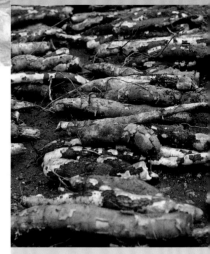

This is a particularly interesting perennial, a shrubby small and quite delicate looking tree that originates in parts of Brazil. There are several varieties of *Manihot*, and ancient rituals and traditions revolve around the genus and the preparation of the root, which is the main edible part, as well as the leaves. From its Brazilian beginnings, thanks to its high nutritional content and the ease with which both the fresh and the dried root, or flour made from the root, could be transported in those early centuries, it was used as trade. It soon spread to the Pacific Islands, Indonesia, the Philippines and New Guinea where it is a staple food, and in later centuries it spread into Africa and India and on into China.

As a staple food it is very carefully prepared as it has poisonous cyanogenic compounds within its exceptionally large roots, which need to be removed by boiling or fermenting. The roots and the leaves are eaten, but are also used as medicine still today in parts of Mexico and Brazil. It literally is a treasure and so easy to grow, I am astonished it is not offered for sale everywhere!

Growing Cassava

It thrives in tropical conditions in well-composted soil and loves heat, humidity and tropical rain, and can take shade and sun. It enjoys a good twice weekly soaking. In colder areas the cassava needs winter protection and it will lose its leaves.

Propagate by stem cuttings – ensure that at least 3 nodes are underground. Within a year the thick tuberous roots will have grown enough to dig up. I have cassava trees that are 8 years old and they form an attractive spreading small tree that I constantly reap cuttings from for new trees, and it continues to send out more little branches. We take several cuttings to over-winter in our protected hot house just to ensure we never lose this fascinating plant.

Using Cassava

It has long been used as a treatment for diarrhoea, stomach upsets, fatigue and for convalescence. A soft porridge made from cassava flour is eaten twice a day with a little honey, and for severe diarrhoea it is eaten without the honey. Warmed mashed root wrapped in soft warmed leaves is placed over an aching back for strains and over swollen ankles and stiff necks to reduce the swelling, pain and stiffness. Cassava cakes baked in the coals were eaten with warm coconut milk to ease insomnia and hot baked roots were mashed and wrapped in leaves to ease arthritic pains, headaches and toothache.

The leaves are fairly rich in minerals and vitamins and high in protein, and are eaten as a spinach when young and tender, often cooked with other greens or thinly sliced and stir-fried, or the older leaves are wrapped around fish or chicken or meat with ginger and chillies, and cooked in a steamer or wok. The older and tougher leaves are used to wrap food when steaming or baking or grilling.

High in carbohydrates, the root has been made into a flour used for baking a kind of flat bread, for stewed meats to thicken the gravy with onions, and fried as a savoury pancake. Cassava flour, dried cassava and cassava paste can be bought from specialist food stores. Tapioca or pearled manihot, made from the roots, is an old-fashioned and much-loved ingredient for puddings. The root is boiled, dried and pounded and the tapioca is rolled into small 'pearls' that are then boiled up in coconut milk with sweet palm sugar as the dessert we all once used to enjoy! Tapioca was one of the first thickeners used in Chinese cooking, long before flour, and the powdered dried cassava became a valuable trade.

Health Note

Cassava is an excellent source of iron, magnesium, vitamin C and potassium, a good source of calcium and phosphorus, and it even has a little niacin.

Preparing Cassava Roots

I was taught by a man who had lived in Mozambique for a long time how to cook cassava. Although the poisonous cyanogenic glycosides are today no longer so prevalent in the sweet varieties, he advised always to cook the peeled roots first: boil up in enough water to cover for 20 minutes, and then discard the water. Boil up again until tender, discard the water and then slice and fry the roots in a little sunflower cooking oil until golden brown with onions, or add it to soups, stews and casseroles.

Caution

Cassava roots contain cyanide – so proper preparation by boiling or fermenting is essential. Although today there are varieties that do not have the poisonous elements, you are still advised to boil up the roots for 20 minutes, discard the water and boil again.

Lucerne
Alfalfa

Medicago sativa

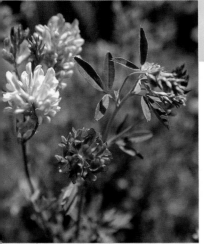

The word 'alfalfa' or 'lucerne' means 'life' in the language of flowers, and this exceptional and extraordinary plant has so fascinating a history, a reputation for building energy, strength, vitality and wellness that absolutely no garden should ever be without it. Pliny the Elder (AD 23–79), records that King Darius the Great, the King of Persia (550–486 BC) introduced alfalfa into his soldiers' diet in an attempt to conquer Athens.

Originating in southwest Asia, lucerne spread via the trade routes across Europe where it became naturalised as a valuable fodder crop and, surprisingly, even then as a vegetable – the young and tender shoots and leaves were added to soups and stews for energy and vitality, and to build resistance to illness.

Grown for forage for livestock in ancient times and stored in bales for winter feeds in snowbound countries, by 1500 the Spanish explorers found alfalfa so valuable as a medicine and a food they took it to South America and around 1736 European colonists introduced it to the United States.

Many stories, myths and legends surround lucerne, and in all its long and fascinating history, it has never lost its popularity. Early on the seeds were sprouted and eaten with gruels and stews, soups and porridge. It is thought that alfalfa seeds were taken on the long voyages and used as sprouted seeds to prevent scurvy, as the tiny seeds travelled so easily.

Growing Lucerne

When I married a farmer in my very early twenties, the first crop I became aware of on a large scale was lucerne. For the milk cows this was a vital crop, and fascinated with the ease that the seed was scattered into most recently ploughed furrows, I started my own row in my newly dug vegetable garden. I added the fresh leaves and flowers to salads and soups – unwilted, I was constantly reminded – and read up everything about lucerne I could lay my hands on in those days.

Sow in full sun, in richly composted, deeply dug, moist soil and water daily until the tiny seeds germinate – in a mere few days – and then water carefully to never let those minute plants dry out. In the intense heat of midsummer sowing the seed in compost-filled bags for planting out later seemed a better bet if the rains were unpredictable, and soon I had a thriving crop and I experimented throughout the year.

In winter I grow delicious alfalfa sprouts and I serve these precious, energy-packed little vigorous scraps of vitality with every salad and savoury dish.

Using Lucerne

Just two or three lucerne plants in the garden will offer you a constant supply of tasty leaves, shoots and flowers. The roots spread deep and wide into the soil to draw up the mass of minerals within the soil.

The array of beneficial compounds lucerne offers is exceptional. Amongst those compounds are the phytoestrogens which play a valuable role in the prevention of osteoporosis, menopausal symptoms, cancer and heart disease. The saponins in lucerne help to lower blood cholesterol without diminishing the beneficial HDL cholesterol and help to exert a protective effect against cardiovascular disease. Lucerne has so great an antioxidant activity it ranks amongst the best known to medical science.

Growing your own sprouts is easy, trouble-free and quick (see instructions alongside). Keep the sprouts refrigerated and rinse extra well before eating and include in the diet often. Add them to soups, stews, smoothies and juice them with carrots, apples, beetroot and wheat grass.

Health Note

Alfalfa is rich in calcium, iron, magnesium, silica, potassium, chlorine, manganese, vitamins A, B, E, D and K, and an excellent source of Vitamin B12.

Sprouting Alfalfa Seeds

For smaller quantities, spread a layer of cotton wool into a tray or flat glass dish and moisten well. Sprinkle the seed quite thickly over the surface. Never let it dry out – a spray bottle is very effective in keeping the sprouts moist and healthy. Pull up when the little leaves form and use in salads and stir-fries.

For larger quantities it is worth investing in a tiered sprouter, available from health shops.

Caution

Although alfalfa sprouts and leaves detoxify and reduce inflammation, they are contra-indicated with lupus and other autoimmune diseases. *Always check with your doctor first before including new foods in your diet.*

Eating wilted leaves and flowers can produce uncomfortable gas – remember cattle eating cut and wilted lucerne can easily succumb to bloat! So always pick and eat as fresh as is possible. Stand the sprigs in iced water in the kitchen and add to the salad at the last minute!

Bitter Melon

Momordica charantia

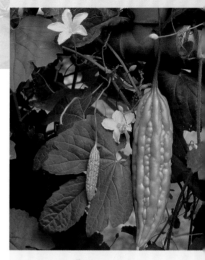

History

This is a really strange and amazing plant that is a fast-growing, tender annual climber that belongs to the cucumber family. Sometimes known as karela or balsam pear or bitter gourd, it is an ancient, much-loved and respected food and medicine that has been used in many cultures since the earliest of days.

Native to India, parts of Africa and Asia, the fruit is now grown in China, Pakistan, Indonesia and Southeast Asia as an important food. A popular vegetable in China, India and Taiwan particularly, it is an acquired taste for most Westerners, but due to its extraordinary medicinal values I must include it here.

Growing Bitter Melon

Sow the seeds in spring in well-dug, richly-composted, moist soil spaced 50 cm apart along a fence for the vines and tendrils to climb upon. It is quick and thrives with a deep, three times a week watering. Solitary yellow 5-petalled flowers appear followed by the 20–25 cm long warty pale green cucumber-like fruits. As the fruits ripen, they turn pale yellow, but usually the fruit is eaten young and green. Split the fruit open and you will be astonished to see bright orange flesh with brilliant red spongy placentas to which numerous light brown seeds are attached.

The vine tips and young leaves are also eaten as a vegetable. The vine will bear sporadically until the frost. Sow fresh seed each spring in newly composted soil.

Using Bitter Melon

A tea made of the leaves (see recipe alongside) is used in India and in Brazil to treat diabetes, as it is a natural hypoglycaemic (blood sugar-lowering agent), and also for infections, worms, parasites, fevers, measles, hepatitis and colic, and as a wash for wounds, rashes, grazes and sores. In India particularly the tea, and adding the fruit to the diet, is used to treat haemorrhoids, to increase scanty menstruation, skin diseases and scabies. In the Philippines it is used to treat leukaemia, asthma, diabetes, coughs, insect bites (the tea is cooled and used as a lotion) and to regulate the menstrual flow.

The Chinese use the bitter melon as a tea and in the diet to treat bronchitis, coughs, throat ailments, gastrointestinal infections, and to combat breast cancer. Even the inner pulp and crushed seeds are used to treat skin ailments and sprains, and in the splints to heal fractures, as well as the fruit, which is included in the diet, and a tea of the leaves.

Ongoing research finds it rich in a protein extracted from the fruit and seed that inhibits tumours, shows antiviral activity against the *Herpes simplex* virus and it has some profound anti-cancer effects, especially against leukaemia, and has shown it can inhibit the HIV/AIDS virus in test tubes.

Health Note

The bitter melon is rich in vitamins A, C and E, folic acid, zinc, potassium, pantothenic acid, copper, magnesium and manganese, and it contains antiviral compounds.

Bitter Melon Tea

Add ¼ cup fresh leaves to 1 cup of boiling water, stand 5 minutes. Strain and sip slowly.

How to Use Bitter Melon

To eat bitter melon, wash well, slice lengthwise and remove the red pith and seeds. To lessen the bitterness, soak slices in salted water for half an hour, then parboil for 5 minutes in fresh water and throw the water away. In fresh cold water, boil up again until tender. Add to a rich curry or stir-fry with onions and potatoes, chilli and cumin seeds, and tomatoes if liked.

Caution

Do not consume excessive amounts as too much can be poisonous!
As a therapeutic dose, take no more than 30 millilitres once a day.
Do not eat if you are pregnant.

Moringa
Spinach Tree ▪ Drumstick Tree
Moringa oleifera

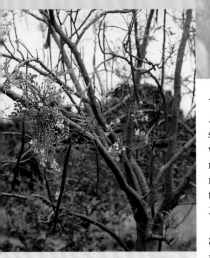

Moringa Tea
Add ¼ cup fresh leaves and flowers to 1 cup of boiling water, stand 5 minutes, strain and sip slowly. This tea is used for a wide array of ailments (see main text) – take 1 cup a day for 7–10 days.

Hint
Moringa has the extraordinary ability to act as a water purifier – the dried, winged seeds are crushed and steeped in dirty river water to clear it. Here is how you do it: The inner white seed kernels are crushed and pounded to a fine powder, then mixed into a paste with water. Usually 2–3 teaspoons of paste will treat 20 litres of dirty river water. Add 2 cups of water to the paste and shake up in a screw-top jar for 5 minutes to activate the 'chemicals' in the seed. Then pour into the bucket of water and stir for 10–15 minutes – this action is vital and a paddle works quickly and well. Then stand at least 30 minutes and you'll find all the particles sink and settle at the bottom of the bucket and clear water can be drawn off. *Note that this water still needs to be boiled if used for drinking water.*

I have grown the moringa for about twenty years now and I never cease be astonished by its sheer tenacity – against the ravages of drought, intense and unbearable heat, the ferocity of devastating storms, sudden cold and although it will not survive below 15 °C, it can take the winter wind if it is well protected – I am in awe of its sheer will to survive. It has been eaten to its very core by mousebirds, monkeys, squirrels and even the porcupines, who savour its luscious 'horseradish-like' roots. I have nearly lost my precious quartet of trees many a year, until I protected them by cages. Now behind the bird-, monkey- and porcupine-proof netting they flourish, trusses of creamy flowers followed by 30 cm long beans, deliciously succulent, and a canopy of extraordinarily pretty fern-like edible leaves.

Indigenous to Northern India and Arabia, this shrubby, quick-growing and beautiful tree can reach 8 metres in height. It is actually a legume and as such adds nitrogen to the soil. It thrives on neglect and in its native India it is a treasured tree as all parts are edible. Young beans are sold in markets in India, Sri Lanka, Reunion Island and the Seychelles, but although it appears in every garden there, it is seldom planted commercially. Ancient and treasured, the heavy, half-ripe pods or beans have been traditionally used to beat the drums in religious ceremonies, hence its name the 'drumstick tree'.

Growing Moringa
Propagation is from seed, ripe and dried in the long pods. Slightly scarify the outer covering by rubbing gently on a rough surface like a flat stone. Immediately plant the seed in a compost-filled bag that has been thoroughly soaked in water, in the shade. Transplant when they are big enough to be hardened off into bigger bags and place in partial shade, moving them into the sun as they grow. Plant out 4 m apart once they reach about 75 cm in height in deep, compost-filled holes with a pipe set at an angle into the root area so that a hose can be inserted into it in order to get water down to the roots. Water deeply once or even twice a week. Give each tree a wheelbarrow load of compost twice a year and you will be rewarded with masses of flowers, leaves and pods.

Using Moringa
The grated root is added to hot water and taken for heart and circulatory ailments. The young, tender green pods are used to treat fatigue, for children failing to thrive and for the elderly, as a general tonic. The leaves and flowers are taken as a tea (see recipe alongside) to stabilise blood pressure, to prevent and clear infections of the chest, throat, lungs and skin, to strengthen the heart, and to ease and soothe stomach ailments. The juice of the leaves and flowers can be applied to skin ailments, acne, pimples and rashes. The leaves, soaked in hot water, are an excellent muscle relaxant and can be used as a poultice over swellings, aching strains and sprains, and to ease a headache.

The tiny compound leaves, stripped off their stems, are cooked with onions and tomatoes, or added to curries, to make the cherished spinach dishes so loved in its native India. Young and tender pods, cut into 2 cm pieces, and steamed or boiled, or added to soups, stews or stir-fries, taste exactly like green beans. The creamy white flowers can be added to curries and stir-fries. The roots contain strong mustard oils that give it a hot and spicy taste, much like horseradish. Carefully dug up, peeled and finely grated, they can be added to sauces, stews and seasonings, or they can be pickled or made into a relish. The oil-rich seeds can be shelled and roasted like peanuts – a popular street food in India. The excellent oil extracted from the seeds is known as 'oil of ben', and can be used for cooking or as a salad oil. It does not turn rancid and it burns without smoking.

Health Note
The green pods are rich in vitamins C, B and E, calcium, iron, potassium, phosphorus and manganese.

Mulberry

Morus nigra

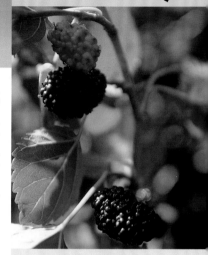

This much-loved fruit – particularly enjoyed by children all over the world – may have originated in the mountains of Nepal or the Caucasus. Its ancient beginnings are truly lost in the mists of time, and there is so much history and legend woven around it that during my research I kept feeling a whole book could be written about this marvellous tree. The little sentence I loved the most that really sums it up, went something like this: 'We humans in our typically egoistical way suppose the God created His fruits for us, the birds, maybe fruit-eating bats – but we have to accept that He created the mulberry for the silkworms!'

Morus alba, the white mulberry, the one preferred by the silkworms, was cultivated in China for the silk industry at least 5 000 years ago. And what is astonishing is that the mulberry tree lives for around 600 years! No one is sure of how and when it reached Europe – it is thought possibly via the Romans – and its spread can to some extent be explained and traced via the silk trade routes. By the 16th century, recipes for mulberry jams and syrups and drinks, and importantly the dye from the brilliantly purple fruits, were so popular that cuttings from the dormant trees during winter were sold in damp sawdust, bundled into thick coarse cloths, at marketplaces across Europe and into the Scandinavian countries and Russia, and as far south as Portugal and Spain, so that today this easy-to-grow and celebrated fruit is an international favourite.

Growing the Mulberry

It is usually thought that the mulberry tree is a huge and spreading tree with a mass of voluptuous branches, covered in huge leaves – and yes, certain varieties are so. Should you live in an area of cold winter frosts, the compact, grey-branched 'English mulberry' would be perfect. We grow what we have come to know as the 'Queensland mulberry' for its large and delicious fruit, usually the length of your thumb. It becomes a really huge and somewhat overgrown specimen with hanging branches reaching the ground, thick with bigger than hand-sized, heart-shaped leaves. Deciduous and a hungry feeder, the spring branches are further weighed down by an abundance of the succulent fruits.

The mulberry is a hungry feeder – be sure to dig a huge hole in full sun and fill it with compost. Plant the tree deeply within the hole and make a large secure dam around it to hold a deep twice weekly watering, once a week in winter. You can prune a mulberry, and often quite ruthlessly. It will recover well. Do it only in midwinter, late June at the latest, as this is one of the first trees to show spring growth.

Using the Mulberry

Morus alba, the white mulberry, has been used as a traditional Chinese medicine since AD 659. All parts are used and are still listed in the Chinese pharmacopoeia, anciently used for elephantitis and tetanus, and still used today. Leaves, roots and bark are processed with honey and are used to lower temperatures and to treat rheumatism. Black mulberry juice is fermented into a wine, which is excellent for coughs and colds, bronchitis, even for tinnitus and postnasal drip.

Mulberries, the black ones particularly, contain resveratrol, which acts as an antioxidant and has been shown to reduce the build-up of plaque in the arteries, thus reducing the risk for atherosclerosis and it even shows some anti-cancer effects and reduced inflammatory reactions.

Mulberry wood is used in ageing balsamic vinegar and for the manufacture of tennis racquets and cricket bats as the wood has an exceptional 'spring' in it.

Health Note

Mulberries are rich in vitamins, especially vitamin C, beta-carotene, potassium, magnesium, phosphorus, calcium and resveratrol (an antioxidant).

Mulberry Smoothie

Eating even just 10 or 12 mulberries a day in season and dried ones out of season, is considered to be a valuable blood tonic for all age groups, especially the aged.

Or try this delicious mulberry smoothie: Whirl a cup of freshly picked mulberries with 1 cup of Bulgarian yoghurt and a little honey in a blender. Pour into a glass and drink immediately. Serves 1.

Hint

Mulberry stains fingers and clothes heavily, so always pick mulberries wearing purple! But seriously, green mulberries help to lighten the stain if quickly and thoroughly rubbed into the spot.

Banana

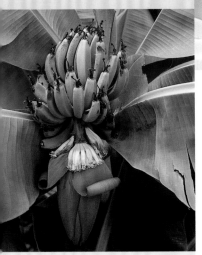

Musa acuminata

I'm quite sure bananas came from Paradise! This exotic-looking, huge-leafed 'tree' grows in tropical regions throughout the world. Records show it's been around for 4 000 years. It is thought that the genus originated in India, and dispersed to Malaysia and the steaming forests of New Guinea, and from there it was taken to Africa probably by the Arabs, and by Captain Cook to Australia, and was spread into the Americas by Spanish and Portuguese explorers around the early part of the 15th century. From then on the world's most loved fruit became an important crop for Brazil, Ecuador, Honduras, Panama, Costa Rica and Mexico, who are the main producers of bananas today, and in Asia and Africa it is a staple food.

The plantain (*Musa paradisiaca*) is the cooking banana, eaten as a vegetable and much loved as a sustaining food in Indonesia and Malaysia.

Growing Bananas

Fast, vigorous and easy, all you need is a hot, frost-free climate, richly composted soil and good rainfall. Suckers with fleshy rhizomes from the parent plant are dug out and replanted continuously, and still today the best, the sweetest, the most vigorous and the largest fruits are chosen to propagate. Huge trusses of male and female flowers form and genetic improvement has now produced the most delicious flavour and sweetness. Bananas thrive in plantations of richly composted soil in full sun, and in the garden as a feature plant, always allowing space for the new plants to form.

Using Bananas

A medium-sized banana provides around 90 calories, 23 g of protein, almost 3 g of fibre and 12 g of natural sugar (which are glucose, fructose and sucrose), a massive 360 mg of potassium, 27–30 mg magnesium and 6–10 mg calcium, which is why they are so good for you! Potassium is one of the most important electrolytes in the body as it controls the fluid balance, regulates heart function, protects against heart disease, strengthens the arterial walls, stabilises blood pressure and protects the body from tension, which could result in a stroke. Bananas in the diet are important as they ease constipation due to their high fibre content, promote and normalise regular bowel function, soothe stomach ulcers and give that energy boost we so often need.

The old Indian folklore says: It is best to eat a banana in the morning to feel like a king! But the most important way of eating a banana is to mash it with a little raw honey and sprinkle it with cinnamon. This will activate the sugars and the potassium and immediately make it available to the body and it will disperse any build-up of phlegm.

Banana leaves are one of the most precious leaves known to mankind. Fish or chicken cooked in a blanket of banana leaves retains all its goodness and the leaves are a source of minerals that act as a healing poultice around wounds, broken bones and painful joints, drawing out infections, inflammation and discomfort. Food is served on banana leaves – no leaf is so tough, so smooth and so important as a banana leaf, and tiny Malaysian babies are washed on a banana leaf to give them health and long life!

Health Note

Bananas are rich in vitamins A, B, C, as well as minerals, particularly potassium (see main text), iron, calcium, magnesium and phosphorus. They are also a good source of dietary fibre.

Fresh Banana Energy Zap

Serves 1

Mash a ripe banana, dribble over it a little honey, sprinkle with cinnamon, and add a dessertspoon each of chopped almonds, sesame seeds and sunflower seeds and mix well. Add a spoonful or two of plain Bulgarian yoghurt and put on your dancing shoes!

Hint

To ripen a bunch of bananas to perfection on the tree, tie a large hessian sack or a strong woven salt bag around it. Within a short while – check them daily – the bananas will ripen to sweet and golden, blemish-free beauties.

Jaboticaba

Myrciaria cauliflora

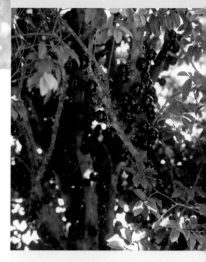

This small-leafed, attractively shaped, evergreen, small tree is fascinating to grow in tropical and subtropical areas. Indigenous to Brazil where it is grown in many gardens as a much-loved fruit, it is included in many traditional dishes. In its native Brazil the tree reaches some 12 to 15 metres in height and it thrives in moist, hot, tropical conditions, even in partial shade.

The most curious aspect of the jaboticaba is that it grows its small, round, black and intensely juicy and sweet grape-like fruits directly on the branches and trunk of the tree. The white or translucent sugary pulp is relished as a drink, a syrupy sauce, as a fermented wine and as a jelly served at celebrations and ceremonies and festivals.

For centuries the jaboticaba has been an important crop in Brazil and was used as trade – its sugary sweetness eagerly searched for by travellers. Jars packed with ripe fruits preserved in vinegar are still today sold in markets for the traditional sweet and sour sauce served with onions and chicken. Traditional recipes are handed down from generation to generation, and the seeds from the mature fruits, ground and pounded, were made into medicines for bladder and urinary ailments – the grandmother of the house being the one to dispense it. In the markets of Brazil baskets of jaboticaba fruits are on sale in early summer like black and glistening cherries, succulent and irresistibly sweet, as they have been through the centuries and are as much loved and cherished today as they were then.

Growing the Jaboticaba

Interestingly, the first jaboticaba fruits I tasted came from a protected, tree-rich garden in Johannesburg – but a hot, moist and tropical climate is actually required for the tree to produce those incredibly delicious fruits. I was fortunate many years ago to be able to get a few small jaboticaba trees from Nelspruit's Tropical Fruit Research orchards. Although slow growing and often only bearing fruit after 7 or 8 years, I have been fortunate to experience the tiny clusters of yellowish, multi-stamened 'knobs' rather than flowers that appear along the thicker branches in spring, to be followed by the clusters of shiny, black, thumbnail-sized fruit. The jaboticaba can be grown from seeds or cuttings, and planted in full sun, or even in some afternoon shade, in a deep, compost-rich hole that can be flooded with water weekly, the trees grow steadily with new reddish spring leaves yearly, and become more shrub-like with multiple stems forming continuously.

Using the Jaboticaba

The flavour of the early summer fruits is said to be a mixture of litchi, grape and very sweet cherry. Squeezed for juice – the pips and skins strained out – jaboticaba juice is luxuriously sweet and full of flavour and can be made into a drink served with ice and slices of lemon and diluted with a little cold water, or made into a jam, or a jelly, or a sorbet. Whole crushed fruits, fermented, make a rich dark red wine which is also taken as an after-dinner drink to aid indigestion, or served warm to ease a cough or feverish cold.

The skins, sun dried and chopped and kept in the kitchen in screw-topped jars, are added to a spicy mixture made with coriander, star anise and ginger, and added to sauces, stews and soups – this delicious mixture crushed with a little salt adds both flavour and colour, and gives sweetness that makes a dish so satisfying.

Health Note

Jaboticaba fruits are rich in vitamins C, D and E, beta-carotene (found in the skins), calcium, potassium, phosphorus, magnesium and fructose.

Jaboticaba Syrup

Slice 20–30 jaboticaba fruits in half. Simmer with 1 cup of water in a heavy bottomed stainless steel pot. Add 2 tablespoons of honey and 2 teaspoons of finely grated fresh ginger root. Simmer 15 minutes, then strain, and serve warm over ice-cream or fruit salads.

Or serve fresh fruits with Bulgarian yoghurt and a little honey, the way they do in Brazil – it is addictive!

Hint

The dried, finely chopped skins can be added to syrups and sugars, or when cooking fruit or rhubarb, to give texture, colour and flavour.

Olive

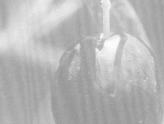

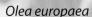
Olea europaea

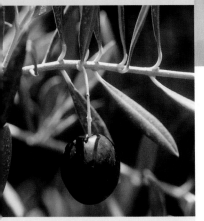

Olive Leaf Tea

Olive leaf tea builds the immune system and can be taken for a host of ailments (see text) – take a cup or two daily for 10 days, then give it a break for 2–3 days, and then repeat.

To make the tea, add ¼ cup fresh leaves to 1 cup of boiling water, stand 5 minutes, strain and sip slowly.

Olive Tissue Oil

Partially dried olive leaves steeped into extra virgin olive oil has been used for stretch marks for centuries! Into a small bottle of extra virgin olive oil press in half the quantity of partially dried olive leaves. Stand in the sun for 10 days, giving it a daily shake. Strain. Use as a tissue oil and to moisturise dry, cracked skin.

A Note on Olive Oil

Always choose cold-pressed virgin or extra virgin olive oil. The very first pressing is referred to as 'extra virgin' or 'virgin' and these oils retain both the flavour and all the goodness of the olives. Refined oil has many of its health-promoting substances removed during the manufacturing process. The oil is extracted under high temperatures, which results in a loss of nutrients. This also applies to seed oils such as canola, sunflower and safflower oils.

An ancient and long-lived and precious tree, the olive is one of the world's most revered and respected trees and perhaps one of the oldest foods and medicines ever known. The history of the olive goes back into the mists of time – we can only imagine its earliest beginnings. The ancient Assyrians, the Romans, the Greeks, the Egyptians and the Palestinians all treasured the olive, and early on began the most valuable extraction of its oil. The olive is mentioned in the Bible and was first cultivated in Crete around 3500 BC. Even then the leaves were used as a wound wash, a burn dressing and to rid the body of parasites. During the Middle Ages, the monks used infused oils as medicine and the olive leaf, pounded and crushed, was added to the oil for wounds and burns, and olive trees were grown in the cloister gardens as a valuable medicinal herb.

An ancient symbol of wisdom, of prosperity, of peace and of plenty, the olive has remained one of mankind's most valuable treasures and today medical research proves its efficacy for many ailments as well as for skincare and cosmetics.

Growing Olives

Specific conditions are needed for fruiting – hot, dry conditions are the first requisite but cold winters, a certain amount of humidity with rain at particular times of the year and experimentation is all that can be counted upon. The Cape grows the best olives in general for South Africa and yet surprising places show promise. In the Herbal Centre gardens we have trialled olives for many years with the very occasional burst of heavily laden fruit after or even during a rainy season, but the valuable medicinal qualities within the leaves make it so worthwhile a tree in every garden, so we grow olives for that purpose alone, and when there is an erratic harvest of fruit we are ecstatic and process it carefully.

Plant the young olive tree – we grow Mission olive – in a 1 m by 1 m hole in full sun, filled with good compost and rich topsoil. Set a pipe into the hole at an angle at least a metre in length so that a hose can be inserted every now and then to get water down to the roots. A barrow load of good compost twice a year and a long deep watering every two weeks in the hot months, less in winter, is all that the olive requires. Occasional pruning in winter to tidy the trees is also worth giving attention to, and every pruned branch can be used in teas and in oils.

Using Olives

Extracts of the leaves, which contain oleuropein and have strong antiviral and antibacterial properties, will help to lower blood pressure, stabilise blood sugar levels and improve the whole circulatory system. A valuable treatment for diabetics over the centuries, the olive leaf is now recognised as an excellent natural medicine. A cup of olive leaf tea (see recipe alongside) a day is excellent for dizziness, disorientation, cystitis and high fevers. As a diuretic and a comforting treatment for chronic fatigue syndrome, multiple sclerosis and ME, and for feelings of utter helplessness and despair, olive leaf tea is proving invaluable. A poultice of fresh leaves crushed into a little oil is excellent for aching muscles, slow-healing wounds, infected grazes and rashes. Apply fresh twice daily until the area heals.

The processed fruit is a much-loved salad ingredient and the oil, monounsaturated and rich in oleic acid, is the best oil for high cholesterol. A simple salad dressing of extra virgin olive oil with freshly squeezed lemon juice is the world's favourite and a health booster beyond compare!

Health Note

Today's research finds olive oil rich in minerals like calcium, magnesium and potassium, in vitamins and enzymes in a unique combination that makes it a superb health food. Include cold-pressed olive oil in the diet every day.

Prickly Pear

Indian Fig•Cactus Pear
Opuntia ficus-indica

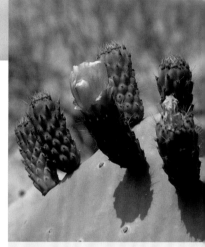

The prickly pear is a fascinating plant. Thick spiny 'pads' form the plant's succulent 'leaves', only leaves are not what they are! The 'leaves' are actually the stems and along the top of the 'stems' the large 'buds' form, which turn into the delicious fruits.

Probably native to South America and Mexico, from prehistoric times the prickly pear was a valuable food, both the thick 'pads' or leaves and the fruit. The Spanish explorers brought it from Mexico into Europe, and the Franciscan monks, who used it as a medicine, introduced it to California. It quickly spread and became a sought-after trade. This rapid spread into the temperate parts of the world was astonishing as no food plant grows with the ease and neglect that the prickly pear does. A mere 'leaf' tucked into the soil, stem end down, and watered once, could easily and quickly become a new plant, and the trade was brisk in those early centuries as the fruit was prized for its sweetness and often came in exciting colours – orange-yellow, crisp and juicy green, and the sought-after deep shocking red! (Today that luscious red prickly pear is known affectionately as 'the Free State ice-cream' as it grew abundantly in the Free State on those huge and isolated mealie farms.)

Growing Prickly Pears
Prepare a large hole, about 1 m wide and 1 m deep, in full sun and fill with compost. Tuck in 3 large 'leaves', stem side down, covering one-third of the leaf with soil, and flood the hole. Water once a week, or once every two weeks in winter or if it rains. Tolerant of both drought and neglect, it thrives in adverse conditions and can become a problematic invader, so take care where you plant it. Note that it is classified as an invader plant in South Africa and planting it is prohibited.

Using Prickly Pears
The Spanish boiled the pulp down to make a paste known as 'queso de tuna' – prickly pear cheese – which was an excellent treatment for bringing down a fever, for using over rashes, scratches and grazes as a comforting poultice, and as a baby food, sieved to remove the seeds. Thin strips of the dethorned leaf, cooked like green beans and then dipped in batter and fried, not only became a reliable famine food, but with its excellent mineral and vitamin content is eaten for energy and vitality and for 'flu and colds, and like the fruit, to bring down a fever.

In the Free State, farmers' wives made excellent jams, syrups and cordials from the sweet fruits, and even pickles using the leaves. I have been fascinated by this extraordinary famine food for many years, and have grown an almost thornless commercial variety in my gardens for those divine Christmas ice-cream dishes we all enjoy. And nothing beats the heat like a bowl of chilled, sliced prickly pear on a summer afternoon!

I learned, as a young farmer's wife, from the farmers of surrounding farms that a couple of prickly pear leaves scored with a garden fork to break the skin so that the juice could flow, could be tossed into a stagnant pool in the river to kill the mosquito larvae – which I patiently did for years. Interestingly, the leaf 'skeletons', fibrous and fascinating, the flesh having rotted off in the river, were washed up for me to collect along the riverbanks. Dried and bleached in the sun, these attractive, rounded leaf skeletons were eagerly bought from my farm cottage industry shop by flower arrangers who bleached or painted them white!

Health Note
Prickly pears are rich in calcium, magnesium, phosphorus and traces of iron and copper, as well as vitamin C and some B-vitamins.

How to Eat a Prickly Pear
Spiny with tiny, hair-like little 'thorns', this is one fruit that needs to be handled with care. Luckily the boxes of prickly pears bought from the greengrocer are 'spineless' or thornless, those skin-irritating little thorns having been expertly rubbed off before sale.

The ripe fruits – at their best from December – are a delicious treat chilled and carefully peeled. With a fork holding the fruit firmly slice off both ends with a sharp knife, then make a slit from end to end in the skin and open the slit with the knife and the fork to reveal an egg-sized succulent and juicy and enticingly sweet fruit which can be eaten as it is or thinly sliced and served with whipped cream.

Note
In South Africa the prickly pear is classified as a Category 1 Invader Plant. It may not be planted in gardens under any circumstances. Commercial plantings have been registered with the Agricultural control bodies.

Pachira Nut
Malabar Chestnut

Pachira aquatica

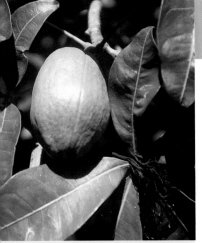

Pachira Ice-Cream

We make this fabulous dessert around Christmas time when the pachira trees are heavily laden with their giant nuts.

2 cups thick cream, well whisked

2 cups ripe mango, well mashed

2 tablespoons runny honey added to the mangoes

4 eggs well beaten with 1 teaspoon vanilla essence (or a vanilla pod carefully scraped out)

1 cup roasted, chopped pachira nuts

Fold the beaten eggs and vanilla into the whipped cream, then fold in the honey and mango mixture, stirring lightly, and finally gently stir in the chopped roasted pachira nuts. Pour into an ice-cream maker or into freezer trays. In the freezer trays whisk it up once it is almost frozen and return to the freezer until set. Serve in pretty glass dishes with a sprinkling of roasted pachira nuts.

Hint

The young leaves make a delicious spinach dish. Simmer 3 minutes in a stainless steel pan with ½ cup water, keeping the lid on. Remove from the heat and let it stand for 5 minutes before serving. This makes the leaves extra tender.

This fascinating, exotic tree frequently starts off as a pot plant! Often with three stems twisted or plaited together, and topped with a cluster of star-pointed leaves, it stands in the indoor section of nurseries and no one ever realises what a treasure it is. A native of the indigenous forests and riverbanks of Brazil, Peru, Ecuador and parts of Mexico, it is a much-loved traditional food. The fruit – a large, green pod – has five or sometimes six segments which, when ripe, burst open to reveal the thumbnail-sized round seeds (or nuts). As the tree grows tall – it can reach up to 18 metres – the fruit obligingly splits open when ripe, causing the seeds to drop to the ground. You just have to be on the lookout for them before the squirrels and the monkeys get them!

Pachira has a long and ancient history as a valuable food source. The seeds were used as barter, roasted and ready to eat, and the raw, fresh seeds quickly exchanged hands. The young seedlings, which needed only water and grew easily in shady places, were taken on board as part of the ship's food store. One can only imagine the places this precious tree was taken, for those fresh, young and tender leaves would have been a valuable food for the scurvy-ridden sailors.

Growing Pachira Nut

Fresh seeds grow easily, virtually germinating 100% in frost-free areas, and the little tree is undemanding, tolerant of poor soils and even short periods of drought. But in deeply dug, richly composted soil with a good weekly watering, our plantings have shown just how beautiful this unusual and exotic tree can be.

The flower never ceases to amaze – its finger-length, pointed bud opens in a burst of succulent, pale-green spirals of calyx to reveal a 'fibre-optic' pale, creamy mass – hundreds of stamens that turn golden as the flower ages. Short-lived and intensely perfumed, this exotic beauty is held upright above the leaves and in 2 or sometimes 3 days it drops and the fruit quickly begins to form. The breathtaking flowers appear all through the spring and summer, and the trees planted close to the buildings in the Herbal Centre gardens are watched in eager anticipation. Visitors are fascinated, and the sale of our baby pachira trees in the nursery is assured. In fact, we never have enough to meet the demand!

Using Pachira Nuts

The seeds need to be planted within a few days of gathering, or shelled and roasted, or eaten fresh. Roasted and sprinkled with a little salt, they are similar in taste to chestnuts, and are a favourite snack that everyone enjoys. In Mexico the shelled nuts are chopped and fried, and served with desserts, or salted and sprinkled over savoury dishes. The nuts can also be ground into a flour, which makes a delicious pancake or a light bread when added to other flours, and in Peru the flour is used for a type of flat bread that is cooked in the sun on a flat rock.

Medicinally, pachira nuts have been crushed and pounded, and mixed to a paste with boiled water as a wound dressing for cuts, grazes and infected insect bites, held in place with a banana leaf bound over the area. The same paste mixed with warmed oil – like maize or sunflower oil – is an ancient beauty treatment for dry, cracked heels and hands, and is even used on the face – especially for the lips. Rich in proteins, amino acids and unsaturated fats, pachira nuts are an excellent tonic for the whole cardiovascular system.

Health Note

Pachira nuts are high in vitamin A and especially vitamin E, and also contain proteins, amino acids and unsaturated fats.

Millet

Panicum miliaceum

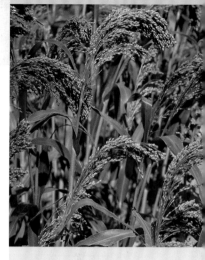

Millet is the name given to a group of cereal grasses which have been used since prehistoric times for brewing as a porridge or gruel across Europe, Asia and Africa. The word 'millet' is thought to have originated from the Latin 'millesimum' meaning 'one thousandth part' – an apt description of the tiny millet seeds. Evidence of the early beginnings of millet, the actual cultivation, was found on an ancient Assyrian carving discovered in an Assyrian palace excavation, although it is believed to have been first cultivated in Ethiopia from where it spread to Arabia and the Persian Gulf, and from there to India, where it has been grown since 2000 BC! From there millet continued its journey via the silk trade route on to China. It is thought from Ethiopia it came south in Africa and the Bantu tribes adopted it, pulverising it into a porridge or a beer brew. Today millet is still grown in Africa and teff – a grass often considered to be a millet in parts of Africa – features as a main ingredient in *injera*, one of Ethiopia's most-loved breads.

The true millet remains a staple food for Africans, Indians, the Chinese and the Russians. The Egyptians made the first 'pita bread' from millet until one day some brewed beer made from millet was accidentally added to it, which made it into the lighter, fluffier bread texture we know today, and after this lucky accident, it is thought, beer instead of water was used to make their millet bread! Millet bread before this was always 'the unleavened bread' known in biblical history and millet remained the key grain until maize and wheat became known.

Growing Millet

An annual summer grass and the main ingredient in commercial birdseed, growing millet is fascinating in its variety. Valuable in that it will grow in climates inhospitable to wheat and barley, today it has become a health food that suits gluten-free requirements and hulled millet is a much sought-after health food.

Millet needs full sun and a well-dug, well-composted bed in full sun. We grow the beautiful foxtail millet for our birdseed ranges as well as the textured golden grain millet and finger millet. Seed for sowing must be unhulled and sowing is from early spring. We water it twice weekly and it survives even hailstorms, strong hot winds and heat up to 38 °C!

Using Millet

Today millet is a valuable health food: is a low-allergy, gluten-free grain, an excellent source of fibre and it offers well-documented protection against heart disease and cancer, and for diabetes it is becoming more important as medical research continues.

In health shops and on the health section shelves in the supermarkets, millet flakes, grains and flours are easily available with instructions on how to use it in baking, porridges and soups. Our own millet range, sold under our 'Nature's Pantry' label, is something we are becoming excited about, as day by day many millet devotees share their health-restoring stories with us. Add millet to muffin, biscuit and cake recipes as well as to soup or serve the cooked grains like rice.

Made into an energy-boosting snack with dates, sesame seeds and almonds, millet can also help to manage those blood sugar levels. Interestingly, millet is recommended for gout sufferers as it is one of the foods lowest in purines, which in abundance – like in meats, saturated fats, anchovies, herrings, mackerel – increase uric acid production. Millet is an excellent source of fibre and so is a good laxative food for those with irregular bowel movements. Cook it as a porridge and serve with plain yoghurt, chopped almonds or pecan nuts, a little raw honey and some grated apple.

Millet Porridge

Serves 4

Our favourite way of eating millet is still as a porridge that gives an energy-giving boost at the start of a busy day, especially served with home-dried fruit and Bulgarian yoghurt.

1 cup dehusked millet seed
1½ cups water
1 cup milk
½ teaspoon salt
2 teaspoons cinnamon

Simmer the millet in the water, milk, cinnamon and salt for 20 minutes, stirring frequently. Add ½–1 cup chopped fresh or dried fruit like apple rings, cranberries, wild cherries (*Prunus capuli*), pineapple or mango slices. Alternatively, eat it as it is with milk or plain yoghurt and a little honey.

Health Note

Both the pulverised grains and sprouted, unhusked millet seeds are rich in iron, vitamins A and B, potassium, phosphorus, zinc, selenium and manganese. Millet is a highly alkaline food, rich in fibre and is known as a low-allergenic food, so it is no wonder millet is becoming the health food of the moment.

Granadilla
Passion Fruit

Passiflora edulis

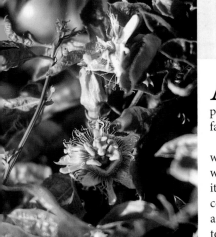

A much-loved vigorous and charming climber, the granadilla or grenadilla, is native to Brazil, Paraguay and northern Argentina. Spanish explorers used both the fruit and the easily grown plants as trade and spread it quickly through the rest of the world. There is no fruit that has quite that fabulous taste of the exotic as granadilla has, and everywhere it went people wanted more!

The passion fruit, as is also known, comes from a large genus of several hundred varieties, and it was so named by the Spanish Jesuit priests using it to explain the passion or crucifixion of Christ when colonising South America, and not, as many people believe, for inducing passion when eating it! The priests interpreted the beautiful and unusual flowers like this: The pillar or column in the centre of the flower represents the cross, the three stamens are the Holy Trinity – the Father, the Son and the Holy Spirit – the five anthers under the stamens indicate the five wounds which nailed Christ to the cross. Beneath the three stigmas is a small swollen seed vessel denoting the sponge soaked in vinegar that was thrust into Christ's mouth. The calyx represents the Halo. The corona of fine purple tendrils represents the blood-soaked crown of thorns; the ten petals are the 12 disciples – excluding Judas, who betrayed Him, and Peter, who denied Him. The three-lobed leaves suggest the hands of the persecutors and the long, green tendrils along the stem are the whips they lashed at Him, and the climbing vine, with its solitary flowers, indicates our aloneness as we climb higher in our seeking of our oneness with God.

This extraordinary plant has been grown extensively through the centuries as both a medicine, calming, soothing and quietening, and as a treasured food in warm and temperate regions all over the world. In the early centuries it was grown around the churches, used in religious ceremonies, and the delicious juice made as a drink of thanksgiving. The Spanish explorers called the fruit 'granadilla' which means 'little pomegranate' and took it with them to cure scurvy and chest ailments and for bladder discomfort. A treasured and adored fruit from long before Christ, it has never lost its popularity.

Growing Granadillas

Frost sensitive, the granadilla is a perennial vine that thrives along a fence or along a wall or over an arch, and produces masses of round purple fruits the size of an egg from midsummer onwards until around May. With its eager tendrils it climbs ever higher and will thrive in full sun in a wide and deep compost-filled hole, spaced 2 m apart. Our most productive vines last about five years and cuttings taken in late summer grow easily. Be sure to water it thoroughly and deeply twice a week, especially in hot weather, and once a week only in the cold months. There are several varieties of *Passiflora edulis*, from the well-known purple-fruited one to a prolific larger red-skinned variety and a bright yellow, sharply sour variety.

Using Granadilla

The Spaniards still today use the leaves, soaked in hot water, bound around aching sprains, bruises, varicosities and swollen ankles – the hot leaves held in place by the vines, twisted around the limb. The monks in medieval times grew the passion fruit vine in their cloister gardens to use in many ways, and for arthritic joints the leaves, warmed and soft, were considered to be invaluable.

The fruit pulp is at its most sweet and delicious when the fruit is wrinkled and mature. The pulp is nothing short of divine in desserts, cake icings, jellies, jams and drinks, and as a coulis for ice-cream. We find it indispensable in our restaurant kitchen and for our jams and jellies and drinks in our shop.

Health Note

The fruit pulp is rich in vitamins A and C, some B vitamins, phosphorus and potassium.

Granadilla Coulis

This is a thick 'syrup' that is simply delicious over ice-cream, sago pudding and rice pudding, or diluted with crushed ice and iced water as a refreshing drink.

20 granadillas

3 cups sugar (less if the granadillas have really ripened and are sweet – more if they are sour)

juice of 1 lemon

Simmer for 30 minutes, taste as you go, then pour into sterilised bottles with a secure screw top. Refrigerate once you've opened it and in hot weather keep refrigerated all the time.

Note: To keep the sugar content down and if it is going to be used immediately, we often add chopped fresh stevia leaves while cooking. It is so worth experimenting with stevia to lessen the sugar content.

Hint

In a liquidiser, whirl 1 cup of sieved fresh granadilla juice with 1 cup of pineapple cubes, 1 cup ripe mango slices and a dribble of honey. Serve with plain vanilla ice-cream or plain Bulgarian yoghurt.

Parsnip

Pastinaca sativa

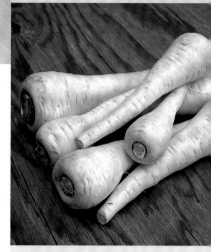

I've never been able to get my children to eat parsnips and I've grown absolute beauties! It has a long, pale, carrot-like root of intense flavour – I've loved it as a soup ingredient in amongst the survivor plants in the heart of winter, even under a blanket of snow. Its tall-growing, green leafy top looks like a coarse flat-leaf parsley and it too is part of the great Umbelliferae family along with carrots, parsley and celery.

Originating in the Mediterranean area, the Romans actually cultivated the wild form and according to Pliny the Elder, Emperor Tiberius held parsnips in such high esteem he had them brought to him from the banks of the river Rhine where they grew prolifically, to Rome where fields of parsnips were successfully reaped. In the Middle Ages the parsnip became the food of Lent for its substantial carbohydrate content – it is a sweet and succulent food, and after the winter its nutritious sugars were sustaining, making it the perfect Lenten food. By the 16th century parsnips were under careful cultivation in Germany, England and to a degree in France and Italy. Then the colonists took them to the New World and parsnips were a major food source, a staple food in Europe and beyond, and in America it became a favourite, not even the potato could upstage it in the 19th century. The colonists enjoyed parsnips in pancakes and puddings, and with the winter freeze turning the starches to sugars, many a pilgrim blessed the parsnip, paired with salted fish, as a lifesaver.

Growing Parsnips

Sow the seed either in spring or in hot areas at the end of summer in full sun in a wide trench that is deeply dug and filled with compost, and that can be flooded with water twice weekly. This is where they will grow, just like carrots, so sow carefully and thinly and cover lightly with soil, then cover with raked leaves to keep the moisture in and the birds out. Parsnips thrive with compost and a deep and slow twice weekly watering, and once a week in the dead of winter.

Using Parsnips

Parsnips are a superb support to the spleen and the kidneys, which they help to flush, and they detoxify and cleanse the entire body. Centuries ago the soldiers and the sailors were given mashed carrots and parsnips as soon as they returned from their battles or their sea voyages. Because carrots and parsnips lasted well they were part of the essential provisions sent with the sailors and the soldiers at that time, for the action on the bladder and the bowel. Only later was it found that these two root vegetables were probable lifesavers!

Parsnips are delicious in soups, peeled and finely grated, and chopped into stir-fries, or served thinly sliced with a cheesy white sauce. Much like a potato the parsnip's texture is improved by mashing with milk or a little cream or with added butter or plain yoghurt, a grinding of coarse sea salt and black pepper and a squeeze of lemon juice. They are at their best cooked with stews, soups and casseroles, and their rich vitamin and mineral content (see Health Note) makes them a valuable tonic to the whole body.

Health Note

Parsnips contain vitamins C, B and E in significant amounts, along with folic acid and potassium, phosphorus, calcium and magnesium – perfectly balanced so as to give a real health boost to a meal.

Roasted Parsnips

Try roasting parsnips in a roasting pan with potatoes, carrots, onions and sweet potatoes, even whole garlic. Cut the vegetables in half, toss in olive oil, salt and black pepper and add a scattering of fresh thyme and about 2 cups of water. Roast slowly and keep the pan well covered. A chicken roasted alongside these delicious root vegetables makes a substantial meal, and one fit for a king, as King Henry VIII will attest – this was his favourite 'rib sticking meal'!

Hint

Parsnip leaves, finely chopped and steamed quickly, are delicious with a touch of butter and a squeeze of lemon juice, and can be mixed with other spinach leaves.

Caution

The leaves contain compounds that may cause skin irritation in people with sensitive skins.

Avocado

Persea americana

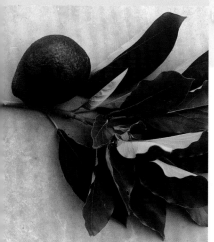

Belonging to the fabulous *Persea* genus of about 150 species of luscious evergreen trees and shrubs indigenous to tropical and subtropical regions of Central and South America and Southeast Asia, the avocado has been cultivated since 8000 BC. Different varieties from Brazil to California, Mexico to Guatemala ensure year-round avocados virtually all over the world.

This precious oil-rich nutritious fruit and its leaves have been used in medicine since the earliest centuries, and it has never, to this present day, lost its popularity. One of the most perfect foods, it is now grown all over the world in warm countries, and it constantly reveals more and more marvellous benefits.

Growing Avocados

Dig a large hole in full sun with good space around it. Fill the hole with rich, well-rotted compost and fill with water. Plant the avocado tree in it and stake it. Make a good dam around it to flood with water once or twice weekly. Cover it with frost protection 'fleece' in winter, and watch the pale yellow sprays of tiny spring flowers form. Some years the crop is huge and others, especially if there has been a cold snap in early spring, the yield may be poor.

Whatever the time of the year, the avocado tree will fascinate you with its big leathery leaves and gnarled fissured trunk. If I could only have one tree in my garden, I would choose an avocado!

Using Avocados

Here is where the real fascination begins. The little fruits start ripening at the end of summer. These fruits are high in monounsaturated fats, the heart-healthy unsaturated fatty acids, and avocado oil is one of the most important plant oils, second only to olive oil. Avocado oil contains oleic acid, linoleic acid and small quantities of linolenic acid, and this exquisite oil is superb in cosmetics as it is a perfect skin moisturiser.

Avocado oil is an excellent carrier oil for essential oils, and aromatherapy oils can be added to avocado oil and used as a soothing and gentle massage oil. Avocado oil can be added to moisturising creams, soaps and shampoos, and a brew of the leaves is an excellent lotion or wash for oily skin and acne, and as a rinse after shampooing the hair. Make at least 6 cups of avocado leaf brew by boiling 3 cups of fresh torn and crushed leaves in 3 litres of water for 15 minutes, cool and strain. Use as a final rinse for the hair and massage it well into the scalp. It clears scalp conditions and stimulates hair growth.

A tea made of 1 tablespoon bark and 1 tablespoon crushed pip in 2 cups of boiling water, stand 5 minutes and strain, is taken ½ cup at a time as a diuretic. Tea of the leaves will help to lower high blood pressure and is also taken for coughs, colds, fever and bronchitis. Add ¼ cup of fresh chopped leaves to 1 cup of boiling water, stand 5 minutes, strain and cool before sipping slowly.

A poultice of leaves warmed in hot water is soothing over the temples for headache, over painful sprains, strains and rheumatic joints, and if the leaves are toasted, the pleasant taste flavours a bean stew!

The best way of eating avocado is sliced thickly on homemade brown bread and butter with black pepper, a little grinding of sea salt and a squeeze of lemon juice. Just taste a complete food!

Health Note

Considered to be the most nutritious of all fruits thanks to it high levels of monounsaturated fatty acids, avocados are also a good source of vitamins A, B3, B6, C, E and K, folic acid, beta-carotene, iron, copper, potassium and phosphorus.

Guacamole

2 ripe avocados
juice of 1 lemon
1 medium ripe tomato, finely chopped
½ cup finely chopped young coriander leaves
1 clove garlic, finely chopped
a sprig or two of parsley
1 teaspoon cumin seed
black pepper and sea salt to taste
Mix everything together smoothly and serve as a dip on biscuits.

Hint

Make an avocado leaf and apple cider vinegar infusion for shiny, healthy hair. Steep fresh leaves in a bottle of apple cider vinegar for 2 weeks. Shake up daily. Add a dash to the final rinsing water after shampooing the hair. It clears itchy scalp too!

Caution

Do not take avocado leaves, seeds or bark if you are pregnant as it stimulates the uterus.

Parsley

Petroselinum crispum

Although parsley is not strictly a food, I include it here because it is so valuable in the diet. A close cousin to both carrots and celery – this threesome is perhaps the most valuable health food combination we enjoy in our daily salad – parsley is the king of herbs, not as a garnish and not only as a medicine, but as a food source of so huge an array of vitamins and minerals it literally can knock your socks off! I grow both the moss-curled parsley and the huge and fabulous flat-leaf Italian parsley in unending abundance in my herb gardens. I plant twice yearly so that I always have masses and I am eternally grateful to the ancient Greeks and the Romans who made it famous.

Ancient, revered and cherished, parsley was held to be a sacred herb, placed in reverence on the tombs of the deceased, and cultivated as a medicine over 2 500 years ago. In the Middle Ages the monks used parsley tea to cure gout, to ease chest ailments, to soothe arthritic aches and pains, to clear bladder and kidney ailments, to clear spotty skin, oily acne and skin infections, as a poultice over infected wounds, burns and grazes and even for hair loss, tooth decay and piles! In fact, parsley was the base of all their treatments and to this day parsley is still growing in many cloister gardens.

As a garnish it was the ancient Romans who used it to decorate the great meat platters of roasted pigs, goats and sheep, served in mighty splendour at celebrations and feasts. Bowls of fresh parsley were placed along the tables to chew between the feasting to sweeten the breath and as a digestive. And to remove foul odours it became a valuable bathing herb. Parsley wine was made as a body deodoriser and every cottage garden grew their own beds of parsley for washing waters.

Growing Parsley

All it asks is a well-dug bed of richly composted friable soil in full sun with a weekly or even twice weekly watering in hot weather. It needs no special attention, it is a prolific biennial and moss-curled parsley makes so neat and uniform a row that the designer show gardens favour it as path edgings and even circling roses. Flat-leaf parsley grows taller and wider, often reaching 30 cm in width and height, but it is equally charming and uniform, its fernlike feathery sprays so pretty you'll be tempted to use it in everything!

Using Parsley

Parsley is an alkaline forming food that cleanses the kidneys, bladder and the whole urinary system. It is a deodorant, and it reduces coagulants in the veins and helps to clear kidney stones. Over the centuries parsley has established itself as a valuable natural diuretic and has proved useful in the treatment of arthritis, gout and rheumatism. Parsley tea (see recipe alongside) is an effective treatment for cystitis, along with celery and fennel. The tea is also useful for cleansing the liver, helping to control high blood pressure, for nausea and flatulence, that feeling of 'liverishness' or slight queasiness, bloating, tummy rumbles, bladder ailments, and for men with prostate problems. Eating finely chopped fresh parsley, and drinking a cup of parsley tea will gently, safely and easily soothe all the above ailments. Parsley contains volatile oils such as limonene, eugenol and myristicin, which have shown strong anti-cancer effects that we should be aware of.

Eating fresh parsley daily will brighten the complexion, clear the skin, heal acne and pimples and with its vitamin A and C content promote elasticity in the skin. A handful of fresh parsley tied in a cloth and used in the bath with soap will tone the skin, remove oiliness, clear infections and give that marvellous alkaline freshness to the whole body. Eat fresh chopped parsley with everything – sprinkle it lavishly on every savoury dish and add it to salads, stir-fries and even tomato and cheese sandwiches!

Health Note

Rich in chlorophyll, vitamins, especially vitamins A and C, B-vitamins, beta-carotene, iron, calcium, magnesium, potassium and folic acid, parsley is actually a multivitamin in a leaf! A mere half a cup of finely chopped parsley contains more vitamin C than 2 oranges, more beta-carotene than 2 large carrots, 20 times more iron than one serving of liver and 10 times more calcium than a cup of milk!

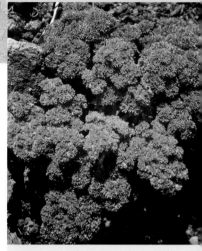

Parsley Tea

One or two or even three cups during the day will gently, safely and easily soothe a host of ailments (see main text).

Add ¼ cup fresh parsley sprigs to 1 cup of boiling water, stand 5 minutes, strain and sip slowly.

Hint

Always eat parsley with food that has been fried in oil or butter, as it literally helps to inhibit the cancer-causing compounds in fried foods. If you have to indulge in fried foods, make this a rule: always sprinkle finely chopped fresh parsley over fried eggs and bacon, or over that plate of chips.

Beans

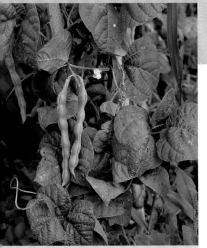

Phaseolus and other species

I have been a bean grower and a bean collector since I was a child, and these rewarding plants never cease to amaze me. This section covers only a few of my collection – the best known and most easily found ones. All belong to the great family of legumes, Fabaceae, or plants that bear their nutritious seeds in pods. What is important is that all the different and fascinating species and varieties have been found to be so rich in vitamins and minerals, particularly iron, that beans have remained one of the world's most cherished, respected and popular foods throughout the centuries.

In the beginning it was thought that the bean originated in India, but by the end of the 19th century it was proved that the common bean or kidney bean, *Phaseolus vulgaris*, originated in America! After exhaustive studies, palaeo-ethnological and ethnographical researchers agreed that the bean existed on the American continent before it appeared in Europe in the 16th century. The French word 'haricot' was part of the language around 1640, but in 1572 the English already called both green beans and the dried 'seeds', haricot or French beans, which had come to England from France!

Commercially, beans are divided into two main categories: *pod beans*, which are marketed and consumed while still unripe as green beans, and *shelled beans*, which are either climbers or dwarf bush beans, and are mostly consumed dried and shelled. There is no real difference between the two categories – the only difference is in the way they are used, and many of the cultivars are almost impossible to define.

Growing Beans

Prepare a bed in full sun by digging deeply. Now spread a thick layer of compost over the area and again dig deeply, working the compost in well, as beans are heavy feeders. Moisten thoroughly by setting a sprinkler over the area, and then mark out lines 40 cm apart where the beans are to grow. Set up trellises or tepees for climbers, or in the case of bush beans, mark out a row. Press the beans, 2 or 3 together, into the soil and keep moist. Spread a mulch of dried leaves over the area to keep the soil cool and moist, and to deter the birds. Water 2 or 3 times a week once the beans are sturdy.

Using Beans

All the beans – kidney beans, butter beans, haricot beans, sugar beans, lima beans and more – are rich in vitamins and minerals (see Health Note), amino acids, protein and carbohydrates. Whichever you choose, they all are extremely valuable, both green and fresh in their pods (sometimes you'll find purple beans like Blue Peter or bright yellow bush ones) or used as dried pulses. Make sure these valuable foods are included frequently in the diet.

High in protein and fibre, beans are an essential part of the vegetarian diet. They are energy boosters in the long term – not just a quick pick-me-up. They build muscle, tone the muscles and restore muscular strength after debilitating illnesses such as tuberculosis, malnutrition, pneumonia and emaciation. They tone and strengthen the whole body system, strengthen veins and soothe haemorrhoids, and act as a tonic to the whole body. They are excellent for treating anaemia and are essential in the diet for treating high cholesterol.

Health Note

Beans in general are a good source of vitamins and minerals, including vitamins A, B, C and E, calcium, phosphorus, magnesium, potassium and iron.

Bean Salad

Serves 6–8

Use any of your favourite dry beans – I like the big white butter beans.

Soak 4 cups of beans overnight in enough warm water to cover. Next morning drain the beans and place in a large, heavy bottomed pot with enough fresh water to cover them, and 2 or 3 sprigs of fresh winter savory. Simmer until soft and tender. Drain and spoon into a glass dish. Make a dressing of 1½ cups finely chopped fresh mint, ¾ cup hot water, ¾ cup grape vinegar and ½ cup raw honey. Mix well and pour over the beans. Keep chilled in the fridge. Serve as a salad or side dish with grilled meat.

Hint

Cook beans with a few sprigs of mint or winter savory to ease any flatulence or discomfort. Serve beans with chopped mint, and a sprinkling of crushed coriander seed and fennel seed. Also chew caraway or fennel seeds or make a cup of mint tea to sip after the meal.

Black-Eyed Bean

Vigna unguiculata

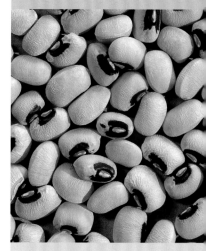

Also called the black-eyed pea, cowpea or the yard-long bean, it is often grown in arid areas, hot and dry and with low rainfall, yet it still thrives, and grown with maize and sorghum and potatoes it is a viable crop that needs to be reintroduced to everyone who has even a tiny portion of land. Originating in Africa where it is today a vital staple food, eaten both matured and dried, and young and green and fresh, the black-eyed bean is believed to have come into Europe from Egypt around the 17th century.

It is adaptable and quick to grow and so is grown commercially all over the tropical parts of the world as a valuable crop that is rich in protein, calcium, potassium, iron, vitamins A, B1, B2 and C, magnesium, phosphorus and folic acid. In parts of Africa the black-eyed bean is ground into a nourishing coffee-like drink. The young leaves and shoots are eaten steamed as a green vegetable and added to curries, stir-fries or relishes, and the young beans are eaten whole as a delicious green bean with mint. The mature pods, filled with ripe beans, are harvested as a winter food and the dried beans form the base for curries, soups, stews and mashes. The mature seeds are made into the popular sustaining and energising dish 'Hoppin' John', a delicious traditional soup that is often served with rice.

Mung Bean

Vigna radiata

Also known as green gram bean, most people think of mung beans as a delicious sprouting seed, but, in fact, cooked, dried mung beans can be ground into a nutritious flour and made into biscuits and breads. The Chinese were the first to sprout it as part of their national cuisine, and today mung beans are still the most important source of beans sprouts, eaten raw in salads or added to stir-fries and many oriental dishes. Mung beans were first cultivated in India, where it is called *dhal*, and the little green beans were used as barter and trade, and in those early centuries it was made into a gruel with rice.

Medicinally, the mung bean is used to treat wasting illnesses and beri-beri. High in calcium, iron, vitamins A, B1, B2 and C, mung beans (along with chickpeas, see page 99) have the highest amount of vitamin A of all the legumes. So they are a very valuable and easily grown food.

Adzuki Bean

Vigna angularis

Native to Japan and cultivated for centuries in China and Korea, both as a medicine and a food, the adzuki bean is particularly rich in protein, iron, calcium, vitamins A, B1 and B2, folic acid, magnesium, potassium and phosphorus. Interestingly, George Oshawa, the founder of the macrobiotic diet, identified the adzuki bean as one of the most important staple foods of the diet.

This is an ancient recipe for a health tonic: Take 2 tablespoons of adzuki beans and soak overnight in water. Next morning, drain the beans and boil in 2 litres of water with 1 stick celery and 1 carrot until soft and half the liquid has boiled away. Divide the liquid into three parts and drink 1/3 in the morning, 1/3 at noon and 1/3 at night for kidney ailments, bladder infections and water retention.

Hoppin' John

Serves 6–8

Hoppin' John is served in midwinter to keep the circulation moving and to thaw frostbite and frozen feet. It is also added to the watchdog's dinner to keep the winter chill away through the long, cold night!

2 cups black-eyed beans, soaked overnight
3–5 tablespoons olive oil
3 cups chopped streaky bacon
2 large onions, finely chopped
2 cloves garlic, finely chopped
2 cups chopped celery (leaves and stalks)
1 tablespoon chopped fresh oregano
1 tablespoon chopped fresh thyme
2 teaspoons mustard powder mixed into 2 tablespoons honey
juice of 2 lemons
salt and black pepper to taste
3 litres good strong chicken stock
½ cup chopped parsley

In a large stainless steel pot sauté the bacon in a little of the olive oil. Once it starts to brown lift it out with a slotted spoon and in its fat sauté the onions and the garlic. Add the rest of the olive oil and the celery and stir until everything is lightly brown. Add the drained beans and stir for 3 minutes. Then add the rest of the ingredients except the bacon and the parsley. Simmer gently, covered, for 1 hour or until the beans are tender. Finally add the bacon and the parsley and heat through. Serve hot, spooned over a bowl of hot cooked brown rice, if liked, or with crusty bread as a nourishing soup.

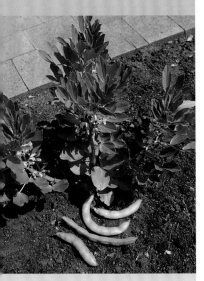

Broad Bean

Vicia faba

A superb winter crop and so easy to grow, no garden should be without these incredible beans. In Brazil the large flat inner seed, matured and dried and roasted, is ground into flour, and in France very young and tender whole pods are cooked. An ancient and respected food source, broad beans or fava beans can be traced back to over 5000 BC and is native to the Mediterranean area. Some ancient types of broad bean have been found in settlements dating back to the Bronze Age, and in Egypt dating back to 2400 BC. In ancient Greece and Italy and during the Middle Ages, the broad bean became a staple food because of its resistance to drought. It is also used as a valuable green manure crop, often ploughed back into depleted soils once the beans have been reaped.

Rich in amino acids and especially vitamins A, B (in particular B6), C and E, as well as calcium, iron, magnesium, zinc, folate and fibre, this valuable food remains today, as it did when cultivated in England in the Iron Age, one of the most important food crops ever known to mankind. Interestingly, broad beans are known to cause a rare allergic disease known as favism, occurring in the Mediterranean region, but only in individuals with a hereditary predisposition.

Jugo Bean

Vigna subterranea

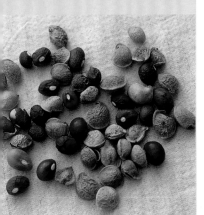

An underground bean, much like the peanut in its growth habit, the jugo bean is a tough annual, and it looks nothing like a bean! It originates in tropical Africa, from West Africa all the way down to South Africa, and is part of an ancient African crop that has been cherished through the centuries. Jugo bean seeds are shiny and hard and come in a range of bright colours, from creamy white to yellow, beige, pink, red and even almost black, and they are covered by a papery husk that washes off easily. The beans ripen in their papery husks and when the leaves just start to brown on the edges, pull up the whole clump and shake off the masses of beans.

Long known as a sustaining whole food, rich in protein, amino acids, minerals and vitamins, the jugo bean is a powerhouse of energy-building properties, especially for stamina, endurance and muscular strength. Given to travellers as 'padkos', lightly salted cooked jugo beans eaten a handful at a time the way peanuts are enjoyed, is considered to be as good as a meal. The ripe seeds are ground into a nutritious flour and can be made into pancakes and fritters, baked as a bread or made into a porridge.

Jugo Stew

Serves 6

This is delicious, nourishing and energy boosting!

Soak 2 cups of jugo beans overnight. Boil for about 2½ hours to soften. Strain and discard the water. Fry 2 chopped onions in 3 tablespoons olive oil until lightly brown. Add the following ingredients:

2 cups chopped celery (leaves and stalks) • 2 cups chopped green peppers • 2 cups chopped fresh pineapple • juice of 1 fresh lemon • 1 tablespoon chopped fresh thyme • 1 tablespoon chopped fresh parsley • 1 tablespoon crushed coriander seed • 3 tablespoons fruit chutney (best is homemade) • 2 teaspoons cumin seed • sea salt and black pepper to taste Simmer 30 minutes. Serve hot with crusty bread.

Hyacinth Bean

Lablab purpureus

A beautiful climbing perennial with bright pink flowers and tender purple pods that mature to reveal flat creamy coloured seeds with a white lip, the hyacinth bean is native to India, Ethiopia and possibly parts of Egypt. It has been a treasured food and medicine in Malaysia and Southeast Asia as well as Africa and India for many centuries. The young leaves can be eaten as a spinach and are delicious in curries and stir-fries. High in calcium, iron, vitamins A, B and C, the lablab bean has played a huge role in times of drought and food scarcity. Soups, stews and gruels made with the hyacinth bean are not only nourishing but energising and for the aged, the hyacinth bean has proven to be not only sustaining, but an excellent tonic for regaining strength and a positive outlook. The hyacinth bean was considered to be so valuable in life that seeds were buried with the dead for the afterlife.

Caution

Do not eat the hyacinth bean raw. It contains glucosides, a poisonous substance, which must be removed by cooking the beans for at least 10 minutes and discarding the cooking liquid.

Date Palm

Phoenix dactylifera

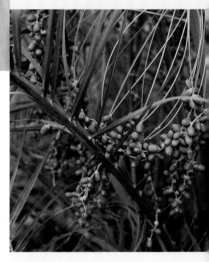

Dates are nothing short of miraculous. Dates contain one of the most extraordinary sugars that nothing has ever surpassed, and the date palm has been a treasured, loved and cherished tree since the beginning of time. The most highly esteemed food in the Middle East and the top of Africa, dates are the precious staple food of the poor.

The cultivation of dates goes back to the times of the Chaldeans. Archaeological excavations have found that dates were used as both food and medicine even before 4000 BC and that in ancient times the date formed one of the four fruits which were renowned as a cure for throat and chest ailments, the other three being the fig, the raisin and the jujube.

Known for surviving in the desert where today both wild and cultivated trees can be found, the date is a superb health food that has attained extraordinary commercial value.

Growing the Date Palm

Survivors in extremely hot, dry conditions – but they need water and this is why they are so well known for being clustered around an oasis. Both male and female trees are needed to produce the fruit. In commercial plantings usually one to two male palms are enough amidst 50 female palms.

Propagation is from the hard seed within the fruit, but commercial propagation is done from the suckers that form around the base of the palm, and in Egypt it is also done with tissue culture. With the right conditions, the palm grows fairly quickly and comes into its fruit-bearing stage between 5–8 years of age, and its best years of production are when it is between 70 and 80 years old! After 80 its production declines slowly, but it is still nurtured for its shade and for the use of its leaves.

Using the Date Palm

The terminal top part of the trunk, where the flowers and new leaves emerge, provides a drink – once fermented it becomes the much-loved 'palm wine' that is briskly traded. The tough, huge leaves are used as thatching and the trunk is used to build shelters.

The ripe dates are packed with nutrients (see Health Note) and have been used for centuries to treat diarrhoea, dysentery and stomach upsets, as well as for chest ailments, asthma, coughing and pleurisy, often combined with finely grated ginger and hot water.

The pips, once the date has been eaten, are given to the camels as fodder, and are a precious fuel, as are the tough stems and the sheath of the inflorescence. In some countries the date pips are ground for a type of coffee. Every part of the palm is used – even the sap is tapped from the growing trunk by piercing the bark, and used as a sweetener for drinks.

Dried dates never lose their sweetness and have been carried all over the world, sustaining many a traveller, and date paste was carried by ancient explorers and is still made the same way today. Interestingly, dates provide 64% more potassium than bananas and contain a soluble fibre called beta-d-glucan which decreases the body's absorption of cholesterol and slows the absorption of glucose in the small intestine thus keeping the blood sugars level. This soluble fibre also acts as a gentle laxative and recent studies show that dates are full of excellent antioxidants that have anti-cancer properties and protect against free-radical damage. So perhaps a date or two a day will keep the doctor away better than we think.

Health Note

Highly nutritious, ripe dates contain vitamins A, B, C and D, folic acid, beta-carotene, calcium, magnesium, phosphorus, potassium, iron, selenium, zinc and beta-d-glucan (an antioxidant).

Date Candies

This is a real health treat and is much loved by children.

1 packet of compressed dates
3 tablespoons butter
3 tablespoons shelled sunflower seeds
3 tablespoons finely chopped almonds
1 tablespoon boiling water
2 tablespoons sesame seeds

Chop the dates, carefully removing any seeds, and place in a double boiler with the rest of the ingredients, except the sesame seeds. Warm through until the butter has melted. Stir well and mix thoroughly. Set aside to cool and when it is cool enough to handle roll into balls in buttered hands and finally into the sesame seeds. Keep in a covered dish in the fridge. For an energy boost this takes some beating.

Hint

When you want sweetness in a dish, add finely chopped dates. Although very rich in natural fruit sugars, they are the ideal sweetmeat!

Cape Gooseberry

Physalis peruviana

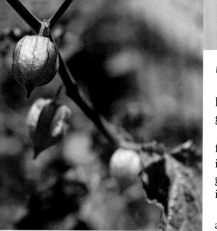

My Grandmother's Gooseberry Tart

This is the tart I always made with my grandmother for a family Sunday afternoon tea – it is in my heart!

½ cup sugar

1½ cups milk

1 level dessert spoon custard powder, mixed with a little cold milk

1 level dessertspoon gelatine

2 cups gooseberries

3 egg yolks, beaten

1 tablespoon butter

¼ teaspoon salt

Start by making the crust. Crush 1 packet Marie biscuits with 6 tablespoons melted butter and press into a pie dish.

Place the gooseberries into the crust. Boil up the milk and beaten egg yolks, salt, sugar and custard powder. Add the butter and boil up. Cool and add the gelatine, which has been dissolved in hot water. Pour over the gooseberries and place in the fridge to set. Serve with cream.

Hint

Freeze Cape gooseberries without their husks for serving in summer fruit juices. They explode their flavour in your mouth!

This softly scrambling, sprawling perennial bush of our childhood, the Cape gooseberry, belongs to the great *Physalis* genus, which is distinguished by its 'gift-wrapped' little fruits in their papery husks. This is a cosmopolitan genus, which around 80 species, amongst them our much-loved, easily grown Cape gooseberry and many others that have excellent medicinal properties.

The Chinese lantern (*Physalis alkekengi*), which also has edible berries but is usually grown as a florist's favourite, and the tomatillo (*Physalis ixocarpa*), which bursts out of its tight-fitting cape and which is valuable in Guatemalan and Mexican cooking and which grows easily in South Africa, are part of this fascinating genus. All have been used as food and medicine for centuries and our own Cape gooseberry is much loved in India, Sri Lanka, Malaysia, China and Hawaii, and is often known as 'poha', the Hawaiian name for it.

The Cape gooseberry originates in Peru and Chile, and it came to South Africa in an early voyage and was established in the first gardens of the Cape around 1670. It became known as the Cape gooseberry from the Cape of Good Hope and it was immensely popular, but some say its name comes from the papery husk that encloses the fruit, like a cape over the shoulders.

Growing Cape Gooseberries

Easy, prolific and self-seeding – once you have it, it seeds here and there and young plants can be easily transplanted. Velvety soft leaves and downy soft stems make picking the ripe fruit a pleasure, and my childhood memories are of creeping carefully through my grandmother's Gordon's Bay garden picking enough fruits to fill any tiny basket for her much-loved gooseberry tart. From those early beginnings my grandmother showed me how you squeeze a ripe fruit onto a piece of blotting paper – today you would use a double thickness of kitchen paper towel – spreading the juicy, seed-laden, soft, ripe, golden flesh evenly, which you then leave to dry. When you need new plants in spring, the piece of paper was laid on a box of moist compost, lightly watered to soften it and then gently covered with a thin layer of compost, and again very carefully watered. We covered the box with a piece of glass so that the warm winds did not dry it out, and watered it very gently every day and kept it shaded and protected. Once the little seeds germinated, the glass was removed and the tiny seedlings were kept moist. When big enough to handle they were pricked out with great care and transplanted into moist, compost-filled bags which were gradually brought out into the sun to strengthen them.

Plant out the little plants when they reach about 12–15 cm in height and space them a metre apart in full sun in well-dug, richly composted soil. The older sprawling branches can be cut back, and new growth will start almost immediately. Although perennial, we set new plants each spring to ensure an abundant crop, as the birds, the squirrels and the monkeys devour the little treasures consistently!

Using Cape Gooseberries

In Hawaii the fruits are eaten fresh as a diuretic, a laxative and to reduce fever and treat kidney and bladder disorders. The leaves, warmed in hot water, make a soothing poultice over arthritic and rheumatic aches and pains, and for lower back pain.

The delicious sweet-sour berries can be added to fruit salads, to smoothies and to syrups, jams, cordials, and homemade ice-cream with honey, fresh cream and finely chopped up fruits. Interestingly, the fruits of the tomatillo are one of the main ingredients in *salsa verde*, which is also taken to relax tension, spasm and rheumatic aches and pains!

Health Note

Gooseberries are rich in the minerals potassium, magnesium and phosphorus, vitamins C, B and E and beta-carotene.

Pea

Pisum sativum

Garden peas, sugar snap peas and mangetout peas, all equally delicious, are so much a part of winter, and now the juicy tendrils, the flowers and the tips of the vines are gourmet salad ingredients – we grow several rows of peas in the Herbal Centre gardens for our winter salads, and we see how the visitors enjoy them!

The exact history of the pea is unknown. The first wild peas may have come from Central Asia and the Near East, and possibly from parts of Africa near Ethiopia. It could have been cultivated near the Burma–Thailand border close to 2 000 years before it became domesticated in the Near East. No one is certain, but the seeds of ancient varieties have been found in excavations of Bronze Age burial sites in Switzerland that date back to over 5000 BC! The ancient Greeks and Romans grew peas and they were the first to use dried peas in their winter 'gruels' or soups. The green pea, shelled and eaten fresh or lightly boiled, only became a food in the 16th century. A French gardener developed the first climbing, tender-podded variety, which became the gourmet food of the court of Louis XIV. The pea was taken to the Americas in 1602 on the *Mayflower* and dried peas became a valuable commodity.

Over the years plant breeders have experimented widely with the garden pea, and by the 1970s the first sugar snap peas emerged with a sweetly delicious, edible pod – a cross between a snow pea and the much-loved garden pea! Dried peas are a huge trade today and 80% of the world crop is turned into dried peas, but in America it is the reverse with fresh, frozen and tinned peas leading the way!

Growing Peas

An annual cold weather crop, peas can be sown 30 cm apart in deeply dug, richly composted soil in full sun in March or early April. Keep them well watered and set a trellis or fence or lattice in place over which they can climb. Watch carefully over the young pea shoots – the birds, the cutworms, the caterpillars, the squirrels and the monkeys *cannot* resist so tender a mouthful!

Help the new little shoots to find their way up the fence or frame – their quick-to-grow tendrils will soon latch on. Twice a week watering, slow and long and deep, will give them a good start and thereafter as the winter days shorten, only once every 8–10 days is sufficient.

Using Peas

Peas have been an ancient medicine for both the liver and the stomach for centuries. Considered to be a good treatment for stomach ailments, fresh green peas, lightly steamed and given for 3 days as a medication, have been found to improve digestion, cleanse and tone the liver, and act as a tonic for the whole digestive system as well as boosting the immune system. Medical research today finds that peas are an excellent treatment for liver damage and over-indulgence and a tea made of the young sprigs as well as the tendrils, enough to fill ¼ of a cup, with 1 cup of boiling water, is still today one of the best liver-cleansing teas, often with some parsley and celery added as well.

Organically grown garden peas eaten fresh in salads have been a gourmet treat for centuries and for the young soldiers going into battle green peas were considered to be so energy boosting and so good for the immune system, they were part of the rations through the ages. For athletes and sportspeople, eating fresh peas is worth looking at for their excellent amino acid, mineral and vitamin content (see Health Note).

Health Note

A *good source of protein and minerals like phosphorus, potassium, zinc, magnesium, manganese and iron as well as vitamins B, C and K, carotenes, folic acid and amino acids, peas are a marvellous health food that should be eaten often.*

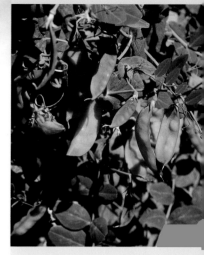

Traditional Liver-Cleansing Pea Soup

Serves 4–6

A bowl of this green pea soup, made with masses of parsley and celery, is today given to clear the liver of toxins as it was centuries ago!

6 leeks, thinly sliced
4 cups fresh peas, shelled
2 cups young and tender pea pods
2 cups tips of the pea vine with tendrils
3 large potatoes, unpeeled, well-scrubbed, then cubed
juice of 2 lemons
2 cups chopped celery, leaves included
1 cup finely chopped parsley
sea salt to taste
little olive oil
about 2–3 litres of water

Fry the leeks in the olive oil until soft and lightly brown. Now add all the other ingredients except the salt and the parsley. Stir well and frequently. Simmer with the lid on until tender. When everything is well cooked, add the salt and the parsley and simmer 5 minutes. Serve in big bowls with crusty bread.

Hint

Serve young tendrils and vine tips in a salad with lemon juice and olive oil – it is a gourmet treat!

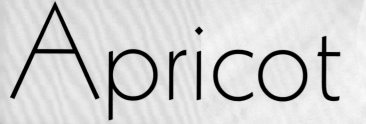

Apricot

Prunus armeniaca

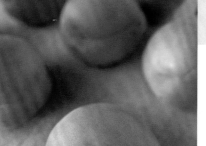

Apricot Health Salad

Serves 4

12 apricots, pips removed and quartered
1 cup celery, finely chopped
1 cup mung bean sprouts
2 cups watercress
1 cup coarsely grated Mozzarella cheese
juice of 1 lemon
a little olive oil

Arrange the first four ingredients in a shallow bowl. Lastly sprinkle the grated Mozzarella cheese over the top. Dress with the lemon juice and olive oil.

Apricot Jam

This is our year-long standby for soups, stews and sauces, so we make several batches.

Choose firm, well-ripened fruit – halve, and remove the pips. Weigh the fruit. Place in a heavy bottomed stainless steel pot with a little water. The ratio is 75 ml water to 1 kg fruit. Cover the pot and simmer for 15 minutes, until the fruit is soft. Now add the sugar and stir in gently. The ratio is 750 g sugar for each 1 kg fruit. Turn up the heat, stirring every now and then as it boils. Skim off any foam that rises to the surface. Test a little on a saucer to see if it sets – it usually takes about 45 minutes. Ladle into hot, sterilised jars and seal.

I sometimes think the apricot is my favourite tree. It has to be the most perfectly shaped spreading umbrella of a tree with the most attractive knobbly beautifully formed dark brown branches, and its thick green summer cloak of heart-shaped leaves offers dense cool shade, and its delicate and exquisite spring blossoms on bare branches are an unforgettable sight. Then think of the luscious golden golf ball-sized fruit in amongst the early summer leaves – a fruit that splits open so easily, is just so juicy and so delicious one could almost write a lyrical poem about it! If you have space for a big and beautiful tree, choose the apricot!

The apricot is thought to have originated in China, and ancient records reveal it has been cherished for literally thousands of years as both a food and a medicine. Alexander the Great brought the apricot from China to Greece and from there it spread into Italy and the rest of the world. But it was only around 1720 that the first apricots arrived in North America, where they flourished in California, and by 1792 the state became world renowned for its superb exported apricots which were sold both fresh and dried. The Arabs spread the apricot around the Mediterranean area where it was used medicinally by the monks for treating constipation and worms, and for obesity, and today's medical research verifies this.

Growing Apricots

Select a site in full sun and dig a huge hole about 1 m deep and 1 m wide. Fill this with first well-rotted manure at the bottom for the first ¼, then add bonemeal and seaweed meal and chopped fresh comfrey leaves, well mixed in, for the next ¼, and then top up with rich old compost. Fill the hole with water and plant the young apricot tree in this. Support with a stake and flood the hole with water weekly. Every spring and every midsummer add at least one barrow load of rich compost and some bonemeal. And sit back and watch it thrive.

Using Apricots

High in vitamins and minerals (see Health Note), the apricot is beneficial in treating chest ailments, catarrh, sinusitis, toxaemia, anaemia, blood impurities and tuberculosis, acne, skin rashes, infectious and inflamed bites, stings, scratches and pimples, and some cases have been reported where apricots removed gallstones. The ancient monks treated both constipation and diarrhoea with apricots, both fresh and dried, and in the diet of those struggling to lose weight the apricot is invaluable. Apricots have a sweet flesh that is low in usable sugars (less than 7%), which is why it is used to treat obesity. Its high vitamin A content is what is really astonishing. It has almost 80% more vitamin A than any other fruit or vegetable when fully ripe. Vitamin A helps with night blindness and combats infections – not even a carrot has this level of beta-carotene.

Seek out organic apricots that are dried without sulphur dioxide or sugar. Every late spring and early summer, look out for fresh apricots as a health booster. They are invaluable for treating heart disease, macular degeneration of the eyes and the circulation, as well as cancer and debilitating illnesses. Dry your own apricots for winter use. Split the apricots in half and remove the pips. Place on trays in the sun, and cover with a net. Turn often – they dry quite quickly. Or invest in a home dryer, as we have. Store in airtight glass jars, and add to stews or eat as a snack.

Health Note

Apricots are rich in B and C, iron, calcium, phosphorus and very high in Vitamin A and potassium.

Cherry

Prunus cerasus • Prunus avium • Prunus capuli

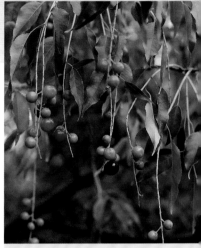

Wild cherry (*Prunus capuli*)

Cherries belong to the same genus as plums, peaches, almonds and apricots, and there are around 500 varieties in the world today. They originate in Europe and Western Asia and during the Roman occupation of Britain in AD 100, cherry trees were brought into England and cultivation began in earnest. Both sweet cherries (*Prunus avium*) and sour cherries (*Prunus cerasus*), the two main groups of cherries and their hybrids, are cultivated on a large scale in Europe today, as well as in Australia and in South Africa's colder areas. Cherries were named after the ancient Turkish town of Cerasus and by 70 BC cherry trees were growing in England, France, Germany, as well as in Rome.

For the past 25 years we have grown from seeds a few great and fabulous trees which we have named the wild cherry (*Prunus capuli*). It is indigenous to Mexico we hear, and is planted as 'the bird cherry' as it draws birds to the garden. Unlike the other cherries, its tiny, sweetly scented, creamy white flowers hang on a single thin stem, so the cherries, have the unusual habit of forming on the same thin stem – a string of them at different stages of ripening. Easily and quickly grown from seed, in the cold areas it is deciduous like most *Prunus* varieties; with us in our very hot more tropical area it keeps its leaves throughout the winter but their colour changes to gold as new leaves push through, so could be almost evergreen in its habit. Pruned and shaped it makes a fabulous spreading shade tree, and it asks for little except a long deep watering when it flowers in October, and by early December cascades of enticingly sweet cherries will ripen. Give it a barrow load of compost every now and then – we find in late winter it sends out new leaves after its compost mulch has been well dug in and watered.

Growing Cherries

Don't even try to grow cherries unless you live in an area that has cold, well below freezing winters. In the intense heat of the Herbal Centre gardens we are only able to grow the lofty wild cherry (*Prunus capuli*) with sprays of sweet small russet cherries that make a delicious jam (see above).

Sweet cherries require cross-pollination to set fruit, so plant two or even three cultivars to ensure this. Sour cherries do not need cross-pollination (nor does *Prunus capuli*, our wild cherry) and a popular variety is the Amarelle cherry, a variety of *Prunus cerasus*. Plant in deep, very large compost-filled holes, in full sun spaced 6–10 m apart and water deeply once a week.

Using Cherries

The juice of the cherry has for centuries been used to treat gout, rheumatism and painful joints, made into a hot toddy with honey. Cherry tea (see recipe alongside) has been used to treat headaches, as an antispasmodic and as a natural antibiotic. Because of their high flavonoid content, the darker the cherry the better. Natural pain-killing ingredients within the fresh cherry make it one of the most valuable fruits we can eat and it offers important anti-cancer protection. Research conducted at Michigan State University isolated perillyl alcohol, a natural compound that has been found to be a cancer cell inhibitor – possibly by depriving the cancer cells of the proteins they need to grow and develop. Breast, ovary and prostate cancers have responded favourably to the cherry treatment.

As well as this, the cherry has been found to have potent antioxidant activity and by eating a cup of fresh cherries daily when they are in season, will help to break down uric acid crystals in the joints, especially in the toe joint causing the intense pain so typical of gout.

Delicious in liqueurs, drinks, crystallised, in jams, desserts and cakes, candied cherries are as much a part of Christmas in the heat of our South African summer as they are in their native cold climates.

Health Note
Cherries contain vitamins A and C as well as minerals like copper, manganese, calcium and phosphorus.

Cherry Tea

This tea was used all over Europe to bring down fevers, to ease pain and discomfort and two to three cups are taken through the day at intervals.

Pour boiling water over ½ cup of stoned sliced cherries with 1–2 fresh leaves (any variety will do the same). Stand 5 minutes. Strain, sweeten if liked with a little honey and sip slowly.

Hint

Make honey and cherry syrup (equal quantities of each simmered until syrupy) and store in the fridge. Take 1 dessertspoon added to a cup of hot water daily when this precious fruit is not in season to treat 'flu and colds.

Look out for sun-dried cherries, unsweetened, for use when fresh cherries are not available. We dry our own wild cherries by removing the pips and spreading the flesh out to dry on trays in the sun. It takes only a day or two, and stored in glass jars they are delicious.

Plum

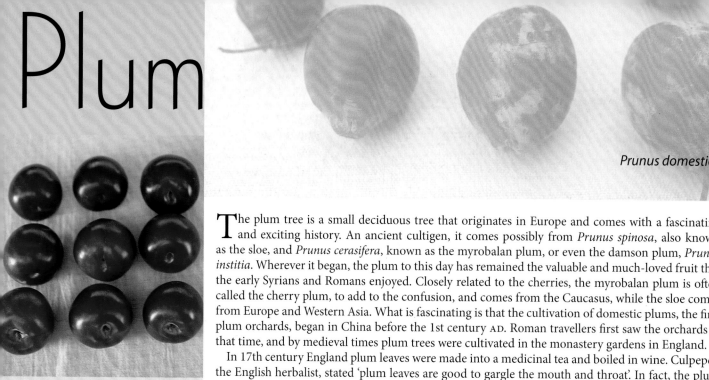

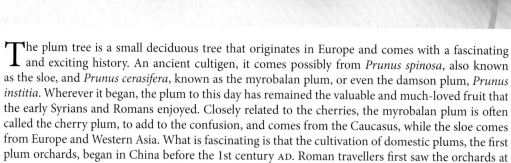

Prunus domestica

The plum tree is a small deciduous tree that originates in Europe and comes with a fascinating and exciting history. An ancient cultigen, it comes possibly from *Prunus spinosa*, also known as the sloe, and *Prunus cerasifera*, known as the myrobalan plum, or even the damson plum, *Prunus institia*. Wherever it began, the plum to this day has remained the valuable and much-loved fruit that the early Syrians and Romans enjoyed. Closely related to the cherries, the myrobalan plum is often called the cherry plum, to add to the confusion, and comes from the Caucasus, while the sloe comes from Europe and Western Asia. What is fascinating is that the cultivation of domestic plums, the first plum orchards, began in China before the 1st century AD. Roman travellers first saw the orchards at that time, and by medieval times plum trees were cultivated in the monastery gardens in England.

In 17th century England plum leaves were made into a medicinal tea and boiled in wine. Culpeper, the English herbalist, stated 'plum leaves are good to gargle the mouth and throat'. In fact, the plum soon became the favourite fruit and espaliering plums against warm south-facing walls in the gardens of England, France and Italy to enable the fruits to ripen to perfection during the summers, became an art. Hot houses became valuable assets and plums flourished in the heat, but require cold winters to do well. So the heat was turned off for the winter for the bare trees to develop buds.

Growing Plums

Although they are amazingly adaptable, the plum loves a hot summer and icy winter. Although they can produce quite good crops in the subtropics it seems that frost and snow on the bare branches does the trick of a really good harvest. With the many varieties on sale in the nurseries in midwinter, it is worth experimenting. Space plum trees 4–5 m apart. Dig a really big deep hole in full sun with space around it and fill with compost. Set a metre long pipe at an angle into the hole so that a hose can be inserted into it to get water to the roots. Often a plum will need staking – do that as you plant it so as not to disturb the roots. Water long and slowly once a week and once every 2 weeks in winter. Make a wide dam around it to hold the water and give it a barrow load of compost twice a year. Prune carefully in the winter before the sap rises – mid-July is best – and prune into a cup shape so that the sun can get to the centre of the tree.

Using Plums

The plum is an extraordinary and valuable fruit that is beneficial for the brain, the nerves and the blood, it helps to lower cholesterol and it is an excellent laxative (especially dried plums or prunes – a mere five prunes with breakfast yoghurt or porridge act as a safe and easy laxative).

Plums made into jams and jellies and chutneys are especially popular and plum puddings and plum cakes became excellent sellers in several countries and remain so today. Not only used in sweet dishes, plums are delicious cooked in stews and casseroles, lending their taste to beef and lamb stews with mouth-watering results.

Sliced plums, the pips removed, laid out on trays in the sun, dry easily. Keep the tray covered with a net as the birds and fruit flies love this feast. Turn every now and then. When dry, store in glass jars. Add a few slices to stews for a rich flavour.

Health Note

Plums are especially rich in vitamins A, C and E and calcium, and also contain folic acid, potassium, iron and beta-carotene.

Grandmother's Plum Pickle

As a child we had two heavily laden plum trees in the garden – one with small sized dark red flesh and pale pinkish skins, the Methley plum, and a Santa Rosa plum. Both were turned into preserves, including this wonderful plum pickle.

8–10 cups plums – small, firm and just ripe
4 cups brown sugar
2½–3 cups brown grape vinegar
1 tablespoon coriander seed
2 teaspoons whole cloves
10 cardamom pods

Tie the spices in a piece of butter muslin. Take the stalks off the plums and prick all over with a fork. Boil up the vinegar with the sugar for 5 minutes with the bag of spices. Then add the plums, and gently simmer for about 10 minutes or until they are tender but unbroken. With a slotted spoon take out the plums and spoon into hot sterilised jars, packed neatly and tightly. Reboil the vinegar and sugar mixture, discard the spice bag and pour it into the jars to cover the fruit. Seal, label and store for 1 month before eating with cold meats or cheeses.

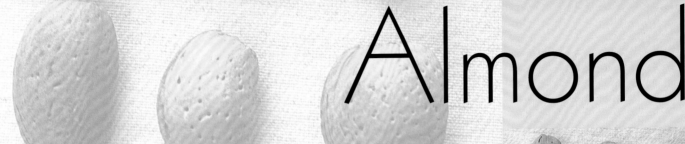

Almond

Prunus dulcis

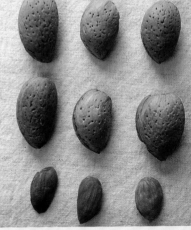

This precious, deciduous tree is thought to have originated in Western and Central Asia and North Africa. Cultivated for literally thousands of years, both as a food and as a medicine, explorers carried almonds on their journeys and this is how the almond spread into the Mediterranean area, particularly Spain and Italy. Known to the Hebrews centuries before Christ, it is thought the Phoenicians brought it into the rest of the world.

Used in ancient Egypt as an ingredient in the energy-giving bread served to the Pharaohs, the almond has been a significant part of history through the centuries. In the Bible Aaron's rod blossomed and bore almonds, almonds were used in religious ceremonies and as barter and trade up to the present day where it is one of the most prized and nurtured commercially grown crops in Spain, Italy, Portugal, California and Morocco. No crop quite exceeds almonds in value.

Growing Almonds

Almonds need cross-pollinating, so choose compatible varieties – for example, at the Herbal Centre we grow 'Papershell' and 'Brits' together. Most nurseries will advise you as to what particular varieties do well in your area.

They need full sun and deeply dug, richly composted holes and a twice weekly watering. The weekly, or twice weekly watering in hot weather, is vitally important and at least 2 wheelbarrow loads of compost per tree is needed in midwinter to encourage the early spring blossoms, and again in midsummer to encourage the swelling of the fruit. Pruning is kept very light to shape the tree and this is done in midwinter before the buds swell. Some growers do not prune at all.

The velvety nuts, encased in a cloak of protection, must only be picked once the outer husk becomes brown and dry. The exquisite petals are edible too and can be added to fruit salads and drinks, and nothing is quite as beautiful as an almond tree in shell-pink spring blossom.

Using Almonds

The actual inner nut is amazingly rich in vitamins and minerals (see Health Note) as well as protein, monounsaturated and polyunsaturated oils, and they are an excellent source of antioxidants, which makes the almond a truly important health food. Eating eight almonds a day – chewing them really well – is an excellent treatment for fighting heart disease, lowering blood cholesterol, and as an anti-cancer treatment almonds are becoming more and more important.

Important for all ages, the sheer nutty deliciousness of almonds can be easily incorporated into almond milk (see recipe), almond paste, almond sprinkles – finely chopped and sprinkled over desserts, stir-fries, muesli, yoghurt, homemade ice-creams and custards, or into breads, biscuits and rusks.

Almond oil is a precious and very useful ingredient in the cosmetic industry. Used as a carrier oil for essential oils, it is soothing, skin softening and moisturising. A dry skin treatment oil can be made by mixing 6 drops of rose essential oil into 2 tablespoons of almond oil (bought from your chemist) and adding 1 teaspoon of flaxseed oil and 1 teaspoon of extra virgin olive oil. Mix well and store in a dark glass bottle. Massage into the skin gently.

Health Note

Almonds are an excellent source of vitamins E, B2 and B3, folic acid, calcium, potassium, magnesium, phosphorus, zinc and protein.

Almond Milk

Serves 1

This is my recipe for those days when there is so much to do and you run out of energy. It is like tiger's milk and it never fails to work to get you feeling good, strong and ready-to-go!

1 cup milk
2 teaspoons raw honey
10 roughly chopped almonds
½–1 teaspoon cinnamon powder
1 small banana
½ cup plain yoghurt

Combine everything in a liquidiser and whirl for 2 minutes. Pour into a glass and drink it slowly. Literally, as you take the last sip you'll find your energy returns and your brain slips into gear and you start running!

Hint

Keep almonds in the fridge in well-sealed containers as their rich oils and proteins can easily become rancid. Sprinkle chopped almonds, with sunflower seeds and flaxseed, over your morning porridge for extra energy and vitality.

Peach & Nectarine

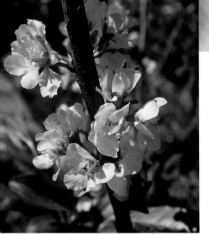

Two favourite summer fruits, loved and enjoyed the world over, with similar health benefits and growing conditions, both the peach and the nectarine – which is merely a smooth-skinned peach, also known as *Prunus persica* var. *nectarina* – have many varieties. The two major types are freestone and clingstone, and each includes fruits of both yellow and white flesh.

Originating in China, the peach and the nectarine were introduced to the Middle East some 2 000 years ago and cultivation spread westwards into places of suitable climate. Thriving in the perfect conditions of Kashmir and Persia, it came to be regarded as a native Persian fruit – hence the specific name *persica*, meaning 'of Persian origin'. The nectarine has a smooth skin and a flavour so delicious it was named for 'nectar', the legendary drink enjoyed by the classical gods! The Spanish were introduced to the peach from China and it was the Spaniards who took the peach to America in the 16th century, and the canning industry started to grow towards the end of the 19th century to preserve that incredible summer bounty. The most famous peach dessert remains 'Peach Melba', created in the late 19th century to honour Dame Nellie Melba!

Growing Peaches and Nectarines

Originally peaches were grown from selected pips; today it is a grafted tree that growers have perfected. Available from midwinter at your nursery, it is self-fertile, and the variety is huge. A small and attractive tree, it needs a huge, deep, compost-filled hole in full sun that can be flooded with water once or twice a week, with the addition of a barrow load of compost in winter after the pruning, and again in midsummer after the fruiting.

Using Peaches and Nectarines

The best way to eat them is tree ripened and succulent, if you can beat the birds! What is extremely worrying though is the frightening poisonous spraying programmes that have become essential in order to even *have* a peach on our dining room table. Organic growers struggle to reap a crop. Long gone are the luscious baskets of peaches picked from our own trees that I remember with such joyfulness from my childhood. Each garden in suburbia had its own little prolific orchard and the favourites were the first pink-and-white-fleshed 'Early Dawn', which fruited before Christmas!

Organically grown peaches and nectarines are vital for our health, so we need to be vigilant about the use of poisonous sprays – even peach leaves, used for centuries in medicines and washes, need to be organically grown. Natural sprays and companion planting is starting to make a difference, so do persist – read my book *Companion Planting*, for more on the organic growing of peaches.

The health benefits are vast: rich in carotenes and flavonoids, like lycopene and lutein, peaches help to prevent macular degeneration of the eyes, cancer and heart disease, and also assist to eliminate toxins, soothe stomach ulcers and colitis as they are easy to digest, and for breakfast with plain yoghurt, peaches are an excellent laxative, and gentle and cleansing for the kidneys and bladder too. Peaches have an alkalising effect within the body, which is vital, for stress causes acidity, and we all suffer from too much acidity.

Note that those with a tendency to kidney stones should limit their intake of fresh peaches. Always wash non-organically grown peaches very well, or soak them in a diluted additive-free soap solution or in an organic vegetable and fruit wash with a few drops of tea tree oil added.

Health Note

Peaches and nectarines are rich in iron, vitamins A, B and C, calcium, magnesium, phosphorus, potassium and manganese.

Yellow Peach Pickle

A delicious sandwich spread and a divine condiment with cold meats, or add it to stews.

3 kg yellow cling peaches, well washed (or peeled), stoned and sliced
3 large onions, sliced into rings
1½ litres white grape vinegar
2 tablespoons coriander seed, crushed
1 tablespoon allspice berries
1 tablespoon black peppercorns
2 tablespoons fresh grated ginger root
2 tablespoons mild curry powder mixed with 1 teaspoon turmeric powder
250 g sugar (preferably soft dark caramel sugar)
2 teaspoons sea salt
5 teaspoons cornflour

Dissolve 100 g salt in 5 litres of water and pour over the sliced peaches and onion rings. Soak for 1 hour, then drain and rinse well in fresh water.

Tie the coriander seed, allspice berries, peppercorns and ginger in a piece of muslin, and boil in the vinegar for 5 minutes in a large heavy bottomed stainless steel pot. Mix the curry powder and turmeric with the sugar, cornflour and sea salt to a paste with a little cold water, and add slowly to the boiling vinegar, stirring vigorously and constantly. Now add the peaches and onions, and simmer for 10–12 minutes. Remove the muslin bag. Ladle hot into sterilised jars. Seal and label.

Guava

Psidium guajava

This pretty, evergreen little tree is indigenous to the warm tropical areas like Peru, Brazil and Mexico, and spread to other parts of South America. The history of the guava is colourful and the earliest recordings of the 'guavavu' were found in Peruvian archaeological sites dating back to around 800 BC. By 200 BC it had spread to Mexico, and European visitors first tasted it when they visited Haiti, known there as 'guavavu' from these early beginnings. It was the Portuguese traders who took it to India, and the Spanish explorers who took it to the Philippines and on into Hawaii where it is still grown commercially today. It has become naturalised in many parts of the world, spread by the birds in most frost-free areas and in some countries, like South Africa, has become 'an alien invader' and has been added to the list of prohibited plants.

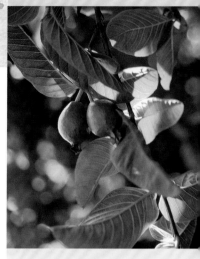

Growing the Guava

For commercial growers permits are needed in South Africa, and there are a few varieties to choose from. Easy to grow in frost-free areas it will thrive in a deep, compost-filled hole in full sun, flooded with water twice weekly. Tie it to a stake to encourage its shrubby growth upwards as it can sprawl. Trim the exuberant branches every now and then and give it a barrow load of compost twice yearly. It will reach a height of 4–5 m and a width of 3–4 m in full maturity.

Using the Guava

Strongly pungent and penetrating, the scent of ripe guavas is unmistakable. In the West Indies a festive party food is still served today from the cooked shells of the halved guavas, seeds removed, and filled with cream cheese – known as 'cascos de guayaba'. The heavy scent of stewing guavas and guava jellies fills the air far and wide, and the festival of dancing and thanksgiving for the precious and abundant fruiting in late summer revolves around this guava feast. Guava drinks, some even intoxicating, guava cakes and ice-cream and sweets are everywhere, and every house has a guava tree bowed down with ripening fruits!

The extraordinary medicinal value of the guava is often overlooked. One of the richest and most easily digested sources of vitamin C and A, eating a ripe organically grown guava is considered to be a premier health food. Rich in antioxidants, the guava is important in lowering the risk of heart disease. Ripe guavas are high in pectin, which helps to lower high blood cholesterol – it is thought that well-chewed fresh guava literally lines the stomach by forming a gel that soaks up fats and keeps them from being absorbed in the bloodstream. In countries where guavas form part of the daily diet cardiovascular disease is virtually unknown.

Medical research points to high blood pressure being significantly lowered by including guavas in the diet or drinking a cup of guava tea daily (steep 2 fresh guava leaves in 1 cup of boiling water, stand 5 minutes, then strain and sip slowly). Guava roots, bark and leaves, even the green fruits, have been taken as a traditional medicine in Mexico, Brazil, India and parts of Africa, for centuries for diabetes, and I am often asked for fresh guava leaves from my trees by visiting sangomas for the treatment of high blood pressure and diabetes as part of their traditional repertoire.

More and more plant research verifies what those ancient and traditional folk medicines proved so long ago. We need to reconsider the guava for this fact alone: Tests recently done in America showed that men eating just half a fresh guava very day (or guava roll, unsweetened, made of sun-dried mashed guavas when the fresh fruits were not in season – see recipe alongside) significantly lowered their risk of a stroke by up to 60%!

Guava Roll

Make your own guava roll by spreading out cooked, sieved guava pulp (no sugar added) on a stainless steel tray. Lightly oil the tray with sunflower oil first, and then spread the pulp evenly and thinly. Cover with a net and place in the sun. In hot weather it will dry in a day. Roll up while still pliable and store in a sealed container in the fridge. This is a delicious chewy snack and lunch box treat!

If you want it sweeter, add fresh stevia leaves while cooking the guavas.

Health Note

Guavas are one of the best sources of vitamin C, which is concentrated in the skin and outer layers of the fruit. They are also a good source of vitamin A, phosphorus and niacin and are low in calories and high in fibre.

Pomegranate

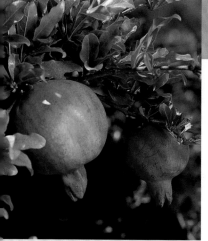

Pomegranate Salad

Serves 4–6

This is our favourite way of eating our big pomegranates.

Lay several boat-shaped butter lettuce leaves on a platter (count on 4 per person!) Deseed 2 or 3 pomegranates. Fill the little boats with pomegranate seeds, and top with small cubes of feta cheese. Pour over this salad dressing:

½ cup balsamic vinegar
½ cup honey
¼ cup olive oil
1 teaspoon mustard powder
1 teaspoon crushed coriander seed

Mix in a screw top jar and shake vigorously. Pour over the pomegranate seeds and enjoy as an aperitif with drinks.

Hint

Taking fresh pomegranate juice, crushed from the bright seeds, is a valuable general tonic drink that is even more popular today. Shake the seeds free of the bitter membranes, place them in a bowl and press down on them with a potato masher. Pour off the juice and chill.

The seeds can be dried on a stainless steel tray in the sun. Use them, crushed or ground, as a spicy flavouring in curries, marinades and sauces.

One of the world's most loved and cherished fruits – like a jewelled apple – the pomegranate has been cultivated, eaten and used as medicine since time began. Pliny the Elder named it 'the apple of Carthage', but records show that long before this it was used in ceremonial rites, and carved in stone at places of worship. A motif often found in Chinese paintings, in carvings and wall paintings in Egypt and Persia, its ancient beginnings are lost in the mists of time. It is thought the pomegranate originated in the Mediterranean area, or even further east towards India. The pomegranate appears in many references in the Bible, and Moses reassured the wandering Israelites of a land of plenty that they yearned for, with 'figs and vines, and wheat and pomegranates'. King Solomon had a pomegranate orchard and drank the cooling ruby liquid crushed from its jewel-like seeds. Wines, jellies, conserves and sherbets have been made from pomegranates for centuries, and great passageways and temple gardens have been planted with pomegranates to symbolise wealth and beauty. India and China, in the early centuries after Christ, had begun the cultivation and the first medicinal records were started then. The Spanish sailors took the pomegranate on their voyages of discovery to North and South America and Mexico. Immediately the seeds were planted, and pomegranate cultivation began in earnest.

Growing Pomegranate

The sturdy little evergreen tree or shrub thrives in full sun in a large, deep, compost-filled hole. Set a pipe into the hole at an angle for a hosepipe to be inserted to get water to the roots, and make a large dam around it so it can be flooded with water at least once a week. In colder areas the little tree, which can grow up to 4 m in height, loses its leaves, so it is recorded as being deciduous. It needs a barrow load of compost in late winter and again in midsummer – the reward is a mass of bright orange flowers in a hard fleshy calyx, followed by the bounty of succulent and beautiful fruits that ripen in late summer.

Using Pomegranate

The bark, branches, roots and fruit rind (known as the pericarp) are all used medicinally. Used as a treatment for diarrhoea in the early centuries, the dried rind of the ripe fruit, taken as a tea, has been a trusted remedy for stomach cramps, colic, digestive disturbances and upset stomachs. Place ¼ cup peeled rind, cut into thin strips, in 1 cup of boiling water, stand 5 minutes, strain, sweeten with a little honey, if liked, and sip slowly. It is soothing, calming and very comforting. The fruit rind was dried and stored in the winter months in sealed canisters, and taken sweetened with honey as a safe and easy method for clearing tapeworm from the body. Rich in tannins and alkaloids, the bark and rind has the ability to cure diarrhoea, and even dysentery, with no side-effects. Interestingly, in classical times the pomegranate became the symbol of fertility, and eating the fruit was considered to be the treatment for infertility.

Pomegranate juice is an ancient beauty treatment applied to oily problem skins, and mashed with the membranes between the bright seeds it was used as a gentle scrub to clear away blackheads and spots. The nails were dug into the inner fleshy rind, and into the bright juicy calyxes of the flowers, to strengthen them and to repair the cuticles. The flowers, boiled in water (10 flowers, finely chopped, and simmered in 2 litres of boiling water for 15 minutes, then cooled until pleasantly warm), were used as a foot scrub for tired, aching feet and for calluses and corns. Fresh leaves softened in hot water made a comforting poultice over painful feet, and stiff, sore backs and shoulders.

Health Note

Pomegranate juice is rich in enzymes, amino acids, vitamins C, A, E and some B-vitamins, as well as several minerals, especially potassium, calcium and phosphorus.

Pear

Pyrus communis

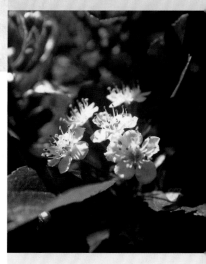

This much-loved fruit is steeped in history. Its beginnings date back to the Stone Age and it has been cherished and nurtured from those ancient days. Originating in Europe and Western Asia its cultivation is thought to have begun 35 to 40 centuries ago. Known as the 'gift of the gods' propagation by seeds and, unbelievably in those ancient days, by grafting and by cross-pollination, were recorded by esteemed writers like Homer, Pliny, Cato, Virgil and later Theophrasus, learned and cultured writers who identified varieties and made careful records which are still used by historians today!

Trade routes bartering ripening pears and grafted small trees in clay containers – the first pot plants – were numerous across Europe and pears became a marketing feat in the early centuries, picked half ripe and nestled in grass and carried in wide flat baskets made of willow. The monks in the Middle Ages realised the pear's potential as a medicinal syrup and one of the first cough and cold syrups was made of pears. Early on, dried slices of pears became the traveller's sustaining energy food.

There are two main species of pear: the well-known European pear (*Pyrus communis*) and the more apple-shaped Asian pear (*Pyrus pyrifolia*), which has a crisp granular texture and somewhat bland flavour.

Growing Pears

A medium-sized, fascinating and beautiful tree, undemanding, attractive, often breathtakingly so, at all times of the year, the pear is a precious asset in every garden. Slow growing and charming at every stage, the great gardens of Europe espalier them across sun-drenched walls to encourage the ripening of fruit and today smaller trees are available for small gardens, growing 1–2 m in width and 3–4 m in height. Pears are mostly infertile so that at least two cultivars should be grown together ideally.

Pear trees need full sun and a huge, deep, compost-filled hole with a large metre-long pipe set in it at an angle for inserting a hose to get the water down to the roots for a good weekly watering. Generally a deciduous tree – although some pear trees seem to retain their dark and glossy leaves – but in spring the blossom, palest pink in some, and pure white in other varieties, exquisitely fragrant, brief and unforgettable, completely pushes the leaves aside!

The European pears can be picked green to ripen later, which is excellent for transport, but the harder fruit of the Asian pear should be left to ripen on the tree. On one of our Asian pear trees the fruit remains on the tree for months, but once cooked it is so juicy and delicious we always wish we had more!

Using Pears

Rich in vitamins and minerals (see Health Note) and low in sodium, the pear is excellent for kidney ailments, even for severe kidney malfunction. Rich too in pectin and dietary fibre, pears are considered valuable in lowering cholesterol levels, and toning and regulating the intestines. Pears are valuable in the hypoallergenic diet and are one of the first fruits introduced to babies for their safety factor in allergic reactions.

A soft and succulent dried pear helps to satisfy a sweet tooth, but it is really its ability to remove toxins from the body as well as being a tonic for the whole body – it not only benefits thyroid function but also acts as a safe diuretic – that makes the pear a wonder fruit. Whether fresh or dried (at home without any preservatives and stabilisers – see page 23) the pear is superb!

Health Note

Pears are rich in vitamins A, B and C, beta-carotene, folic acid, iodine, potassium, iron, calcium, magnesium and phosphorus.

Spicy Pears

This is delicious served with cold meats, cheeses, Christmas turkey, sausages or grilled steak.

about 1½ kg fresh firm pears
20 cloves
500 ml water
400 g soft brown caramel sugar
500 ml white grape vinegar
3 thumb-length pieces fresh ginger, thinly sliced
1 stick cinnamon
10 cardamom pods

Peel the pears with a potato peeler. Cut in quarters and press 2 cloves into each piece. In a stainless steel pot bring the water to the boil, add the sugar, and stir to dissolve. Add the vinegar, ginger slices, cinnamon stick and cardamom pods. Stir well. Add the pears and cook for 10 minutes. Remove the pears with a slotted spoon and pack into sterilised jars. Reheat the liquid and boil for 20 minutes. Pour the hot liquid over the pears, covering them completely. Seal immediately, label and store.

Hint

The best way to eat pears is fresh, cut into wedges with a little lemon juice squeezed over it to keep it from turning brown.

Radish

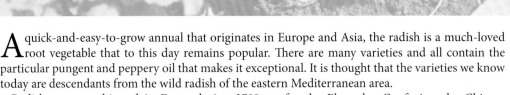

Raphanus sativus

A quick-and-easy-to-grow annual that originates in Europe and Asia, the radish is a much-loved root vegetable that to this day remains popular. There are many varieties and all contain the particular pungent and peppery oil that makes it exceptional. It is thought that the varieties we know today are descendants from the wild radish of the eastern Mediterranean area.

Radishes were cultivated in Egypt during 2780 BC for the Pharaohs. Confucius, the Chinese philosopher, recorded their medicinal use in 479 BC and the ancient Greeks and Romans cultivated fields of radishes for their feasts and celebrations. By 1547 the radish was taken to Britain – the seeds fetching a good price – and by 1598 at least four varieties were recorded in Britain. By the 1700s radishes in several varieties were introduced to the New World and trade in radish seed became lucrative.

The leaves and green seed pods are also favourite vegetables in many countries and it is so treasured in Mexico that an annual festival – 'La noche de los Rabanos' (the Night of the Radishes) – celebrates the introduction of the radish to the New World by the Spanish colonists, with radishes carved into exquisite shapes depicting scenes from the Aztec legends, history and the Bible.

Growing Radishes

Foolproof, rewarding, fascinating and delicious, the radish is one of the first food crops sown by children and by those beginning their vegetable gardens. A mere packet of inexpensive radish seed – and there are several varieties to choose from – will give you an endless interest and a quick health-boosting crop that you'll be constantly sowing.

A well-dug, richly composted furrow that can be gently watered by a hose running in at one end, will ensure a luscious reward. The seeds, thinly sprinkled and carefully covered with soil – just a light blanket – will germinate within a few days if kept moist and shaded, and can be sown all through the year except in the coldest months. They mature quickly and can be pulled up as soon as the little root swells.

Using Radishes

Used as a medicinal food for centuries, the radish contains several natural compounds that increase the flow of bile, flush the liver, cleansing and repairing it, and also act as a tonic on the gall bladder and improve the digestion. Lightly steamed baby radishes, leaves and all, served with lemon juice are an excellent tonic for the liver and the digestive system, and were used by the ancient healers throughout Europe and Asia as a tonic taken during the cold winter months to boost the whole system, to resist chest ailments, to act as a diuretic, an expectorant and a digestive, and to relieve flatulence, colic and heartburn. Fresh radish, finely grated, and finely chopped green leaves were served with rice and mashed vegetables frequently to treat all the above ailments.

Both the leaves and bulbs are highly nutritious and lightly steamed or finely chopped into stir-fries they are a good source of vitamins and minerals (see Health Note). Make it a habit to eat four radishes a day with a little parsley, fresh from the garden. This acts as a quick tonic, and is particularly valuable if you have over-indulged in rich foods, as it clears the liver of overload.

The daikon radish, Asia's predominant variety, remains one of Japan's most cherished vegetables and pickled daikon is the top seller in Japan to this day, forming part of the traditional diet. The Chinese grate daikon radish into flour to make a delicious cake and stir-fry thinly sliced or grated radish into a variety of tasty dishes.

Health Note

Radishes are a good source of vitamin C, calcium, copper, folic acid and potassium.

Radish Stir-Fry

This is a quick and easy supper dish that is so tasty you'll be trying all sorts of vegetables with it.

2 or 3 cups thinly sliced fresh radishes and some chopped radish leaves
2 cups onions, finely chopped
2 cups mushrooms, thinly sliced
2 cups potato, peeled and grated coarsely
1 cup chopped green pepper
juice of 1 lemon
sea salt and black pepper to taste
½ cup finely chopped parsley
olive oil for frying – about ½ a cup
dash of soy sauce
2 teaspoons finely grated ginger
2 teaspoons honey

Start by frying the onions in the hot oil. Let them start to brown, then add the mushrooms and potatoes and keep stir-frying. Now add the radishes, the green peppers and the lemon juice, stirring all the time. Add the rest of the ingredients except the parsley, and about 1 cup of water. Stir well and cover for about 5 minutes – shake the pan so as not to let anything stick or burn. Serve with brown rice, sprinkled with fresh chopped parsley.

Rhubarb

Rheum rhabarbarum

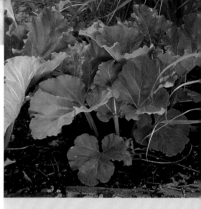

Rhubarb is an ancient plant that originates in Northern Asia – from Mongolia to Siberia, to the Himalayas and on to East Asia. Records going back over 2000 BC showed it was used as a medicine rather than a food. Around 200 years BC the Chinese began a remarkable trade with rhubarb as a medicine to Western Asia and the Arab countries. By the 16th century the 'crowns' or the 'roots' of various rhubarb species reached Europe and England and it was grown as a curiosity and as a medicinal plant, and only around 1783 did the first recipe using the stems become public knowledge in a book written by John Farley, called *The London Art of Cookery*. By 1861 the much-respected Mrs Beeton had introduced rhubarb jams, pies and even rhubarb wine in her cookery books. From then on rhubarb became known as a food, and its medicinal beginnings were lost in the mists of time.

A fascinating accident occurred one winter in the Chelsea physic garden hot house in London, in the early 19th century. A large clay pot had been accidentally overturned over a crown of rhubarb and, unnoticed, the plant flourished underneath it, producing by midsummer a mass of curly sulphur yellow leaves and tender pink stems, so sweet and mild that the gardeners repeated the 'accident' in their rhubarb hot houses the next winter. And so the 'forcing method' was born!

Growing Rhubarb

Rhubarb thrives in cold climates. It cannot take the heat of the summers in Africa, and its crowns need the frozen soil of the Siberian winters, the snow of the Himalayas, and as much as we love rhubarb and search for the crowns, it does not really do well in any climate above 24 °C. Where you do find rhubarb growing in the colder parts of our country, it still does not quite have the taste, the vigour and the quality of the rhubarb of the lands of its birth, but it is still worth trying to grow it.

It needs full sun for those giant leaves to unfurl and for the stems to become thick and sturdy. The crowns need to be planted out in late winter into deep, compost-enriched, well-dug trenches so that watering can be slow, thorough and deep. It should not ever fully dry out. The clump becomes large so space each plant 1–1½ m apart and pick the outer stems by carefully pulling them from the base or cutting them with a sharp knife right at the base. The purists say only pulled stems, *not* cut stems, are good for the plant. A heavy feeder, rhubarb needs lots of compost and water throughout summer, and in the hot summer, shade in the afternoons.

Using Rhubarb

One of rhubarb's earliest uses was in a wine, and specialist growers with knowledge of the forcing method could produce a sweet and superior stalk for wine-making purposes. It was once used as a laxative, and its high vitamin C content made it a valuable treatment for coughs and colds. A syrup made with honey is still used in the countries of its origin today. (To make rhubarb syrup, gently simmer equal quantities of thinly sliced rhubarb stems and honey and a stick of cinnamon for 15 minutes, or until the stems are tender. Mash and pour into sterilised jars. Take a teaspoon at a time for coughs and colds.)

The huge leaves, discarded due to the high levels of oxalic compounds, were used in mulches to shade and cover tender seedlings and to keep insects away. Rhubarb leaves were made into an effective 'spray' to keep whitefly and aphids away from tender vegetables, and the cut leaves were wrapped around rhubarb stems to protect them. Today rhubarb leaves are still used in insect-repelling sprays (make your own by steeping roughly chopped leaves in boiling water overnight).

Health Note
Rhubarb stalks are rich in vitamin C and K and folic acid.

Rhubarb Crumble

This is a classic dessert: warm, spicy and delicious.

3 cups rhubarb stalks, cut into 1–2 cm pieces (peel away any skins)
1 cup water
¾ cup soft brown caramel sugar

Boil the rhubarb pieces with the water and sugar. Simmer 10 minutes. Spoon into a baking dish and cover with the following topping:

1 cup cake flour
½ cup butter
pinch of salt
¼ cup oat flakes
½ teaspoon cinnamon powder
1 dessertspoon finely grated fresh ginger
½ cup chopped pecan nuts
1 tablespoon honey
1 tablespoon coconut flakes

Mix together the flour and butter until it resembles fine breadcrumbs. Add the rest of the ingredients and mix well. Spread over the cooked rhubarb and bake at 180 °C for 30–35 minutes or until it lightly browns. Serve hot.

Caution

Only the stalks are eaten. Do not eat rhubarb leaves – they are poisonous! Rhubarb contains high levels of oxalic acid and consuming too much can interfere with the absorption of calcium and iron in the body. Do not eat it if you have a tendency for kidney stones.

Watercress

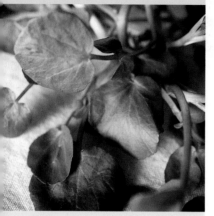

Native to Europe through to Central Asia, this delicious aquatic annual or biennial herb has floating stems that root all along the muddy edges of streams or ponds, producing tiny white, four-petalled, edible flowers which turn into tiny oblong pods as soon as the weather warms up, and which seed readily. Easily spread along furrows and watercourses it has now become a cosmopolitan weed, but its early beginnings and recordings have been found in ancient Persian, Greek and Roman writings as one of the much revered ancient medicines for treating a host of illnesses.

'Physic gardens', which were the 'gardens of medicine' in the Middle Ages, grew watercress in shallow trays at the edges of the streams and ponds all year round, protected from the winter snow and freezing waters by covering the trays with coarsely woven cloths made from flax stalks. The plantings were tended by the monks for making into a valuable syrup boiled up in honey to treat respiratory ailments, blood disorders and liver problems.

Watercress seed, taken on the voyages of discovery, was eaten by the sailors with mustard seed to prevent scurvy, and it is thought that this was the way it spread to the rest of the world.

Growing Watercress

If you are lucky enough to own a property where a river runs through it, watercress will perhaps already have found a home in these perfect circumstances. Today's rivers are so polluted that commercial watercress is grown in areas where water from a safe source can be gently flooded through a shallow pond and recycled – it does not grow in stagnant water, it needs moving water in which to thrive and is particularly succulent in dappled shade.

Grown in this way, and usually only from early spring to midsummer, sprigs are packaged into cellophane bags, well washed and wet, and kept refrigerated. The chilled pack only lasts a few days, so be on the look out for watercress at your local greengrocer and eat it quickly!

Growing your own in winter is well worth trying, even without a river. I grow it from seed every year in May in shallow trays that I fill with compost and flood with water very gently every day or even couple of days. Although I watch over it with great care, it is never anything as big or as luscious as the watercress growing on the river edges. But I get enough salad pickings and sandwich fillings to satisfy that craving, and often enough to make my much-enjoyed watercress soup. By midsummer it becomes too hot for watercress, so gather the seeds and store in sealed bottles for May sowing. It will reseed itself along the rivers.

Using Watercress

Just think about this: today's medical research finds watercress to be excellent for treating catarrh, chronic sinus, blocked nose and postnasal drip, wet coughs, bronchitis, phlegm, anaemia, rheumatism, chronic coughs, low immunity, gall bladder problems, coughs, colds and 'flu, it breaks up kidney stones, it clears bladder stones, treats bladder ailments, purifies the blood, acts as a safe diuretic, especially combined with celery and fennel, and it has a high iodine content, so it stimulates the thyroid. And as an expectorant it clears the whole respiratory system. How did those ancient healers know all this?

Try to include watercress in your diet whenever you can. But caution is advised: gathering the leaves from river edges is extremely risky, due to the danger of contamination by agents that cause waterborne diseases. Never just pick and eat – be safe and grow your own!

Health Note

Rich in calcium, magnesium, phosphorus, potassium, iron, iodine, beta-carotene, vitamin C and amino acids, watercress is literally power packed! It clears toxins from the body and is a superb tonic and an excellent digestive.

Watercress and Potato Soup

Serves 4–6

This soup with a little grated ginger added is so comforting if you have a cold or a cough.

4 cups potatoes, peeled and diced
3–4 cups fresh green peas, shelled
4–6 cups fresh watercress sprigs, lightly chopped
2–3 cups finely chopped onions or leeks
½ cup olive oil
sea salt and black pepper to taste
juice of 1 lemon
about 2 teaspoons of lemon zest (but only if the lemon is organically grown)
2 tablespoons honey
1 litre milk
1 litre good strong chicken stock
fresh sprigs of watercress for serving

In a heavy bottomed pot fry the onions in the olive oil until lightly browned. Then add the potatoes and stir-fry with the onions for a few minutes. Add the peas and stir-fry 1 minute, then add the chicken stock. Turn the heat to low and simmer gently until the potatoes are tender, adding a little water or more stock if needed. Keep stirring with a wooden spoon. Now add the milk, the watercress, sea salt and freshly ground black pepper to taste, the honey and the lemon juice and zest. Stir well to prevent any burning and keep the heat on low. Simmer for 10 minutes. Pour into a liquidiser to purée the soup. Serve in bowls with sprigs of fresh watercress.

Rose Hip

Rosa species

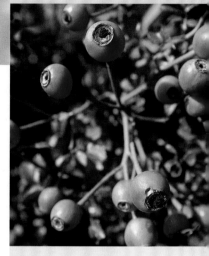

The rose hip is the bright orange or red seed capsule that forms once the rose has faded. Once a treasured food and medicine, its origins are ancient, revered and cherished, and today research has proven the value of the rose hip ripened by the sun – so rich in health-building vitamins and minerals it is no wonder that this could have been one of nature's first medicines.

The great *Rosa* genus contains over 125 species, some Asian in origin, some American in origin, some European in origin, and some African in origin – all have curious names, and are the parents of the roses we know today. Many rose varieties bear hips and all hips are edible, some are just juicier and sweeter than others. I grow hedges of *Rosa rugosa* and to this day I grow the apple-scented *Rosa villosa* and *Rosa canina* and *Rosa damascena*, and I love their ancient 'moss rose' look – my grandmother called them 'briar roses'. Their petals are edible too and delicious in homemade ice-creams.

The monks and the first healers created medicines from the hips, and through the centuries ways of cooking them, preserving them and using them in medicine were handed down from generation to generation – each country keeping its own recipes closely guarded, ancient and precious.

My grandmother came from Scotland and her rose hip syrup was our winter standby as a cough mixture, and she made it from the same recipe *her* mother had given her family whenever anyone had a cough or a cold. I made it for my children, and grow roses with big hips still today for this wonderful mixture. Whenever I make it, I think of those ancient hedgerows where the hips were picked, even before the Middle Ages, and I am so grateful that under the heat of the African sun we too can grow those ancient roses.

Growing Rose Hips

Plant roses in a deep, compost-filled hole in full sun and give them a large dam able to hold a thorough weekly watering, and twice weekly in the heat of midsummer. Roses need a good bucket or two of strong, rich compost twice a year and frequent attention. At the end of the summer, do not deadhead any longer so that a mass of hips can form. Leave the hips to ripen as the winter days set in. When they are richly coloured pick them for processing. Prune the roses after midwinter – around the last 10 days of July is ideal.

Using Rose Hips

Rose hips are bursting with vitamin C and during the Second World War school children in England and parts of Europe were sent out to gather the hips to be made into rose hip syrups, which the government donated to all the schools to keep winter coughs, colds and 'flu, and bronchitis at bay. My grandmother's rose hip syrup (see recipe alongside) was so delicious we took a teaspoon every morning after breakfast all through the winter. We had an old-fashioned mincer with sturdy blades that could mince the well-washed hips that had been 'topped and tailed'.

Interestingly, the rose hips are rich in nutrients (see Health Note), with lycopene and beta-carotene as well as fruit sugars as valuable components. Wild roses gathered in the cold areas of the country are used in many ways, and the crushed seeds yield the extraordinary rose hip oil, which is a treasured beauty treatment, used in cosmetics, in skin-softening creams, in lip balms and in ointments for cracked heels.

Our row of 'rose-hip-roses' is never enough for all we want to do with them! We use the petals in salads, jams, cakes, juices, ice-creams and in the making of rose petal conserve. The precious rose hips go into syrups, and many young mothers ask for it for their babies, remembering their own childhood spoonfuls of health-boosting syrup. Each season we promise ourselves we'll grow more rose-hip-roses as the demand increases. Do yourself a favour, grow roses for the hips – the demand for old-fashioned medicines is increasing daily!

Rose Hip Syrup

Rose hip syrup diluted with iced water makes a nourishing 'cool drink' for thirsty children, and for rose growers all over the world the promise of rose hip syrup, rose hip jelly or jam is an assured sale!

4 cups minced ripe rose hips
2 cups sugar (we use soft brown caramel sugar)
juice of 2 lemons
about 3 teaspoons of lemon rind
8 cups of boiling water

In a heavy bottomed pot with no lid on, simmer everything together very gently on low heat until tender – about 40 minutes. Stand aside 10 minutes, then pour through a strainer, mashing out the seeds carefully. Take out a cup of the hot syrup and pour through the sieve again, mashing out the seeds, and repeat again and again until most of the pulp is worked through. Bottle the syrup into sterilised screw-top bottles and label and store in a cool dark place. The seeds are discarded.

Health Note

Rose hips have very high levels of vitamin C and also contain vitamins D and E, beta-carotene, calcium, magnesium, potassium, zinc and phosphorus.

Blackberry
Bramble

Rubus fruticosus

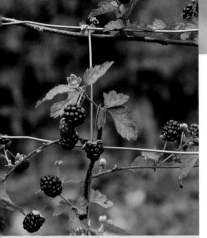

Blackberry belongs to a fascinating genus of prickly shrubs that originates in Europe, parts of North America, Britain and the Mediterranean region, and has become naturalised in many countries. Ancient and respected, the bramble was planted in the early centuries around holy places to protect them from intrusion, and today many ancient sites where churches once stood are still covered in brambles. Through the centuries the blackberry has been both a food and a medicine, and the monks grew blackberries in the monastery gardens to make into jams, jellies, wines and cough syrups.

Growing Blackberries

They are unfussy as to soil type and are fully hardy. They take frost, snow, heavy rain, strong winds and searing heat and, I have found, can even withstand long periods of drought. Look out for thornless varieties like 'Loch Ness'.

They send up suckers everywhere which can be dug up (water them well first) and immediately transplanted into richly composted, moist soil, and you will find they just keep going. Don't let them dry out in their early stages. Set up fences or long wire frames as supports as they are vigorous climbers, and tie up and neaten as they send out long vines. The fruit is borne on new stems each spring. Every winter dig in lots of compost and water it in well, and trim and tidy, being mindful that those long summer vines will bear the spring fruit.

Using Blackberries

From medieval Europe and Britain, an ancient gargle recipe has been handed down through the centuries, and this is how it was made: Ripe berries were crushed and pounded into honey with a few flower petals and the very tips of the vines. Boiling water was added to make a thin syrup, and cooked for about 15 minutes. It was then left to cool, strained and sealed. It was taken as a gargle and a mouthwash for sores in the mouth, and for sore throats and coughs.

Through the ages it has been found that the human body really benefits from eating fresh blackberries – because of their exceptionally high mineral and vitamin content the body absorbs the fruit well. In the early centuries blackberries were eaten to cure quinsy and other throat infections, also snakebite, for dissolving kidney stones and easing bladder and kidney infections. Blackberry leaf tea was taken to treat diarrhoea, dysentery and cystitis. To make the tea, take ¼ cup fresh leaves and pour over this 1 cup boiling water. Stand 5 minutes, strain and sip slowly. Interestingly, medical science today actually supports those ancient findings, as the blackberry is found to be rich in vitamins and minerals (see Health Note).

The leaves were boiled in water to make a rinse after shampooing the hair, for crusty, scaly, dry scalp, skin eruptions, and dull, lifeless hair. The blackberry brew was massaged into the scalp, and used as a daily lotion dabbed onto the scalp, to clear up the dryness. An excellent hair tonic can be made by adding 2 cups fresh rosemary sprigs to 2 cups fresh blackberry vines and leaves, and boiling everything in 6 cups of water for 20 minutes. Cool and strain. Add some to the rinsing water after shampooing the hair, and comb into the hair daily.

The most delicious way of all to eat blackberries is fresh with sugar and thick cream, and they are worth growing for just that incredible springtime feast!

Health Note

Blackberries are rich in vitamins A, B, C and E, calcium, magnesium, iron, phosphorus and beta-carotene.

Blackberry Cordial

This is an ancient gypsy drink and one that is so loved it has withstood the test of time.

6 cups fresh blackberries (remove stalks and calyxes)
1 cup honey
½–1 cup brown sugar (the ancient recipes suggest 1 cup molasses instead of sugar)
a squeeze of lemon juice
3 thin parings of lemon rind
1 stick cinnamon
2 cups of water

Simmer very gently until the sugar and honey have dissolved and the fruit is soft, stirring frequently, usually about 15 minutes. Strain and pour into a pretty decanter or bottle with a well-fitting lid and keep refrigerated. Pour about ¼ of a glass of cordial and top with iced water and crushed ice. Serve with a sprig of mint and 'sip slowly for a spring in your step', the gypsies say.

Hint

Set up a tunnel made of wire in full sun for growing blackberries. Train the vines over it – you'll be surprised by the abundance of fruiting tips. Hang tin foil flags to keep the birds away.

Raspberry

Rubus idaeus

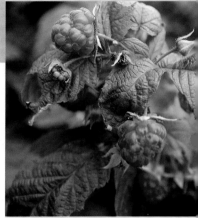

Indigenous to Europe and Eastern Asia, the raspberry has a long and intriguing history. Myth and legend intertwine around its bristly stems, and from Scandinavia to Scotland, from Germany to Greece, Russia to Yugoslavia, England to Poland, the raspberry remains to this day an enviable trade. Made into syrups, jams and jellies, vinegars, 'sweetmeats', dried raspberries and raspberry wines, liqueurs and brandies – the raspberry has never lost its appeal. From the Middle Ages onwards, monastery gardens grew raspberries for teas, for laxatives, coughs and colds, to clear mucus and to soothe rheumatism. Warriors in the early centuries took dried raspberries and leaves with them on their journeys to use as a tonic, a wound wash and to treat 'soldier's diarrhoea'. The ancient healers prescribed raspberry leaf tea for eye ailments, for throat and chest infections, to ease childbirth, and today's medical research verifies all this, and the raspberry retains its status as a medicinal herb of note, as it has for centuries.

Growing Raspberries

Raspberries need a cool climate and neutral to slightly acid soil. A long, deep, well-drained trench in full sun, filled with compost and with bonemeal added, with a deep and thorough weekly or even twice weekly watering in very hot weather, will ensure good, strong canes and aid fruiting. Set a fence up along the furrow of about 1 m in height, and plant the canes 1 m apart. Tie the canes up the fence to make picking easier and prune out non-fruiting canes. Mulch the furrow in the midsummer heat to keep the roots cool. Raspberries fruit from midsummer to late autumn, clusters forming on the tips of the sprawling stems on new wood. It is therefore vital to prune back the long stems in winter and to give copious amounts of compost after pruning to ensure a good crop the following season.

Using Raspberries

Rich in vitamins, minerals and other compounds (see Health Note) and low in calories, a bowl of raspberries is a real health booster and just half a cupful of mashed raspberries will help to eliminate toxins, clear phlegm, relieve menstrual cramps and flush and clear the kidneys and bladder.

Raspberry leaf tea (see recipe alongside) has been taken over the centuries as a treatment for coughs and colds, and late in pregnancy to prepare for childbirth. The same tea makes an excellent mouthwash and a gargle for mouth ulcers, gum ailments and throat infections. The cooled tea can also be used as a wash for wounds and it remains a favourite treatment for varicose veins – pads of cotton wool soaked in the warm, *not* hot, tea and applied to the area have astringent properties and will soothe the veins, as well as being an excellent treatment for thread veins on the face. Use the cooled tea as an eye-wash to treat pink eye and as a lotion for freshening the face, refining large pores and removing oiliness.

Probably the world's favourite fruit, our plantings have become so valuable to our kitchens as well as to our cosmetic products that we constantly extend our rows by propagating new little root runners in August from our sturdy mother plants. Sales in our little herb nursery are so quick and so much in demand that we find we never have enough, and we urge our visitors to try several varieties for their particular area. 'Autumn Bliss' has been our best variety, but newer varieties now more freely available that are worth considering include 'Raspberry Heritage' and 'Raspberry Glen Prozen'.

Health Note

Raspberries are rich in vitamins A, B, C and E and a host of minerals, including calcium, phosphorus, magnesium, iron and potassium. They also contain valuable flavenoids, mainly the anthocyanins, which are responsible for the brilliant red colour and which are powerful antioxidants, as well as ellagic acid, a proven cancer fighter.

Raspberry Leaf Tea

Add ¼ cup fresh raspberry leaves to 1 cup of boiling water, stand 5 minutes, then strain and sip slowly. This tea makes an excellent mouthwash and a gargle and a lotion with a host of uses (see main text).

Caution

Be aware that this tea is a uterine stimulant! Only take the tea during the last stages of pregnancy, and only under your doctor's guidance.

Raspberry Vinegar for Salads

In a large glass bottle filled with apple cider vinegar, drop in at least 2 cups of freshly picked raspberries and 6 fresh leaves. Place in the sun and give it a daily shake. Do this every day for 10 days. By now it will be bright red. Strain, taste and repeat if the flavour is not strong enough. Pour into a pretty bottle, add a fresh leaf or two, label and store in a dark cupboard and serve with salads. This is a gourmet delight!

Hint

Pick raspberries early in the morning to keep the fruit firm and luscious and be gentle and quick, carefully cupping the hand or the punnet under the cluster of ripening fruit, as handling the fruit softens and breaks the juice-laden 'drupes' as it is pulled away from its central cone.

Sorrel

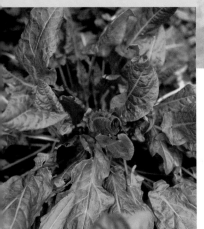

Rumex acetosa

As a salad ingredient sorrel takes some beating, and it is such an easy plant to grow it should form part of the perennial vegetable section in every garden. Indigenous to Europe and parts of Asia, it was treasured by the ancient Greeks, Romans and Egyptians, mainly as a soup ingredient but also as a diuretic, astringent, cooling herb, and served in salads and egg dishes. Closely related to sheep sorrel (*Rumex acetosella*) and found as a wild herb, the Romans and Greeks grew it around their banqueting halls to offset the richness of the foods – baskets of fresh sorrel leaves wrapped in wet cloths were placed on the long tables for guests to pick out and eat whenever they needed to 'refresh the palate'. The word 'sorrel' is derived from the Greek word for 'sour' and this sour and delicious taste was much sought after in those ancient days.

Growing Sorrel

Propagation is from seeds, which germinate readily in seed trays and, kept moist, quickly grow into sturdy little plants which can be pricked out and planted into compost-rich bags to mature before planting out into their final place in the garden. Plant them in full sun (although they can take partial shade) in a deeply dug, richly composted bed, spaced 75 cm to 1 m apart. Water long and deeply twice a week in hot weather and once a week or even every 2 weeks in winter, and twice yearly give it a large bucket of compost dug in around it. A clump or two is enough for the household. Undemanding and attractive, the clump reaches about 45 cm in height and width but with good water and rainy summers grows even bigger, with large and lusciously succulent leaves. Occasionally pull off the larger leaves as they dry in maturity, to neaten and tidy up, and cut off the flowering head as it forms. For the most part it needs very little attention and remains a neat and fascinating lime-green focal point in the garden.

Using Sorrel

Grown in the cloister gardens in medieval times, sorrel was an important medicinal herb that the monks dispensed. Warmed sorrel leaves were used as poultices over slow-to-heal wounds and over cuts, grazes and scrapes – a sorrel poultice, bandaged into place, with its astringent properties, soon stopped the bleeding and kept the area safe from infection.

Sorrel salad with watercress and leafy greens became so popular it became a celebration dish – perhaps one of the first salads as we know them today.

Of the great *Rumex* genus of over 200 species, the most popular is *Rumex acetosa*. Its sour qualities curdle milk and those same sour qualities are still today considered to have blood-building, blood-cleansing properties, and with its high vitamin C content it helps to clear skin rashes, infections and acne.

Well known today as an ingredient in Rene Caisse's 'Essiac' (Caisse spelled backwards) cancer treatment, sheep sorrel (*Rumex acetosella*) is an important ingredient and one that gave garden sorrel (*Rumex acetosa*) new exposure and new interest.

Health Note

Sorrel has high levels of vitamins A and C and is also rich in magnesium and potassium.

Caution

Like rhubarb and spinach, sorrel is high in oxalates, which if taken in excess, can exacerbate rheumatism, arthritis, kidney ailments, kidney stones and over-acidity. Large doses may, in fact, be dangerous and damaging to the kidneys. So remember, a little goes a long way.

French Sorrel Soup

Serves 4–6

Taken as a summer soup occasionally, this 'French sorrel soup' is delicious and one that King Henry VIII would have enjoyed!

2 cups fresh chopped sorrel leaves, stalks removed

2–3 cups thinly sliced leeks

4 large potatoes, peeled and cubed

1 cup parsley

juice of 1 lemon and a little lemon rind, finely grated

1–1½ litre good chicken stock

½ cup olive oil

½ litre full cream milk

2–3 cups thinly sliced lettuce (we use butter lettuce)

sea salt and freshly ground black pepper to taste

Fry the leeks in the olive oil until golden. Add the potatoes and stir-fry a few minutes. Then add all the other ingredients except the parsley. Stir well. Simmer for about 30 minutes until the potatoes and leeks are tender. Whirl in a blender. Serve hot, sprinkled with the chopped parsley.

Hint

The juice of the succulent stems has been used through the centuries to remove rust, to clean silver, to remove mould stains and ink stains from linen and to brighten and clean wood and wicker.

Sugar Cane

Saccharum officinarum

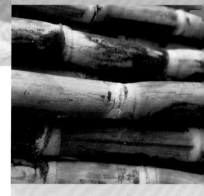

Is cane sugar a food, really? It is so extraordinary a plant with an even more extraordinary beginning, and it is one of the most gigantic businesses in the world that I am unsure if within these pages I can do it justice. *Saccharum officinarum*, a huge perennial grass, is a descendant of an ancient grass which, it is thought, originated in New Guinea. Now extinct, the sugar cane we know today was cultivated in Asia, India and China, in ancient times since before 2500 BC. The earliest written reference to sugar cane was found in the *Atharva-Veda*, a sacred Indian text. The Greek historian Herodotus in the 5th century BC recorded it, and by 327 BC Alexander the Great introduced it to Europe from India. One could say the sugar cane took the world by storm! No one could get enough of it and in 510 BC a Persian tablet describes the boiling of the sweet juice to make a solid sugar, from the Indus Valley. India today still produces that same raw solid sugar – unrefined and rich in flavour – known as *jaggery* or *gur*. It was the Persians in the 7th century who further refined the processing of sugar, and they added lime to remove impurities.

Sugar cane reached high prices and cultivation soon spread from the Mediterranean area both north and south and many trials were planted. The Venetians set up trade routes to supply Northern Europe with crude sugar and by 1493 Columbus took the plants to the Caribbean. In that warm and stable climate it soon became the main cultivated crop and the economy thrived. As it spread into suitable areas, prices began to drop and the processing and refining became so competitive that whole industries were developed around it. Stems cut as close to the ground as possible where the intense sweetness occurs, were crushed by simple ox-driven weights to press out the juice, and the juice, boiled in shallow pans, had lime added to help it to coagulate. The scum of impurities was skimmed off and the boiling process finally produced sugar crystals. Those first solid crystals, moist, brown and tasting of molasses, became the base from which the refining process developed in earnest.

'Loaf sugar' was easier to transport and conical moulds were made that were re-dissolved, re-refined, re-purified and double refined, making it a highly valued commodity. The first 'lump sugar' was made by sawing up the 'loaf sugar', and it fetched ever higher prices! Today, with modern machinery, that long and colourful and very sweet history has been so changed, and all vestiges erased of what was once a truly remarkable, even healthy food (think of blackstrap molasses). We are left with a refined product that is most certainly not health building and with the alarming increase of diabetes worldwide we need to stop, re-think and curb that sweet tooth and become seriously aware of the 'hidden sugars' in many processed foods. (See also the box on page 33.)

Growing Sugar Cane
Sugar cane requires a warm, frost-free, humid climate with high rainfall, and friable, well-dug and richly composted soil in full sun. The canes are pressed into furrows – long, deep and moisture-holding – spaced 1 m apart. Left to mature, the clump forms untidily with dry elongated leaves as the cane grows taller. Watering is essential and the furrows are flooded once a week.

Using Sugar Cane
Sugar comes in many forms today. Fresh cane juice – ideally crushed fresh from the sugar cane – is the very best way to taste sugar at its purest, other than chewing the cane, with very strong teeth! Sugar is used for jam making, confectionery and as a preservative, and sugar is added to processed foods of every description. It is an essential grocery item in the kitchen cupboard, but nevertheless, too much sugar is dangerous to our health, to our teeth and to our general well-being!

Know Your Sugars
Molasses is a thick, dark syrup that is a by-product of the sugar refining process. It consists of sucrose (about 30%), glucose and fructose (around 15%), water (about 21%), other sugars and gums, traces of B vitamins and calcium, magnesium, iron, phosphorus, silica and potassium. Blackstrap molasses is the molasses that remains after the maximum quantity of sugar has been extracted from the sugar cane and would be the healthiest way to eat sugar.

Brown sugar is a soft, dark caramel sugar that has still a small percentage of molasses in it. It is made up of sucrose (around 95%), glucose, fructose, small quantities of calcium, magnesium, potassium, iron, phosphorus and some water. Probably the best sugar for us, if 'best' is the right word!

White sugar is the highly processed granulated crystals used as a sweetener in confectionery, one of the most widely used of all sugars.

Castor sugar is refined white sugar that has been re-milled to a fine powder. It is used mainly in confectionery and has the same 'properties' as white sugar.

Icing sugar is even more refined! It has a small quantity of calcium phosphate or cornstarch, sometimes both, blended into it as an anti-caking agent to extend its storage life.

Cane syrup is produced by evaporating sugar cane juice so that a very sweet, thick syrup remains.

Golden syrup is made from sugar syrup which has been processed so that some of the sucrose is converted into fructose and glucose (which crystallise less readily than sucrose). It also contains water and traces of sodium potassium.

Elder

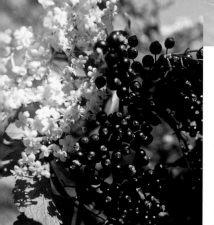

Sambucus nigra

My perennial passion for the elder tree has never abated – I am just mad about elders! I brought my first elder sprig, a mere 10 cm long bare twig, into South Africa around 40 years ago with my first imports of herbs. They remained so long in customs that I feared they were all lost, but that tough little twig survived and the luscious elders I grow and sell in my nursery today come from that one berry-bearing little twig, and I never cease to be amazed. Indigenous to Europe, Britain and Asia, 'the medicine chest tree' has been used for centuries and had been introduced to most parts of the civilised world by the 17th century, mainly as food but traditional medicine played a huge role in its extraordinary journey.

Growing the Elder

Propagation is by cuttings – pencil thin twigs with at least 3 nodes are pressed into bags filled with a mix of light soil and compost. The base node is where the little roots will form and it needs to be well pressed into the soil. Keep shaded and moist and wait at least a year before planting out, as the forming roots need to be sturdy. Plant the elder in a deep and wide compost-filled hole in full sun and flood with water once a week. In bitterly cold areas protect from winter frost by making a tent of hessian or straw over it for its first three to four winters. Thereafter it grows fast and sturdily and forms a multi-stemmed shrub or small tree that takes heat and cold equally well.

It literally needs no maintenance apart from a barrow load of compost once (or even twice) a year – late winter is a good time to encourage the mass of creamy white flower heads that appear in October. Prune long branches every now and then to shape the little trees and plant it where you can see it every day. It is fascinating the way it changes and the birds love it too. Use the leaves, which are poisonous, for sprays for aphids and white fly.

Using the Elder

On a breathtakingly beautiful summer morning in Kent, England, I once joined a group of elderflower pickers in an elder orchard to hand pick the masses of flower heads for the popular commercially produced elderflower cordial. The sweet smell of the flowers, which we picked and tossed into great flat stackable trays that summer morning with the larks singing, the bees all around us and the chamomile and red Flanders poppies between the rows of elders, will forever remain in my heart. The pickers were mostly students and for lunch we sat together in the shade of the elders and ate cheese sandwiches and drank ice-cold elderflower cordial and talked of elderflower fritters and elderberry jam and elderberry and honey cough mixture that had been part of everyone's childhood, and I was entranced. It was then that I decided I'd grow elders for my children and make cordials and syrups and jams. Sandy's dream is to have an elder orchard and to make elderflower champagne and cordial and elderberry wine commercially – we're getting there slowly and our rows are growing well under the heat of the African sun, so far from the cool moist meadows of England.

We make elderflower face creams and elderflower lotion for problem skins from the ancient recipes the monks used, and we add the flowers to soaps and bath salts, scrubs and extracts, and never seem to have enough. Elderflower fritters have long remained one of the highlights in our restaurant and the laden elder trees in our kitchen garden in front of the restaurant are continuously picked. Cooked with apples, elderberries make a glorious jam that is a best seller in our shop, if we can get there before the birds and the squirrels! The berries cooked with honey to a syrup (see recipe alongside) is taken for coughs, colds, 'flu, sore throats, anaemia, insomnia, anxiety, neuralgia, mouth infections and even epilepsy and kidney ailments, and is a patent medicine in Europe.

Health Note

Elderberries are especially high in vitamin C and also provide vitamin A, several B-vitamins, calcium, iron, magnesium, potassium and phosphorus.

Elderberry Syrup

A teaspoon of this syrup can be taken at a time several times a day for a host of ailments (see main text) it can be added to crushed ice and chilled water for a tonic drink.

Boil 4 cups berries removed from the stalks (be diligent, it's only the berries that is needed) with 2 cups of raw honey. Simmer in a double boiler. Add 2 tablespoons of water if needed to start the syrup. Simmer for 2 hours with the lid on. Pour into screw top sterilized bottles or jars (to sterilize stand the jars and lids in boiling water for 15 minutes). Seal and refrigerate.

Elderflower Cordial

20 elderflower heads (remove tough stalks)
4 litres boiling water
juice and finely grated zest of 4–6 lemons
4 cups sugar

Simmer the sugar, water, lemon juice and zest for 15 minutes. Add the elderflowers and simmer 5 minutes. Cool overnight. Next morning strain and bottle. Serve (if liked) with ice and a little cold water. Float a few flowers on top.

Marula

Sclerocarya birrea subsp. *caffra*

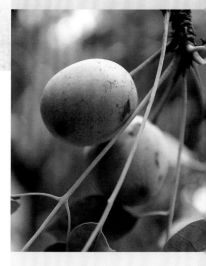

I think I love marulas the way I do because I live amongst these great trees and I watch their seasonal changes with such endless fascination. I am always so overcome by their midsummer bounty – the ground is literally covered with butter-coloured, amazingly scented fruits that drop enticingly when they are ripe. Many legends are woven around this precious tree – the stories are filled with myth, magic and medicine. It is found in frost-free tropical and subtropical areas in Africa and it grows into a beautiful shape – wide and spreading – up to 20 m in height. It needs space and male and female trees are separate (often the biggest and most spectacular tree is the male tree). The female tree bears masses of sweetly scented, creamy yellow and pink sprays of flowers, which are followed by the heavy, juicy and extraordinary fruits that ripen and fall around February and March. The greater part of the fruit is taken up by the seed, which is a skull-shaped 'stone' with usually 3 holes. Within each hole is a delicious oblong, soft, protein-rich 'nut' that is covered by a small 'door'. So not only is the juicy flesh and flavour-filled juice the part that is eaten, but also the 'nut', which is tricky to access.

Growing the Marula

Although we have bagged and sold in our small nursery, many small marula trees dug out from our compost heaps, we are largely unsuccessful in propagating the seeds. It is thought that the seed needs to pass through the gut of an elephant or a baboon first in order to make them viable!

Should you have the right space and the right climate, this is a superb and fabulous tree to grow. Plant in a huge compost-filled hole with a thick pipe set in at an angle into which the hose can be inserted to enable water to reach the roots. It needs a deep and thorough weekly watering until it is well established and thereafter once a fortnight, even once a month in winter or in the rainy season. A barrow load of compost twice yearly in early spring and in midsummer will ensure quick and abundant growth. Other than that it requires nothing – no attention other than marvelling at its fascinating growth and development.

Using the Marula

Zulu women pound the seeds into pulp and boil it up with water until an oily residue emerges. Strained and bottled, this precious substance is used to rub into animal skins, belts and reins to soften them, and is also used as a beauty treatment for dry cracked heels, ageing dry skin and cracked lips! The bark is considered to be one of Africa's superb medicines and a brew made of 1 cup of shaved bark gently simmered in 3 litres of water for 3 hours, is taken in small doses to treat dysentery, gonorrhoea, malaria and diarrhoea, or used as an enema for abdominal upsets. For malaria, ground powdered bark is taken a teaspoon at a time in water, but no medical evidence supports this treatment. The inner bark, boiled and mashed, is used as a poultice over ulcers, skin ailments, rashes, grazes, cuts, and in some distant areas even for smallpox pustules.

The fruits are fermented into an intoxicating and nourishing beer, and the Tswana and Venda have 'marula binges' during the time of the ripening fruit that can last weeks! The fruits are also made into marula jams, jellies, desserts and sweets. A commercial drink – a liqueur known as 'Amarula' – has become well known worldwide and is made from the juice.

The Zulus and the Tswanas in rural Africa use the fruit boiled in water as an insecticide over tick-infested cattle or goats. It is thrown over and rubbed in as a drench. The marula bark exudes a gum rich in tannin. If the gum is dissolved in hot water and mixed with soot, it makes a natural ink for writing and drawing.

The marula seed, with its 'eyes' removed, and the delicious and precious inner nuts, so rich in protein and oils, picked out, is scrubbed and dried, and hung on a thin thong as a symbol of good luck. It is often given to visitors or friends as a memento or talisman to wish them good fortune or a safe journey.

Marula Jelly

Here is our well-known marula jelly recipe we make every year.

Wash about 3 kg of ripe marulas. Slit a gash or two into the skin, submerge in enough water to just cover them and simmer gently for 2–3 hours. Strain, pour off the fragrant juice and measure it. Discard the seeds and work the skin through a sieve to extract the pulp.

For every 1 litre of juice add 2 cups of sugar. Simmer with grated lemon zest – 1 tablespoon per litre – and the juice of 2 lemons per litre. Simmer until dark red and thick. Pour into sterilised bottles and seal and label.

Serve with cold meats, use as a marinade for fish, meat and poultry, serve with cheese or dribble over hot scones. We add marula jelly to our tomato and onion pastas to give it that delicious taste of sweetness from the African bush!

Health Note

The fruits are exceptionally rich in vitamin C and also contain beta-carotene, calcium, magnesium, phosphorus and potassium.

Rye

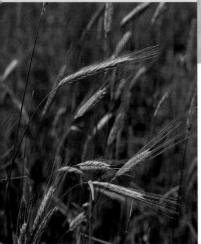

Secale coreale

Native to Central Asia where it has been cultivated for thousands of years, rye is one of those ancient grains around which history revolves. A wild grass that can today still be found growing in certain areas, it spread amongst the fields of wheat and barley. Often growing in poor soil, rye stood out as it was taller than the wheat and barley. Because of its long stems, rye straw was used to weave hats, baskets and bags, and during the Iron Age was used as bedding on the floors of the caves to protect against the winter cold.

For centuries rye has been cultivated in Asia and Central Europe, later spreading into Southern Europe and the Mediterranean area. Used to make breads and whiskey, it has been a valuable crop and is still today so much a part of tradition that each country has its own recipes and rituals revolving around it. Pumpernickel bread is one of the traditional recipes that is still baked today.

Because rye grows well in poor soils and moist climates, it was in the distant past – especially during the Middle Ages – susceptible to the ergot fungus which grew on it. Ergot was the cause of epidemics known as 'St Anthony's fire', characterised by circulatory disorders and intense pain in the extremities along with mental derangement and often followed by gangrene. Today ergot compounds are used in very small quantities in certain medications. Modern farming practices have completely removed the ergot fungus and today's best rye crops come from Russia, Poland, China and Denmark, and it is a common crop in many other countries across the world.

Growing Rye

Sown in well-tilled fields to which masses of manure and compost have been added, in full sun and kept moist, rye is a valuable commercial crop that needs a long, hot summer to ripen it to perfection.

Using Rye

Rye is rich in minerals and vitamins (see Health Note) and rye grains, soaked overnight then rinsed and boiled into a porridge or used to thicken soups and stews, have been a great part of ancient health-building recipes handed down from generation to generation. A packet of rye flour added to the same quantity of wheat flour, forms the base for an excellent loaf that has been found to ease arthritis, stiffness and swollen joints and has become a bestseller in many health shops today.

Once 'rye berries' – the cleaned thrashed grain – made a sustaining 'soldier's gruel' or 'rice'. The rye grains were soaked in warm water overnight, then well rinsed and simmered for 1 hour – 1 part rye to 3 or 4 parts boiling water with a little salt. Walnuts and raisins were sometimes added, and it became a favourite dish. Rye berries today can often be found toasted as a 'granola' in health shops and 100% rye loaves are available in most bakeries and supermarkets today. Rye bread is considered to be a slow release energy food, particularly if eaten with mashed avocado.

Rye cleanses and rejuvenates the arteries, it cleanses and tones the liver, and it removes arthritic stiffness and pain and loosens up the joints. Perhaps this is why the 'soldier's gruel' was so popular. We should be looking at rye as an energy food, as a de-stressor and as a snack – think for example of rye biscuits with mackerel pâté, to replace chocolates and sweets. The pancreas will be so grateful!

Health Note

Rye is high in vitamins B, E and K, calcium, iron, phosphorus, potassium, magnesium, zinc, manganese and selenium.

Sweet Potato Crumble with Rye

Serves 4

Excellent for soothing the digestive tract and stomach ulcers, why not try this easy-to-make dish as a lunchtime pick-me-up.

Peel and slice 3–4 large sweet potatoes, boil until tender, drain and return to the pan. Add a tablespoon of olive oil, 1 teaspoon of freshly grated nutmeg and a pinch of salt. Mash well and spoon into a baking dish.

Crumble 2 slices of 100% rye bread and stir-fry in a little olive oil in a pan on top of the stove until golden. Sprinkle on top of the sweet potatoes, and bake at 180 °C for about 20 minutes. Serve hot sprinkled with freshly chopped mint and a squeeze of lemon juice.

Hint

Bread made with 100% rye flour is accepted by the body that shows wheat and gluten intolerance. Health shops and some supermarkets stock rye flour, which can be used to make pancakes, biscuits and breads.

Su-Su

Chayote

Sechium edule

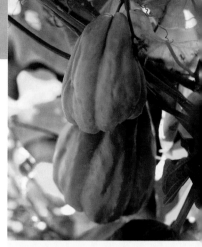

The su-su is a vigorous vine that produces large, pear-shaped 'marrows' in spectacular summer abundance. A perennial vine, it dies down in the winter with new luscious tendrils appearing in spring for another season of mile-a-minute growth! Originating, it is thought, in Central America in prehistoric times, it spread into Mexico and later to the West Indies. The single-seeded fruit could be carried far – remaining fresh and edible for long periods. Travellers took it on their journeys and the ancient Aztecs used it as both a food and a medicine, and they named it chayote. It was introduced to the Mediterranean area by the early traders and the sailors who ate the vine tips to treat scurvy. Early white settlers took it to Australia where it is known as 'choko'. It grows wild down the mountainsides in the volcanic ash on Reunion Island where it is known as *le chou-chou* and there it is cooked in 100 ways – even crystallised su-su can be bought in the marketplace. Hats and baskets woven from the vines are a tourist attraction as are the cakes, the tarts and the tender green vine tips cooked in curries. The islanders say proudly no one ever starves on Reunion Island – *le chou-chou* is available in abundance to everyone. It has been grown all over Africa for over two centuries at least, and is included in many traditional dishes.

Growing Su-Su

The vine emerges from the fruit tip in spring, so place the whole fruit in a compost-filled hole and half cover it so that the roots, which form as the vine tip extends, can easily settle into the ground. Keep it moist and protected. It needs a fence or a pergola to grow over and it needs full sun and a deep weekly watering. The vine growth is rapid – so check it frequently to train it up. It will quickly shade an area and by Christmas time the new little fruits, the tips of the vines and the young leaves are ready for picking. The underground tubers are also edible and can be dug up in the winter once the vine has died back.

Often the large, single seed within the fruit germinates while the fruit is still hanging on the vine in late summer. These can be tucked into large compost-filled pots to overwinter, the young tender new vines twisted around a pair of support sticks stuck into the pot. Keep the pot in a protected sunny area to overwinter and plant out, 2–3 m apart, once the weather warms up.

Using Su-Su

In Mexico and in the West Indies fresh slices of the fruit are placed over minor burns and rashes, scratches, grazes, sunburn and infected insect bites. Baked su-su is an ancient treatment for bringing a boil to a head – the fruit is split open, the single seed removed and the pulp is mashed, spread as hot as is comfortable over the boil, covered by a leaf or two soaked in hot water, then held in place by a bandage comfortably bound over it. This was done until the boil came to a head and burst. Interestingly, the vines, softened in hot water, have been used for centuries to bind bandages or to hold splints in place or to hold warmed leaves over aching feet.

In the kitchen the su-su is an absolute joy! Grate young and tender fruits into stir-fries, into pancake batter, into fritters with mince, onions and grated potatoes, cook with rice or steam quartered like a squash and serve with butter, salt, brown sugar and a squeeze of lemon juice, or add it to stews, to soups, to casseroles, fry it with onions and fish, add it to jams and cakes – replace carrots with su-su in a favourite carrot cake recipe – and grate it fresh into a salad served with lemon juice. As it gets older, peel off the slightly hard skin – it sometimes has a few prickles on it – and grate the now quite big fruit coarsely into soups and casseroles. There is no end to this marvellous plant's versatility!

Health Note

Su-su is a good source of B-vitamins (especially B3), magnesium and potassium, and an excellent source of vitamin C and K, folic acid, zinc, copper, manganese and dietary fibre.

Chicken and Su-Su Hot Pot

Serves 4–6

This is a delicious and satisfying stew that everyone enjoys.

1 organic chicken
olive oil
6 large, young and tender su-su
4–6 large potatoes
4–6 large carrots
4 sticks celery, leaves included
4 large onions
juice of 2 lemons
sea salt and black pepper to taste
3 tablespoons apricot jam (preferably homemade)
3 tablespoons fresh thyme, stripped off their stalks

Peel and chop the vegetables into chunks. In a large heavy bottomed pot, brown the chicken in the olive oil, turning it frequently. Add the onions to the pot and brown them. Now add 1 litre of water and all the other ingredients. Turn the chicken and cook it breast side down. Add more water to cover everything. Simmer 1½ hours or until the chicken and vegetables are tender. Serve hot with rice.

Sesame

Sesamum indicum

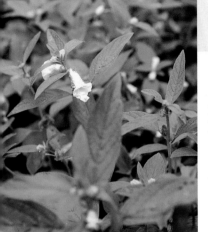

Sesame Spread

Better than peanut butter, this paste is like gold as it is so rich in vitamins, minerals and amino acids.

In a seed grinder grind 1 cup of hulled sesame seeds with ½ cup sunflower seeds and ½ cup flaxseed. (Mix together and grind a little at a time.) Mix in 2 teaspoons of cinnamon powder and a pinch of sea salt (Himalayan rock salt is best if you have it). Add a little raw honey, just enough to make a paste and about 2 teaspoons of sesame oil. Spread it on home-baked bread or biscuits as an energy-boosting snack or mix a spoonful into breakfast porridge.

Hint

The sesame plant contains insect-repelling compounds that can be used in the same way as the pyrethrins in insect sprays. Pour 1 bucket of boiling water over ½ bucket crushed stalks, leaves and seedpods. Stand covered overnight. Next morning strain, add ½ cup soap powder and mix well. Splash or spray onto aphid-infested plants.

Sesame, it is thought, originates in Africa, India, Indonesia and the Middle East. It was recorded by the Assyrians and the Greeks in ancient times, has been cultivated in Indonesia for over 4 000 years and sesame crops grown in the Tigris and Euphrates River Valleys date back to 1600 BC! A plant of myth and legend – think of Ali Baba and the 40 thieves – it is recorded in ancient Sanskrit, Egyptian and Hebrew writings, and so steeped in history, mystery and magic that its journey remains one of the most speculated. Marco Polo wrote that the sesame oil he tested on his travels through Persia was the most extraordinary oil he had ever encountered. Cleopatra probably used it on her legendary beautiful skin and sesame seeds were found in Tutankhamen's tomb. During the Babylonian era (2100–689 BC) sesame oil was used to make the first exotic oils and perfumes, mixed with jasmine, rose petals and violets. The Egyptians used sesame as a medicine from 1500 BC and this became so valuable that it was found in the burial chambers of the pharaohs. Europe was introduced to sesame, imported from India in the 1st century AD, and in the 17th century the African slaves took the seeds with them on their anguished journey to America.

Growing Sesame

Sesame is a pretty pink-flowered annual that grows into tall and almost fragile 1–2 m high stalks, rich in seed capsules. In spring scatter unhulled seeds (the creamy-white hulled seeds we buy in health shops will not grow!) in a shallow furrow in full sun that has been deeply dug and enriched with compost and moistened lightly. Rake them in and set a gentle sprinkler over the area to really soak the seeds into the soil. Check and water lightly daily. Once the little seeds have sprouted keep them moist as they grow quickly and sturdily. They are tender and fragile, so keep the soil damp. The tubular flowers appear as the tall stem matures. Once the seed capsules form they need to be watched as the seed ripens quickly. The entire plant is pulled up just as the first pod splits. Tied in bunches and hung over floors spread with cloth – as the ancient Egyptians did, nowadays plastic is used – the ripe seeds drop. New varieties have a pod that ripens after harvesting, and are laid on floors out of the wind and sun so that the crop can be easily gathered.

Using Sesame

Sesame seeds have been taken since ancient times for constipation, to remove worms from the body, to aid digestion, stimulate blood circulation and to soothe and calm the nervous system. Eating sesame frequently – a mere tablespoon sprinkled onto porridge or plain yoghurt or a mashed banana with cinnamon – will stimulate breast-milk production in new mothers, strengthen the heart, lower blood pressure, cleanse the kidneys and bladder, and detoxify an overloaded liver. The root can be made into a tea – ¼ cup chopped root and 2 teaspoons of seed boiled up in 2 cups of water for 15 minutes, then strained – and taken as a medicine for coughs, respiratory ailments, asthma, dizziness, tinnitus (ringing noises in the ears), for blurred vision due to anaemia, and as a general tonic.

Toast sesame seeds by lightly and quickly frying dry in a pan – tossing and stirring for a minute or two. Add to stir-fries, pancake batter, breads and salad dressings, stuffings and porridges, savoury biscuits and make into a delicious paste by grinding in a seed grinder and mixing with a touch of sesame oil as a butter substitute. Rich in polyunsaturated and monounsaturated fats, sesame seeds are the main ingredient in tahini, hummus and halvah. Sesame oil is an ingredient in many Chinese and Arab recipes and can be stored for long periods as it is slow to turn rancid. Sesame oil is superb for dry, sun-damaged skin, for cracked lips, cracked heels, itchy flaky skin and especially for ageing skin. Used through the centuries to treat dry scalp and falling dry hair, problem skin, brittle nails and for a youthful appearance, sesame oil takes some beating. Use as a weekly facial massage and watch the wrinkles disappear!

Health Note

Sesame seeds are rich in vitamins E, B1 and B2, copper, magnesium, iron, zinc, calcium and phosphorus and a lignan called sesamin, which displays excellent antioxidant and cholesterol-lowering effects.

Brinjal

Eggplant ▪ Eggfruit ▪ Aubergine

Solanum melongena

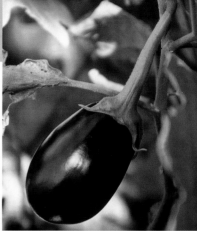

Originating in India from a small, prickly, grey-leafed plant, the brinjal has been grown in Southeast Asia, Turkey and China since 500 BC. Eaten cooked or raw, the skin was eagerly saved to make a black dye to stain the eyelids and the teeth – then considered to be a fashionable beauty aid by the young ladies! It arrived in Europe only by the 17th century and much later reached the Americas and Australia. The French and the Italians were the first to grow it as a commercial crop by the 18th century, ever improving the strains, and from then on this extraordinary vegetable became increasingly popular. Varieties abound – from the early white 'eggfruits' the size of a jumbo egg, to the finger-thin Japanese aubergines to the small, green Thai 'pea aubergine', to the lusciously purple, giant, globe eggfruit we know today, available in every supermarket and greengrocer.

Growing Brinjals

Try as many varieties as you can find, as they are all prolifically beautiful in the garden! I have planted them in flower borders in front of purple heliotrope and purple irises and as fascinating borders along paths. They are never without fruits and the abundant crop inspires the invention of many a gourmet dish! Start off with seedlings and plant out in well-dug, richly composted rows 40 cm apart in full sun. Water deeply twice weekly and pick the fruits when they are large and glossy. The more you pick the more the plant produces.

Using Brinjals

An anthocyanin flavonoid called nasunin is found in the skin of the brinjal. This is a potent antioxidant and free radical scavenger and is known to protect cell membranes from damage, but it also cleans the blood, literally removing toxins, and helps to protect arteries that are damaged by cholesterol. Research on nasunin proves that it helps to remove excess iron in the body by binding with it. Excess iron promotes free radical production, and increases the risk of heart disease. Post-menopausal women, and men, can accumulate excess iron, which is difficult to excrete. By helping to bind the excess iron, nasunin lessens free radical formation with numerous beneficial results. In tests it was found that eggplant juice lowered high cholesterol in rabbits, especially in the aorta to the heart. The results were put down to nasunin and other phytochemicals in eggplant known as terpenes.

To get the full benefit of the brinjal's cholesterol-lowering properties, steam slices of brinjal, skin and all, and season with fresh chopped basil, celery and parsley. This is also an excellent recipe for releasing the pain of arthritic joints, and for lessening and preventing cellular free radical damage in the joints. In China eating aubergine daily is considered to be an important energy-building food – it often replaces meat – and in Italy, a divine tomato, onion and aubergine dish is served almost daily as a tonic.

In Greece, moussaka remains a favourite dish and there are many varieties of this popular dish, which includes onions, peppers, garlic, tomatoes and thin slices of mutton. In South Africa the brinjal is known commonly as 'vleisvrug' and is eaten often in place of meat. A favourite way is to bake it cut into thick discs, with tomatoes and onions and a squeeze of lemon juice.

Health Note

Versatile, delicious and good for you, the brinjal contains potassium, calcium, phosphorus, folic acid, beta-carotene, vitamin C, iron and niacin.

Baked Aubergine

The French bake aubergines unpeeled, cut in half, lightly brushed with olive oil and sprinkled with a little salt, flat, cut side up, on a baking tray for 20–30 minutes until tender. Baked this way and *not* fried in oil and butter, it is a superb dish for treating high cholesterol.

Hint

Slice the brinjal after thoroughly washing it and sprinkle the slices with salt and allow it to rest, covered for 30 minutes. This method pulls out any bitter compounds and a lot of the water. Rinse, pat dry and steam or lightly turn in just a touch of olive oil, both sides. Serve with lemon juice and black pepper.

Fruit Salad Plant

Melon-Pear ▪ Pepino *Solanum muricatum*

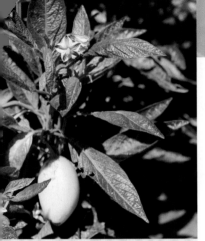

Easy Ideas With the Fruit Salad Plant

For a summer barbecue treat, make skewers – soak the sticks in water first to quickly turn on the braai – with cubes of fruit salad plant, onion, red peppers, tomato and pineapple that have been sprinkled with coarse salt mixed with coriander, cumin and oregano. Turn them frequently on the braai, just to soften. Serve with fresh lemon juice squeezed over them.

Our favourite is the quartered fruits steamed with thin slices of fresh ginger, dribbled with honey, served as a dessert with vanilla ice-cream. Or try steaming it sliced with dates in a little apple juice and served with custard and cream as a lovely autumn pudding.

It is delicious added to a tomato bredie, or steamed with green beans and served with mint sauce, or thinly sliced into chicken salad, or eaten with cheese.

In a fruit salad the sliced or diced pieces of ripe melon-pear are superb – try it with spanspek or the green melon, with sweet grapes and whipped cream.

The fruit salad plant is indigenous to the temperate Andean region of South America. Known to the Bolivians as the 'pepino', it has played a huge part in their history and is depicted in their paintings, their pottery and in their woven garments. It belongs to the great nightshade family, and from the early centuries began to make its name as a valuable medicinal plant, mainly for the efficacy of its thin slices that were applied warmed to boils, pimples and rashes, and it was grown in every town as a valuable medicinal herb as well as a food. Like the potato and the tomato, it is part of the *Solanum* genus and it is thought that its spread from Bolivia, Peru and Chile was due to its trade value, as it bears fruit throughout the warm months, offering flush after flush of ripening mini-melons. Introduced into Florida around 1880 it became an instant success and spread quickly. Currently Australia is growing it abundantly, and in many tropical and subtropical countries far from its native Peru, Chile and Bolivia it is thriving.

Growing Fruit Salad Plant

This is a fascinating plant to grow – a tumbling, spreading, metre-high perennial shrub with branches that often root where they touch the ground and fruits that hang voluptuously and heavily abundant at all stages of ripening. The egg-shaped fruits are shown off to their best in a huge pot where they hang invitingly over the sides, ripening to a soft yellow apricot shade, often with purple streaks.

It thrives in full sun in a deeply dug, compost-filled hole that has a substantial dam around it so that it can be flooded twice a week in summer and once a week in winter. If it is in a big pot it will need more frequent watering and feeding with an organic supercharger or a spade or two of rich compost every month. As it is such an abundant producer of the beautiful dangling fruits it needs lots of nourishment! In the garden, feed it 3 or 4 times a year with a good few buckets of compost and a regular deep watering.

It multiplies by cuttings, which can be rooted in moist sandy soil in bags. In late winter prune it to shape and replant rooted shoots in compost.

Using the Fruit Salad Plant

The ripe fruits are likened to a melon, not as sweet as a melon but certainly the same texture. It is as refreshing as a cucumber and is equally delicious in salads and if you smell it, it has the definite scent of a ripe pear smothered in honey!

In Peru and Bolivia thin slices of the fruit are used on burns, over scratches and grazes, as a dressing, and finely grated as a soothing sunburn treatment gently smoothed on. A whole fruit warmed in the oven and cut in half, is placed over boils and abscesses as hot as it can be tolerated – test carefully first – and held in place with crêpe bandages.

In Hawaii it is mashed with fresh pineapple juice and applied as a treatment for oily problem skin. The fruit is grated, mixed with grated pineapple and its juice and used as a scrub and a mask. Done once or twice a week it is a popular beauty treatment among teenagers, both boys and girls. According to an ancient Brazilian recipe, a fruit cut in half and baked until it is soft and while still hot is smeared over greasy, oily skin with acne. The pulp is left to dry on the skin and finally washed off with warm water, leaving the skin soft, cleansed and smooth. It is grown in commercial plantations in Australia and New Zealand not only as a table fruit, but also as an ingredient in soaps and cosmetics!

Health Note

The fruit salad plant contains vitamins A and C in high quantities and it also provides calcium and iron.

Nastergal
Black Nightshade ▪ Msoba

Solanum nigrum • Solanum retroflexum

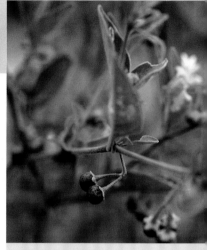

The nastergal is so much a plant of Africa and yet its origins are believed to be European, but it has become naturalised in many parts of the world and is often known as black nightshade. On the farm we grow 'umsoba' or 'msoba' (*Solanum retroflexum*) for making the most delicious jam from the tiny ripe black berries that form in clusters along the stems. Planted out from seedlings gathered in the wild, we are constantly on the lookout for the tiny seedlings, as many visitors to our nursery want plants for their gardens. *Solanum nigrum* is a taller, paler, smooth-leafed plant that grows to a height and often a spread of over a metre – and is also a potherb. The leaves can be eaten as a spinach. The garden huckleberry is also part of this family, often known as *Solanum nigrum* var. *guineense*, and much history surrounds these fascinating plants and their journey from Europe to Africa.

Growing Nastergal
We grow it easily – it could be said to be a fairly common weed – and we transplant small self-sown plants into either compost-filled bags for sale in our nursery or into well-dug, richly composted beds in full sun spaced 1 metre apart. It seeds everywhere easily. Treat it as an annual, and start up new plants every year, discarding the old ones on the compost heap.

Using Nastergal
A tea made of the leaves – ¼ of a cup to 1 cup of boiling water, stand and steep for 5 minutes, then strain – is sipped frequently for stomach ulcers, to treat fevers, convulsions, for malaria, headaches, dysentery, diarrhoea, as a sedative, and as a wash for wounds, skin ulcers, infected bites, rashes, grazes and scratches. Leaves softened and warmed in hot water are used as a soothing dressing for haemorrhoids, varicosities, and for bruises and severe sprains. Recently I learned from a highly respected Muslim doctor that the tea and the ripe berries are beneficial for severe kidney ailments, taken 3 or 4 times a day in monitored doses – but this must only be taken under your doctor's supervision.

The cooked leaves eaten as a spinach are considered to be blood cleansing, revitalising and energising, cooked on their own or combined with stinging nettle and amaranth leaves, as well as other leaves from well-known weeds such as purslane, sow's thistle (*Sonchus oleraceus*) and fat hen (*Chenopodium album*). The Xhosas and Zulus often dry the leaves for winter use to add to stews and soups after first soaking the leaves in hot water, and find it nourishing and delicious.

A strong brew of the ripe berries steeped in brandy, then a spoon or two of this mixed with honey and added to hot water as a gargle, was the early colonists' effective treatment for a sore throat. Many tribes still use the ripe berries mashed into honey as a cough mixture, a teaspoon taken at a time and held in the mouth so as to trickle gently down the throat.

The ripe fruit mixed with honey has been a traditional medication for chest ailments, postnasal drip, to clear sinuses, tuberculosis, and a constant cough. Interestingly, 1 tablespoon of ripe fruits crushed and mixed into ½ cup of hot water is sipped slowly to treat heart ailments, liver ailments, eye problems and diseases, and it is enjoyed as a general tonic! This pleasant-tasting tea can be taken twice or even three or four times a day if the condition is acute.

Health Note
The berries are high in vitamin C and beta-carotene, and contain several minerals, especially calcium, magnesium, iron, potassium and phosphorus.

Msoba Jam
This jam is delicious on hot buttered toast on a winter's morning; or add a small spoonful to oats porridge as our grandmothers did … or try it on rice pudding with cream.

Simmer gently on very low heat equal quantities of nastergal berries and sugar (or use just a little less sugar, if possible, as the fruit is so very sweet). Stir often and thoroughly and carefully. The secret is *slowly*, as this is what makes it so special. (And as the farmers' wives in the 'Orange Free State' did so long ago – stir in a prayer!) When it thickens and gels – just a drop or two on a cold saucer – it is ready to be poured into hot sterilised bottles with good screw tops. Label and store.

Caution
Be very careful not to eat the green berries, which are highly poisonous. The green berries contain toxic alkaloids and eating a mere 4 or 5 green berries could kill a child. Pick only the fully ripe berries.

Potato

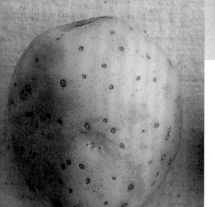

Solanum tuberosum

This outstanding staple vegetable originates from Chile and the Andean region of Bolivia, Ecuador and Peru, where it has been in cultivation for over 7 000 years. Wild species of potato still grow here today and the South Americans had already been cultivating this valuable crop for centuries when Spanish explorers arrived in 1537. Spanish sailors took the potato back to Spain and Portugal and in the mid-16th century Sir Francis Drake is credited for discovering it in Chile and he took it home to England. Sir Walter Raleigh took the potato to Ireland, as its nutritious value was so astounding, and cultivation began in earnest. It was brought into the United States in the early 18th century by Irish immigrants who came to settle in New England after the terrible Irish potato blight and famine of 1846–1850 took about a million lives, changing so profoundly the future of the Irish that emigration began in earnest. By the 19th century the potato was extensively cultivated in many countries and today it is the most popular of all vegetables. And it is a viable crop – for example, 40% of potatoes grown in the United States are sold to fast-food outlets like McDonald's for French fries. Other main producers of potatoes today are China, India, Poland and Russia.

Growing Potatoes

If you've never grown your own potatoes, start now – this is a fun crop and a dish of freshly harvested baby potatoes with their skins on and butter and parsley, is a gourmet treat that nothing surpasses!

Dig a wide and deep trench in full sun and fill it with lots of compost, the older and richer the better. Mix it with a little topsoil and soak it thoroughly. We have a trench always ready for those sprouting potatoes at the back of the vegetable rack that somehow get forgotten. You merely tuck them into the compost, cover them completely and flood the trench with water once a week. The only time the potato does not grow is in the winter months.

When my children were little we made 'potato tyres' by setting three tyres, one on top of the other, and filled the hollow centre with rich soil and compost mix. As the potatoes grew we added another tyre to the heap and topped up with soil. We circled the space between each tyre with a tight plastic band to keep the water in, as you need to top up with a gentle hose every second day. Once the pretty mauve flowers stop and the leaves turn yellow you can dig them up, or for the children's tyre potatoes, just lift off a tyre to expose the treasure within!

Using Potatoes

One of the most useful and delicious of all vegetables, I constantly find new ways of using potatoes. Mashed potatoes with milk or a dash of cream and chopped chives remains a family favourite as does roast potatoes, and baked potatoes with butter. In gluten-free diets, potato flour is used for baking breads, biscuits and also even porridge.

Interestingly, besides being a valuable food the potato has several other uses. It is grown for forage, particularly in Europe, and it is used in the production of alcohol. Polish vodka – famous for its purity – is distilled from potatoes. In Third World countries, potato skins peeled off boiled potatoes are an effective wound dressing where skin grafts are not available. A research study done at a children's hospital in Mumbai, using a dressing made up of sterile potato peelings attached to a sterile gauze bandage, confirmed the excellent healing effect on burns and wounds the potato peel dressings had in keeping the wound clean, with no bacterial infection, less pain for the patient and faster healing!

Health Note

The potato is packed full of goodness: it is rich in vitamin C and several of the B-vitamins, calcium, potassium and iron. It is also a source of lysine, an essential amino acid, as well as valuable dietary fibre.

Potato Bake

Serves 6

This is a favourite dish that Sandy created and it is served in our restaurant constantly.

6 large potatoes
2 cups cream
2 eggs beaten into 1 cup of milk with
*   2 tablespoons flour whisked into it*
sea salt and freshly ground pepper
2 teaspoons crushed coriander seed
2 teaspoons crushed caraway seed
2 teaspoons fresh thyme

Peel the potatoes and boil them (or, if preferred, boil them in their skins). Once soft, drain and cool. Slice and arrange the potatoes in a greased glass baking dish so that the slices overlap. Mix the cream with the milk mixture. Add the rest of the ingredients and mix everything together well. Pour over the potatoes and bake at 180 °C for about 25 minutes, or until the creamy sauce is thick. For a change, sprinkle with grated cheese before putting it in the oven. Serve hot.

Caution

Avoid ageing sprouting potatoes or potatoes with a green colouring as this points to the presence of solanine, a toxic element that can cause poisoning in people.

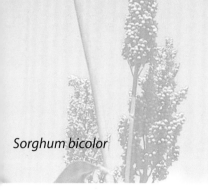

Sorghum

Sorghum bicolor

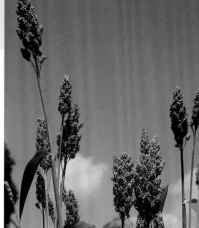

Sorghum is a robust annual grain, indigenous to Africa and grown in Ethiopia as a crop over 5 000 years ago, from where it spread to India and on into Asia over 3 000 years ago. It remains a staple food in several countries and it is the fourth leading grain crop in the world today. So precious was sorghum in the early centuries that it has been found in archaeological sites, in burial chambers and in the earliest writings and paintings. A hugely valuable and popular trade, four varieties of sorghum are cultivated today from those ancient beginnings: grain sorghum grown for grain production, grass sorghum grown for animal silage and feed lots, sweet sorghums which are similar to sugar cane and which are processed into sweet syrup, and broom corn sorghum, a stiff and tough variety which is grown to make broom bristles.

A fascinating 'grass' to grow with its large head of closely packed round 'seeds' or berries which range in colour from dark red to black to grey, bronze, yellow and white, depending on the variety. The white-berried sorghums were developed in Africa and in India, and have been made into 'mabela' porridge and flat breads for centuries. Recently new varieties of sorghum have come onto the market with high levels of wonderfully beneficial phytochemicals, antioxidants and flavonoids for cereals, snack foods and baked foods, and for the nourishing and much-loved traditional beers!

Growing Sorghum

I still grow sorghum not only because I was once a 'farmer' and I grew it for my children's bantams and pigeons and for the wild birds, but because it is so attractive and interesting in our food gardens, and we teach visitors how to grind it and make flat breads and porridges. The kernels or berries can be crushed, flaked, popped, puffed, or added to biscuits, breads, muffins and cakes. We still have the hollow stones which were once used to crush the seeds or 'berries'.

Dig a long trench in full sun, fill it with compost and water well. Sprinkle the seeds sparsely into the trench and cover with more compost. Keep it watered and moist, covered with a thin layer of leaves so as to keep the birds out and watch the sturdy little shoots emerge. Water twice a week. Like a mealie it grows tall quickly, and as the cluster of berries or seeds start to ripen, cover with a paper bag tightly tied on or the birds and the squirrels will completely denude your crop.

Using Sorghum

We grow the white sorghum for our pancake mixes and the red sorghum for popping and for our popular 'bird seed mix' which includes linseed, sunflower seeds, millet seed, sesame seed and sorghum. It is worth investing in a 'stone mill' for grinding your own organically grown sorghum as this spectacular grain is loaded with valuable micronutrients and phytochemicals and phenols that block the onset and the progression of cancers – colon, lung, liver, pancreas and breast cancer. It contains potent antioxidants that protect against these cancers and against cardiovascular disease. The anthocyanins contained in sorghum are strong antioxidants that scavenge the free radicals, especially in lung tissue, and they inhibit tumour growth, reduce cholesterol, and strengthen collagen in the skin and the artery walls.

Sorghum contains no gluten so for those on gluten-free diets this is an excellent treatment for gluten intolerance allergies, coeliac disease, even autism and mood swings and for children with poor eating habits sorghum is extremely important.

Boil the grain like rice and serve it with a hearty stew or add it to vegetable soups, use it as a thickener in sauces and dips, and add ground flour to pancake batter and brownies!

Health Note

Sorghum is a good source of the B-vitamins, in particular thiamine, riboflavin and niacin, as well as calcium, iron, phosphorus and potassium.

Sorghum Hot Pot

Serves 4

This is particularly delicious with grilled fish or chicken.

400 g cooked sorghum (see Hint below for instructions on how to cook sorghum)
a little olive oil
2 large onions, finely chopped
4 large tomatoes, chopped
2 green peppers, finely chopped
2 tablespoons soft brown caramel sugar
1 litre good stock, or water
sea salt and black pepper to taste
juice of 1 lemon

Fry the onions in the oil until golden brown. Add the tomatoes and green pepper and stir-fry briefly. Add the rest of the ingredients. Simmer for about 10–15 minutes, stirring frequently, to allow the flavours to blend and some of the liquid to evaporate. Serve like rice as an accompaniment to meat or fish.

Hint

The different varieties of sorghum have different cooking times. The basic ratio is 1 part sorghum grains to 2 parts water, with a pinch of salt. Cover tightly and simmer very gently for 1 hour, but keep checking and add more water as needed. The grains should be soft and separated, like cooked rice.

Spinach & Swiss Chard

Spinacea oleracea • Beta vulgaris var. cicla

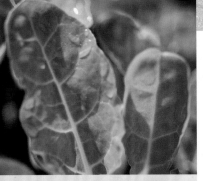

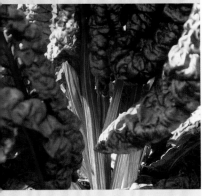

When we say 'spinach' South Africans generally think of 'Swiss chard', which belongs to the same great family – the Chenopodiaceae – as the 'real spinach' or 'baby spinach' does, but Swiss chard is a close relative of beetroot, the leaves of which are also eaten as a spinach. Swiss chard originated from the wild sea-beet, which grew abundantly along the coastal regions of Western Asia and in particular around the Mediterranean area. The ancient Greeks and Romans used it to treat congestion and to neutralise acidity and as a laxative. The flatter, smaller-leafed 'real spinach' originated in southwestern Asia and Persia and has been cultivated by the Chinese for at least 2 000 years! Cultivation in Europe began much later – in the 11th century when the Moors introduced it to Spain – and for some time spinach was known as 'Spanish greens' or 'Spanish vegetable' in Britain. During the Middle Ages both spinaches became popular vegetables and have remained so through the centuries. Today spinach is grown commercially in temperate climates throughout the world.

Growing Spinach

An easy-to-grow annual, both spinach and Swiss chard can be started in seed trays for pricking out once they reach a size that is easy to handle. Plant them out in full sun in a well-dug, richly composted bed, spaced 30–40 cm apart. The softer more tender spinach does best in the cooler months and both can take a fair amount of cold. Both need a good twice weekly watering, the more tender baby spinach even three times a week in very hot weather.

Using Spinach

Spinach was fed to the soldiers, the stone quarry workers and the field workers, and the historical beliefs that it gave energy, health, strength, restored vitality and improved the blood have today been verified by medical science. It is true that spinach contains a lot of iron, and yet spinach is an alkaline food, clearing acidity from the body. Spinach is high in lutein, which is needed for healthy eyesight, and helps to prevent macular degeneration, cataracts and weakening eyesight.

The old adage of 'eat your greens' that parents drummed into their children really was and is good advice: spinach is a superb antioxidant, it protects against cancer, research has identified around 13 different flavonoids and a host of vitamins and minerals (see Health Note), all of which regulate blood pressure, boost the immune system and build bone health. Spinach is a powerful anti-cancer food rich in phytochemicals, valuable for treating colon and digestive tract cancers, and for maintaining bone health – thanks to the vitamin K content which activates osteocalcin, which anchors calcium in the bone.

Easily and quickly cooked – steamed for a few minutes or eaten raw in a salad – spinach and Swiss chard are a vital part of a healthy diet and it should feature often. Even the thick white stems of Swiss chard are delicious quickly chopped and steamed, and served with a dab of butter, a grinding of black pepper and a squeeze of lemon juice. A dish of spinach topped with a poached egg is an old favourite for a light supper dish, and creamed spinach in a cheesy white sauce is an easy way to get spinach into the pickiest of eaters. Or use it in quiches, tarts and phyllo pastry rolls, in salads, in stir-fries and in pastas.

Quick Spinach Stir-Fry

Serves 2

1 large onion, finely chopped
4 cups fresh spinach
little olive oil
½ cup pecan nuts
½ cup sesame seeds
sea salt and black pepper to taste
2 cups chopped and sliced mushrooms
liberal squeeze of lemon juice

Brown the onions in the olive oil, add the mushrooms and stir-fry. Add all the other ingredients and stir-fry quickly. Serve piping hot with crusty bread.

Caution

Swiss chard is high in oxalates – those with a tendency towards kidney stones should avoid Swiss chard.

Health Note

Both spinach and Swiss chard are packed with nutrients, including vitamins A, B, C, E and K, folic acid, beta-carotene, iron, calcium, magnesium, potassium, manganese, phosphorus and zinc.

Stevia
Sweet Herb

Stevia rebaudiana

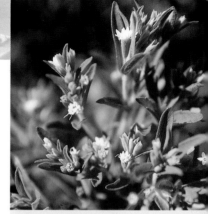

Although stevia is not really a food as such, it is so extraordinary a natural sweetener it needs to find its place within these pages for the role it plays as we search for *natural* sugar-free sweeteners in the daily diet.

A herb of ancient beginnings, it is indigenous to South America, Paraguay in particular, where it is known as the 'sweet herb' or 'honey leaf'. Research on stevia began in 1937 when two French chemists, Bridel and Lavielle, isolated a compound within the leaves that they named 'stevicide'. They found it to be 300 times sweeter than sugar, and in 1941 it was grown in trials in Kew Gardens in England, and was declared safe for sweetening beers and drinks for diabetics, and was immediately put to use, but it became impractical, as the demand grew and importing it was erratic. So it got somewhat lost as cheaper artificial sweeteners were developed. Interestingly, when the Japanese started banning artificial sweeteners 30 years ago, their food industry included stevia as a natural sweetener and favoured it over other sweeteners because of its stability when heated.

Growing Stevia

Stevia needs full sun and compost-rich soil. Propagation is both by seed and thumb-length cuttings. Keep the cuttings moist but not sodden. Seeds are erratic to germinate but tender perennial plants, once established, prove to be quite tough. We plant out well-established plants that have been hardened off in full sun into deeply dug, richly composted soil and plant them 1 m apart as, once it is a couple of years old, the tall flowering sprays can reach 1 m in height, and we find it does not do well crowded together. The tiny white flowers produce feathery seeds that blow away easily if the ripening spray is not covered with a paper bag or picked before the seeds have gone into the wind. Cut the old seed sprays back to the ground to make way for new tufts of leaves in spring. It is completely dormant in winter, and the soft and luscious new little leaves in spring seem extra sweet.

Using Stevia

Harvest the fresh leaves frequently and dry some for winter use. Use them fresh for the best flavour – chopped or added to stewed fruit, custards or porridge while it is cooking. Remember it is 300 times sweeter than sugar, so go slowly! Stevia is heat stable so you can add finely chopped fresh leaves to baked biscuits and muffins and cakes. You can fill a pepper grinder with dried stevia leaves and grind it over your porridge or fruit salad or into your tea.

I boil up stevia leaves in water to make a sweet liquid which I use for drinks, teas and to cook with. Simmer 1 cup of fresh leaves in 2 litres of water for 15–20 minutes with the lid on. Strain and keep it in the fridge, adding a tablespoon to a cup of tea, or use the water to cook porridge with or to stew fruit in. Or add freshly squeezed lemon juice and lemon slices to the chilled liquid for a refreshing lemonade.

Stevia is a safe sweetener for diabetics, but discuss it with your doctor and in no way replace the medication you are currently on without your doctor's advice. Modern research has found that stevia has beneficial effects on high blood pressure, high blood sugar levels and blood cholesterol levels. Stevia is used in toothpastes and mouthwashes where it helps to tighten up the gums, soothes and clears bleeding gums, and eases sore throats and fever blisters, as it is a natural antibacterial!

It is thought to have a strengthening effect on the heart and the whole cardiovascular system, and just a cup of stevia tea, hot or cold, a couple of times a week will surprise you so pleasantly with its beneficial effects you'll be as excited as I am about this truly extraordinary plant.

Stevia Spice Cake

⅓ cup sunflower cooking oil
1 tablespoon finely chopped fresh stevia leaves
2 eggs (jumbo size and free range)
½ cup plain Bulgarian yoghurt
½ cup milk or soya milk
1 cup apple sauce (see instructions below)
¾ cup Nutty Wheat flour
¾ cup cake flour
2 teaspoons baking powder
1 teaspoon cinnamon powder
1 teaspoon allspice powder
pinch of salt

To make the apple sauce: Peel and thinly slice 6 apples, boil up in a heavy bottomed pot with 1 tablespoon of honey and 1½ cups of water. Simmer gently until tender and mash well.

Preheat the oven to 180°C. Oil a cake pan with a loose bottom. Beat the oil, apple sauce and the stevia leaves until well mixed. Add in the eggs, one by one, and beat until fluffy. Now add the milk to the yoghurt, beat well and add to the mixture. Sift the two flours and the baking powder and salt together with the spices. Stir into the wet ingredients and mix gently until well blended. Pour into the cake pan and bake until cooked through and golden brown, about 35–40 minutes. Test by gently pressing on it – it should feel springy. Cool on a wire rack. Serve with extra apple sauce, whipped cream and a dusting of ground cinnamon.

Rose Apple
Jambos ▪ Malabar Plum *Syzygium jambos*

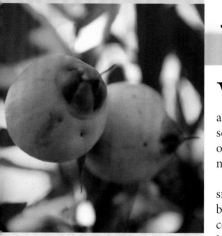

Visitors to our gardens are amazed at our big trees of rose apples, hanging in clusters, pale, creamy yellow with the texture of an apple, crisp and juicy and sweet, and yet the unmistakable fragrance and taste of the rose! A large evergreen tree that can reach well over 10 metres in height, with honey-scented, creamy white, powder-puff flowers borne on the tips of the branches in clusters, the jambos or rose apple is indigenous to Southeast Asia and India, where it is a much-loved delicacy sold in the markets in bunches.

Grown for centuries in its native India as a popular fruit and traded and sold in street markets as a snack for travellers, it has remained a favourite. A distilled 'brandy' or wine made from the fruits has been taken as a medicinal wine to ease rheumatism and arthritis, and with honey and mint to soothe coughs, colds and bronchitis in its native India and Asia. The name *jambu* is of Sanskrit origin and in Malaysia and Indonesia can be applied to different fruits, but the true rose apple is also known as the 'Malabar plum' and has been cultivated for centuries in plantations for the making of jams and jellies, 'sweetmeats' and syrups, so valuable it is used in religious ceremonies and thanksgiving festivals.

Growing the Rose Apple

Propagation is quick and easy from the pip merely pushed into a bag of compost and kept moist. It can be planted out when it is about 30 cm high and it needs a large, deep hole filled with compost in full sun and into which a wide pipe about 1 m in length is pushed at an angle to allow a hose to be inserted so that water, once a week, can be funnelled down into the roots.

It grows quickly and easily. It makes a good shade tree and its long shiny leathery leaves and powder puff multi-stemmed flowers are a perennial delight. It only fruits on the tips of the branches, so keep pruning and clipping to a minimum. Give it a barrow of compost twice yearly and a good long weekly watering and you'll reap basketsful of the delicious rose apples as a reward!

Using Rose Apple

In ancient days ripe thinly sliced rose apples were preserved in honey with lemon rind and thinly sliced ginger for coughs, colds, bronchitis, 'flu, sore throats and for ear infections. Made by the elders of the village this was one of the first 'medicines' available in rural India and Asia. I am always intrigued by the ancient uses – how did they know that the rose apple has so high a vitamin C content that it could boost the immune system? And combined with lemon, honey and ginger makes the perfect medication for the coughs and colds and 'flu's that have plagued mankind?

Eating the crisp pale yellow fruits – they reach about the size of a litchi – when fully ripe, is an experience. You need to watch them carefully, as overripe fruit will buzz with fruit flies. The fruit ripens midsummer and can be made into a delicious pie filling cooked with apples, or into syrups and jams with other fruits like pears, apples, melons, peaches, pineapples. Cooked up finely and sieved with red rose petals (we use Crimson Glory) and a little sugar and fresh sliced ginger, we make an exciting jelly-like jam that is divine on toast or served with cheese on scones. In the cooking the rose apple retains its shape and crispness. It is so versatile you'll be able to add it to your favourite jam and apple recipes with success. Add finely chopped rose apples to fruit salads, custards and to stir-fries the way the Malaysians do, and cook it in coconut milk for curries.

Health Note

Rose apples are rich in vitamins A, C and E, as well as calcium, phosphorus, potassium and magnesium.

Creamy Rose Apple and Pear Dessert

Serves 4

12–16 thinly sliced rose apples, pips removed

6 large pears, peeled, cored and sliced

2–3 cups water (just enough to cover the fruit)

½–¾ cup honey

6 cloves

1 tablespoon finely chopped fresh stevia leaves

¼ cup sesame seeds

1 cup whipped cream

ground cinnamon

In a heavy bottomed pan, simmer the sliced fruit in the water. Add the honey, cloves, stevia and sesame seeds and simmer gently, stirring often, until the fruit is tender. This will take about 10–15 minutes. The rose apple will remain slightly crisp. Mash the pears lightly with a fork, and with a slotted spoon, remove the fruit and place in a glass bowl, draining off any water. Let it stand to cool and then lightly fold in the whipped cream. Sprinkle with cinnamon just before serving.

Hint

The rose apple makes a tall and thick hedge that takes clipping easily, and the bonus is the fruit! Planted 2 m apart and kept pruned, this makes a stunning feature in the garden.

Tamarind
Indian Date

Tamarindus indica

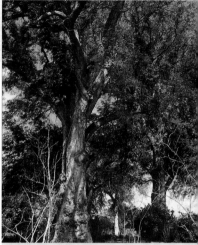

The tamarind is an exquisite evergreen tree that reaches 25 m in height, with fine, compound leaves and yellow and orange flowers that turn into long, bean-like fruits. An ancient tree, it is thought to be native to tropical North Africa, from where it spread via the trade routes to India and Asia. The Arabs took the seeds from India to Europe and from there to tropical America. The name 'tamarind' comes from the Arabic word *tamar*, which means date, and the Indian word *hindi*, which means from India – so 'Indian date' is the name it is still known by today.

Many centuries ago it was taken as a trade to Malaysia and Indonesia where it has formed a part of the culture and the diet, and all parts of the tree are still used today for food and medicine following ancient traditions. In many parts of the world the tamarind is a tree of ceremony and thanksgiving, and in many countries it is believed that chopping down a tamarind invites bad luck!

Growing the Tamarind

Propagation is from ripe seed and it is slow but it is steady. Start them off in deep, compost-filled bags and never let them dry out and keep them protected and shaded. In tropical areas propagation is by grafting or layering or by cuttings of growing tips. Once the little seedling is over 40 cm in height, plant out in full sun in an extra large, compost-filled hole. Give it a lot of space as it grows into a huge spreading tree! Water deeply twice weekly and protect in winter. It is a tropical tree so it will not survive temperatures lower than 10 °C.

Using the Tamarind

The uses are ancient and much respected, handed down from generation to generation. It has become so integral a part of traditional dishes that keeping tamarind in the store cupboard is vital. The pods can be preserved in syrup, in sugar or in a savoury paste or kept dried in a glass jar for long periods. Ripe tamarind pods are made into chutneys, spreads, syrupy desserts and confectionery, and whole industries are devoted to tamarind products. Picked ripe from the tree, the pod, finely chopped, seeds and stalks and outer shell removed, are used as sour seasoning for meat and bean and fish dishes, or they can be cooked with apples or quinces or mangos and mashed into a chutney or jam. A mere teaspoon of this paste will enhance any dish.

Children in India and Malaysia push the mature but not fully ripe pods which they call swells, into the hot coals to bake. The seeds bubble and froth and are raked out of the fire, carefully cooled, peeled and eaten with salt as a snack. Street vendors sell 'swells' at the markets.

Fresh and dried fruits, thinly sliced, can be made into a delicious 'lemonade', boiled up with sugar and diluted with crushed ice and water. In some countries the creamy yellow, red-veined clusters of flowers and the young new leaves are fried in olive oil mixed with sunflower oil as a snack or served on top of soups, stews and stir-fries, and pancakes drenched in tamarind syrup are served on religious holidays and celebrations.

Medicinally tamarind tea (see recipe alongside) or syrup has been taken to bring down fevers, to treat catarrh, jaundice, liver ailments, nausea, morning sickness during the first months of pregnancy, and for asthma, dysentery and as a gentle laxative tamarind is a valuable medicine. Tamarind contains a complex volatile oil that shows traces of limonene, geraniol, safrole, cinnamaldehyde, menthol and methyl salicylate (wintergreen). It is a tonic herb, an anti-ager, it lowers fevers, eases and improves the whole digestion, it is a safe and gentle laxative and it has strong antiseptic properties!

Health Note

Tamarind contains some B-vitamins and also vitamins C and A, as well as a high amount of calcium, phosphorus and iron.

Tamarind Tea

This tea is taken for a host of ailments (see main text) and ½ a cup can be taken at intervals through the day.

Take 1–2 teaspoons tamarind pulp or 2–3 slices of ripe peeled pod, and pour over this 1 cup of boiling water, stand 5 minutes, stir well and sip slowly ½ a cup at a time. Sometimes a fresh leaf is added to the brew. Add a little honey, if liked.

Tamarind Paste

This gives a rich and exotic flavour to savoury dishes.

Remove the outer shell of the pod and finely chop the flesh, removing and discarding the seeds. You need enough to fill 2 cups. Add 2 tablespoons of honey and mix well. Now add 2 tablespoons of chopped fresh ginger, 2 teaspoons crushed coriander seed and 1 teaspoon crushed allspice berries and mix well. Spoon into a screw-top jar. Add 2–3 teaspoons of the paste to meat dishes, chicken dishes or to vegetarian stir-fries.

Dandelion

Taraxacum officinale

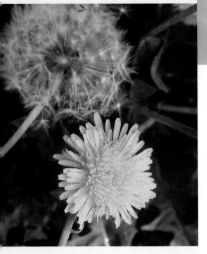

Perhaps the dandelion is the world's commonest and best-known weed! It has a worldwide distribution – usually an unwanted, tenacious and tough survivor weed, but nevertheless a most valuable and quite amazing medicinal and food plant. A hardy perennial, it originated in Europe mainly but was originally found in all temperate areas of the Northern Hemisphere.

Dandelion is part of history, part of legend. Theseus ate a dandelion salad after killing the Minotaur, and the Roman armies ate dandelion daily to give them vigour and strength, as did the Gauls and the Anglo-Saxon tribes, and the sea explorers took the roots and dried leaves on their voyages to treat scurvy. The first writings of its virtues and wonders were recorded around 980 BC and many monastery gardens all over Europe grew it in the early centuries to treat the sick, believing that a leaf shaped like the tooth of the lion – *dent de lion* – had enormous health-building and disease-fighting powers! In the early centuries it was taken mainly as a medicine for its diuretic, cleansing effects, and was taken to treat liver, kidney and bladder ailments, as well as any number of other common ailments – coughs, colds, skin ailments and even falling hair! By the 18th century it became a food, and less bitter varieties gradually were grown for their salad leaves and their root, which was roasted, ground and made into a delicious drink – dandelion coffee! Dandelion wine, dandelion sherry and even dandelion stout became such popular beverages that dandelion fields were planted, and a brisk trade was done with the biggest, most tender and least bitter leaves. I like to think that the huge and beautiful dandelion plants we grow for salads at the Herbal Centre today from the seed I imported from Europe 40 years ago came from those dandelion fields grown in the 18th century in England's green and pleasant farmland!

Growing Dandelion

Nothing is easier – it comes up everywhere! But I urge every gardener to root out the common small lawn invaders and search for the big succulent and beautiful often 30 cm high plants that have evolved from those bitter and really unpalatable beginnings. Sow the seed in trays and transplant when big enough to handle into bags to establish well before planting out into the garden. Plant out in full sun in well-composted, moist soil and flood with water once a week. Seedlings that come up all over the garden transplant well when they are small (it has a long tap root).

Using Dandelion

Dandelion is quite a miraculous plant for its incredibly high vitamin and mineral content (see Health Note) and is one of the most vital body 'toners'. It is thought that the digestive tonic properties it possesses are due to its taraxacin content, which has intestinal antiseptic and antibacterial effects. Perhaps the best liver cleanser known, it promotes the flow of bile and improves liver function, like congestion of the liver, hepatitis and jaundice, as well as gallstones – it has a direct effect on the gall bladder. Used as a weight loss treatment due to its diuretic ability, the French call it *pissenlit* – wetting the bed!

Dandelion root contains up to 40% of inulin, an indigestible carbohydrate that is a food source for the friendly digestive bacteria *Bifidobacterium* and *Lactobacillus*, which act like a natural protective antibiotic within the colon and normalise the intestinal flora, especially after taking antibiotics. Inulin also regulates and improves blood sugar control and diabetes, and raises the beneficial HDL cholesterol within the blood. The benefits of eating fresh dandelion greens are huge and vital to building health.

Health Note
Dandelion is rich in vitamins A, B6 and C particularly, as well as copper, magnesium, manganese and iron.

Dandelion Salad

Serves 4

4 cups of dandelion leaves
1 small butter lettuce
2 cups cucumber slices
2 cups chopped green peppers
2 cups croutons fried in a little olive oil
juice of 1 lemon
1 cup feta cheese, cut into small cubes
sea salt and black pepper to taste

Mix all the salad greens in a bowl, and top with the croutons and feta cubes. Squeeze over the lemon juice and season with salt and pepper. Serve chilled.

Hint

Dandelion root makes a delicious coffee with many health-giving properties. See page 231 for instructions on how to process the root for coffee. And dandelion is good for teeth, bones and nails!

Cacao Tree
Cocoa Tree

Theobroma cacao

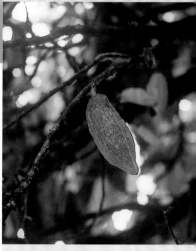

This fabulous 'food' needs to find a place in this book! Chocolate is produced from the beans of the cacao tree, named *Theobroma cacao* by Linnaeus in the early centuries. It is believed to originate in the Amazon basin in Brazil, although some say it comes from the Orinoco Valley of Venezuela, and others believe it originates in Central America. Wherever it comes from, history indicates the Mayans and the Aztecs enjoyed this precious cacao bean over 5 000 years ago! Cacao pods were carved as a symbol of life on ancient stone temples, and used in rituals and ceremonies literally as 'food for the gods'. By the 6th century BC the Aztecs were making a drink from the nourishing seeds they called 'xocoatl' – spicy, bitter and rich – and since sweeteners were still unknown, they flavoured it with chillies and 'corn meal' made from the first mealies ever grown, and this potent brew was considered to be a valuable health elixir. By 1200 BC the Aztecs conquered the Mayans and used their *xocoatl* recipe, which the Aztecs called 'shocolatle', and so valuable was this drink, that the Aztec Emperor Montezuma drank it from golden goblets, considering it to be more valuable than the golden goblet itself, and so the cacao bean became currency. The Emperor became so addicted to it he was probably the first chocoholic!

Columbus in 1502 was the first explorer to come in contact with the cacao tree, and from then on it became known in the New World. The Spaniards in 1519, led by Hernando Cortes, murdered Emperor Montezuma and presented the cacao beans to King Carlos of Spain, stating that the drink helped to build up resistance and fought fatigue. Sugar, spices and wine were added for the Court of Spain, and cacao plantations were begun. Cacao drinks became popular in Europe long before tea and coffee, and cacao powder and slabs of chocolate later appeared on the scene and the rest, as they say, is history!

Growing the Cacao Tree

A true rainforest tree, the cacao needs high humidity, high temperatures never going below 24°C, and a constantly high rainfall. It the rich forest soil some trees can live for more than 200 years, but usually after 25 years its fruit production starts to decline. Cacao plantations usually grow two or three varieties, the commonest being 'Forastero' which gives around 90% of the world's cacao crop.

One mature tree produces around 15 to 30 oval pods per year. From each pinkish-red pod are scooped out around 20–30 cream-coloured beans. After a period of fermentation, the beans are carefully roasted, then cooled and their thin brittle outer shells broken away. The kernels, called nibs, consist of around 45–50% pure cacao butter and are the basic chocolate ingredient.

Using Cacao

The health benefits of chocolate come from the flavonoids, the proanthocyanidins, which are similar to those found in red apples, cherries and red grapes. Medical research has found dark bitter chocolate benefits cardiovascular disease – the saturated fats found in dark chocolate do not elevate cholesterol levels, and the antioxidants in it help to keep the arteries clear of cholesterol 'clumping'. Dark chocolate contains the amino acid arginine, which helps nitric oxide to dilate the arteries and which helps to prevent the platelets aggregating. Research also confirms the ancient belief that chocolate is a mood-lifter, an antidepressant and even possibly an aphrodisiac!

Health Note

Cocoa beans are rich in essential minerals, including magnesium, calcium, iron, zinc, copper, potassium and manganese and also contain vitamins A, B1, B2, B3, B5, C and E.

Chocolate and Banana Smoothie

Serves 1

Chocolate nibs or the fine powdered nibs in their raw state (without the milk solids and the sugar, which make it addictive) are health boosting and can be added to desserts, drinks and smoothies for that wondrous get-up-and-go feeling!

1 cup plain Bulgarian yoghurt
1 banana
1 tablespoon pure chocolate nibs
1 tablespoon sunflower seeds
1 tablespoon chopped almonds
1 teaspoon raw honey
1 peeled, quartered and cored apple (crisp red apples are best when you can find them)

Whirl everything together in a liquidiser, drink it down and watch your speed!

Hint

The raw cacao beans before being roasted are an almost perfect food with incredibly high levels of antioxidants, minerals, natural proteins, trace elements, enzymes and vitamins, and can be sprouted as one of the most precious health-boosting foods known to mankind, or they can be ground up into a drink – should you be lucky enough to find them!

Fenugreek

Trigonella foenum-graecum

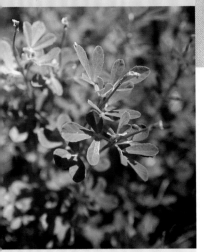

Spicy Curry Mix

This can be changed and adapted and it is simply delicious! Crush a little at a time in a mortar with a pestle to really grind down the seeds.

½ cup fenugreek seeds
½ cup coriander seeds
½ cup cumin seeds
1½ tablespoons paprika powder
1 tablespoon turmeric powder
½ tablespoon cayenne pepper
1 tablespoon crushed dried chilli (with
  the seeds if you want it hot)
1 tablespoon powdered ginger
1 tablespoon mustard seeds

Mix together very well. Be careful not to inhale over it – it's hot! Store in a screw-top glass jar. Crush in a mortar and add a teaspoon at a time to soups, stews, savoury dishes, tasting as you go.

Caution

Fenugreek seeds induce childbirth so do not eat them if you are pregnant. Also, do not eat the fresh leaves, for they too may have an effect upon the uterus.

One of the oldest foods and medicinal plants used by the ancient Assyrians and indigenous to the Mediterranean area and North Africa, the prolific annual fenugreek has a long history. Seeds have been found in Egypt at Tutankhamen's gravesite dating back to 1325 BC – so valuable was this plant that in the afterlife it too had its place. A favourite with both the Egyptians and the Arabs, fenugreek was not only an important food, but the roasted seeds made a nutritious and tasty coffee which is still a favourite drink today. An Egyptian papyrus dating from 1500 BC records medical uses of fenugreek and showed that it was important for inducing childbirth, as a wound and burn dressing and as a quick-acting digestive. Dioscorides in the 1st century AD recommended eating fenugreek leaves and seeds for all gynaecological ailments and Hippocrates in the 5th century recommended it for treating inflammations, dyspepsia and ulcers. Fenugreek has been around a long time and it has never lost its popularity!

Growing Fenugreek

A quick, easily germinating annual crop, the pungent oddly shaped seeds can be sown throughout the year except in the coldest months. For a continuous supply, sow every 3–4 weeks. Sow the seeds where they will thrive in the sun, in richly composted, well-dug soil in narrow drills that are shaped with the end of a rake so that they can be kept moist. Cover with a little soil and a light layer of raked up leaves and sprigs to shade the row.

Seedlings can be pulled up and added to salads at any stage, and for a quick crop of sprouts the seeds can be sprouted on wet cotton wool on a sunny windowsill at any time of the year, even during the cold months. Fenugreek is also an excellent green manure crop dug back into the soil, and the seeds self-sow easily, so it is an economically viable crop to grow.

Using Fenugreek

For centuries it has formed part of Indian, Egyptian, Ethiopian and Arab cookery. The protein-rich seeds are cooked the same way as lentils, the salt added at the end of the cooking time. In several countries ground, mashed and sieved fenugreek seed is used to feed babies as a milk substitute, and fenugreek flour is cooked with sugar and oil to make a nourishing pancake-like dish for women while breastfeeding to increase breast-milk production.

All parts of the plant are used – the leaves are rich in minerals and vitamins, as are the nondescript pale flowers, and even the young soft green pods. These are all added to salads, sauces, stir-fries, soups and marinades. Old recipes suggest that this acts as a tonic to the whole body.

Once the seeds have ripened they can be rubbed in the hands to release them from the pods and stored in glass jars. Fenugreek is now being tested as it may have anti-diabetic properties, as well as the ability to lower blood cholesterol levels. A warmed paste of cooked fenugreek seeds makes an excellent poultice over abscesses, boils, rashes, ulcers and suppurating sores and infected insect bites.

A tea made of 1 teaspoon of fenugreek seeds in 1 cup of boiling water, stand 5 minutes then strain and sip slowly, is excellent for period pains, stomach upsets, fevers, diarrhoea and importantly for anorexia. The seeds are so nourishing they help to stabilise and encourage weight gain.

Chewing a couple of fenugreek seeds will sweeten the breath and seeds added to coarse sea salt in the bath clear the skin of greasiness and help to soften and clear cellulite, if tied in a cloth and soaked in warm water and gently massaged over the area. Use ½ cup of fenugreek seeds to 1 cup of sea salt.

Health Note

Fenugreek seeds are a good source of iron and also contain B-vitamins, magnesium, copper and manganese.

Wheat

Triticum aestivum

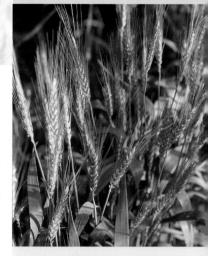

An ancient, precious grain, wheat originated in the Middle East as a wild grass and was used as a food over 28000 years BC – one of mankind's most ancient and valuable foods that has remained part of the world's staple diet for so many centuries its very beginnings are shrouded in mystery. By around 7000 BC domesticated grains appeared, cultivated in the Fertile Crescent in southwestern Asia and then in Egypt. Two varieties, emmer wheat (*Triticum turgidum*) and einkorn wheat (*Triticum monococcum*), were first planted over and over again, and the wheat we know today started its life in Egypt, then in Turkey and Mesopotamia and parts of Iran during 7000 to 5000 BC, with constant selection of the best quality. From there it spread into Asia, Europe and China. A decisive factor in the development of civilisation, wheat has remained the most precious food in the world with over 22% of arable land throughout the world devoted to this 'king of grains'.

Growing Wheat

The secret of successful wheat growing is to dig or plough a field with as much compost as you can find. Wheat needs full sun, rich, loose soil and a thorough weekly soaking. Wheat is a winter annual, so sow the seeds in autumn before the first frosts.

The fast pace and the increased stress of daily life as we know it today, opened the door to the value of wheat grass juice. I grow winter wheat in every space I can and reap the 10–15 cm high succulent shoots for my now famous wheat grass juice, but I also grow it all through the year in special windowsill troughs and trays. This is how you do it: Fill a trough or a deep tray with moist compost. Sprinkle the wheat seeds in it (do the same with barley seeds), cover lightly with compost and water well. Do not let it dry out and keep it in the light, but not in full sun. Within a few days the first pale sprouts appear. Move it into the sun and keep it watered every day. Once it reaches 10–12 cm in height you can cut it off with scissors and push it through a juice extractor with a centrifugal action – it is that spiral twist that gets every drop of the potent and amazing juice out. I find the wheat grass continues to grow for another cutting, and I have several troughs and trays that I sow every 2 or 3 days so that I have a continuous supply.

Using Wheat

Around 1977 I learned of 'wheat berry sprouting' and I began my sprouting career in earnest, much to the consternation of all my friends! I learned early on that the sweetness of just sprouted wheat gave energy and vitality, but only years later did I discover the wonders of wheat grass. Rich in antioxidants, vitamins, minerals and enzymes, chlorophyll and carotenoids, proteins and peptides – wheat grass is a complete life-sustaining food. A mere tot of wheat grass juice a day will repair the DNA; rebuild the blood and increase the production of haemoglobin; alkalise the blood, removing acidity; neutralise toxins and eliminate parasites; cleanse an overloaded liver and the colon; chelate out heavy metals; heal wounds, grazes, scratches and infections; and stimulate enzyme activity, literally rejuvenating and revitalising the entire body.

Fibre-rich sprouted wheat, whole wheat and cracked wheat will reduce the incidence of colon cancer and breast cancer, promote regular bowel function and build energy. But beware of white flour. This has been so refined, all the goodness has been removed from it. No wonder so many people are gluten intolerant, but organically grown, stone-ground brown flours are health boosting and wheat grass has got to be nature's finest and most dynamic medicine. Don't delay – grow it today!

- -

Health Note

The wheat seed or 'berry' contains vitamins B1, B2, B5, B6, E and folic acid, calcium, magnesium, iron, copper, phosphorus, zinc and manganese.

Wheat Grass Energy Drink

Serves 1–2

This *really* gives you wings! I think it is my favourite energy booster of all time and as a mid-afternoon booster, especially in the heat, it literally makes you dance!

3 cups fresh wheat grass
1–2 organically grown carrots, peeled
2 small organically grown beetroots
1 stick celery with leaves
1 handful fresh parsley
1 cupful of fresh lucerne sprigs
1 large apple, peeled and quartered

Push everything through the juice extractor and sip slowly.

Hint

Planted in trays or pots, wheat grass needs sun to keep it from becoming mildewed. So, once it has sprouted, bring it out in the sun and keep it moist. The sun also helps the chlorophyll to develop, and a vibrant crop of brilliant green and healthy wheat grass is the result, just awaiting the juicing process!

Blueberry

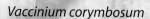

Vaccinium corymbosum

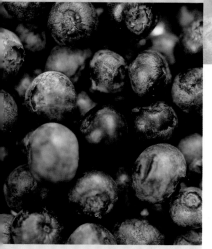

The relatively recently introduced blueberry is becoming more and more available, and it is fast gaining popularity worldwide. Indigenous to mainly the eastern parts of the United States and Canada, where it grows in acid soils, blueberry farming has been attempted in several countries and highbush blueberries, a cultivar derived from *Vaccinium corymbosum*, are now being grown on a fairly large scale in Australia, New Zealand and at last, on a smaller scale, in South Africa.

The *Vaccinium* genus consists of some 450 species of evergreen often berry-bearing shrubs – the cranberry included – and several have been used for centuries by the Native Americans as superb medicines. How did those early healers know that blueberries, with their high levels of anthocyanosides, have extraordinary and potent antioxidant effects? The blueberry today is considered to be one of the most important health foods, and how lucky we are to find them fresh at certain times of the year at specialist greengrocers and in the freezer departments at the supermarket. Look out for South African blueberries that have been grown in the acid soil along the southern slopes of the Simonsberg near Stellenbosch, and in the cooler Sabie area in Mpumalanga.

Growing Blueberries

Blueberries are cultivated from cuttings or tissue culture (the Highbush blueberry does well in South Africa) but the requirements of this somewhat tricky plant need to be thoroughly understood first.

The first requirement is acid soil, and they do not tolerate too much heat and drought – be guided by your local agricultural experts before starting out. To my intense disappointment my own plantings have succumbed to the searing summers we have been experiencing, and the long periods of rain scarcity. So temperate, cool mountain breezes and steady rainfall periods will ensure a crop.

Using Blueberries

Ancient folklore remedies for blueberries abound, and they were used for treating diarrhoea, poor circulation, menstrual disorders, poor skin conditions, constipation, anaemia, inflammatory conditions and even dysentery. Later, medical science proved that blueberries help to unblock blood vessels, even in the eye, so helping to prevent macular degeneration, and can combat diarrhoea and even kill infectious viruses.

'Blueberry Soup', a hot blueberry drink, is served on the European and Canadian ski slopes as a cold remedy, and in Quebec crushed blueberries have been taken for diarrhoea for many decades, and it is still the most popular treatment today!

Blueberries have antiviral and antibacterial compounds, and the blueberry, along with Europe's blackcurrant, are the two fruits that contain the highest levels of anthocyanosides, which have proved lethal to several types of bacteria, even *E. coli*, often the cause of infections, diarrhoea and urinary tract infections.

Latest medical research shows that blueberries counteract some of the ill effects of atherosclerosis brought on by a high-cholesterol diet, and the natural chemicals in blueberries treat hardening of the arteries effectively, as well as varicose veins and haemorrhoids, and improve blood flow to the skin, eyes and nervous system, and so help to prevent microcirculatory deterioration, slowing down ageing, both mental and physical. The blueberry is important – let's get to know it and eat it often!

Health Note

Blueberries are rich in vitamins C and K particularly, vitamins E and A, beta-carotene, as well as calcium, manganese and phosphorus.

Blueberry Muffins

Makes 12

These are our quick and easy favourites.

2 cups Nutty Wheat flour
4 teaspoons baking powder
1 large egg
1 cup full-cream milk
¼ cup honey
½ cup sunflower oil
1 cup of blueberries

Place the flour and baking powder in a mixing bowl. Beat the egg with the milk and honey and sunflower oil. Add the blueberries to the flour mix and mix lightly. Then add the liquid and mix lightly. Spoon into greased muffin tins, only two-thirds full, and bake at 180 °C for about 20 minutes. Serve warm.

Hint

Eating blueberries fresh is best, but they are often not available and frozen blueberries are the only ones we can find. Just before eating, let the berries defrost slowly at room temperature. Then rinse briefly under the cold-water tap to wash away some of the ice, before serving with plain Bulgarian yoghurt.

Cranberry

Vaccinium macrocarpon

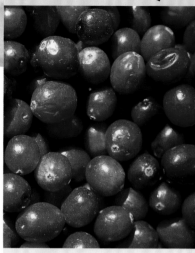

Although the cranberry, a creeping perennial, grows nowhere else easily except in sandy, marshy areas of Northern Asia, North America and parts of Canada, and it does not adapt to any other places in the world, it is so important as a health-boosting food that it finds its way into this book. It is one of the most precious berries known to mankind, but remained as a purely wild-harvested American fruit for centuries, until towards the end of the 20th century when it literally exploded onto the health food scene.

The North American cranberry has a fabulous history! Native Americans used it as both food and medicine. Commercially, its journey began with the first cranberry vines (it needs marshy conditions) planted in Cape Cod in 1816. By 1820 the War Veteran Henry Hall was shipping his cranberries to New York City and Boston. Favoured by millions for the refreshing taste, soon all Massachusetts had cranberry growers and the industry was in full swing. Many other countries have tried to create cranberry bog plantings but the bulk and the best remains in America. Around 154 thousand metric tons of fresh cranberries are harvested annually. Massachusetts still reaps half of that vast amount.

Growing Cranberries

Grown close to the sea in marshes that have specific tidal sands, the cranberry has proved to be a difficult crop for those who do not have the perfect conditions. Luckily the rest of the world is able to import dried cranberries, and at times, if you're very lucky, fresh ones, but at a price.

Using Cranberries

Cranberries have been eaten to treat and prevent urinary tract infections and genital herpes, and will assist in building good heart-protective HDL cholesterol. An American university ran a comprehensive study on women who struggled with constant cystitis attacks and gave them 1 small glass of cranberry juice daily and found those who had the juice had 42% fewer infections than those who did not take it. Several other studies have verified this, some getting over 50% fewer infections.

Cranberries have also been found to protect against *E. coli* infections, and for kidney stone prevention cranberries are proving formidable. They contain an acid, quinic acid, which is not metabolised by the body, so it is merely flushed out in the urine unchanged. This then increases the acidity in the urine so that insoluble calcium and phosphate ions are prevented from forming.

Another astonishing fact is that cranberries contain five times the antioxidant content of broccoli due to the high concentration of anthocyanidins in them. These anthocyanidins inhibit the development of heart disease, cancer and other serious diseases. The deep red colour pigment of the fruit indicates the presence of these anthocyanidins, so eating cranberries fresh or drinking cranberry juice in unsweetened fruit drinks, would be the ideal way to consume this exceptional fruit.

Dried vacuum-packed cranberries can be bought at health counters, and if kept in sealed jars maintain their chewy texture for a long time. Buy cranberries whenever you see them and serve them in snack bowls with almonds or walnuts or pecan nuts. Children love chewing dried cranberries mixed with sun-dried sultanas, and this makes a healthy lunch box snack.

Health Note

Cranberries are rich in potassium, manganese, beta-carotene, copper, iron, zinc and vitamin C, and contain so high a level of phenols they far outclass any other fruit.

Cranberries on Ice

Cranberries are tart and are best added to apple or pear juice.

In your liquidiser blend a cup of dried cranberries that has been soaked in a cup of unsweetened apple juice or pear or even peach juice overnight. Whirl briskly and if it is very sour add a touch of honey, but usually it is delicious served chilled over crushed ice unsweetened.

Caution

If you are on Warfarin do not eat a lot of cranberries, as they are known to enhance the effect of Warfarin. Cranberries also contain low levels of oxalate, which may increase the risk of kidney stones in susceptible people. Always talk to your doctor first before beginning a home treatment, especially if you suffer from kidney stones!

Grape

Vitis vinifera

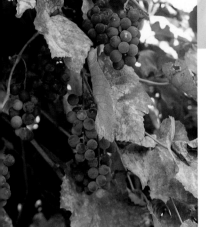

One of the most ancient, most treasured of all fruits known to mankind, the grape is thought to have originated in the Caucasus and parts of Asia. It is also found growing wild in southern Europe and North Africa. There is a slip skin grape (*Vitis labrusca*) indigenous to North America, and the well-loved cultivated black 'Concorde' grapes so popular today in America come from this original species. Now it is estimated that there are around 10 000 varieties of the original *Vitis vinifera* grown for both eating and wine making, but the medicinal value is all but forgotten. In ancient times the grape harvest was extremely valuable as a medicine and as sugar syrups, made by boiling down grape must, which is fresh unfermented grape juice. Grape syrup is still made today in the Levant where it is known as 'dibs'. Verjuice, which is the juice of unripe grapes, was used as a souring agent in European cookery and was used in great quantity until vinegar became more popular.

The first recordings of wine making were made in Mesopotamia and Egypt 3000 BC, where it was used in religious ceremonies, in temples and in sacrificial ceremonies. During this time the Chinese were making wine from grapes grown on rootstock that went back before the Ice Age. In Europe, the Greeks and Romans made wine and introduced it into Britain in AD 10, and the Roman monasteries continued to cultivate the precious vines even after the fall of the Roman Empire. Today many countries are producing superb wines. South Africa, too, holds a marvellous and outstanding collection, and our table grapes, introduced by the Dutch to the Cape of Good Hope in 1655, rank amongst the best in the world.

Growing Grapes

No garden should be without a vine or two. Grow your grapevines in deep, compost-filled holes in full sun spaced 1 m apart. Flood the vines with water twice a week, and train the branches up a pergola or over an arch. Prune and tidy the vines in winter and add a barrow of compost to each vine.

Using Grapes

The tendrils, the vine tips and the leaves were used in ancient times to relieve conditions associated with excessive heat, chronic congestion, toxicity, 'liverishness', overloaded liver, excessive obesity and sluggish metabolism. Resveratrol, a flavonoid found in grape skins, has anti-cancer properties, and grape seeds contain active phenols that are excellent antioxidants. The stems yield drops of liquid which can be diluted with sterile water as an eye wash for red, tired, inflamed eyes.

The benefits of drinking a glass of red wine a day for maintaining cardiovascular health have been well documented, and today researchers find taking grape seed oil, or chewing grape seeds, is beneficial for retarding the ageing process. Eat fresh grapes for varicose veins, heavy and uneven menstruation, for hypertension, poor circulation, high cholesterol, bladder and kidney ailments, menopause (fresh grape juice is excellent for hot flushes), as a diuretic, for reducing inflammation and to clear toxins, and for their anti-cancer properties.

The grape has to be one of the most versatile and valuable crops to grow. The fruits are used to make wines, juices, sherry, liqueurs, vinegars and spirits. The dried fruits make energy-giving and sugar-rich raisins and sultanas, and the seeds yield a superb polyunsaturated oil for both beauty and cooking. Use chopped tendrils in salads and young leaves in teas and in stir-fries, and crush the seeds with coriander and black peppercorns and eat sprinkled over meats, fish and poultry. Put the leaves, tendrils and the fresh grapes through a juicer with carrot, beetroot and celery for a superb detoxifier and cleanser, and add grape seed oil to cosmetics and hand and nail creams, and cook with it!

Health Note
Grapes are a good source of vitamins C and K and also contain B-vitamins, calcium, iron, magnesium, phosphorus, potassium, manganese and copper.

Grape Juice

Our Catawba vines hang heavy in midsummer with succulent black grapes that make a superb juice. Crush through a strong sieve and serve fresh with ice for the utmost benefit – unsweetened and uncooked. The fruit-sugar content of grapes is very high, so diabetics should avoid drinking this juice.
We also grow 'green Catawba' vines, which are equally flavour-filled and delicious and easy to grow.

Hint

In winter, new vines can be started from hardwood cuttings. Cut pieces of stem, with 6 or 7 nodes, and press into moist, compost-filled bags, deep enough to cover 3 nodes. Keep shaded and moist. Roots will start to develop around the nodes, and the plants need to become strong and sturdy before being planted out.

Maize
Corn ▪ Mealie

Zea mays

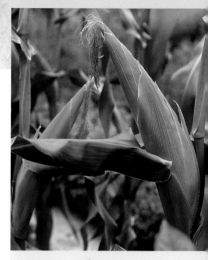

Probably the world's most treasured grain, ancient and steeped in the history of several countries, its earliest beginnings date back to around 5000 BC in Central America and Mexico, and it was and still is a staple diet for many. Maize has adapted to different climates and soil types with such diversity, it has become endemic to many areas. First taken into China around AD 1550 and planted where the rice paddy fields could not thrive, maize became a valuable staple food, but it was found, although a healthy food, it is not nutritionally complete. Those subsisting solely on maize run a risk of developing pellagra, which is a vitamin B3 (niacin) deficiency. Pellagra is characterised by lack of energy, skin rashes, poor and painful digestion and enormous lassitude. Long before Christ, the Native Americans observed this and learned quickly to cook their maize meal with a little limestone that was burned to an ash. Thanks to those early beginnings, today we know that the limestone ash helps the body to absorb the valuable niacin properly – how clever of those ancient growers – and today we should still take note to vary the diet so that there are no deficiencies, particularly if mealie meal forms the major part of the diet.

Growing Maize

One of the easiest and most rewarding of all annual crops to grow, 'green mealies' is everyone's favourite. A row in the garden creates much interest and much discussion! In spring, dig a trench in full sun about 30 cm wide and 50 cm deep and fill in with rich compost and set the hose at one end to flood it thoroughly. Then space the seeds about 30 cm apart, pressing them well into the moist trench. Flood the trench every 3 days or so, so as not to let the area dry out at all. Once the little seedlings become sturdy, flood the trench twice weekly depending on the rain. I have also been successful in planting a row of green mealies in midsummer as the cobs have time to ripen before the winter, so stagger the plantings to have green mealies all through the summer.

Using Maize

The maize flower – the tassels at the top of the up to 3 m high stem – and the silk within the cob, have been used as a diuretic tea for centuries to treat bladder and kidney disorders as well as cystitis, and the 'silk' within the husk of the cob is a valuable tea for treating disorders of the prostate gland, and to reduce swelling. Because of its abundance of healthful fibre, excellent carbohydrate content and essential fatty acids, maize remains a valuable food source worldwide. Rich in carotenoids, it protects against macular degeneration of the eyes (due to its high lutein content) and it is an excellent food for the brain, the nervous system, and for the skin, especially for eczema – ancient writings reveal mashed cooked young green mealies were used through the centuries as a soothing poultice over eczema and psoriasis.

Tests have found that green mealies particularly, but also mealie meal is a valuable anti-cancer food. Yellow mealies have higher beta-carotene levels and the colourful ancient Indian corns, although not easily available today, show even more anti-cancer activity. Popcorn – salt and sugar free – is a healthy snack food for children and in adults it is beneficial for arthritis and rheumatism.

Without doubt the best way to eat mealies is fresh from the field, quickly pushed into a pot of boiling water, then served immediately with a dab of butter and a light sprinkling of salt. No one can resist that 'corn-on-the-cob' summer feast. And for that alone it is worth growing your own row of mealies!

Health Note

Maize is a good source of vitamins A, B1, B2, B3 and B6, as well calcium, potassium, phosphorus, magnesium, iron, zinc, manganese and selenium.

Maize Silk Tea

Use ¼ cup of maize silk taken from inside the husk, or ¼ cup of the 'tassels' from the top of the maize plant, and pour over this 1 cup of boiling water. Stand 5 minutes, then strain and sip slowly. Take 2 cups a day.

Green Mealie Stir-Fry

Serves 4–6

This is delicious served with chicken.

8 young and tender green mealies
2 large onions, chopped
2 green peppers, chopped
1 finely chopped stalk of celery, leaves included
2 cups sliced mushrooms
sea salt and black pepper to taste
1 teaspoon crushed coriander seed
juice of 1 lemon
olive oil

Boil the green mealies until tender and cut off the cob. In a large, heavy bottomed pan, fry the onion in a little olive oil. Add the green peppers, celery and mushrooms and stir-fry. If necessary, add ½ cup water. Add the lemon juice, coriander, salt and pepper and stir-fry. Finally, add the cooked mealies and stir-fry. Serve piping hot with a sprinkling of chopped parsley and another squeeze of lemon juice.

Ginger

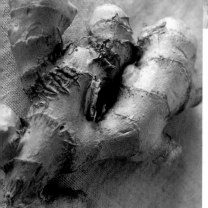

Native to Southern Asia, India and China, ginger is, and always has been, an important and much-loved part of the diet in those countries, and it features prominently in their ancient medicinal, traditional texts and pharmacopoeias. The ancient Romans traded with China over 2 000 years ago primarily for the valuable ginger root and carried ginger in their medical supplies when they invaded Britain in AD 431. It spread quickly throughout the Mediterranean area and by the 9th century Spanish explorers used ginger as trade, introducing it to the West Indies, Mexico and South America in an effort to increase the availability. By the 16th century ginger became more common as the West Indies and South America began exporting it back to Europe, and ginger became quite popular in medieval times. It was one of the medicines used against the plague, and to this day it retains its precious medicinal status.

By the 19th century pub keepers in England started a new craze of sprinkling a dash of dried finely ground ginger into the beer – this was the beginning of ginger ale, which has never lost its popularity. Today the best commercial ginger is grown in Jamaica, India, Fiji, Indonesia and, surprisingly, Australia. Never has it been more popular than it is now, as modern-day medical research proves its efficacy as a remarkable and valuable medicinal plant for a number of different ailments.

Growing Ginger

Ginger is so easy to grow! The thick underground tuberous rhizome is branched and on each of the smaller branches an 'eye' or growing tip is visible. Once the root is mature these smaller 'branches' can be snapped off and planted in moist, compost-rich soil in full sun. The succulent leafy stalk with smooth pointed leaves emerges and can grow up to 1 m in height. Plant the rhizomes 30–50 cm apart and only when the plant dies down at the end of the summer can the roots be lifted. White fragrant flowers in summer are a bonus and these have been used through the centuries to decorate churches, and for religious ceremonies, and the leaves are used to line baskets and dishes.

Using Ginger

Ginger is an excellent carminative, relieving heartburn, colic and intestinal gas, it relaxes and soothes the whole digestive tract and it prevents motion sickness, seasickness, nausea and intense indigestion, burping and sour flatulence. It literally soothes, smoothes and releases the spasm. The doctors call it 'intestinal spasmolytic effects', which a cup of ginger tea magically alleviates. To make ginger tea, thinly slice a piece of ginger root, usually 4 or 5 slices are sufficient, enough to equal between 2 and 4 teaspoons. Pour over this 1 cup of boiling water. Stand five minutes, then sweeten, if liked, with a little honey and stir well. Sip slowly. Leave the slices in the tea and chew a little of the root while drinking the tea. You will feel warm and relaxed very soon.

This same tea is excellent for coughs, colds, 'flu, bronchitis, lack of energy, poor peripheral circulation, nervous exhaustion, diarrhoea and even the nausea associated with chemotherapy. New medical tests prove ginger helps to lower high cholesterol, vomiting and nausea associated with pregnancy, and it contains potent anti-inflammatory compounds, called gingerols, which help to alleviate osteoarthritis and rheumatoid arthritis and improve mobility. The gingerols inhibit the formation of inflammatory cytokines, which reduces the pain and the swelling. Drinking a cup of ginger tea daily – doctors say even 500 to 1 000 mg of ginger a day – will make a huge difference in elimenating the pain and inflammation. Talk to your doctor about this natural treatment – it is well worth trying.

Search out all the ginger recipes you can lay your hands on and try them out. Old-fashioned ginger teas and drinks, even crystallised ginger, still remain favourite health builders today, and add grated ginger to stir-fries and stews, salads and desserts, and literally feel the goodness.

Spicy Ginger Tea

Serves 2

*6 slices ginger root (about
   2 tablespoons)
2 cardamom pods, crushed
2 sprigs of mint
2–3 thin parings of lemon rind (about
   2 teaspoons)
½ teaspoon freshly grated nutmeg*

Pour 3 cups of water into a stainless steel pot. Add all the ingredients to the water and simmer for 10 minutes with the lid on. Stir every now and then. Stand 5 minutes. Strain, sweeten, if liked, with a little honey and add a good squeeze of lemon juice. Serve hot, or chilled on a hot summer day.

Hint

Fresh ginger can be bought virtually all year round in greengrocers and supermarkets and it stores well in the fridge. Powdered ginger is delicious in home-baked puddings and biscuits made with honey and whole-wheat flour. To dry and powder your own ginger, wash the roots well, peel thinly and grate on the fine side of the grater. Spread on a stainless steel tray in the sun, and stir now and then with a fork to make sure all parts are dry. Once fully dry, spoon into a glass screw-top jar and label.

A–Z Ailment Chart

Abscesses & Boils

These are raised hot, sore bumps that can appear anywhere on the body. Boils usually occur under the arm or on the buttocks. They may be accompanied by a fever and the area may be swollen and tender. Usually takes around 2 weeks to come to a head. They are caused by a depleted immune system, zinc deficiency, toxic overload, and a diet high in sugar. Diabetics and overweight people are more at risk.

The danger foods

Sugar, coffee, tea, carbonated drinks, processed foods, especially meats, excess salt, pork products high in salt.

The superfoods

Raw fruits and vegetables, especially parsley, dandelion, apples, lemons, barley, carrot, celery, fennel and beetroot. Drink 1–2 glasses daily of the following juices: wheat grass, carrot, parsley, lucerne, apple, beetroot, celery. Eat garlic daily – it is a natural antibiotic – with lots of parsley. Eat papaya, prunes and flaxseed – ½ a cup of seeds soaked in warm water and then ground – to act as a gentle, cleansing laxative. Drink at least 8 glasses of water a day.

Tissue Salts: No. 3, 5 and 12 (2 of each sucked frequently).

Acidity

Symptoms of over-acidity in the body include overstress, irritability, exhaustion, aches, pains, headaches, insomnia, sour belching, indigestion, flatulence, spotty skin, acidic sweatiness (notice jewellery turns black and green on the skin), fever blisters.

The danger foods

Sugar, white bread, white flour, cakes, biscuits, buns, coffee, tea (except rooibos), carbonated fizzy drinks, sweet fruit juices, processed meats, red meat, smoked foods, eggs, dairy products (except plain Bulgarian yoghurt), excess salt.

The superfoods

Eat two fresh salads daily with lemon juice as a dressing only. Drink wheat grass juice with apple, carrots, beetroot, celery and parsley. Drink herbal teas throughout the day – fennel, celery, parsley, basil. Replace black and white pepper with cayenne pepper.

Take 2 teaspoons apple cider vinegar in a glass of water twice daily. Bath in a warm bath with ½ a cup of Epsom salts dissolved in it to help alkalise the skin, with a cup of oats (use large, non-instant flakes) tied in a muslin cloth as a scrub all over.

Tissue Salts: No. 2, 8 and 10 (2 of each taken 3–4 times a day).

Acne *see* Skin Problems

Ageing

Know this: you can be bright, happy, active, positive, vital, enthusiastic about life, healthy and clever – yes clever – all the days of your life, but you need to work at it! When I was 16, my marvellous father uttered these words: 'There are three things you need in life: determination, persistence and enthusiasm.' I have lived with these three powerful words all through my life and now, in my golden years, they thread through each day. I now know they have made me who I am and I am so utterly grateful for those precious words!

Old age is not for sissies, they say. My mother at age 90 said: 'Old age has nothing to recommend it!' and she said 'The more the years add up, the more you need to build up muscles, strength, stamina and expand your mind and set free your soul!' I think of how she went for her daily walk, of how she gardened and planned the next season's planting, how she painted her exquisite flower paintings and how, even in her last days in Frail Care, she asked for her painting table to be placed near her bed as the Iceberg roses at the sliding door into the garden just off her room were coming into their full glory and she wanted to record that beauty!

We can make old age something to look forward to, we need to know, we do not have to live in a degenerative state, we do not have to be subjected to the ills and woes of a deteriorating body. Ageing is a multidimensional process and it can be kept at bay with careful nourishment, the right antioxidants, vitamins, minerals and tissue salts, exercise and the right mindset!

The body changes constantly, the cells change, and a diet of fresh fruit and vegetables, less animal protein and absolutely no processed foods of any kind will slow down the ageing process.

The danger foods

All refined foods – white bread, white sugar, white rice, white flour, cakes, biscuits, sweets, chocolates, sugar in any form; carbonated drinks; fried foods; alcohol; instant coffee and even filter coffee as it can over-stimulate the heart.

Avoid all processed foods and all instant foods – forget that instant soup and make your own! Forget that instant oats porridge and make your own large-flake, non-instant oats porridge daily. Processed and packaged foods are full of chemicals – anti-caking agents, stabilisers and those ominous E-numbers, which on the packaging verify the presence of not-good-for-you-chemicals (see box).

Food additives by the number

Here is a list of ingredients in a chewy chocolate bar, a popular and much-loved treat for children and the elderly, available at every sweet counter, café, supermarket and corner store. Look at the poisons contained in it (you'll need a magnifying glass to read it and the E-numbers are abundant!):

Chocolate flavoured coating 22%, sugar, whey powder, glucose syrup*, vegetable fat (partially hydrogenated*), wheat flour (gluten), flavourants not specified, raising agents: E500, E223, Emulsifiers E322, E476, E471, Acidifiers E330, E334, Colourants E104. Allergens: This product may contain traces of peanuts and tree nuts.

* See pages 33 and 34 for information on these danger foods.

Now take a look at some common food additives (and known allergens) found in many processed foods:

E210: Benzoic acid – a preservative in drinks, sugar products, processed meats, sauces, spreads, cereals which is also present in many cosmetics and which can cause asthma, rhinitis, hay fever, urticaria, skin weals and in some cases induce severe allergic reactions.

E621: Monosodium glutamate – a controversial flavourant that appears in many foods. It is a neurotoxin which causes vomiting, migraine, asthma attacks, nausea, tight chest, disorientation, long-term eye damage including macular degeneration.

E310: Propylene glycol – a solvent and a wetting agent used in foods, cosmetics and in some cleaning products. Irritates the mucous membranes causing itchy red eyes, hay fever and asthmatic attacks. Found in chocolate products, ice-creams, beverages, baked goods.

E104: Quinolene yellow – a colourant – may cause rashes, asthma, hyperactivity. Banned in several countries. If you are sensitive to aspirin you must avoid it.

E223: Sodium metabisulphite – can provoke gastric irritation, nausea, diarrhoea, vomiting and asthma attacks. Destroys vitamin B1. Must be avoided by people suffering from emphysema, impaired kidney function, conjunctivitis, bronchitis, bronchial asthma or cardiovascular disease.

E322: Lecithin – allergic reaction in sensitive cases.

E330: Citric acid – can cause indigestion, heartburn, asthma attacks.

E334: Tartaric acid – can cause digestive disturbances.

E471: Mono- and diglycerides of fatty acids – possible digestive irritation.

E476: Polyglycerol polyricinoleate – emulsifier and stabiliser – possible allergen.

E500: Anti-caking agent – possible allergen, digestive irritation.

Isn't this quite a shock? A small treat full of 'poisons' that we give to our children?

The full list of E-numbers looks like this:

E100–E199: Food colourants

E200–E299: Preservatives and acids

E300-E341: Acidity regulators and antioxidants

E400–E499: Thickeners, stabilisers and emulsifiers

E500–E599: Acidity regulators, mineral salts and anti-caking agents

E600–E699: Flavour enhancers (there are some natural ones, but mostly these are chemicals)

E700–E799: Antibiotics

E900–E1599: Miscellaneous chemicals, including waxes, glazes, sweeteners, improving agents and foaming agents

Note that not all the E-numbers are 'poisons'. Some, like E100 which is curcumin, comes from the turmeric plant, but it can also be artificially produced and any adverse effects are not specified. Not all E-numbers have been tested fully and conclusively for safety, so it is impossible to say which are completely safe and which are not. Because I want to be as close to nature as I can, I avoid all products that have E-numbers, for as we age we need to be even more aware of building up our health and not breaking it down further.

The superfoods

Eat a wide variety of superfoods daily to include all the precious nutrients we need: brightly coloured berries, fruits and vegetables, lots of orange and red and purple.

Drink wheat and barley grass juice with carrots, kiwifruit, beetroot, lucerne leaves, parsley, celery, apple and pineapple. Get to know smoothies: make your own combinations – try papaya, guava, granadilla and pomegranate juice for a real taste of paradise! Drink lots of water.

The following vitamins, minerals, antioxidants and enzymes top the list! Be sure these are included in the diet every day and talk to your doctor about supplementing.

- Vitamin A and beta-carotene are excellent for the respiratory system.

Caution: Consult with your doctor before you embark on any form of self-diagnosis or self-treatment.

- Vitamin C is a great protector and at least 1 000 mg daily needs to be taken with breakfast. Vitamin C builds collagen, keeps the skin free of wrinkles and flakiness, protects the eyes against degeneration and cataracts, prevents the growth and development of tumours, boosts the immune system, protects the liver and is a general anti-ager. Increase Vitamin C for fighting any infection, especially sore throats, coughs and colds, and eat foods rich in vitamin C daily (see page 13).
- The B-vitamins – balancing and mood lifting – all are valuable.
- Vitamin E is vital for the cardiovascular system, it protects the eyes against age-related degeneration, and it keeps the body fats from becoming oxidised – vitamin E literally protects the brain! Include nuts in the diet to get lots of vitamin E (see page 13 for other foods rich in vitamin E).
- Selenium is a powerful antioxidant that aids in both repair and growth of the cells of particularly the skin, the hair, the nails and the bones. We need selenium to support a healthy immune system and also to tone and strengthen the eyes and the heart. Selenium also develops antioxidant enzymes within the body.
- Coenzyme Q10 strengthens the heart and the whole arterio-venus network and keeps the brain alert and quick.
- Turmeric – along with ginger and garlic – shows valuable protective and curative qualities. It stimulates the brain cells; its consumption literally keeps age-related deterioration at bay, like Alzheimer's disease, speech impediments, forgetfulness, uncoordinated movements and intellectual impairment.
- Rosemary is also a brain power plant and a cup of rosemary tea 2 to 3 times a week helps to prevent Alzheimer's disease and forgetfulness.

Take good exercise daily. Start a new hobby or enrol in a course on a topic that interests you, and work at being positive and useful and interested in everything around you! Take all 12 Tissue Salts, but not No. 12 if you have an implant.

Aids see HIV / Aids

Alcoholism

This is becoming more and more prevalent in our stress-filled environment. Symptoms of alcoholism include drinking too much, too often. Not being able to get through the day without a drink. Liver damage, high blood pressure, behavioural problems and aggression, malnutrition, cardio-vascular ailments, osteoporosis, hallucinations, convulsions, insomnia.

The danger foods
Sugar, refined carbohydrates, white bread, buns, cakes, sweets, chocolates, fast foods, all fried foods – your liver is far too damaged to cope with these too. The most damaging are fried chips, fried bacon and fatty fried meats. Avoid sweetened carbonated drinks of any kind. Replace with your own smoothies, and freshly squeezed fruit and vegetable juices. Coffee in any form (because of the caffeine, which will lead to cravings which, in this case, will lead to alcohol). Replace with dandelion coffee (see page 231) or rooibos tea.

The superfoods
Alfalfa sprouts, fresh lucerne leaves, abundant fresh fruits, vegetables and lots of salads! Celery, parsley and basil to clear the toxins; vegetable juices with wheat grass and barley grass; oily fish to replace red meat; sunflower seeds, sesame seeds and pumpkin seeds to replace salted peanuts.

At least 8 glasses water a day. Barley water to flush out the poison alcohol puts into your body and herbal teas to rehydrate.

Other recommendations
Speak to your doctor about taking a good multivitamin to replace the nutrients alcohol leaches from the body. The B-vitamins, magnesium, zinc, calcium are especially valuable.

Tissue Salts: No. 5 and 8 (take 2 of each, up to 10 times a day).

Join a support group and Alcoholics Anonymous. Avoid places and activities which lead to drinking – this means 'drinking buddies' and bars! Do not smoke!

Take up new hobbies and learn new skills. Try hypnosis, kinesiology, anything that can literally save your life.

Allergies see Food Allergies

Alopaecia see Hair Loss

Alzheimer's Disease

The main symptom is forgetfulness – this tragic disease affects the memory, usually the short-term memory and impairs the intellectual capacity. Factors that play a role include ageing, stress, an unhappy environment (for example lack of caring, lack of a loving family, death of a spouse), poor diet, loss of interest in life, genetic predisposition.

The danger foods
White bread, buns, pastries, cakes, biscuits, white rice, white sugar, jams, coffee, especially instant coffee, and all forms of alcohol.

Be aware of the aluminium content in processed foods like cheeses, pickles, cake mixes, and even our familiar baking powder can have aluminium in it. Avoid taking antacids as many contain aluminium. Rather take mint, fennel or aniseed tea for digestive complaints. Beware of aluminium in beauty and grooming products such as shampoos, soaps and deodorants – use natural products.

Be aware of mercury fillings in the teeth and replace them if possible.

Manage your stress, which is the trigger to so much anger, irritation and helplessness.

Keep your brain active: read, do crossword puzzles, take a walk to the library, study a new language, force yourself to participate in exercise, in discussions and keep a daily journal.

The superfoods
Include whole foods like sprouts, berries, fresh fruits and vegetables in abundance. Nourish the brain by eating sunflower seeds, pumpkin seeds, flaxseed, fish, chicken, sardines, tuna, eggs, horseradish, avocados, garlic, lots of lentils, chickpeas, dried beans, brown rice, millet, amaranth, walnuts, pecan nuts, buckwheat, rye, barley, wheat grass and barley grass, rooibos tea, turmeric, soya products like tofu, oats porridge with ground

Caution: Consult with your doctor before you embark on any form of self-diagnosis or self-treatment.

nuts and seeds (see page 26) every morning, nourishing home-baked breads (see page 35) and biscuits with oats, sesame, sunflower seeds, coconut, flaxseed. Include red clover, stinging nettle, gingko biloba teas and capsules in the daily diet.

Use sunflower cooking oil and, with your doctor's guidance, take DHEA oil supplements (DHEA is a hormone which declines as we age; low levels are linked to memory loss). Other supplements to consider are the B-vitamins, zinc, soy, lecithin and omega-3 oils.

Tissue Salts: No. 6 and 12 (avoid No. 12 if you have implants). Eat foods and herbs rich in silica (see box on page 253).

Never cook in aluminium pots and pans and avoid using aluminium foil.

Anaemia

Anaemia is a reduction of red blood cells, so that not enough oxygen is carried through the circulatory system. Possible causes include pregnancy, ageing, heavy menstruation, not absorbing enough iron from the food, liver damage, surgery, bleeding ulcers and nutritional deficiencies. Young children on milk diets without minerals and fatty acids are prone to anaemia. There are various types of anaemia, for example pernicious anaemia, sickle cell anaemia, megaloblastic anaemia and thalassaemia – let your doctor guide you on the correct nutritional therapy.

Anaemia is far more common than we think. Symptoms include fatigue; dizziness; rapid heart rate; pale nails, skin, lips; sensitivity to cold; poor appetite; slow-healing wounds, grazes, scratches, bites, cuts, etc.; fuzzy thinking; breathlessness with light exertion; constipation; indigestion; muscle weakness; compromised immune system; falling hair; lacklustre hair; pale, enlarged, flabby tongue.

The danger foods

Tea, coffee (especially instant coffee), rhubarb, wheat bran, spicy foods, fast foods, fried foods, fatty foods, alcohol, beer, chocolates, sweets and sugary snacks, confectionery, carbonated drinks, ice-cream (unless homemade) Avoid all processed foods: the additives in these foods interfere with the absorption of iron.

The superfoods

Lentils, chickpeas, beans (haricot, butter and sugar beans), peas, nuts (almonds, pecans, cashews, Brazil nuts, walnuts), molasses, oily fish, barley grass and barley grains, sesame seeds, sunflower seeds, amaranth, figs, apricots, cherries, pears, dates, mangoes, grapes, blueberries, raspberries, lettuce, watercress, spinach (not Swiss chard), kale, cabbage, broccoli, beetroot, celery, tomatoes, fenugreek, ginger, anise, cumin, mint, parsley, caraway, thyme, cinnamon, nettles, dandelion, red clover, alfalfa sprouts and fresh lucerne, freshly squeezed orange or naartjie juice, fresh lemon juice.

A daily salad of raw beetroot grated with apple served with chopped parsley and celery.

Include stinging nettle tea and chamomile tea daily in the diet.

Cook in iron pots to increase the iron content of a vegetable stew or soup.

Supplements: Take iron supplements only under your doctor's supervision. Do not take calcium, vitamin E and zinc at the same time as you take iron supplements as they interfere with the absorption of the iron. Also take vitamins C and B-complex.

Tissue Salts: No. 2, 4 and 9 (take 2 of each, 5–6 times a day).

> **Caution**
> Have blood tests done to confirm that you are in fact anaemic, as too much iron is as bad as too little. Ask your doctor to prescribe an iron supplement as many have toxic effects. It is often better to concentrate on the iron-rich foods rather than take iron supplements.

Anorexia

A worrying and often defeating ailment that means dramatic weight loss for someone who actually denies themselves food. Being 15–25% below the normal weight is considered to be anorexic. Anorexics have a largely irrational fear of being overweight. They wear loose clothes; obsess about food and make a thousand excuses for not eating; show signs of malnutrition and failing health; show nutrient deficiencies like lack of zinc, B-vitamins, etc.; show white spots on the nails; have emotional imbalances, have relationship problems and feel powerless; show loss of sexual desire; become obsessive about exercise; and have low self-esteem, often because of a culture where 'the thinner the better' is considered to be beautiful.

The danger foods

The danger foods are critical. Avoid every kind of processed food; avoid fried foods except nourishing stir-fries with a little olive oil; avoid commercial salad dressings, sauces and pickles, packets of crisps and salty, fried snacks. Avoid white bread, buns, cakes, sweets and chocolates; cut down on sugar and salt, use only a little honey daily. No coffee, tea, alcohol or energy drinks and especially no carbonated drinks – these are dangerous.

The superfoods

You need to work with your doctor and nutritionist, and you need concerned and loving support with three good meals a day that include at least eight different vegetables and fruits. Also include avocados, bananas, watercress, the omega-3 oils, brown rice, oats, chicken and fish (especially herring and mackerel).

Juices are of vital importance: beetroot, carrot, apple, celery, parsley, fresh lucerne or alfalfa sprouts with wheat grass and barley grass *daily*. Grow your own wheat and barley grass (see page 29).

Smoothies are nutritious and easily digested. Whirl fresh fruits with sunflower seeds, pecan nuts, almonds and flaxseed in a blender as a mid-morning snack. Try a banana with plain yoghurt, berries, a peach, pecan nuts, pumpkin seeds, sunflower seeds, sesame seeds and almonds for a mid-afternoon tea.

Talk to your doctor about supplements: probiotics, digestive enzymes, a good multivitamin, zinc and magnesium.

Tissue Salts: No. 6 and 9 (take 2 of each, up to 10 times a day).

Athlete's Foot

This is a fungal infection of intense irritation, usually found between the toes. Highly infectious!

Caution: Consult with your doctor before you embark on any form of self-diagnosis or self-treatment.

Symptoms include severe itch, sore, scaly, scratchy, red skin, cracks and fissures. Localised infection that loves the warmth and moisture of closed shoes and socks. Usually the infection is picked up after a visit to a public swimming pool, a spa or using public showers at the gym, or walking barefoot at the gym.

The danger foods
A diet high in refined carbohydrates, sugary buns, sweets, sugary instant coffee, white bread and cakes creates the ideal environment in which a fungal infection such as this can thrive. Avoid carbonated drinks, alcohol and dairy products (except plain Bulgarian yoghurt).

The superfoods
Include lots of fresh fruits and vegetables in the diet to boost the immune system, especially foods rich in vitamin C. Eat lots of garlic, parsley, celery, lemons and fresh green salads.

Other recommendations
Speak to your doctor about supplements: extra vitamin C (up to 5 000 mg a day); increase your zinc intake and take probiotics (these boost the beneficial bacteria in the digestive system – take them until the infection has cleared).

Tissue Salts: No. 7 and 11. Take frequently, also make a lotion of it and apply to the area.

Make a lotion and a tea of fresh tea tree sprigs or add drops of tea tree oil to hot water in which to rinse the feet. Drink pennywort (*Centella asiatica*) tea – ¼ cup fresh pennywort leaves to 1 cup of boiling water, stand 5 minutes, strain and sip slowly. Use the cooled tea as a lotion in which to soak the feet or to dab on with cotton wool. (The tea tree lotion and tea can be made in the same way.)

After a shower, dry the feet well and dust with cornstarch powder to ensure the area remains dry. Wear cotton socks only, or open sandals.

Attention Deficit Disorder (ADD)
Also known as attention deficit hyperactivity disorder (ADHD), this is far more common than we are aware – and not only in children. ADD is a 'new' condition that has in recent years become so prevalent that the tendency is to immediately medicate with drugs like Ritalin. But what about diet? For virtually every case there has been a marked difference in merely changing the diet and avoiding in serious earnestness the danger foods.

Symptoms and causes include:

Allergies that can easily cause sensitivity, like wheat and dairy and gluten intolerance, or allergies triggered by sugar or food additives such as colourants and flavourants.

Unstable blood sugar levels where mood swings are noticeable like crying fits, unreasonable behaviour, poor concentration, temper tantrums, and in adults, road rage, quick 'short fuse' behaviour and rude uncooperativeness.

Cravings for fast foods, snacks, sweets, chips, crisps, chocolate with resulting nutritional deficiencies, especially zinc, vitamin B6 and magnesium.

Also consider these: oxygen deprivation during the birth process; fluorescent lighting, which could cause over-stimulation; dental fillings for example amalgam; and pollution – smoke, dust, pollen, carbon, roadside pollution fumes and so on.

The danger foods
It is vitally important to eliminate the following from the diet: sugar and sugary foods, salt, soft drinks of every description (especially brightly coloured ones!), processed foods (especially processed meats), chips, fast foods, instant coffee, tea, chocolates and sweets, cakes, icing sugar.

Avoid all foods with artificial colourants and flavourants and preservatives. Get to know them, read the labels on packaged foods and become alert and aware. Be especially careful of sulphites – sulphur dioxide found in dried fruits is a dangerous aggravator – and also benzoic acid.

> ### Foods to monitor
> It has been suggested by some doctors that you monitor these foods. It is interesting to note that they all contain salicylates which have been found to aggravate ADD in some children. So test by eating one at a time at least a day apart and eliminate from the diet those that cause a reaction:
> Almonds, apples, apricots, blueberries, cherries, cucumbers, grapes, oranges, peaches, peppermint, plums and prunes, raspberries, strawberries, tomatoes.

The superfoods
Small regular snacks are important: carrot sticks; lettuce; sprouts like lucerne (alfalfa) and mung beans; nuts like pecan nuts, walnuts, macadamia nuts; seeds like sunflower seeds, sesame seeds, pumpkin seeds. Use flaxseed oil in salad dressings.

Green vegetables like spinach, cabbage and broccoli; fish, meat (*not* processed – no sausages, viennas), stews and grills, organic chicken; whole grains and legumes, for example chickpeas as a snack (see page 99), lentils, beans; fruit, especially figs, pomegranates, pears, avocados, papayas, melons, banana, mangoes, litchi.

Learn to bake your own oats crunchies and cookies, include a little honey as a sweetener with stevia, or a little fructose. Make your own snacks, crisps and tasty lunchbox snacks. Use a herb mix to lessen the salt, for example thyme, oregano, coriander seeds, cumin seeds, celery and celery seeds (see also page 35).

Often correct eating and *lots of water* will change the behaviour patterns drastically!

Consider the following supplements: magnesium, vitamin C, vitamin B-complex, zinc, fish oils, evening primrose oil.

Tissue Salts: No. 2, 6 and 8, taken 2–4 times a day (see also page 24).

Autism
Some of the characteristics of autism are: non-reaction to the usual stimuli, like lack of facial expression and lack of eye contact; limited and often difficult speech; withdrawn, distancing from others; hyperactivity; over-sensitivity to loud sounds, strong smells or too many stimuli; obsessive compulsive behaviour; loud screams and scrambled words; head banging; uncontrollability; poor social interaction.

Parents seek answers so intensely and the explanations listed here are only a few of the most common ones. There

Caution: Consult with your doctor before you embark on any form of self-diagnosis or self-treatment.

is sometimes a family history and the following list that may indicate part of the explanation and a plan of action: impaired immune system; migraines; allergies (not only food allergies but to many other causes, for example bee stings, heat rash, perfumes, etc.); exposure to chemical poisons, for example crop spraying with organophosphates.

This is a difficult journey, but one that can be greatly eased by carefully keeping a notebook on the corrective eating habits.

The danger foods
Gluten and dairy foods – following a gluten- and dairy-free diet has been often a lifesaver. (See page 218 for more on gluten intolerance.) Avoid food plants with solanine in them like tomatoes, green peppers, brinjals, potatoes (sweet potatoes are fine). All belong to the nightshade family and may cause reactions in an autistic child. Yeast can also affect autistic children, so avoid breads, cakes and biscuits, rolls and anything with yeast in it, even pizzas – bake your own. Avoid also chocolate, soya in any form, citrus fruits, any preserved food, processed foods, all sweeteners, especially chemical ones, cut down on sugar and avoid all carbonated sweet drinks, including diet colas, which are pure poison to an autistic child.

The superfoods
Include lots of seeds like sesame seed, pumpkin seed, flaxseed, sunflower seeds; legumes such as beans, peas, chickpeas, lentils, butter beans; brown rice; avocados; bananas; pears; papaya; melons; nuts like pecan nuts, walnuts, macadamia nuts, cashew nuts; sardines and mackerel, which are rich in omega-3 fats.

Other recommendations
Consider the following supplements: vitamin B6 or a good vitamin B-complex; magnesium; probiotics; omega-3 fatty acids – this will aid easier sleep patterns, eye contact, more sociable behaviour.

Tissue Salts: No. 3, 8 and 11 are good starting points with No. 9 as a daily dose. Note also the foods in which these salts appear and introduce those accordingly (see *Tissue Salts for Healthy Living* for more information.)

An Epsom salt bath twice a week has been proved to be a useful little exercise: 1–2 cups of Epsom salts in a warm bath can increase both the magnesium and the sulphur levels in the body which seem to be short.

Most valuable of all will be a food diary. Keep notes of foods that cause trouble and reintroduce foods that previously caused trouble, update the list on a monthly basis.

Bruising
Symptoms are dark purple marks after a fall or a bump or in some cases just a light knock that causes a large and painful haematoma. Bruising can be made worse by anaemia, smoking, vitamins C and K deficiencies and blood-thinning drugs. If the bruise does not heal within a few days you do need to see your doctor.

The danger foods
Fried and fatty foods, fast foods, alcohol, carbonated drinks and sugar in all its forms; aspirin and anti-inflammatory medications may also cause bruising.

The superfoods
Eat berries of all types – mulberries, strawberries, raspberries, elderberries – kiwifruit; onions; apricots; lucerne and alfalfa sprouts; green peppers; citrus fruit (and scrape some white pith from their inner skin); lots of buckwheat greens as well as flowers and the seeds added to breads and stews, as buckwheat contains rutin; also foods rich in vitamins C and K: asparagus, broccoli, cabbage, cauliflower, stinging nettle greens, egg yolks and oats. Also include red clover and lucerne daily in the salad, both leaves and flowers.

Tissue Salts: No. 4 and 12 (2 of each, taken 3–4 times a day).

Burns
Burns and scalds, even severe sunburn, cause much pain and skin damage. Burns are classified according to the extent and severity: first degree burns are lighter with unbroken skin, second degree burns are when the skin is blistered or broken and third degree burns are when the burn is so severe it needs to be treated in hospital.

The danger foods
Alcohol, as it suppresses the immune system and dehydrates and slows the healing process; fatty foods, fried foods, processed foods, sweets, chocolates – avoid these, as you want to boost the immune system to speed up the healing.

The superfoods
In order to assist the healing process once the burn has been treated by a doctor:

Firstly drink lots of water. Twice a day drink ½ a glass of fresh carrot juice with beetroot and wheat grass and parsley and apple and celery. Rich in vitamins and beta-carotene, this precious juice will aid the quick healing. Consider investing in a powerful juice extractor.

Eat lots of berries, blueberries included, broccoli, cabbage, green peppers, kiwifruit, cucumber. Rich in vitamins and antioxidants, these help the skin to heal.

Raw fruits and vegetables and lots of salads will boost the immune system.

Other recommendations
To help the healing process and lessen scar tissue formation once the burn is clear of infection and the skin is regrowing, use aloe vera juice and pulp directly from the freshly cut leaf and also the juice and pulp from bulbinella (*Bulbine frustescens*) leaves. Once the burn has grown new tissue over it, then you can apply healing creams in a non-oily base. Keep up the diet of raw fruits and vegetables.

Tissue Salts: No. 3, 4 and 5 (taken 5–6 times a day in the early stages).

Bursitis
Bursitis is the inflammation of a bursa (bursae are fluid-filled sacs that protect the tendons near the major joints). Depending on where it occurs in the body it is also commonly known as **tennis elbow** or **frozen shoulder** or **bunions**.

An inflammatory condition, it is characterised by pain on movement, swelling and tenderness, usually caused by an injury or wear and tear like a heavy tennis schedule, lifting

Caution: Consult with your doctor before you embark on any form of self-diagnosis or self-treatment.

heavy weights, overweight and standing or walking for long periods of time – sometimes called the 'chef's bunions'!

The danger foods
Fatty foods, fast foods, sugar, chocolates, white bread, sweets, biscuits, carbonated drinks and salty snacks. All these will aggravate the inflammatory condition. Replace with plenty of fresh fruit and vegetables and lots of plain water.

The superfoods
A doctor and a physiotherapist need to guide you through your medical treatment. I am a physiotherapist and have been so successful in treating stubborn painful stiff elbows and shoulders, I urge you to follow the course of treatment.

But also include these valuable and very necessary antioxidants and anti-inflammatory foods in the diet: Lots of raw juices, raw fruits and raw vegetables for repairing injured tissue.

Anti-Inflammatory Juice

This juice is invaluable – it is so rich in antioxidants.
In a juice extractor push through:
1 cup parsley
1 cup celery
1 cup carrots, peeled
1 cup beetroot, peeled
1 cup pineapple, peeled and cubed
1 cup fennel, stems and bulb
1 apple, peeled
2 cups barley grass
Drink immediately and slowly, and do this every day.

Eat nuts like pecan nuts, walnuts, macadamia nuts, as well as pumpkin seeds, sunflower seeds and oily fish for their anti-inflammatory effects. Add fresh pineapple to the diet, especially eat the core – it contains bromelain which acts as a strong anti-inflammatory – and eat lots of papaya and papinos!

Make teas of stinging nettle and celery and fennel to flush out the acidity and add turmeric to the diet in stir-fries of fresh vegetables.

Vitamins B12, D and E, and magnesium and calcium are excellent for reducing inflammation.

Tissue Salts: No. 4 and 5, and No. 2, 8 and 10 for the acidity (2 of each taken at least 3 times a day).

Cancer
Never has there been so much cancer suffering as there is at present! There are so many factors that come into play with breast cancer, bowel cancer, prostate cancer and lung cancer as the most common, and with the right eating and lifestyle changes, like avoiding smoking and following a healthy diet, positive outcomes are now more possible.

Factors that seriously contribute to the carcinogen factor and proliferation of cancer cells include: diets high in saturated fats, processed meats, fast foods, carbonated drinks, red meat, alcohol, radiation – for example excessive use of cell phones and living close to cell phone masts – microwaves, smoking and passive smoking, industrial chemicals and pollution.

Symptoms to be aware of include lumps in the breasts, swollen lymph nodes, weight loss, chronic fatigue, anaemia, poor appetite, general malaise.

The danger foods
Avoid the following: all processed foods; fast foods; fried foods, especially burned or blackened barbequed fatty foods; all refined foods, including white rice, white sugar, plain pasta; refined flour products of all descriptions, for example biscuits, buns, cakes, white bread; block margarines (become aware of saturated fats, hydrogenated fats and trans fats – see also page 34); artificial sweeteners, alcohol, coffee, especially instant coffee.

Replace sugar with honey or stevia leaves (best is fresh or air-dried stevia leaves, not the powder) and eat sun-dried dates and raisins (free from preservatives like sulphur dioxide) to satisfy that sweet tooth. Cut down on salt in the diet.

The superfoods
Fresh fruits and vegetables organically grown in abundance are a priority. *Raw food* is essential. Or lightly steam vegetables or add to soups, stews and stir-fries.

Include in the diet daily:

Fresh, raw juices: wheat grass and barley grass with fresh lucerne, red clover leaves and flowers, apples, carrots, beetroot, celery, parsley.

Salads of thinly sliced organic tomatoes, celery, basil, red peppers, dandelion, cabbages, broccoli, kale; sprouted seeds, especially organic sprouted broccoli; cereals, legumes and seeds, for example brown rice, millet, lentils, chickpeas, peas and split peas, flaxseed, oats, sesame seed; flaxseed oil; raw almonds; spinach; garlic and lots of fresh fruit – apples, apricots, organic grapes, papayas, berries of all sorts, figs, pomegranate, lemons, melons – make a selection and prepare as much fruit salad and salads as you can enjoy every day.

Green tea is excellent, and so are peppermint and melissa tea, ginger tea and a selection of fresh herbs from the garden to boost the digestive system.

Other recommendations
Buy natural cleaning products – many chemicals used routinely in the home are hazardous! Use natural and organic toiletries and cosmetics – avoid those that contain petrochemicals and parabens. Avoid paints, toxic weed killers, sprays, fumigants, insect repellents and chemical fertilisers. Read the labels and become aware of additives, stabilisers, colourants, chemicals (denoted by E-numbers – see also page 210). Make this a mission – become aware of the chemical world we live in and fight it!

Grow your own organic herbs and fruits and vegetables. Plant vines – grapes, su-su, granadillas, peas and beans of all descriptions. Set up the most beautiful vegetable garden possible and give it your full attention and work in it yourself! Set up wheat grass and barley grass trays for daily juicing (see page 29). As your interest grows so will your health!

Speak to your doctor about supplements: vitamins C, B-complex, D and E, coenzyme Q10, selenium, cancer bush (*Sutherlandia frutescens*) in capsule form.

Tissue Salts: The cancer formula is No. 3, 4, 5, 6 and 7 (take 2 of each, 6–8 times a day).

Caution: Consult with your doctor before you embark on any form of self-diagnosis or self-treatment.

Chemotherapy

This seems to be the first step in treating cancer, yet it is a seriously debilitating treatment and often tumour cells develop resistance to it, and so promote, instead of suppress, the growth of cancer cells. Chemotherapy and radiation therapy can activate certain enzymes, known as COX-2 enzymes, and an inflammatory condition, which is present in most cancers, can be further activated and aggravated.

But certain phytochemicals that are found in green tea, garlic, fresh ginger, soya beans, grapes, anise, basil and turmeric, as well as mustard greens and lemons, have been found to deactivate or certainly reduce the activity of the COX-2 enzymes as well as other molecules, which will make the cancer cells sensitive to both radiation therapy and chemotherapy, strengthening their therapeutic action. So these valuable cancer fighter foods must be included in the daily diet with diligence. Talk to your doctor and oncologist about this.

Candida

Candida is the name given to an excess of yeast in the body which leads to thrush or vaginal infection or itch and hot swelling and discomfort. Often certain situations or events seem to set it off, for example stress, anxiety, major life changes (such as loss of a loved one, divorce, job loss), birth control pills, menopause, pregnancy, poor diet, prolonged use of antibiotics and liver damage.

Symptoms include premenstrual tension; insomnia; night sweats and discomfort; bloating and indigestion; constipation and / or diarrhoea; dry, flaky and itchy skin; headaches and migraines; exhaustion and constant fatigue; athlete's foot, easy bruising; excessive mucus, blocked sinuses, hay fever and sinusitis; certain food allergies that were not there before; low blood sugar (hypoglycaemia); tongue sore and often burning; unexplained, persistent cough; brain fog, confusion and mental dullness; loss of libido.

The danger foods

Liver health is vital, so drastic changes in the diet are needed.

Start gradually by eliminating the following foods: anything made with refined flour and anything with yeast in it, such as bread, buns, doughnuts, biscuits; sugar in any form, including sweets, chocolates, honey, fructose, maple syrup and replace with stevia; dairy products; mushrooms; coffee and tea – replace with herb teas or rooibos; carbonated drinks of any kind; orange juice, especially bottled orange juice, concentrated orange juice and commercial fruit juices of any kind; alcohol of any kind.

Cut down on the following foods: red meat – replace with chicken, fish and eggs; tomatoes; all nuts for at least one month; any pickles, sauces and vinegars; potatoes and sweet potatoes; fruit – due to the fruit sugars – for a month, then gradually reintroduce berries, pears, melons, papaya, apples (make a note of any adverse reactions).

The superfoods

Your aim is to boost the immune system, cleanse and stabilise the liver, eliminating the symptoms. Include in the diet: raw vegetable salads; steamed vegetables; wheat grass and barley grass juiced with parsley, celery and fresh red clover leaves; vegetables like Brussels sprouts, cabbage, kale, cauliflower, radishes, watercress, dandelion greens, green beans, Swiss chard, squashes, pumpkins, onions, lots of garlic, spring onions; ginger; amaranth, both leaves and seeds; buckwheat greens, flowers and the seeds (use buckwheat flour for pancakes – see page 124); millet, rye (try 100% rye bread or rye crackers). Use fresh oregano and thyme as flavourants. Within the first month you'll start to feel better.

Other recommendations

Speak to your doctor about supplements: blue-green algae supplements, zinc, selenium, magnesium plus calcium, a good multivitamin, and milk thistle. Within two months, friendly bacteria can be introduced like *Lactobacillus* – follow your doctor's advice.

Tissue Salts: No. 5 is particularly helpful, taken up to 10 times a day.

Canker Sores or Mouth Ulcers

More and more people are plagued by these painful mouth ulcers (do not confuse them with cold sores or fever blisters which are recurring and caused by the *Herpes simplex* virus).

These usually small, shallow, flat, painful ulcers occur in the soft tissue inside the lips, on the gums, tongue, inside the cheeks – anywhere in the oral cavity – and they usually clear up in about 10–20 days. Caused by stress, food allergies, fungal and viral infections, nutrient deficiencies (especially vitamin C), lactose and gluten intolerance and sensitivity, they can be recurrent. Interestingly, the lining of the mouth is one of the first places to show nutrient deficiencies.

The danger foods

Dairy products; wheat products; sugar; acidic fruits and vegetables like tomatoes, citrus fruits, chilli peppers, plums; spicy foods; pickles and very salty foods; coffee, tea and alcohol; fast foods, fried foods and processed foods; artificial colourants, flavourants and preservatives.

The superfoods

Include in the diet lots of red and yellow fruits and vegetables like pumpkins, mangoes, carrots, squashes, marrows, watermelon, beetroot (including the leaves); legumes like beans, peas, lentils, chickpeas; freshly juiced celery, wheat grass, barley grass and lucerne; white meats like chicken and turkey; white fish; wholegrain cereals like rye, oats, millet, brown rice and buckwheat; cucumber; lettuce; cauliflower; cabbage and amaranth.

Keep a diary to record the best and the worst foods and concentrate on boosting the immune system by careful food choices.

Other recommendations

Take supplements under your doctor's supervision: look at the B-vitamins, especially folic acid, B1, B6 and B12, check for an iron deficiency and include probiotics daily.

Tissue Salts: No. 3 and 12 (take 2 of each frequently).

Make a mouthwash by adding 2–3 drops of tea tree oil to ½ a glass of water and gently swish out the mouth, at least three times a day.

Caution: Consult with your doctor before you embark on any form of self-diagnosis or self-treatment.

Cardiovascular Disease *see* Heart Disease

Carpal Tunnel Syndrome

This is caused by pressure on the nerves of the wrist, often brought on by repetitive movement like computer use or exercise, or injury to the wrist, sprains, strains, and also, surprisingly, nutrient deficiencies of vitamin B6 and the omega-3 fats. Tendonitis, arthritis, fluid retention, diabetes, circulatory problems, even menopausal symptoms may be contributory factors.

Symptoms include numbness, pain, burning sensation, tingling in the fingers and hand and wrist, often worse at night. The wrist movement becomes tight and sore and the pain often goes up the arm.

The danger foods

Sugar, salt, coffee, tea, alcohol, processed foods, salty snacks and food additives (these can interfere with the body's absorption of vitamin B6). Too much meat aggravates the condition, and so do food colourants like tartrazine. Oxalic acid, found in spinach, Swiss chard, rhubarb and asparagus, should be carefully avoided. Also be aware of the number of eggs you eat – more than three a week could be part of the problem.

The superfoods

Oily fish to get those omega-3s; turmeric contains curcumin, which has good anti-inflammatory action (add it to brown rice and millet, stir-fries, lentil and bean dishes); brewer's yeast; bananas; pumpkin seeds, flaxseed and sesame seeds (grind them together with sunflower seeds and sprinkle over porridge, soups and stir-fries or add to smoothies). Grow alfalfa sprouts and eat fresh lucerne sprigs in the daily salad.

Include foods rich in vitamin B6: walnuts, green peas, soya beans, fish (sardines, mackerel, trout, herring). Eat fresh pineapple as it contains bromelain, which is a known anti-inflammatory. Eat it with freshly grated ginger, avocado, fennel, celery and parsley. All have cleansing diuretic properties, which help to remove toxins from the body.

Tissue Salts: No. 2, 4 and 8 (2 of each taken at least 4 times a day).

As a physiotherapist I always took extra care to look at how the carpal tunnel patients sat at their desk or what position they slept in to ensure no pressure disturbed the nerves and circulation at the wrist. Just changing your position at your desk or in front of the computer could alleviate a lot of discomfort.

Thinking About Tartrazine

An approved food additive, tartrazine is a bright yellow, orange or red dye labelled E102 and it is found in sweets, beverages, desserts, cakes and custards. It is widely regarded as an allergen that sets off asthma attacks, causes skin rashes, changes behaviour, leads to hyperactivity, alters perception, and actually turns a peaceful child or teenager, or even the elderly, into a rude, difficult and often impossible person! It interferes with the digestive system, with the metabolism of certain enzymes, vitamins and minerals, and has been banned in the Scandinavian countries and is restricted in Germany and Austria.

What are we waiting for? Read all labels carefully and look out for additive E102, also sometimes called 'Food Yellow 4' or 'FD&C Yellow' or 'C1 Acid Yellow'. It is bad news for everyone, but especially for carpal tunnel syndrome sufferers.

Cataracts *see* Eye Ailments

Cellulite

That dreadful dimpling orange peel appearance on the thighs and buttocks sends many of us into a tailspin! The uneven lumps are fatty deposits under the skin that have accumulated, and not metabolised, along with waste products and fluid into lumps and bumps that are difficult to remove.

It is caused by an overworked liver and strained circulation. The lymphatic system is under strain because of not enough water. Usually 6–8 glasses of water a day would greatly assist it. Poor diet, and saturated fats in particular, is the main contributory factor and being overweight adds to the condition. Hormone balance also needs to be checked. Avoid all alcohol.

The danger foods

Caffeine, coffee (especially instant coffee), tea and carbonated, sugary drinks are some of the worst offenders. Avoid sugar (cakes, biscuits, sweets and chocolates) and trans fats (found in fried foods, chips and fast foods). Processed, refined foods and saturated fats trigger hormonal imbalance. Eat red meat only once a week, preferably mutton with all visible fat removed. Keep an eye on your salt intake and have your blood pressure and blood cholesterol levels checked. Check dairy products for intolerances.

The superfoods

Make sure you drink enough water – the ideal is 2 litres through the day.

Include in the diet daily: lecithin, which repairs tissue damage and lifts fatty deposits; raw and lightly steamed cabbage, broccoli, kale, cauliflower, Brussels sprouts, turnip (roots and leaves), radishes (roots and leaves), mustard leaves and flowers, horseradish (grated finely with apple cider vinegar), watercress, parsley, celery, fennel, buckwheat leaves, dandelion leaves, wheat grass and barley grass juice, and sprouted broccoli, alfalfa and buckwheat seeds. All these will assist with the detoxification of the liver and so will antioxidant-rich, detoxifying fruits like berries (all kinds), apple, melons, pineapple, papaya, grapes, pomegranates and figs.

Sprinkle nuts (pecans, walnuts, almonds, Brazil nuts) and seeds (flax, sunflower, sesame and pumpkin seeds) milled in a coffee grinder over non-instant oats porridge or over fruit salads.

Eat a whole grapefruit daily with some of the pith to clear the liver and take a milk thistle supplement to clear the liver.

Pennywort (*Centella asiatica*) is an excellent circulatory herb and will hasten the break-up of fatty deposits. Take as a tea once a day – 3 fresh leaves in 1 cup of boiling water, stand 5 minutes, strain and sip slowly. Take only one cup a day; after 2 weeks give it a 3–4 day break, then start again.

Caution: Consult with your doctor before you embark on any form of self-diagnosis or self-treatment.

Other recommendations
Avoid smoking, even passive smoking.

Take salt baths: tie 1 cup of coarse, non-iodated sea salt mixed with fresh pennywort leaves in a face cloth. Stand in the bath, wet it thoroughly and with circular movements massage slowly and deeply over the thighs and buttocks, then lie back in the bath and massage the thighs in the water. This helps to loosen the cellulite.

Use a cellulite cream to rub into the area, massaging it in deeply after the bath (we post this countrywide – see our website www.margaretroberts.co.za).

Tissue Salts: No. 9 and No. 11 (take 3 tablets 3 times a day).

Cervical Dysplasia
In the last three years I have had so many queries on how to treat this condition naturally – always under the doctor's supervision – that I include it here briefly. Detected only by a pap smear, this is the appearance of abnormal cells on the wall of the cervix. Although it is not cancerous, if ignored it can become a cancer within the cervix.

It is caused by the human papilloma virus (Hpv) and risk factors include intercourse at an early age, multiple sexual partners, the *Herpes simplex* virus type 2 (genital herpes), deficiency in vitamin A and folic acid, using contraceptive pills and smoking, especially smoking from an early age. Smoking in young girls and being promiscuous is not clever! The price of such behaviour is becoming frighteningly high!

The danger foods
The greatest risks are alcohol and smoking, which is the major risk factor for incubating Hpv, as smoking compromises the immune system, depleting the body of vital vitamin C and the inhaled smoke concentrates the carcinogenic compounds in the soft wall of the cervix.

Fast foods, trans fats, fried foods, carbonated drinks, diet drinks, sugar in all its many forms – sweets, chocolates, cakes, energy drinks, all make the body pay too great a price.

The superfoods
Fresh fruits and vegetables, especially broccoli, cabbage, kale, radishes, turnips and turnip leaves, lettuce, fennel, celery, orange, green and yellow fruits and vegetables like bell peppers, berries, citrus fruit, carrots, tomatoes, chickpeas, baked potatoes, sweet potatoes, and also whole grains like non-instant oats, nuts, sunflower seeds, sesame seeds. All these foods will help the immune system fight the cancerous cells.

Take folic acid and a vitamin C supplement.

Tissue Salts: No. 3, 4, 5, 6 and 7 (take 2 of each at least twice a day).

Cholesterol *see* High Cholesterol

Chronic Fatigue Syndrome
Also known as ME or myalgic encephalomyelitis, its basic characteristic is intense fatigue that is not restored by rest, preceded sometimes by a bout of 'flu or glandular fever, but it could be many other causes. Some people have it for around 6 months at a time, others have it in shorter bouts, while others can have it for years.

The most common symptoms are exhaustion, depression, headaches, fever, body aches and pains, general lassitude, swollen glands, poor concentration and brain fog, loss of appetite, indigestion, constipation or diarrhoea, dipping in and out of sleep (left alone this sleep pattern could continue all day), adrenal fatigue, impaired immune system, hormonal imbalances, anaemia, chronic stress, new food intolerances, for example gluten intolerance.

The danger foods
A poor diet, low in fresh fruits and vegetables, is a major factor. Avoid the following diligently: sugar, refined flour, alcohol, carbonated drinks, fast foods, salty snacks. Avoid caffeine – both coffee and tea – and instant coffee is banned! So is alcohol – not even a sip! Change to rooibos or herb teas.

The superfoods
Start with getting proper medical help: weekly consultations are essential to ascertain exactly what the problem is.

Search out organic foods. Toxic chemicals can cause too much damage in an already compromised system. Include lots of fresh fruit and salads in the diet; eat at least 6 servings of a variety of fruit every day. Be diligent in juicing your own freshly grown wheat and barley grass. Grow your own sprouts and eat them in salads.

Drink water and herbal teas daily – at least 2 litres. Water is of the utmost importance. Juice wheat grass, barley grass, carrots, celery, beetroot, radishes, cabbage, add apples for taste, and include fennel, parsley, lucerne leaves and sprigs. Ring the changes and add pineapple, ginger, peaches or nectarines. Have half a glass mid-morning and mid-afternoon. Juice it freshly each time.

Replace tea with rooibos or herb teas like pennywort (*Centella asiatica*), rose geranium (*Pelargonium graveolens*), sacred basil (*Ocimum tenuifolium* – once known as *Ocimum sanctum*), all picked fresh from your garden – ¼ cup fresh herb (do not mix them, drink separately), pour over this 1 cup of boiling water, stand 5 minutes, strain and sip slowly. Take 2 or 3 cups of different teas throughout the day to increase your water intake.

Put sunflower seeds, flaxseed, almonds, sesame seeds and pumpkin seeds through a seed grinder or coffee grinder and sprinkle on oats porridge or on plain yoghurt with fresh berries, kiwifruit or pears. Eat mackerel, sardines or trout three times a week – avoid red meat and seek out organic chicken.

Speak to your doctor about vitamin and mineral supplements, especially the B-vitamins, vitamin C and magnesium, coenzyme Q10 and spirulina. Take milk thistle tablets or capsules to clear the liver and regenerate it.

Tissue Salts: No. 1, 2, 9, 10 and 12; No. 6 to combat fatigue from the computer screen.

Use natural cleaning products in the home and for personal grooming. Pace yourself and make sure your bowels work well.

Cirrhosis of the Liver *see* Liver Damage

Coeliac Disease
Coeliac disease is a digestive disease that occurs in the small intestine and interferes with absorption of nutrients from food. People who have coeliac disease cannot tolerate gluten, a protein found in wheat, rye and barley. It is therefore also commonly referred to as **gluten intolerance**.

Caution: Consult with your doctor before you embark on any form of self-diagnosis or self-treatment.

A sensitivity to gluten that is often only diagnosed in the forties, coeliac disease is characterised by bloating, inability to gain weight in children, discomfort, abdominal swelling, muscle and joint pain, fatigue, irritability, pale stools that float and diarrhoea.

Once a baby is introduced to his first cereal, gluten intolerance could be diagnosed at this stage, but often the symptoms are not clearly definable. The baby does not thrive and as the child grows the symptoms become more noticeable.

Become aware of gluten-rich foods and change the diet. Also consider lactose intolerance as these two often show up together.

The danger foods

Cereal grains that contain gluten: wheat, rye, barley, spelt, oats, and sometimes buckwheat and millet are also included in this list; alcohol, especially beer, wine, vodka and malt, as these have a grain base; packaged foods, instant soups, thickeners, ice-creams, seasonings, sauces and spreads, as these often contain flours; dairy products in some cases, for lactose intolerance.

What is gluten?

Gluten is a type of protein found in most grains, cereals, and breads. It is composed of glutenins and gliadins, and gliadins are the activators of the symptoms of gluten intolerance. Rice and maize, for example, contain very few gliadins and although buckwheat is not in the grass family and millet is closer to the rice family, both contain prolamines, which are similar to the gliadins in wheat and therefore also trigger the symptoms of coeliac disease.

The superfoods

Rice, brown rice, wild rice, rice cakes, amaranth, quinoa, sorghum, mealie meal, samp and usually millet, but check each one by having a little at a time. Buckwheat greens are valuable. Include beans, nuts, seeds like flaxseed, pumpkin seed, sesame seed and fresh fruits and fresh vegetables in abundance. Bananas and papaya and papino are particularly good for babies and children. Choose lean white meats, fish and eggs and organically raised chicken.

Check if juiced wheat grass and barley grass are acceptable, as these are excellent energy foods with carrots, beetroot, apple, fresh lucerne leaves and flowers, and parsley.

Interestingly, the protein-digesting enzyme in papaya and papino known as papain has the ability to break down gluten. So including papaya in the diet would be beneficial and a papain supplement, usually 500–1000 mg taken with meals – ask your pharmacist – has often been found to be helpful.

Do not neglect taking a vitamin B-complex supplement. Vitamin B6 is particularly valuable, also zinc, spirulina and green foods like avocados, leafy green vegetables, kale, broccoli, lettuce, spinach, sweet potato leaves, beetroot leaves, alfalfa sprouts and mung beans.

Slippery elm powder for constipation is a soothing bowel treatment that has been found to be a great help through the decades. Ask your pharmacist to order it for you.

Cold Sores *see* Fever Blisters

Common Cold

The most debilitating, wretched and distressing common ailment has to be the common cold! And almost no one escapes it! In order to conquer it we need to boost and maintain a good immune system. Our bodies, under so much stress, with lack of sleep, too much sugar in the diet and lack of good ventilation, are under constant attack and succumb easily to the onset of the common cold.

Dry, sore throat, runny nose, sneezing, lethargy, dull headache, aching body, discomfort are the initial symptoms.

The danger foods

Sugar, sugar, sugar! Chocolates and sweets, carbonated drinks, white bread, sugary buns, cakes, biscuits, fast foods, fatty foods, salty snacks, chips, crisps, dairy products and alcohol.

The superfoods

Chicken soup – this is not just a fable, it is the first line of defence (see box for recipe!). Eat lots of salads, also wheat and barley grass juiced with celery, lucerne, parsley, carrots, apples and beetroot. Add fresh radishes and green peppers to the salad and dress with a squeeze of fresh lemon juice.

Chicken Soup for a Cold

Take one organic chicken, cut into pieces, and brown in a little olive oil with lots of onions, leeks and garlic. Add grated carrots, thinly shredded organically grown cabbage, especially the dark green outer leaves, kale, broccoli, grated sweet potato, split peas or fresh peas, chopped green peppers, and season with lots of chopped celery, parsley, lemon juice, cayenne pepper, and a grinding of sea salt. (If you enjoy hot chilli, add some chopped finely.)

Add chicken stock and simmer until the chicken is tender. Have a big bowl for lunch and for dinner.

Herbal teas – ginger, peppermint, thyme, sage and mullein (*Verbascum thapsus*) – are helpful taken at intervals through the day, one cup of each per day, and only one herb at a time. (¼ cup herb to 1 cup boiling water.) Ginger slices with honey and lemon juice are particularly soothing, especially for a cough.

Drink lots of water and stay in bed for at least 2 days. Sleep is the best treatment, and if you eat only fresh fruits and vegetables and that famous chicken soup, your cold can be gone in 4 days!

Steam blocked sinuses with eucalyptus oil – about 10 drops added to a bowl of boiling water and make a towel tent over the head. Close your eyes and inhale the steam.

Increase your vitamin C intake substantially, up to 5 000 mg through the day with food; also zinc and vitamin A for the first 3 days then stop (do not take vitamin A if you are pregnant).

Tissue Salts: No. 1, 2, 3, 4, 5, 7 and 9 (take 2 of each, up to 6–8 times a day for 4 days).

Caution: Consult with your doctor before you embark on any form of self-diagnosis or self-treatment.

> ### The Value of Vitamin D
> Increasing vitamin D daily throughout the winter is as effective as the 'flu injection. Research has proven that vitamin D's effectiveness protects against all strains of 'flu and is important for adults as well as children who come in contact with many strains of 'flu in the workplace and in the classroom. There are three forms of vitamin D and vitamin D3 is the most effective form of vitamin D. Speak to your doctor about it.

Conception

Too much stress is part of all our lives and for young people today tension, stress and anxiety often show up as the 'inability to conceive', but with a healthy eating plan the impact on the reproductive system can be often dramatically improved. Malnutrition is a word that is used in many instances, but for young people ready to start a family it is not often considered. The nutritional state of both men and women in the six months before conception is vital to their health as well as the health of the foetus (see Pregnancy, page 256). A sound and careful diet and, under your doctor's supervision, the right vitamin and mineral supplements can enhance fertility in both men and women.

The danger foods

Topping the list are the unhealthy fats – fatty meats, margarine, fried foods and snacks, fast foods – and the next is sugar (see pages 32 and 33 for more on sugar and fats). Cut down on sugar (change to stevia and a little honey only) and watch out for hidden sugars in fast foods and processed foods. Avoid refined carbohydrates in any form: white flour and white sugar drain energy and vitality, deplete vitamins, minerals and enzymes in the digestion process, and white flour has been stripped of all the health-boosting nutrients that are vital to the reproductive system (like vitamin E, zinc, magnesium for starters) that you cannot afford even a slice of white bread.

Avoid alcohol and caffeine in any form – coffee is the worst, especially instant coffee, but also tea (change to rooibos), cola drinks, carbonated drinks, chocolates and energy drinks. Alcohol and caffeine are the greatest danger when conception is being considered.

Cut down on meat, as meat is often full of hormones, steroids and antibiotics. Seek out free-range chicken, organic free-grazing mutton and cut out beef altogether. Remember, animal and chicken feeds are treated with a vast array of chemicals in order to keep the animals in 'good health' and to reach their market weight quickly. When trying to conceive, it is preferable to avoid all red meats and processed meats, and replace with free-range, grain-fed poultry, fish and legumes (especially chickpeas, see page 99).

Radiation is a very real presence. Avoid using the microwave even just to warm up food (especially milk, which is the worst!), or to defrost or cook food. Even sitting in front of the computer all day, or the television or keeping a cell phone in a pocket or under the pillow at night exposes the body to devastating radiation, often making conception impossible. Think about this and never be tempted to use it again.

The superfoods

Include lots of vegetables: carrots, green leafy vegetables, avocados, alfalfa sprouts and lucerne, fenugreek sprouts and leaves and sprouted mung beans, wheat grass and barley grass juices, peas – both sprouted and fresh green pods and leafy tips of the vines – onions, chives, spring onions, celery, parsley, baby spinach, green beans, green mealies, mustard greens, dandelion greens, lettuces, all members of cabbage family. Grow your own salad garden – the daily salad is vital and variety is important.

Include the following fruits: dates for sweetness, sun-dried raisins, lemons (oranges, naartjies and mandarins occasionally), apricots, peaches, cherries, all the berries, pineapple (delicious in salads), strawberries and figs, prunes and papaya daily to help the bowels stay regular.

Choose wholegrain foods: buckwheat, millet, whole wheat and wheat germ (rich in vitamin E), oats porridge daily (sprinkled with finely ground flaxseed, almonds, walnuts, sesame seed, sunflower seeds and pumpkin seeds), maize and mealie meal porridge or pancakes, or learn to make green mealie bread.

Snack on walnuts, hazelnuts, almonds, pumpkin seeds, chestnuts and cashew nuts but *avoid peanuts*! Make soups with lentils, chickpeas, butter beans, black-eyed beans, haricot beans, split peas, sweet potatoes, pumpkins and all the greens you can find, like celery, parsley, turnips and turnip tops, mustard leaves. Make it fresh twice a week and keep extra in the fridge for quick snacks or lunches and have a cup of your own soup mid-morning when energy flags.

Avoid all processed foods: learn to bake your own bread and to make your own sauces, mayonnaises, fruit smoothies and drinks. Wheat and barley grass juiced with organic carrots, beetroot, celery, parsley, lucerne sprigs, apples and pineapple is a fabulous daily tonic. Invest in a good quality juicer (I use the Oscar juicer) to process the wheat and barley grass – it is so worth it! Use only extra virgin olive oil and, if you can get it, cold pressed sunflower oil and flaxseed oil.

Eat free-range eggs only, and oily fish like mackerel, sardines, salmon and tofu (soya bean curd).

Tissue Salts: All 12 (can be bought as 'Combin 12') twice a day.

Conjunctivitis *see* Eye Ailments

Constipation

Our bowels need to work every day – even better, twice a day – without straining. If you do not have a regular bowel movement or if you need to sit on the toilet for a long time trying to press out something, it means your liver is also congested and this can be the beginning of a battle for good health.

Symptoms are sluggish bowels due to poor eating habits, hard stools that often are painful to evacuate, haemorrhoids (piles). The main causes of constipation are not drinking enough water, lack of exercise and lack of fresh fruits and vegetables in the diet.

The danger foods

Sugar, including sugary drinks, carbonated drinks, sweets, chocolates, white bread, biscuits, buns, bread rolls; fast foods; fatty foods, red meat and saturated fats; caffeine, especially instant coffee; sweetened custards, sweetened yoghurts, milkshakes and milk; spicy hot foods.

Caution: Consult with your doctor before you embark on any form of self-diagnosis or self-treatment.

The superfoods

Soaked prunes, papayas, papinos, mangoes, soaked flaxseed, ground flaxseed, flaxseed oil. Interestingly, 5 soaked prunes (soak overnight in a little warm water) with the water in which they were soaked and mashed into a cup of papaya (or mashed into plain yoghurt) with 1 tablespoon crushed flaxseed or 1 tablespoon psyllium husks, has remained the favourite breakfast of those who have really struggled with constipation.

Fruit smoothies with mango, papaya, peaches, or apples and carrots with celery, or strawberries and papaya and nectarines, or soaked prunes with pears, etc.

Include lots of fresh fruits daily, and your own freshly squeezed fruit juices about three times a week. Eat vegetables daily: raw and steamed, especially cabbage, kale, radishes, cauliflower, broccoli, dandelion leaves; also vegetable soups made with pumpkin, marrows, spinach, cabbage, kale, beans and chickpeas – have a big bowl every day.

Eat high-fibre foods like brown rice, oats (not the instant kind), buckwheat, pumpkin seeds, sesame seeds, bran (in homemade breads), and plain Bulgarian yoghurt for its balancing of the beneficial bacteria in the digestive tract.

Drink at least 6 glasses of water a day. Herb teas of fenugreek or nettle are also helpful.

Speak to your doctor about supplements: magnesium is excellent at night; also vitamin B-complex, vitamin C, spirulina and psyllium husks.

Tissue Salts: No. 1, 3, 9, 11 and 12 (2 of each taken twice a day).

Constipation Remedy

Many years ago while working in a big hospital, a doctor gave us this recipe for the patients he sent to us in the physiotherapy department. It was so helpful to everyone and I share it with you here as it helps to train the bowel to become regular. Take it for breakfast each morning – all of it – then after 10 days take it alternate days for 10 days. Thereafter twice a week for 2 weeks and finally once a week for a month and by then most patients had regular daily good bowel movements.

2 tablespoons each: digestive bran, skim milk powder and sunflower cooking oil. Mix everything together and eat with mashed papaya, grated apple or soaked prunes, sprinkled with sesame seeds, or mixed into oats porridge sprinkled with crushed flaxseed, served with plain Bulgarian yoghurt with a touch of honey.

Corns and Calluses

Thickening of the skin on the feet or on the hands due to excessive manual work can be caused by wearing badly fitting shoes or by pressure or by excess acidity. Strangely enough, it is the body's acidity that actually makes those painful hot and inflamed corns, a debilitating and often crippling nuisance (see also page 209 for more on dealing with acidity)!

The danger foods

Wheat is considered to be the big culprit, so avoid bread, cakes, buns and sugary biscuits; also fast foods, spicy foods, carbonated drinks, alcohol, instant coffee and sugar.

The superfoods

Include in the daily diet: sunflower seeds, nuts (walnuts, pecan nuts, almonds, cashew nuts, macadamia nuts), avocados, oily fish like mackerel for the essential fatty acids, sprouts (especially alfalfa, buckwheat and millet), lots of fresh raw fruit to clear the acidity, artichokes (both Jerusalem and globe artichokes) and lots of green vegetables.

A daily salad of greens is vital – lettuce, spinach, thinly shredded kale or cabbage, dandelion leaves, buckwheat leaves, lucerne leaves, parsley, celery, fennel. Mix and serve with fresh lemon juice and crushed coriander leaves, seeds and flowers.

Use apple cider vinegar as a salad dressing and drink a teaspoon of apple cider vinegar in a glass of water every day – I find it very refreshing on a hot afternoon served with ice.

Tissue Salts: No. 2, 8 and especially No. 10, which is an acid neutraliser.

A footbath to soften the corns can be made with ½ a cup of Epsom salts with ½ a cup of apple cider vinegar in enough warm water to cover the feet. Relax for 15–20 minutes.

Softening Massage Oil

1 tablespoon almond oil
2 teaspoons vitamin E oil
1 teaspoon pure lavender essential oil

Mix well and massage into the hard sore areas daily after your bath. This will help to soften and soothe. Visit a chiropodist once you have softened the corns and calluses.

Cramp

There is no pain quite like a middle of the night cramp that pulls the feet and legs into such tight spasm you don't know where to put yourself! Causes include either not enough exercise or too much exercise, poor circulation, dehydration, vitamin and mineral deficiencies especially lack of magnesium, old age, pregnancy or certain medications.

The danger foods

Seriously, if you have constant painful cramps, you need to look at the diet. Avoid coffee, especially instant coffee, and tea. Replace tea with rooibos tea or herb teas. Avoid all alcohol, sugary carbonated drinks, sweets, chocolates, cakes, buns and doughnuts, and lessen the sugar in every way you can. Replace with stevia.

The superfoods

Nuts (almonds, pecans, walnuts) and seeds (sesame, pumpkin, sunflower, flaxseed); include lots of green fresh salads – especially parsley, celery, mustard greens, rocket, watercress, cabbage, broccoli, kale, dandelion leaves, turnips, amaranth, buckwheat leaves; lots of legumes (lentils, peas and beans in as many varieties as you can); and lots of fresh fruit like apples, kiwifruit, berries of all kinds, bananas, peaches, plums, melons, cherries, grapes (and the vine tips and tendrils).

Beetroot and carrot, celery and parsley, apple and peach juices with wheat and barley grass are excellent.

Make fresh ginger tea sweetened with a touch of honey, oat straw tea, red clover tea and include fresh chopped basil and fennel and parsley mixed with a little olive oil, cayenne pepper and garlic and lemon juice every day with your salad.

Caution: Consult with your doctor before you embark on any form of self-diagnosis or self-treatment.

Speak to your doctor about supplements: magnesium or a combination of calcium and magnesium, which works well.

Tissue Salts: To ease the pains in the legs tissue salts can be given frequently through the day. No. 8 (Mag.Phos.) is especially effective and just 2 under the tongue every 5 minutes will immediately ease away the cramps. Also helpful are No. 2, 4 and 6.

Cramps in Children

Little children often wake at night with cramp-like pains in the legs. Our grandmothers referred to this as growing pains, but we need to take notice and realise this is a sure sign of mineral deficiencies like magnesium, manganese, zinc, calcium and even the B-vitamins like vitamin B6. Talk to your doctor about this, as these deficiencies could lead to spine problems like scoliosis and hip problems later on as the child grows. Include Tissue Salts daily.

Crohn's Disease

In a nutshell, Crohn's disease is a chronic inflammatory condition of the whole digestive tract which flares up every now and then, causing flatulence, bloating, indigestion, colic and abdominal cramps, both diarrhoea and constipation, weight loss and lethargy, discomfort and depression.

The diet needs to be carefully monitored as there could be food intolerances, an imbalance of the good bowel bacteria – so probiotics could be considered – and even nutrient deficiencies. Stress can trigger this easily, as well as emotional upsets and anger and feelings of rejection. Steroids and anti-inflammatory drugs seemed to be prescribed frequently but today a wheat-free, dairy-free, sugar-free diet is a better way to go, choosing organically grown foods or growing your own wherever this is possible.

The danger foods

Avoid the following with great care and dedication, never allowing yourself to slip up: gluten-rich breads, cakes, pastries, pies, biscuits, etc.; dairy products, as lactose intolerance is a big factor; yeasts – so no products like pizzas or bread rolls, even 'health breads' that have yeast in them; sugar; citrus fruits and tomatoes; too much salt (replace salt with a mixture of celery seeds, dried home-grown thyme, oregano and coriander seed). Avoid all carbonated drinks, alcohol, processed foods, additives, artificial sweeteners (use stevia leaves instead), pickles, spreads, vinegars, commercial sauces. Make your own with mint and coriander, caraway seeds and cumin seeds.

The superfoods

Flaxseed; herbal teas: oat straw tea, mint tea (try different kinds of mint), melissa tea, chamomile tea, ginger slices in tea, and grated ginger – just a little in the food.

Freshly squeezed juices: carrot, apple, beetroot and celery with parsley, and fresh pineapple for its bromelain compounds.

Talk to your doctor about supplements: vitamin B-complex, spirulina and probiotics with acidophilus and bifido bacteria (these are the beneficial bacteria the digestive system needs for good working order and they also regulate bowel movements).

Tissue Salts: No. 2, 8, 10 and 12 taken 3–5 times a day.

Yoga has been found to be extremely helpful in many cases of Crohn's disease, to reduce stress and anxiety.

Keep a notebook on food preferences and intolerances – this will become your own personal health diary, making Crohn's disease something of the past.

Cystitis

This painful inflammation of the urinary tract and bladder is caused by a bacterial infection. Symptoms are frequent intensely burning urination and pain in the bladder area. Thrush can be the cause or, if cystitis is chronic, it could be part of the problem, or a bacterial infection. In men enlargement of the prostate gland could cause the irritation and pain and slow urination, and dehydration could add to the discomfort.

The danger foods

Spices and spicy food, alcohol, acidic foods, fruit juices, coffee, tea, processed foods (study the list of ingredients on all processed foods and avoid preservatives, stabilisers, emulsifiers, colourants, flavourants and sweeteners), refined carbohydrates, sugar, milk, ice-creams, sweetened yoghurts, milkshakes, all soft drinks, especially carbonated colas and bright orange cool drinks, energy drinks, even chlorinated water, and avoid, at this time, swimming in a chlorinated pool.

Chillies and pepper will further irritate the already inflamed mucous membranes; also avoid red meat, asparagus, spinach, potatoes, tomatoes, strawberries and citrus fruits.

The superfoods

Alkaline urine and dehydration caused by excess ammonia being flushed out of the body due to an acid-forming diet are risk factors – so during this time concentrate on bland foods: brown rice, millet, oats, barley and barley water (see recipe on page 135). Avoid all acidic fruits and vegetables and stick with the bland ones like pears, papaya, kiwifruit, sweet potatoes, onions (boiled, for their antibiotic properties). Also include lettuce, parsley, fenugreek, dandelion, cinnamon, ginger, celery, beetroot, carrots, squashes, su-su and green beans.

Cranberries, blueberries and sugar-free cranberry and blueberry juice can be helpful. Drink lots of filtered water, at least 2 litres a day. A drink of 2 teaspoons of apple cider vinegar in a glass of water is beneficial; also add a dash or two of apple cider vinegar to the bath.

Talk to your doctor about supplements: vitamin C, E and A (but not if you are pregnant). If you need to go onto an antibiotic, take a good probiotic with it. The enzyme bromelain found in pineapples is also helpful, but pineapples may be too acidic. Sometimes you can find bromelain supplements – so ask your chemist.

Tissue Salts: No. 4, 5, 7, 10 and 12. Take No. 7, 11 and 12 if there is a yellow discharge. Take 2 of each 6–8 times a day.

Use a non-scented soap, and avoid bubble baths and bath oils, wipes, deodorants; avoid tight-fitting jeans or slacks at this time, and wear cotton underwear. Exercise helps to activate the immune system but gentle walking is best at this time. If there is no improvement within 48 hours, see your doctor. Watch out for nausea, fever and pain over the kidneys. Keep a food diary, as certain foods can worsen the condition.

Dandruff

Surprisingly, dandruff – those little flakes of dried skin that accumulate on the scalp and hair with often oily hair – could

---

Caution: Consult with your doctor before you embark on any form of self-diagnosis or self-treatment.

be caused by a fungal infection or a vitamin deficiency or a hormonal imbalance. In spite of all the hype around antidandruff shampoos, just using a shampoo often will not get rid of the problem, but eating correctly will!

The danger foods
Sugar, refined carbohydrates, carbonated drinks especially bright orange drinks, alcohol, yeast and dairy products (these can increase the activity of the fungal condition), fast foods, processed foods, will all aggravate the problem.

The superfoods
Eat sunflower seeds, pumpkin seeds, sesame seeds, flaxseed daily – sprinkle finely ground onto oats porridge or over millet or brown rice, at least 3 tablespoons a day.

Include spinach, Swiss chard, fresh lucerne and alfalfa sprouts in the diet with raw garlic, soya beans and edamame (fresh, green soya beans), Brazil nuts, broccoli, mushrooms, oily and white fish, cabbage, kale, Jerusalem artichokes, chicory and sweet potatoes. Many of these foods contain zinc and biotin, which help to stop the formation of dandruff cells on the scalp. Make your own juices from fresh fruits.

Tissue Salts: No. 3, 5, 7, 10 and 12 (2 of each taken daily).

Talk to your doctor about supplements: zinc, selenium vitamin C and probiotics, which repopulate the digestive system with good bacteria.

Dandruff Remedies
Interestingly, our grandmothers used **plain yoghurt** to massage into the scalp. After shampooing once and rinsing, cover the head with a square of plastic to keep the yoghurt in place and then wrap in a towel. Leave on for 15–20 minutes then rinse in warm water to which a **rosemary infusion** has been added: boil 3–4 cups of rosemary sprigs in 2 litres of water for 20 minutes. Cool until pleasantly warm. Strain, add to the rinsing water and soak the hair and the scalp in it, massaging it gently in.

Another helpful treatment is **flaxseed oil**. Shampoo the hair once, then work in 1 tablespoon of flaxseed oil into which 1 teaspoon of tea tree oil has been mixed into the scalp. Massage in gently and thoroughly, cover with plastic and a towel for 15–20 minutes, then shampoo it out.

A shampoo and conditioner with **tea tree oil** in it and no harsh chemicals (parabens, petrochemicals, etc.) is helpful. Also add a little **apple cider vinegar** to the final rinsing water.

Depression
Is this debilitating sense of helplessness and despondency a sign of the times as it is so prevalent and so common an ailment in this century? Symptoms include mood swings, crying, lack of motivation, lack of self-worth, lack of energy and vitality, lack of interest, a deep sadness, not finding pleasure in anything.

Causes can include shock, bereavement, a major life change (loss of a loved one, divorce, losing a job or home), illness, alcoholism, thyroid problems, adrenal exhaustion, liver problems, vitamin deficiencies, especially the B-vitamins, emotional stress, some medications, low blood sugar, hereditary ailments, poor diet,

especially too much sugar (chocoholics beware!) and even seasonal affective disorder or SAD where the lack of sunlight, especially in fluorescent-lit buildings with air conditioning, is a factor. There could be many other factors – your doctor must examine you thoroughly!

The danger foods
Alcohol, caffeine, especially instant coffee, sugar, cakes, biscuits, sweets in any form, diet drinks, carbonated drinks, energy drinks, fast foods, fried foods, processed foods (anything with additives – artificial sweeteners, flavourants, colourants, stabilisers and preservatives). Interestingly, it is being found more and more that chemical additives actually depress the vital forces within the body.

The superfoods
Blackberries, raspberries (make a berry hedge in your garden as even the leaves are positively health boosting), black and red grapes, strawberries, blueberries. Make your own sun-dried raisins for the winter along with raspberries, strawberries and apple slices (see also page 23).

Wheat grass or barley grass juice with carrots, beetroot, fresh lucerne, parsley and apples daily – at least 2 tots (it is essential to buy a good juicer that can process the grass) and made fresh every time you need it.

The daily salad is vital, made with all the organically grown greens you can find: dandelion leaves, rocket leaves, watercress, fennel, turnip roots and leaves, buckwheat leaves and flowers, parsley, avocado, broccoli, kale leaves thinly shredded, radishes and radish leaves.

Also flaxseed, sunflower seeds, sesame seeds and pumpkin seeds (these can be finely ground, see page 26), Brazil nuts, almonds, cashew nuts, walnuts, mangoes (fresh and home-dried, not with sulphur), dates, kohlrabi, tomatoes, potatoes, sweet potatoes and leaves, lentils, chickpeas, peas and pea tendrils, beans of all kinds. Make soups with beans, peas, lentils, pumpkin, sweet potatoes, cabbage, cauliflower, celery and parsley.

Include fish in the diet – cut down on red meat and go two days a week on a vegetarian diet. Eat chicken, bananas, wheat germ, brown rice and eggs often (these foods contain beneficial enzymes which lift the mood). Flavour foods with cumin, ginger, cardamom, freshly ground black pepper, basil, rosemary, fresh bay leaves, celery and fennel seeds.

Speak to your doctor about supplements: selenium, spirulina, omega-3 fatty acids and vitamin B-complex. Milk thistle, St John's Wort, gingko biloba, stinging nettle tea and pennywort (*Centella asiatica*) are excellent mood lifters.

Tissue Salts: No. 2, 4, 6, 9 and 11 (2 of each at least 3 times a day).

Eat small meals often – just a salad and a cup of herb tea are often enough – and keep a food diary. Mood swings can be stabilised by a handful of nuts or a smoothie of fruit and nuts or a tot of wheat grass juice. Get to be a clever eater – food and mood go hand in hand!

Dermatitis *see* Eczema

Diabetes
Today diabetes mellitus – which is high blood sugar – is quite commonplace, even, shockingly, in dogs! It is caused by an

---

Caution: Consult with your doctor before you embark on any form of self-diagnosis or self-treatment.

insufficient supply of the important hormone insulin, or by the body's inability to efficiently use the insulin that is produced. The body is unable to regulate the blood sugar and glucose levels go haywire – as a result glucose is not moved from the bloodstream into the cells. Raised blood glucose levels can be destructive, leading to complications in the heart and circulation, the kidneys and the eyes in particular.

What are Type 1 and Type 2 Diabetes?

Type 1 Diabetes is insulin dependent and requires the person to inject with insulin daily or several times a day. Often known as juvenile-onset diabetes, this is where the pancreas cannot manufacture insulin. It affects both adults and children. This type of diabetes needs a carefully monitored diet plus monitored exercise daily.

Type 2 Diabetes or late- or adult-onset diabetes usually occurs in adults over 40 years of age. Also called obesity-related diabetes, today's over-indulged diet of sweets and refined carbohydrates and sweetened carbonated drinks has resulted in many young people being diagnosed with Type 2 Diabetes. In this form of diabetes the pancreas is still able to produce insulin but the body is unable to utilise it, or the pancreas is unable to produce enough insulin. It is normally treated with medication or, sometimes if needed, with injections. With an extra careful diet, exercise and weight loss, Type 2 Diabetes can be lessened or even reversed.

Symptoms include fatigue, irritability, blurred vision, constant thirst and frequent rushing to urinate, excessive hunger, wounds that heal slowly, numbness in the feet and sluggish circulation.

The risks of getting diabetes are being overweight and over-indulging in sugar and sugar-laden foods. High blood pressure and high cholesterol also pose risks, as do long periods of severe and unrelenting stress, poor diet and lack of exercise.

Caution

Please consult with your doctor before following any of the dietary or other advice offered here!

The danger foods

Everything and anything that contains sugar! Read labels and choose foods that say 'unsweetened' or 'no sugar added' or 'natural sweetener'. Watch out for hidden sugars – things like lactose (which is a milk sugar), golden syrup, honey, treacle, maple syrup, glucose, maltose, dextrose and fructose (which is fruit sugar). Be careful of dried fruits and fruit juice and glacé fruit, as these are high in sugar. Avoid all biscuits, cakes, buns and refined carbohydrates like white flour and white rice – these will all raise the blood sugar too fast. Avoid fried foods and cut down on saturated fats like those found in meat and dairy foods. Do not skip meals. It is essential to eat small meals frequently.

Cut down on salt and use herbs or a salt substitute (see page 35) to flavour foods. Kick the caffeine habit – coffee, tea, cola and energy drinks. Avoid alcohol and do not smoke. Avoid all carbonated drinks.

The superfoods

Wholegrain cereals, like brown rice and wild rice, oats (the non-instant kind), whole wheat (choose home-baked brown and seed breads – see page 35). Vegetables (raw or lightly steamed); when eating 'sweet' vegetables like carrots, beetroot, parsnips or potatoes serve them with low-GI foods like beans, chickpeas or lentils so that the sugars in them are released slowly (see also page 29). Eat onions, courgettes, apples, asparagus, garlic, soya beans, fish and beans (kidney beans, haricot beans, butter beans, mung beans and sprouts) – all these slow down the digestion of the carbohydrates preventing blood sugar spikes. Blackberries and blueberries are both low in sugar. Eat oily fish, steamed white fish, lots of dark, leafy vegetables, especially amaranth, dandelion, baby spinach and Swiss chard.

Flaxseed oil is excellent and ground flaxseed and nuts, like chestnuts, pecan nuts, almonds, walnuts, macadamias and sesame seeds, in small quantities take away the desire for something sweet.

Interestingly, prickly pear leaves or pads (the thorns carefully removed) have been found to reduce blood sugar levels. Slice thinly and serve as a vegetable with a little lemon juice at one meal during the day (they taste just like green beans!).

Take herb teas like pennywort (*Centella asiatica*), tulsi or sacred basil (*Ocimum tenuifolium*), stinging nettle (*Urtica dioica*) and include lots of cinnamon in the diet, and also cinnamon tea. Bitter melon in the diet is an age-old remedy.

Include supplements under your doctor's guidance: vitamins A, B-complex, C and E, magnesium, zinc, alpha-lipoic acid, sometimes chromium.

Tissue Salts: No. 9 and 11 in drop form; No. 8, 9 and 11 for late-onset diabetes, taken at least twice daily.

Get to know stevia! It is 300 times sweeter than sugar – a smallish leafy perennial with zero sugar in it. Its sweetness comes from 'stevicide', an enzyme within the leaves. It is an amazing herb that eases a number of conditions (see page 197).

Watch your weight, take daily exercise (walking, swimming, yoga, etc.), drink plenty of water, get enough sleep and watch your stress levels.

Diarrhoea

Commonly referred to as 'runny tummy', diarrhoea is characterised by frequent watery stools, tummy upsets and cramps. It may be caused by several things: food poisoning, food intolerances, gastritis, poor diet, traveller's diarrhoea (ingesting food or water that is contaminated with bacteria), overactive thyroid, chronic conditions like coeliac disease (see page 218), Crohn's disease (see page 222) or diverticulitis (see page 225), too much caffeine, too much sugar or an overloaded liver.

The danger foods

Alcohol, carbonated drinks, caffeine, especially instant coffee, dairy products, meat, rich fatty foods, fried foods, fast foods, spicy foods, processed foods and sugar.

The superfoods

Brown rice, oats or cooked dehusked buckwheat; bananas and a soft-boiled egg on toast with salt and no butter. Eat peeled raw grated apple that has been allowed to go brown.

Increase your fluid intake. Most important, drink plenty of water as you cannot allow your body to dehydrate. Drink juiced

Caution: Consult with your doctor before you embark on any form of self-diagnosis or self-treatment.

A–Z Ailment Chart

224

carrots, celery and apples or blueberry juice. Barley water and black rooibos tea are soothing and calming. Raspberry leaf tea and melissa or lemon balm (*Melissa officinalis*) are helpful as these herbs soothe the digestive tract beautifully.

Go on a strict bland diet for two days and it will give the whole digestive system time to rest. Take probiotics as a supplement to replace lost beneficial bacteria. If after 48 hours there has not been an improvement go to your doctor.

Tissue Salts: No. 3, 4, 8, 10 and 12; bad smelling – No. 6; sour smelling – No. 10; watery, painless – No. 9 and 11; yellow – No. 7 and 11 (2 of each taken frequently).

Diverticulitis

A debilitating and uncomfortable condition, diverticulitis is an inflammation of the small pouches that form in the membrane of the intestines. Waste products and partially processed and digested food accumulate within these pockets, stretching the bowel wall and causing discomfort and often intense inflammation. It usually occurs in people over fifty.

Both diarrhoea and constipation are experienced with bloating, flatulence, severe cramps and often fever. It has been suggested that diverticulitis is caused by smoking; also hot, spicy foods like chillies and curries; a diet low in fibre and high in refined foods and fatty foods.

The danger foods

Dairy and wheat products; sugar, spicy foods, processed foods, deep-fried and fatty foods, nuts, seeds, skins of fruits that can be caught in the pockets, some raw foods, and animal protein as it putrefies in the pockets.

The superfoods

Take herb teas of fennel, melissa, fresh ginger, elderflower, peppermint, chamomile, lemon verbena and stinging nettle (¼ cup fresh herb to 1 cup boiling water). Drink vegetable juices with wheat and barley grass, carrots, apples, celery, parsley, fresh lucerne leaves and flowers, buckwheat leaves and flowers. Make fresh apple purée with a little ginger and grape juice. Make vegetable soups and steamed mashed vegetables. Eat mashed papaya between meals and drink cranberry, blackberry and pomegranate juice.

Drink a lot of water and eat fresh fruit on an empty stomach. Millet and brown rice are good colon cleansers.

Keep a notebook on what fruits and vegetables irritate, for example grape skins or tomato pips or sesame seeds.

Speak to your doctor about supplements: probiotics, vitamins and minerals, especially vitamins A, C, E & K and zinc.

Tissue Salts: No. 3, 4, 8, 10 and 12 for diarrhoea; No. 1, 3, 9, 11 and 12 for constipation; No. 8 for cramps; No. 4 and 9 for fever.

Dry Skin *see* Skin Problems

Eczema

Sometimes known as **dermatitis**, eczema is a skin condition that shows as dry, patchy, often red, itchy and weepy, even inflamed, weals and rashes that can bleed if scratched. It varies in severity and all age groups can be affected by it. Eczema can usually be found on the neck, insides of the elbows, behind the knees, around the ankles and between the fingers, and it is worth getting tested for allergies – cow's milk, nuts, eggs, wheat, soya and shellfish are often the most common triggers. Eczema is also linked to yeast overgrowth, *Candida albicans*, so discuss this with your doctor.

Types of Eczema

Atopic chronic eczema is the most common eczema and is considered to be hereditary; other causes are allergens such as dust, pollen, animal hair or bird feathers, dietary allergic responses or an overactive immune response. Soaps and creams can intensify the condition and stress can exacerbate the condition. It is often accompanied by hay fever and asthma.

Allergic contact eczema is caused by allergic reactions to soaps, detergents, chemical additives in lotions, medications, creams and beauty products (shampoos and conditioners included), all of which can irritate sensitive skin. Washing powder used in the laundry can even cause a rash from the sheets or shirts washed – so systematic lists should be kept to ascertain what is causing the irritation.

Seborrhoeic dermatitis in infants, commonly known as cradle cap, is also a type of eczema and usually clears up within a few months. Adult seborrhoeic dermatitis can start on the scalp – as a dry dandruff – and can affect the ears and even the face.

Discoid dermatitis is a round spot of red itchy dry skin and usually appears on the legs.

The danger foods

Dairy products, fried foods, fatty foods, processed foods, fast foods, salty snacks, chips. Look carefully at hydrogenated fats and oils as these could intensify the condition. Avoid all caffeine, alcohol, sugary snacks, sweets and cakes. Cut down on red meat and salt and keep a food diary to list trigger foods.

The superfoods

Oily fish, mackerel and sardines are hugely beneficial. Eat lots of fresh fruits and vegetables. The daily salad is vitally important – include fresh lucerne or alfalfa sprouts, avocado, carrots, beetroot (raw and grated), celery, lettuce, green peppers, radishes and lots of fresh parsley. Apples and pears are excellent for the skin and freshly squeezed lemon juice is the perfect salad dressing.

Whole grains are essential, for instance non-instant oats (a soothing poultice can also be made of oat flakes soaked in hot water and applied to the area when comfortably warm, to relieve itchiness and rashes). Millet, sorghum, mealie meal and seeds such as sunflower seeds, flaxeed, sesame seeds, pumpkin seed, ground together and served over oats or mealie meal porridge daily, are excellent. Ground almonds or pecan nuts are excellent too if there are no allergic reactions to them.

A food diary is essential, especially for children.

Herb teas are hugely valuable, especially stinging nettle tea and pennywort tea (*Centella asiatica*) and the cooled unsweetened tea of both these herbs is a comforting lotion. Milk thistle tea (or supplements) to cleanse the liver is important and fresh fennel,

Caution: Consult with your doctor before you embark on any form of self-diagnosis or self-treatment.

aniseed and parsley tea with celery are excellent detoxifiers. Drink lots of water daily: 6–8 glasses are ideal.

Speak to your doctor about supplements: vitamin C, the B-vitamins, zinc, omega-3 fatty acids and evening primrose oil. Biotin and probiotics may help to reduce allergic reactions by maintaining bowel health.

Be extra careful in your choice of soaps, cosmetics and moisturising lotions. I have through the years perfected a chemical-free aqueous cream and lotion and a natural, chemical-free unscented soap, made from only palm oil, that has proved to be soothing and comforting (we post these countrywide; see the website margaretroberts.co.za).

Tissue Salts: No. 3, 6, 7, 10, 11; for chronic eczema, try No. 3, 5, 9; for itching and weeping try No. 9. Remember that crushed tissue salts mixed to a paste can be applied externally as well.

Emphysema

More and more people are becoming affected with emphysema due most often and with alarming frequency to smoking or even more worrying, passive smoking. The lungs have become compromised with lack of elasticity which aids the inhalation and the exhalation process. Also known as **chronic obstructive pulmonary disease**, emphysema is debilitating and as stale air cannot get out of the lungs and inhalation is impeded, breathlessness, coughing fits, intense distress and exhaustion make this a difficult condition to cope with. As a physiotherapist I was intensely involved with hospitalised emphysema patients and under the doctor's supervision breathing exercises were of the utmost importance to regain some mobility of the lungs.

The danger foods

Avoid all dairy products, processed and tinned foods, fried foods, red meat and processed meat, refined white flour, sugar, cakes, breads, junk food in any form – all these are mucus-producing which exacerbate the problem within the lungs. Stay away from carbonated drinks, tinned drinks, energy drinks, cool drinks, especially those preserved with sulphur dioxide or benzoic acid. Cut down on salt.

Avoid public places that are smoke-filled and avoid all chemicals in household cleaning products, air fresheners, perfumes, insect-repelling sprays, paint fumes, diesel fumes, all cosmetics with perfumes, talc powder, vacuum cleaners that exude dust, washing powders and solvents, dry-cleaning clothes – anything that may cause irritation to the lungs. Most important of all **never ever** smoke again or go near anyone who smokes!

The superfoods

Chlorophyll helps lung function, so look for everything green and use only fresh lemon juice with a touch of olive oil as a salad dressing. Include lettuce, lucerne and alfalfa sprouts, dandelion leaves, wheat grass and barley grass juice, spinach, broccoli, cabbage, cauliflower, radishes, fennel, rocket, salad leaves of all descriptions, including mustard, watercress, celery and parsley.

Eat lots of yellow and red fruits and vegetables too, like papaya, pumpkin, plums, radishes, apricots, figs, and so on. Fresh juiced carrot and beetroot with celery, apples, lucerne, wheat and barley grass and parsley is a must every day – at least ½ a glass, but even better ½ a glass morning and afternoon.

Add watercress in season and young lettuce leaves too! Drink mucous-reducing mullein (*Verbascum thapsus*) tea and at least 6 glasses of water daily. Speak to your doctor about supplements: coenzyme Q10, vitamins C and B-complex, magnesium, selenium, zinc and bioflavonoids.

Tissue Salts: No. 1 and 5 taken up to 10 times a day.

Endometriosis

Endometriosis is a chronic, often genetic, ailment that shows abnormalities of the inner layer of the uterus wall. I hesitated before writing on this ailment until I got a string of e-mails and phone calls, all begging for help! Most women had spent vast amounts of time and money going from specialist to specialist and all asked for a helpful diet. Ask your doctor to guide you carefully, as hormonal imbalance is a critical factor with possibly high oestrogen and low progesterone that is fluctuating and which needs to be monitored.

Symptoms are painful menstruation, excessive bleeding, lower back pain, bleeding between periods, sometimes rectal bleeding, constipation and painful bowel movements, difficulty in conceiving and painful tension during sex. The symptoms are often exacerbated by environmental toxins, stress, caffeine addiction, iodine deficiency, candida, liver ailments and tenderness around the abdomen.

The danger foods

Alcohol, red meat, white flour (beware of bought bread!), sugar (including cakes, biscuits and sugary drinks, especially carbonated drinks), energy drinks, diet drinks and all types of coffee – these all hinder the absorption of valuable minerals. Be careful of dairy products – keep a careful list here as most dairy could cause allergic reactions. Plain Bulgarian yoghurt may be favourable. Avoid tinned foods, fast foods, fried foods, processed foods, especially salty snacks – too much salt will add to the discomfort. Cut down on salt and use herbs instead for flavouring.

The superfoods

The secret is to eat as consistently and carefully as you possibly can, choosing organic, natural foods. Focus on magnesium-rich foods: leafy green vegetables, lightly steamed or raw in salads – spinach, kale, cabbage, dandelion leaves, celery, Swiss chard, lettuce, watercress, parsley, lucerne leaves and alfalfa sprouts, broccoli, Brussels sprouts, cauliflower, salad greens, mustard leaves, turnip leaves – also artichokes, avocados, lemons, apples, figs, plums, prunes, nuts like Brazil nuts, cashew nuts, almonds, macadamia nuts.

Beta-carotene is essential, so include the bright red, yellow and orange fruits and vegetables daily: sweet peppers, pumpkins, squash and pineapple (which is an excellent anti-inflammatory food and a good digestive), sweet potatoes, carrots, apricots, peaches, cherries, strawberries, blueberries, raspberries, gooseberries.

Include legumes such as soya beans, lentils, peas and beans of all kinds (broad beans, black-eyed beans, haricot beans, etc.), also seeds (flaxseed and flaxseed oil, pumpkin seeds), brown rice, millet, oats, ginger and turmeric. Learn to bake your own bread and go carefully with wheat flour. Try baking with mealie meal, potato flour and rice flour.

Caution: Consult with your doctor before you embark on any form of self-diagnosis or self-treatment.

Get to grow and enjoy herb teas like red clover tea, basil tea (especially tulsi or sacred basil), mullein tea (*Verbascum thapsus*), lemongrass tea and rose geranium tea. Standard brew: ¼ cup fresh leaves to 1 cup boiling water, stand 5 minutes, strain and sip slowly.

Check for iodine deficiency and if so, add seaweed to soups and stews (seaweed is used in sushi and can be found in Chinese or speciality food shops). Take the B-vitamins daily (a good B-complex capsule is essential), and magnesium and zinc supplements are valuable – your doctor will guide you. Take probiotics to help get the 'good' bacteria into the digestive system.

Wear cotton underwear and do not dry-clean your clothes – the chemicals used in dry-cleaning may cause allergic reactions.

As a physiotherapist I found a gentle abdominal and lower back massage helped to release pain and discomfort. Light and slow, in circular movements eased the tension. Using lavender oil diluted in almond oil, warmed by placing the bottle in hot water, helped to break up adhesions and soothed and comforted the patient. Consider this with a physiotherapist under your doctor's supervision and remember stress adds to the discomfort!

Tissue Salts: No. 1, 2, 4, 5, 6, 7, 8 and 9 taken frequently.

Epilepsy

Epilepsy is an almost electrical-like spasmodic disturbance of energy that causes a seizure at any time, with loss of consciousness. The doctor needs to monitor any epileptic patient on a regular basis, but there are foods that can help to build up the health.

Types of Epileptic Seizures

Petit mal seizures are lighter, smaller fits often characterised by the person staring into space, completely unaware of what is happening around him or her and not responding. These smaller seizures last about a minute and are most often caused by outside stimuli – a flickering TV or computer screen, stress, fatigue, even sugar overload.

Grand mal and temperate lobe seizures are more severe and they, too, can be triggered by heat, noise and confusion, crowds and action, flashes from cameras, sugar overload, stress overload and frights or shocks.

The danger foods

Alcohol of any description, coffee, tea, sugar, artificial sweeteners, diet drinks, refined foods, fried foods, sugary cakes, biscuits, instant foods, energy drinks.

Very important: pesticides, sprays for ants, mosquitoes and flies, chemical additives, cleaning materials, solvents, air fresheners, soaps, perfumes and cosmetics that are rich in chemical additives. All these seriously and dangerously affect the central nervous system. Become diligent, aware and informed in your choices. Also avoid smoking and passive smoking!

The superfoods

Choose organic foods and grow your own wherever possible. Grow all the fruits and vegetables you can. Start with lettuce, spinach, dandelion leaves, kale, cabbage, radishes and their leaves, mustard leaves, celery, parsley and watercress. All these are vital for their magnesium content, as magnesium steadies and calms the nervous system. Grow beans, lentils and chickpeas for their potassium content. Grow your own grapes, melons, papayas and berries – make a berry hedge and plant strawberries, granadillas and kiwifruit. Make it a mission to create a wellness garden, and plant the companion plants next to each other so that no pesticides are used.

Include nuts and seeds in the diet: sunflower seeds, pumpkin seeds, sesame seeds, hazelnuts, pecan nuts, macadamia nuts, Brazil nuts and cashew nuts – they all are rich in vitamin E, which can reduce the occurrence of the attacks. Replace salty snacks with these unsalted nuts and seeds. Also include sesame oil, grape seed oil and olive oil with lemon juice and fresh chopped herbs for salads and eat unsweetened fruit salads daily. Cut down on salt and use thyme, coriander leaves and seeds, oregano and celery to flavour the food.

Eat a bowl of oats (not instant oats) daily for breakfast and have a cup of aniseed tea mid-morning. And have melissa (lemon balm) or chamomile tea to reduce stress levels.

Do not cook in aluminium pots and do not cook in aluminium foil or cover foods with it. Aluminium can upset brain function. Add a cup of Epsom salts to the bath on alternate nights to help increase the magnesium in the body. Use a loofah to gently scrub off dead cells and relax in the warm water for a while.

Speak to your doctor about supplements: the B-vitamins, vitamin E, magnesium and in some cases coenzyme Q10 can be of great value.

Tissue Salts: No. 4, 6 and 12. Take 2 of each at least 6 times a day. Avoid No. 12 if you have implants.

Eye Ailments

Always be extra careful of your eyes. Do not put anything into them unless it is prescribed by your doctor, not even drops for red, sore or tired eyes.

Bloodshot eyes

The inflamed whites of the eyes could be caused by irritation or allergy to pollen, dust or air pollution, eyestrain from working at the computer, rubbing itchy eyelids, stress, overwork, fatigue, hangover, high blood pressure, high cholesterol, too much reading late at night.

The danger foods

Alcohol, fatty foods, fried foods, foods that cause allergic reactions like peanuts, certain fish, very rich foods, sugary foods, cakes, buns, white bread, sweetened carbonated drinks, too much meat, fat and alcohol, especially at a braai!

The superfoods

Berries of all kinds will benefit the eyes. Vegetable juice of cucumber, celery, parsley, melon, beetroot and carrots with fresh wheat grass and barley grass acts as an eye cleanser and revitaliser. Include salads and fruit salads to detoxify the body. Drink lots of water and have a daily cup of stinging nettle tea.

Stay away from alcohol for at least a week to give your system time to clear and eat only salads, fruit salads and vegetable soups (homemade with no flavourants).

Tissue Salts: No. 4 and 6.

Caution: Consult with your doctor before you embark on any form of self-diagnosis or self-treatment.

Cataracts

Cataracts are opaque, cloudy blemishes over the lens of the eye that build up slowly and can appear at any age. Age-related or senile cataracts often appear when the body's normal protection from free radicals is diminished. Loss of vision can be slow in forming or it can happen relatively fast with obvious progressive cloudiness over the eyes. If you experience blurred vision, loss of vision or partial loss of detail and colour, have your eyes checked, for cataracts are the major cause of blindness but can be successfully treated if diagnosed early.

Causes include ageing, vitamin deficiencies (especially vitamin B2), diabetes, too much sunlight exposure, smoking or exposure to cigarette smoke, poor lighting in the workplace, poor diet and lack of antioxidants, and it can even be hereditary.

The danger foods

Fast foods, sugar and sugary foods, too much salt, junk foods of every description! Cut down on sugar and avoid preservatives, processed foods, carbonated drinks, energy drinks, alcohol (not even a glass of wine!), saturated fats, margarines, rancid foods and fried foods, milkshakes, dairy foods (in some cases the milk protein is not easily absorbed and processed).

The superfoods

Foods high in antioxidants: leafy greens – cabbage, spinach, celery, lettuce, fennel leaves, parsley, lucerne leaves, red clover leaves, broccoli and broccoli leaves, kale and sweet potato and its leaves; also avocado, carrots, beetroot, tomatoes, cucumber, pumpkins, squashes, apricots, pomegranates, cherries. Eat two fresh salads daily, dressed with freshly squeezed lemon juice and a little olive oil, and also fruit salads that include oranges, pineapple, apples, pears, melons, mangoes, papayas, lots of berries – all kinds, but especially blackberries and blueberries – grapes, prickly pears, kiwifruit, and so on. Sometimes there is a vitamin C and E deficiency, so include foods rich in these vitamins in the diet (see page 13).

Eat leafy greens, spinach, peas and pea leaves and tendrils, rocket, mustard, lettuce, kale, as all these contain the essential compound lutein, which is needed for eye health. Add turmeric to the diet every day. Have a cup of pennywort (*Centella asiatica*) tea daily, as well as gingko biloba tea or supplements for good blood circulation. These herbs also act as an excellent tonic for the eye. Also include cooked chickpeas, sprouts and wheat and barley grass juice with carrot, beetroot, apples, celery, parsley and lucerne every day.

To prevent the formation of cataracts, it is important to keep up the levels of glutathione, which is found in strong concentration in the lens of the eye where it acts as an antioxidant. This can be done by eating plenty of fresh fruits and vegetables daily – the glutathione levels in these foods is high and immediately available to the body. Dark glasses from your optician are important.

Speak to your doctor about supplements: particularly vitamin C (at least 1 000 mg a day but up to 3 000 mg per day), vitamin E (600 iu per day), wheat germ oil, selenium, beta-carotene (400 µg per day).

Tissue Salts: No. 2, 6, 9 and 12 (take 2 of each, 3–6 times a day).

Conjunctivitis or Pink Eye

This is a highly contagious infection with swollen red eyelids, itchiness, weepy eyes and generally irritating and debilitating, caused often by a bacterial or viral infection, an allergic reaction or even certain vitamin deficiencies if it recurs frequently.

The danger foods

Every kind of junk food consumed, which includes fast foods, sweetened carbonated drinks, synthetic orange juice, chocolates, sweets, crisps, also refined carbohydrates, sugar and white flour – all of these undermine and compromise the immune system.

The superfoods

Fresh fruit and vegetables and smoothies made with fresh fruit. Red, orange and yellow fruits and vegetables – these are high in beta-carotene and help to boost the immune system. Make carrot, beetroot, pineapple, apple, parsley, celery and wheat and barley grass juices and take ½ a cup at least daily. Sprout your own seeds, like alfalfa and mung beans, and eat lots of raw foods. Add zinc-rich foods to your diet, especially chickpeas, sunflower seeds and pumpkin seeds.

Take a good multivitamin and ask your doctor to prescribe medicated eye drops. Thin slices of cucumber over the eyes will help to soothe the itchiness and redness.

Tissue Salts: No. 1, 2, 3, 4, 9 and 10 (2 of each taken up to 6 times a day).

Dark rings under the eyes

These are linked to kidney problems, allergies or fatigue.

The danger foods

Salty foods: processed foods, fried foods, processed meats, snack foods, salty biscuits; also carbonated sweet drinks as well as diet drinks and artificial sweeteners. Replace with plain water! Just consider your daily diet – you will be astonished at how little water you drink. Dehydration is often a cause as the kidneys are put under strain. Instant coffee is poison.

The superfoods

Barley water to flush the kidneys (see recipe on page 135); unsweetened berry juices, especially cranberry and blueberry juice. Include fennel tea daily and basil, parsley, celery and fenugreek fresh in vegetable soups (chop in just before serving). A big bowl of vegetable soup is vital to rejuvenate the kidneys and repair the damage. Make it with barley, beans (mung beans, butter beans, haricot beans or kidney beans), onions, garlic, leeks, grated ginger, carrots, pumpkin, sweet potatoes and lucerne. Flavour with lemon juice and fresh thyme, cumin seeds, coriander seeds and fresh oregano to lessen the salt.

Eat magnesium-rich foods daily: steamed cabbage, spinach, kale, pea sprouts, leaves and tendrils, watercress, celery in salads with lemon juice. Drink lots of water. Get enough sleep and take a magnesium supplement at night. Every day, make a different salad and keep a food diary.

Tissue Salts: No. 1, 2, 6, 9, 10 and 12.

Floaters

These are black flecks within the eye that move. They often bother the elderly as well as the short sighted, and can be caused by candida, diabetes, lack of the good bacteria in the digestive system, wrong eating, liver ailments or simply by the ageing process. Interestingly, if we change the diet these floaters often disappear.

The danger foods
Avoid processed foods, especially processed meats, fatty foods, margarines, fried foods, fast foods, alcohol, yeast (breads, buns, bread rolls, any food containing yeast) and refined carbohydrates; also coffee, chocolate and dairy products, especially butter and cream. Avoid peanuts!

The superfoods
Berries, especially blueberries, blackberries, raspberries and strawberries; liver-cleansing foods like celery, basil, parsley, dandelion leaves, alfalfa sprouts, lucerne, watercress as well as green vegetables – eat them raw, thinly shredded in a salad, like cabbage (especially the outer leaves), lettuce, celery leaves and fennel served with lemon juice. Globe artichokes, served with lemon juice and no butter, are valuable in the diet and so are apricots, pomegranates, grapes, apples, pineapple (juiced or eaten fresh), papaya, kiwifruit, nectarines, prickly pears and cherries. All these foods will help to flush out toxins from the liver and kidneys. Add nuts, sunflower seeds, flaxseed and sesame seeds – grind to a powder and sprinkle over porridge or fruit salads.

Take liver-cleansing herbs in supplements like milk thistle, gingko biloba and burdock, as well as probiotics to restore a healthy balance in the digestive system.

Tissue Salts: No. 2 and 6 taken at least twice a day.

Macular degeneration of the eyes
This is one of the main causes of blindness. It starts with a blind spot or blurred vision, usually in the centre of the field of vision – what happens is that the small blood vessels behind the eye that supply the blood to that part may leak or swell. Much research is being continuously done as the main aim is to protect the eyes to prevent further degeneration and certain foods and herbs have been found to be helpful.

The danger foods
Stay away from alcohol and caffeine in any form, especially instant coffee. Saturated fats are a great danger – fast foods, fried foods, margarines, processed foods, fatty processed meats (for example salami, polony, meat loafs, ham), salty snacks, pickles and salty condiments, salted nuts and peanuts. Also have your blood pressure checked often and avoid any foods that are high in salt. Use celery, coriander seeds, thyme and oregano instead to flavour foods.

The superfoods
A healthy, colourful and varied diet is vital: include foods rich in lycopene (for example, tomatoes and watermelon); other carotenes such as lutein and zeaxanthin are also proving valuable. The carotenes prevent oxidative damage to the retina – the part of the eye that is responsible for fine vision. So choose all the vividly coloured fruits and vegetables you can – papaya, star fruit, kiwifruit, strawberries, oranges, pomegranates, persimmons, raspberries, peaches, red grapes, cabbage, broccoli, kale, mustard, turnip greens, spinach, red peppers, yellow peppers, pumpkin, carrots – and talk to your doctor about bilberry extract and drink blueberry juice and eat blueberries often. Also include sunflower seeds, pumpkin

seeds, wheat grass and barley grass juice; as well as omega-3 fats – eat oily fish 2–3 times a week.

Tissue Salts: No. 1, 2, 6, 7 and 11 (take 3 times a day).

Fever Blisters
Fever blisters or **cold sores** are caused by the *Herpes simplex* virus, which can remain dormant in the body for many years and then suddenly flare up causing a hot sore blister around the mouth and nose and sometimes around the eyes. Painful and super-sensitive, it breaks out with redness and swelling, a hot hard core that blisters, weeps and cracks, causing absolute misery!

Aggravating factors include exposure to the sun, stress, low iron levels, poor diet, low immune system, even hormonal imbalances or following a cold. It is very contagious – so keep cups, glasses, spoons, forks, towels and facecloths away from the rest of the family. Don't kiss anyone with a cold sore and don't share food or drinks.

The danger foods
Without doubt there are foods that make the condition worse: sugar, coffee, especially instant coffee, alcohol, fried foods, fast foods, sugary drinks, carbonated sweet drinks, diet drinks, energy drinks, artificial sweeteners. Avoid chocolates and peanuts – both these are rich in the amino acid arginine, which actually strengthens the virus. So avoid these if you are prone to fever blisters. Other foods that contain arginine include wheat products, soya products, oats, pineapples, tomatoes, gelatine, shellfish, nuts (almonds, cashews, walnuts, Brazil nuts, hazelnuts), saturated fats and dairy products.

The superfoods
Look for foods rich in lysine – this amino acid will boost the immune system and inhibit the growth of the *Herpes simplex* virus. So include lots of fresh fruit juices and vegetable juices and masses of fresh salads and fruit salads (but avoid tomatoes, pineapples, mung beans and mung bean sprouts). Eat chicken, brown rice, fish, pumpkin seeds, sesame seeds and garlic. Drink lots of water – at least 6 glasses a day.

Look at immune-boosting supplements and include peppermint tea (*Mentha piperita nigra*) and elderflower tea (*Sambucus nigra*) daily in the diet. Use ¼ cup elderflowers or peppermint sprigs (fresh or dried) and pour over this 1 cup of boiling water. Stir, stand 5 minutes, strain and sip slowly. Drink unsweetened. A cup a day for 14 days, give it a 4–5 day rest, then start again, helps to destroy the *Herpes simplex* virus in the body.

I suffered terribly from fever blisters and tried the peppermint and elderflower tea – I dried both for winter use – and I kept it up for 6 months. I hardly ever have a fever blister nowadays and should one come along after a particularly stressful time, it is small, short-lived, not painful and hardly noticeable. So I believe in a careful diet, as well as the peppermint and elderflower tea and I take Tissue Salts constantly, especially No. 3 and No. 9, both as a preventative and as a cure.

Speak to your doctor about a lysine supplement; and also vitamin C and zinc to boost the immune system.

Fibrocystic Breast Disease
This is characterised by small lumps or cysts that form on the breasts in various places under the skin that have a 'moveable' or loose feeling and that can also change in size. The breasts

Caution: Consult with your doctor before you embark on any form of self-diagnosis or self-treatment.

feel tender and uncomfortable, especially pre-menstruating, and the lumps often swell during that time of the month. It is easily diagnosed by means of a needle biopsy (the doctor will insert a needle into a clump to withdraw some fluid) and is not considered to be a cancerous growth but it needs to be diagnosed correctly. Possible causes are an under-active thyroid or an iodine deficiency, or a hormonal imbalance where there is too much oestrogen in the body. It is exacerbated by a diet high in sugar and refined carbohydrates, and by an overloaded, sluggish liver.

The danger foods

Sugar and refined carbohydrates (white bread, cakes, biscuits, snacks, fast foods, sweets and chocolates), caffeine (especially instant coffee) and alcohol – all of which increase blood sugar levels – and the most dangerous of all: carbonated sweet drinks, diet drinks, energy drinks, especially in tins, or wines and juices in aluminium-lined boxes.

Excessive salt, salty snacks, processed meats (bacon, ham, salami, vienna sausages, polony), all non-organic meat, chicken or eggs as the hormone count is too high, refined oils, fried or fatty foods and dairy products – all these can upset the hormone balance and thus exacerbate the problem.

The superfoods

All meals and all snacks should be made up of fresh fruit and vegetables. Include celery, parsley, basil, fennel, fresh dandelion leaves and buckwheat in the diet every day. Eat small and regular meals, breakfast on fruits like papaya and prunes and oats porridge sprinkled with a powdered mixture of almonds, sesame seeds, sunflower seeds, flaxseed and pumpkin seeds, mixed with Bulgarian yoghurt.

Wheat grass and barley grass juice with fresh carrots, beetroot, celery, parsley, apples, kiwifruit and melons will give energy and vitality and help to reduce the lumps. Check the lumps frequently and include oily fish in the diet at least twice a week for their essential fats, and talk to your doctor about whether you need an omega-3 supplement.

Drink lots of water and rooibos tea, and get to know herb teas. There are many that are not only refreshing, but also cleansing, calming and revitalising. Drink tea of fresh fennel leaves and grow your own parsley, celery and dandelion for fresh pickings twice a day.

Try to find cold-pressed sunflower cooking oil or olive oil, as vitamin E and B-complex are essential for hormonal balance. Speak to your doctor about supplementing these, and also about evening primrose oil, which helps with hormone balance.

Tissue Salts: No. 1, 2, 6, 8, 9 and 12; and No. 3, 10 and 11 to cleanse the liver (2 of each twice daily).

Regular exercise is essential – consider a brisk 15–20 minute walk daily to aid the clearance of toxins. Do not be tempted to take even a sip of wine or alcohol!

Fibroids

Many women suffer with fibroids, which are generally non-malignant cysts that form internally and sometimes on the external wall of the uterus and which can cause heavy menstruation and frequent menstruation, often with big clots. The heavy bleeding can lead to exhaustion and anaemia and the fibroids, which can vary in size, may put pressure on both the bowel and bladder.

Often constipation becomes a problem. Sometimes surgery is needed, usually in women who are in their thirties and forties, but often the fibroids are small and go undetected. Heavy and frequent periods must be checked out by a gynaecologist. High oestrogen levels are thought to be the cause of fibroids and the balance between oestrogen and progesterone is compromised.

The danger foods

All foods that raise the oestrogen in the body, like non-organic meat, chicken, eggs, even non-organic milk and dairy products. Caffeine is dangerous, so avoid chocolate, cola drinks, tea, coffee, especially instant coffee with sugar and milk. Also avoid all alcohol. In some cases wheat products, especially bread, will exacerbate the problem, and refined flour is taboo! Fast foods, fried foods and processed meats spell danger.

The superfoods

Liver-cleansing herbs like parsley, celery, fennel and milk thistle help quickly. Fruit and vegetable salads, oats, brown rice, lentils and chickpeas are essential. Flaxseed, sesame seeds, pumpkin seeds, sunflower seeds, ground with almonds, are an excellent breakfast treat sprinkled over papaya or grated apple and berries, or over a fruit salad. Eat fresh dandelion leaves, watercress, parsley, buckwheat leaves and celery daily.

Take kelp supplements under your doctor's care and eat oily fish twice a week. Stinging nettle tea daily will help to restore the mineral balance lost through heavy bleeding. Have regular check-ups and follow your doctor's advice on supplements you may need, for example evening primrose oil, magnesium, vitamins E and B-complex and milk thistle (an excellent liver cleanser).

Tissue Salts: No. 1, 2, 6, 8, 9 and 12. Take 2 of each frequently. Avoid No. 12 if you have implants.

Fibromyalgia

This is muscular pain – chronic, debilitating and exhausting and far more common than ever before. Usually worse first thing in the morning, it is characterised by pains in specific muscles, stiff aching back, neck and shoulders are the most common, also the legs, especially after a long walk, all with tender points. Headaches are common, along with dizziness, palpitations, depression, a feeling of overload and not thinking clearly, sleeplessness, indigestion, constipation, colic, flatulence and food intolerances.

It is thought to be linked to chronic fatigue syndrome or to candida, food allergies or viral infections, heavy metal toxicity, high acidity, low thyroid function, sleep deprivation, fluctuating blood sugar levels, and even a compromised immune system. It is most common in women between twenty and thirty-five who are under stress or emotional trauma or who have suffered severe shock (think hijacking or armed robbery incidents!) or prolonged grief. Magnesium and serotonin deficiency may be a trigger and supplements, under your doctor's guidance, are vital.

The danger foods

Wheat and gluten-rich foods like oats, rye and barley grains (this may be a major cause), also refined carbohydrates, especially sugar, dairy products, eggs, soya products, tomatoes and citrus fruits. Also avoid aspartame and MSG, and processed foods of any description, saturated fats (found in processed meats, cheeses, margarines), charred or burnt food, fried foods, heated vegetable oils, caffeine, especially in carbonated drinks, alcohol of any description, instant coffee, teas, also iced teas. All these add toxicity and are stimulants, which can change sleep patterns. Consider what you drink last thing at night. Avoid green peppers, tomatoes and potatoes, as these contain enzymes which can cause muscle pains.

The superfoods

Anything the colour green! Juice wheat grass or barley grass with parsley, celery, apples, beetroot and beetroot leaves. Eat lettuce, spinach, cabbage, kale, Swiss chard, watercress, buckwheat leaves, broccoli, dandelion leaves, Brussels sprouts, seaweeds, lucerne, mung bean sprouts and alfalfa sprouts. All are rich in magnesium and so valuable for the muscles and nerves.

Make sure the daily salad is rich in diversity. Eat nuts like walnuts, pecans, almonds and Brazil nuts as snacks. Include brown rice, millet, apricots (fresh and sun-dried), pumpkin seeds, sunflower seeds and turkey in the diet. Replace red meat with organic chicken or try vegetarian combinations, for example sweet potatoes with brown rice. Vegetable soups with peas and lentils are great comfort foods. Increase your intake of the omega-3 fats – eat oily fish at least twice a week. Sardines and salads make an excellent lunch dish. Include freshly squeezed juices, smoothies or fruit salads daily: berries, apples, carrots, pineapple, kiwifruit, peaches, mangoes, papayas, figs, bananas – create your own exciting combinations.

Herb teas are helpful – stinging nettle, chamomile, scented geranium, lavender and melissa all relax and calm. Ginger tea will ease spasm (¼ cup fresh herb to 1 cup boiling water).

Ask your doctor about supplements like fish oils, magnesium citrate, vitamin B-complex and probiotics to ease and benefit the digestion.

Tissue Salts: No. 4, 6 and 8 (2 of each taken frequently).

Drink lots of water to flush out toxins and eat frequent small meals or healthy snacks. Take gentle exercise – easy walking, stretching, even yoga, to keep the muscles moving.

Fluid Retention

Also known as **oedema** or **swelling**, fluid retention is a very real problem for many people and one that is far more common than ever before. Swelling occurs mostly around the abdomen, ankles, lower legs, fingers and around the eyes, but it can even affect the jaw line, the breasts and the arms.

The many factors causing fluid retention can be so varied you need to consult your doctor to pinpoint the cause. Possible causes include: food allergy or intolerance, liver problems like overload or toxicity, too much salt in the diet (which leads to the retention of water), high blood pressure, thyroid imbalance, vitamin B6 deficiency, urinary system ailments and hormonal imbalance (especially premenstrual), blood sugar imbalance, overuse of laxatives or even taking diuretics.

First of all you need to be sure of the cause and then be guided by your doctor. Certain foods can trigger allergies and intolerances – so watch the diet with great care.

The danger foods

Top of the list is often gluten intolerance, yeast intolerance and dairy products – the stomach area feels uncomfortable with bloatedness, flatulence, colic and gassy burping. Keep a food diary and note the symptoms.

Avoid caffeine – found in tea, coffee (especially instant coffee – replace with dandelion root coffee, see box), cola drinks, carbonated drinks, energy drinks – as well as too much sugar.

Be careful of foods containing additives (colourants, flavourants and artificial sweeteners): diet drinks, brightly coloured fizzy drinks (orange, red, lime green and especially blue drinks!). Avoid alcohol (especially champagne or sparkling wines or alcohol with ginger beer), refined carbohydrates like white bread or rolls, hot and spicy pickles, pickled onions, rich spicy sauces, salty processed foods, especially processed meats, cheeses and salty snacks, dips, mayonnaises and hard-boiled eggs and dried bean dishes. Cut down drastically on salt and use herbs or a salt substitute to flavour foods (see recipe on page 35).

The superfoods

Bland vegetable soups flavoured with celery, parsley or fennel (all are rich in vitamins, minerals and potassium, which will flush out high levels of sodium). Include globe artichokes in the diet – boiled with no salt and no butter, just fresh lemon juice! Add fennel bulb, thinly sliced, to salads of celery, parsley, basil, dandelion leaves, watercress, asparagus and raw carrots.

Make fresh carrot, celery, parsley and lucerne juice with apple and beetroot – this is an excellent flush for toxins, and for getting the circulation moving.

Herbal teas are valuable to flush out the kidneys and bladder: stinging nettle tea, fresh ginger tea, the silk from green mealies (this makes an excellent and comforting tea, especially for pressure around the prostate), celery tea made from fresh leaves and seeds, dill tea made from dill seeds, flowers and leaves (¼ cup fresh leaves with seeds, pour over this 1 cup of boiling water, stand 5 minutes, strain and sip slowly).

Ask your doctor about a vitamin B-complex supplement, especially with vitamin B6 which helps to normalise the body fluids.

Tissue Salts: No. 12; ankles – No. 9; feet and hands – No. 4; limbs generally – No. 9. Take 2 of each at least 3 times a day.

Some health shops sell dandelion coffee – try it out (or make your own, see box). This has been a much-loved beverage for centuries and is still around today as a health drink.

> ### Dandelion Root Coffee
>
> Learn to make your own dandelion root coffee: In a food processor finely chop up fresh dandelion roots that have been well washed and scrubbed with a stiff bristle brush. (Keep them in the fridge for 2 days after reaping, sealed in a plastic bag – this makes them crisp and easy to process.) Spread into a glass lasagne dish and roast in the oven on medium heat, shaking up and stirring constantly. The thinner the ground up roots are spread the quicker and more evenly they will dry. When they reach a crumbly dryness remove from the oven. You'll notice they change colour to a darker brown. Spoon into a sterilised, screw-top jar and store in a dark cupboard.
>
> To make the coffee: Use a coffee filter or boil up 2 or 3 tablespoons in 2 cups of water, simmering gently for 10 minutes, then taste and simmer longer if liked for more taste. Sweetened with stevia and flavoured with a squeeze of lemon juice and fresh ginger slices, this becomes quite an exceptional health drink and the more you have it the more you will enjoy it.

Caution: Consult with your doctor before you embark on any form of self-diagnosis or self-treatment.

As a physiotherapist we were taught about skin brushing to get the circulation going. Choose a natural bristle brush firm enough to be pleasantly stimulating. Brush towards the heart – for example start at the feet and brush upwards, or at the fingertips and brush upwards, from the buttocks and thighs brush up towards the neck. A long-handled brush works well and it is worth trying as it gets the circulation going, the lymph moving and it clears sluggishness.

Last but not least – take brisk walks twice or even three times daily, up and down a hill if possible.

Food Allergies

There are two types of food allergy. The first is an immediate reaction to a food consumed, for example peanuts, certain shellfish or pineapple. It is an extremely serious condition that can lead to anaphylactic shock and death. Rush the person to a hospital or doctor for immediate treatment. The second type is a slower, delayed reaction, which can occur from 1 hour to 48 hours or more, even up to 72 hours later, for example a food intolerance which produces a slower response.

Common allergens include dairy foods (see page 244), wheat (see page 218), nuts, citrus fruit, yeast, pineapples, fish, *peanuts*, chemicals added to processed foods, breads, cakes, cheeses and fried foods.

The symptoms can occur within minutes of consuming the food and include rash, red swelling and hot itchiness, wheezing, shortness of breath, throat closing, palpitations, asthma, ears ringing with itchiness, nose running, hay fever, nausea and vomiting, fatigue, irritability, aches all over the body and diarrhoea.

The danger foods
Mucus-forming foods, fast foods, refined carbohydrates, additives in processed foods (colourants, flavourants, preservatives), processed meats, fried foods (especially in oils like peanut, sesame or walnut oil), tea, coffee, alcohol, sugar (which suppresses the immune system), some Chinese foods (they are high in an additive, MSG), foods preserved with sodium benzoate or sulphur dioxide.

Keep a food diary and become alert to anything that may be a trigger. Become an avid label reader.

The superfoods
Eat immune-boosting foods, especially red, orange and yellow foods. Eat lots of fresh fruits and vegetables: green salads that include lettuce, broccoli, cabbage, celery, fennel, spinach, green peppers and parsley. Eat foods rich in vitamin C: apples, onions, parsley and buckwheat. Beetroot, sprouted barley grass, wheat grass, carrots, blueberries, blackberries, avocados, pears, red grapes and pomegranates are all particularly beneficial. Bake your own bread (see page 35). The classic anti-allergy diet includes lamb, peas and pears – test this under your doctor's supervision.

Drink water – up to 2 litres a day. Make a tea of stinging nettle – this helps to normalise the histamine production within the body. Include probiotics in the diet.

Tissue Salts: No. 9, 3 and 7 (take 2 of each frequently).

What are Probiotics?
The word 'probiotic' means 'for life' and probiotics are the beneficial bacteria that live in the digestive system where they help to maintain a healthy intestinal tract and fight illness and disease. Probiotics benefit our health by inhibiting the growth of harmful bacteria that cause digestive problems, improving digestion of food and absorption of vitamins, and boosting the immune system. Unfortunately stress and the use of antibiotics and the contraceptive pill can upset the delicate balance of these beneficial bacteria. In this case, we need to replenish the 'good' bacteria in the gut – this is easily done by taking a supplement in capsule or tablet form. Talk to your pharmacist and your doctor.

Fractures

Cracks or breaks in the bones are not only painful but put us out of action. They may be due to osteoporosis (see page 252) or to an accident or fall. Swelling, numbness and pain are part of the picture but there are measures we can take to ease the healing process.

The danger foods
The very worst are carbonated drinks, the colas and energy drinks, the brightly coloured, super-sweet bubbly drinks so loved by young people. Other culprits are red meat, fast foods, fried foods, fatty foods and junk food – all these are high in phosphorus and other compounds which seriously interfere with the body's uptake and absorption of precious calcium, which is needed to repair the bones. Avoid coffee, especially instant coffee, tea and sugar in all its forms, including cakes, sweets and chocolates, also alcohol, salt, processed foods, salty snacks, crisps, chips and instant foods.

The bones need the best possible nutrition at this time. Be strict with yourself and build bone health with dedication or the whole system will weaken.

The superfoods
Juices and smoothies are an excellent starting point – carrots, wheat grass, barley grass, apples, beetroot, celery, parsley, fresh lucerne and buckwheat leaves, all juiced together (half a glass daily). Pineapple eaten fresh and raw (including the core) or juiced with fresh lucerne, parsley, fenugreek leaves, celery, a good handful or two of sprouted seeds (mung beans, alfalfa or sunflower seeds), apples, strawberries or any fruit in season will help to clear toxins. Adding a little powdered cinnamon will ease the digestion and the healing of the fracture will begin immediately.

Eat foods rich in calcium and vitamins C, D and K: dandelion leaves, green leafy vegetables, tofu, sesame seeds, beans, lentils, almonds, Brazil nuts, turnip greens, amaranth, Bulgarian yoghurt, mackerel, sardines, broccoli – as many of these as you can daily to repair the joints and bones.

Speak to your doctor about supplements: calcium, magnesium, boron and zinc and go to a physiotherapist for careful exercise and movement to keep the muscles fit and strong.

Tissue Salts: No. 1 and 2 (2 of each at least 4 times a day).

Caution: Consult with your doctor before you embark on any form of self-diagnosis or self-treatment.

The herb comfrey is also known as 'knitbone' and a daily cup of comfrey tea is an ancient remedy for broken bones. However, a compound in comfrey is regarded as carcinogenic (it caused liver damage and tumours in rats), so *take comfrey only under your doctor's supervision*. To make the tea use ¼ cup fresh torn-up leaf and pour over this 1 cup of boiling water, stand 5 minutes, strain and sip slowly. Take only one cup a day for no longer than 7–10 days and *only with your doctor's permission*.

Gall Bladder Disease

Nothing is quite as intense as the pain from a gall bladder problem. The role of the gall bladder is to concentrate the bile in the digestive tract to assist with the digestion of fats in food. Gallstones are composed of fatty cells or cholesterol that harden into stones of varying sizes, from the size of a pea to the size of a marble. These are the result of too much saturated fat in the daily diet and not enough dietary fibre to digest the foods adequately. Interestingly, both vitamin C and a compound in lecithin help to ward off the attacks and to reduce the formation of the gallstones.

The danger foods

Food allergies and fatty foods like pork, bacon, fried onions, fried eggs or oily chips can set up an aggravation within the gall bladder and with margarine, these are the most common offenders. Too much sugar in the diet has been found to cause gall bladder attacks and coffee, especially instant coffee, has been found to stimulate gall bladder contractions. Skipping meals adds to the problem as the gall bladder's role is to produce bile acids which dissolve the cholesterol in food.

Avoid the following foods: fatty fried foods, fatty meats, animal fat, processed cheeses, snacks, margarines, dairy products, pastries, chips, crisps, alcohol, caffeine (instant coffee is lethal!), sugar and refined carbohydrates such as white bread and buns, cakes, doughnuts, sweets and chocolate – all these put a huge strain on the liver, on the gall bladder and, in fact, the whole process of digestion within the digestive tract.

Chewing gum can be seriously damaging to the gall bladder. The chewing action stimulates the secretion of digestive juices in the mouth, which are then swallowed, but because there is no food in the mouth with which to mix them, the hydrochloric acid and bile acids in the stomach mix only with the sweet gum-scented saliva. The mixture irritates the stomach lining and the endless gum chewing sets up a vicious cycle of undigested acid, which easily aggravates the gall bladder.

The superfoods

Fresh fruits and vegetables are top of the list with salads, fruit salads, smoothies and juices. Oat bran, flaxseed, lentils, peas, mealies, cherries, pears, apples, oranges, parsley, radish, watercress, artichokes, spinach and turmeric discourage the formation of stones and cleanses the liver. Low fat Bulgarian yoghurt, extra virgin olive oil and almonds are excellent additions to the diet. Artichokes are rich in the compound cynarin, which regenerates the liver – eat them with lemon juice only, and no butter!

Juice carrots, beetroot, celery, parsley, apple and wheat grass daily for that energy fix. Freshly juiced apple is high in pectin and a soluble fibre that can break down cholesterol quickly. Dandelion coffee made of roasted dandelion root (see page

231) is safe and easily digested and rich in nutrients. Use stevia to sweeten and both will ease the whole digestive tract.

If the gall bladder has been removed, turmeric added to casseroles helps the digestion. Also ask your doctor about a digestive enzyme called 'lipase' that breaks down fat.

Take lecithin granules twice daily, sprinkled onto food or added to smoothies, to help break down and emulsify fats. Eat small meals and snacks so as to lessen the strain put on the liver. Ask your doctor about milk thistle supplements for liver health.

Tissue Salts: No. 4, 10 and 11; for gallstones take No. 10 and 11.

Gingivitis

Also called **gum disease**, gingivitis is an inflammatory condition of the gums, which are swollen, inflamed and bleed easily, often receding and accompanied by halitosis. Proper brushing and cleaning of the teeth, check-ups every 3–6 months at the dentist and the right diet will prevent gum disease which, if left untreated, affects the surrounding tissues and can in time invade the bones of the jaw. It is often caused by too much sugar in the diet, which increases plaque formation.

The danger foods

Sugar, refined carbohydrates – white bread, pastries, cakes – sugary icings, chocolates, sweets, ice-creams, carbonated drinks, sweetened fruit juices, fast foods, processed foods, especially processed meats, fatty meats, fatty cheeses. Coffee, tea, cola drinks, alcohol and energy drinks all exacerbate the problem.

The superfoods

Change the diet drastically! Include lots of fruits, fresh vegetables, salads, berries, Bulgarian yoghurt, low fat milk and fish. Make juices with apples and carrots, eat fresh black grapes, include leafy green vegetables in the diet, especially cabbages, lettuce, broccoli, cauliflower, kale, parsley, spinach, Swiss chard and celery and chew fresh carrots, apples and celery sticks every day to cleanse the gums and revitalise them.

Drink herb teas, especially pennywort (*Centella asiatica*), chamomile, lemongrass or thyme tea and drink green tea. Use the teas to gargle with too and to swish out the mouth. Drink different ones throughout the day, unsweetened, with a squeeze of lemon juice.

Replace sugar with stevia for sweetening (never artificial sweeteners) and speak to your doctor about supplements: coenzyme Q10, vitamins A, C and E, calcium, folic acid, zinc and magnesium.

Tissue Salts: For bleeding gums take No. 2, 9 and 12 daily (under your doctor's supervision); take No. 1, 2, 3, 4 and 6 for spongy gums; No. 4 and 9 if there are ulcers. Take 2 of each at least twice daily.

Pure coconut oil to which a drop or two of tea tree oil has been added makes an excellent oil massaged well into the gums at night after brushing the teeth with a good toothpaste recommended by your dentist.

Glandular Fever

A debilitating fatigue and fever caused by the Epstein Barr virus, which affects the glands, liver, spleen, lymph nodes and muscles, glandular fever is no joke and the sore throat, muscular aches and pains and the wretched weakness often bring about

Caution: Consult with your doctor before you embark on any form of self-diagnosis or self-treatment.

fear and depression. It is also sometimes referred to as 'yuppie 'flu' because it often attacks the young and the fit out of the blue. Candida (see page 216) is often a symptom after glandular fever, so be aware of this and follow your doctor's advice and appropriate vitamin therapy. The key word is rest – don't try to push yourself – and cleansing the liver and strengthening the immune system is the first step.

The danger foods

Not surprising the trigger is sugar, which compromises the digestive system. Totally delete sugar from the diet. Also avoid carbonated drinks, energy drinks, caffeine (especially in coffee and instant coffee), processed foods (especially processed meats), salted meats, fried foods, fast foods and sweetened cakes, biscuits, pastries, white bread, buns, and anything fried in butter or oil – doughnuts are lethal! Avoid alcohol in any form, not even a sip of wine! It depresses the immune system and the nervous system and overtaxes the liver.

The superfoods

Although you won't feel much like eating you'll have to nourish the system and fruit and vegetable juices, smoothies and vegetable soups are the way to revitalise. The top of the list is wheat grass and barley grass juice with fresh lucerne, parsley, celery, buckwheat leaves, carrots, beetroot, apples and pineapple. Squeeze through the juicer (a spiral action juicer will get every drop of juice out of the precious wheat grass and barley grass) and drink half a glass twice a day to bring back that lost energy.

Focus on berries, peaches, sprouts (especially sprouted broccoli), fresh dandelion leaves, all members of the cabbage family like kale, broccoli, cauliflower (steamed or in soups), onions, leeks, parsley, celery, lentils, peas, beans, chickpeas, squashes, watercress and stinging nettle tea, as well as brown rice, rice cakes and organic chicken or fish and you will be happily surprised at your quick recovery.

Speak to your doctor about supplements: milk thistle, vitamin C, coenzyme Q10, probiotics and blue-green algae supplements.

Drink lots of water and take Tissue Salt No. 5 and No. 1, 2, 9, 10 and 12 for fatigue (take 2 of each up to 8 times a day). Avoid No. 12 if you have implants.

Gluten Intolerance *see* Coeliac Disease

Gout

Gout is a very real, very painful condition of uric acid crystals that form deposits around the joints, often the big toe joints or the fingers or the knees. Normally uric acid is excreted in the urine, but due to specific causes – often dietary causes like insufficient water in the diet, nutrient deficiencies, disturbance in the metabolism, crash diets, high alcohol and high red meat intake – the elimination of uric acid does not occur. The urine becomes strong smelling, scanty and the crystals form.

The danger foods

Alcohol, red meat, fried or barbequed, processed meats (polony, salami, ham, bacon), biltong, sausages – all are high in purines, a substance which builds up uric acid, and these will be the first foods your doctor will insist you remove completely from the diet. Also avoid refined flour products like white bread and bread rolls, doughnuts, sugary buns and any foods containing yeast. Cut down on salt and sugar as these foods boost the sodium urate crystals with intensity and speed.

Salty foods, chips, fast foods, fried foods and saturated fats all increase the inflammation, the hot, red swelling and the intense pain and discomfort. Avoid sardines, anchovies, salty spreads, dips, flavourings high in MSG and everything that has purines in it. Surprisingly, tomatoes, potatoes, bell peppers, chillies, fruit salad plant and brinjals – all belonging to the nightshade family – are also on the banned list as these increase the intensity of the uric acid crystal formation.

Smoking is also considered to be detrimental to the condition, as tobacco's solanine content easily increases the whole inflammatory condition, and drinking coffee, even filter coffee, adds to the pain and discomfort.

At this point most men throw up their hands in horror, complaining that every little pleasure in their lives has just been outlawed, and they limp off to go and see their doctors again for a magic pill that will just take it all away. A few weeks later they come limping back, almost crying for help. There is no short cut and yes, you do actually have to rethink your eating habits and your lifestyle. Smoking and drinking and red meat and fast food fry-ups are out, but there is much to be excited about ...

The superfoods

First you need to flush out all the toxins, the uric acid and the build-up of inflammation within the body by drinking lots of water: 6–8 glasses is the absolute minimum spread throughout the day. This will save the kidneys and the whole urinary system.

Next you need to clear the acidity. This is done by means of vegetable and fruit juices and you need every bit of alkalinity you can get. Rich in antioxidants, a half a glass of freshly processed vegetable juice twice a day is like a panacea. Here is what you do:

In a spiral action juicer push through 2 cups of wheat grass or barley grass, 3 sticks of celery (including the leaves), 1 cup of parsley, 2 carrots, ½ a fresh pineapple, ½ a lettuce, 2 cups of fresh lucerne sprigs and 2 cups of fennel leaves, leaf bases, even fennel flowers. Sip immediately for breakfast and repeat in the afternoon.

Eat a vegetable salad and a fruit salad daily and vary the ingredients. Choose grilled chicken or fish seasoned with very little sea salt, celery seeds, crushed coriander seeds, fresh thyme and chopped parsley and lemon juice. Eat with salads (no tomatoes) of dandelion leaves, celery, cucumber, grated fresh beetroot with apple, lettuce of all colours, kiwifruit, star fruit, pomegranate seeds, sprinkled with flaxseed, pumpkin seeds and sesame seeds, and a simple dressing of lemon juice and a little olive oil.

Vegetable soups made with pulses like chickpeas, lentils and split peas, barley, masses of finely shredded cabbage, broccoli, kale, celery, spinach, onions, buckwheat leaves, grated carrots, sweet potatoes and pumpkin, flavoured with herbs like thyme, parsley, basil, oregano, coriander seed and a little sea salt, will quickly flush out the system. Artichokes without the salt and butter are also excellent for cleansing, and use apple cider vinegar as a salad or vegetable dressing, and 2 teaspoons of apple cider vinegar in a glass of cold water will soon replace the need for a beer or carbonated drink.

Stinging nettle tea (see page 235) and pennywort tea (*Centella asiatica*) are both superb cleansers of uric acid in the joints. Have 2 cups of each through the day, spaced apart.

Caution: Consult with your doctor before you embark on any form of self-diagnosis or self-treatment.

Ask your doctor about supplements like folic acid to help lower uric acid levels, the omega-3 oils, vitamin C, probiotics to re-establish the friendly bacteria in the digestive system, 'devil's claw', that marvellous arthritis and gout plant remedy from Namibia, and also milk thistle to cleanse the liver.

Use Epsom salts in the bath to clear toxins from the skin – a cup of Epsom salts 2–3 times a week – and use a luffa with a natural soap (we have a pure, unscented palm kernel oil soap that washes away toxins from the skin beautifully that we can post anywhere). Hot and cold showers – first hot then cold then hot then cold – help to clear the toxins too, using the luffa sponge dipped wet into Epsom salts with natural soap to rid the skin of toxins. You'll emerge glowing!

Start taking moderate exercise daily under your doctor's guidance and weigh yourself regularly on your now perfect diet. You'll find you're not only losing weight but also the pain, bad tempers and impatience!

Tissue Salts: No. 1, 4, 10 and 11 (2 of each frequently).

Stinging Nettle – Not Just a Weed

A well-respected and valuable medicinal plant, stinging nettle (Urtica dioica) was one of the first medicinal plants to be registered in the ancient pharmacopoeias. A waste ground weed, we have a stand of nettle that we nurture for our compost heaps, for our soups and stews – as it is incredibly rich in vitamins and minerals – and for treating gout, arthritis, cleansing an overloaded liver, reducing fluid and detoxifying, for bronchitis and congested lungs, jaundice, infertility, anaemia, sciatica, to improve breast-milk production and to ease hay fever, eczema and itchy insect bites. It is a well-established treatment for an enlarged and painful prostate and it helps to expel kidney stones and clear blockages in the urethra.

Nettle tea is an exceptional tea and its uses are well established. For treating all the above ailments, pour 1 cup of boiling water over ¼ cup of stinging nettle sprigs and leaves, stand 5 minutes, sip slowly. Take 1 cup a day for 10 days, then give it a break for 2–4 days, then start again. For intense pain in gout, take the tea 2–4 times a day for 4–5 days, and then stop.

Caution

When picking nettle wear gloves. Once it is submerged in boiling water, the formic acid in the hairs is dissolved. Should you get stung, apply the juice of aloe vera or bulbinella (Bulbine frutescens).

Grave's Disease *see* Hyperthyroidism

Haemorrhoids *see* Varicose Veins and Haemorrhoids

Hair Loss

The scholarly name for hair loss is **alopaecia** and there are several forms of it: alopaecia totalis is baldness, loss of hair on the head, even eyebrows; alopaecia areata is patches of hair loss; and alopaecia universalis is loss of all body hair, including on the head.

Hair loss is a distressing condition that is linked to high stress levels, grief, loss and severe shock. Other causes include chemotherapy, hormonal imbalance in women, thyroid imbalance (usually under-active), rapid weight loss, diabetes with fluctuating insulin levels, nutrient deficiencies, chemicals in hair dyes, cosmetics and shampoos, ringworm, eczema or psoriasis on the scalp, menopause, iron deficiency, ageing, excessive dieting, over-supplementation of vitamin A, the contraceptive pill, or even an overactive or under-active immune system.

First consult your doctor to find out the cause and then follow the doctor's prescribed treatment. Iron, thyroid, hormones and vitamin deficiencies all play a major role, but the diet too, is extremely important.

The danger foods

The biggest enemy is sugar and artificial sweeteners, and refined carbohydrates. By raising the blood sugar and insulin levels we cause untold problems and this we need to address. Caffeine, especially instant coffee, tea and cola drinks lessen the absorption of valuable minerals in varying degrees – so these must be avoided. Drink herb teas like rosemary, pennywort (Centella asiatica), cinnamon, ginger and rooibos instead. (Avoid Centella asiatica if you have thyroid condition.)

The superfoods

Include in the diet: seaweed, dark green leafy vegetables, lots of cabbage, kale, spinach, parsley, celery, watercress, dandelion, mustard greens, turnip leaves, buckwheat leaves, sweet potato vine leaves, pumpkin vine tips and tendrils, young grape leaves and tendrils, sprouts, lucerne leaves, fenugreek leaves and wheat grass or barley grass juice with carrots, beetroot, celery, parsley, lucerne and apples. Make smoothies with fresh fruit, especially berries, pineapples, peaches, pears, cherries and grapes.

Have a cup of rosemary tea daily for 10–14 days, then stop for 3 or 4 days and resume for 10–14 days: ¼ cup fresh rosemary sprigs in 1 cup boiling water, stand 5 minutes, strain and sip slowly. Do the same with stinging nettle tea as an alternative.

Strengthen the immune system. Take extra vitamins under your doctor's supervision: magnesium, probiotics (digestive enzymes to aid the absorption of nutrients).

Tissue Salts: No. 2, 3, 6, 7, 9 and 12. We even have a combination of tissue salts for 'Hair Loss' in one tablet.

Rosemary Hair Rinse

Boil up fresh sprigs of rosemary, enough to fill a big pot, cover with water and simmer 15–20 minutes with the lid on. Strain, use the fragrant dark mixture to rinse the hair with after shampooing, massaging it gently into the scalp. Comb in some of the rosemary brew every day, massaging it into the scalp lightly and gently. Any excess can be kept in the fridge and warmed for comfort. Make a fresh batch every 3–4 days to keep those strong oils in the rosemary active.

Do not treat your hair roughly, do not rub with a towel to dry it, rather bind the head in a towel after shampooing and rinsing well to absorb the moisture.

Caution: Consult with your doctor before you embark on any form of self-diagnosis or self-treatment.

Heart Disease

Heart disease remains a leading cause of death worldwide. It is actually an umbrella term for many different conditions that affect the functioning of the heart. Here are a few of the most common ailments that affect the heart:

Angina pectoris, or more commonly known as **angina**, is severe chest pain that occurs when the heart is not receiving enough oxygen-rich blood. It may be precipitated by stress, exertion, a large meal, emotion, shock, intense fear, distress and nutritional deficiencies.

Coronary thrombosis, also called a **heart attack** or **infarction**, is when the coronary arteries, which nourish the heart, become narrow or blocked by a blood clot. The result is often a sharp pain in the centre of the chest or down the left arm, which could recede when the person comes to rest. It is a serious condition which must be attended to by a doctor immediately and then monitored carefully. Twice yearly checkups are vital! The problem may not be in the heart itself, but in the arteries which feed the heart. If the arteries have hardened, it is called **arteriosclerosis** and with high cholesterol the blood flow may become blocked.

Atherosclerosis is a build-up of plaque within the arteries which leads to a lack of oxygen supplying the vascular tissue, which will extend to skipped heartbeats, chest pain, dizziness and shortness of breath, high blood pressure, leg pains, arm pains and even jaw pains. **High blood pressure** is often caused by stress, enzyme imbalance, nutritional deficiencies or it may be a hereditary condition. So look at your family history and lessen the salt in your diet and monitor it regularly!

Arrhythmia is an irregular heartbeat. **Palpitations** are irregular or even regular, pounding heartbeats. **Tachycardia** is when the heart races while it is resting. **Bradycardia** is when the heart beats too slowly when it is resting. **Ectopic beats** or **skipped beats** are beats that are premature with a longer rest period following the beats which are not in rhythm. Some moments of rest between the beats are longer than others. **Fibrillation** is literally a quivering or twitching instead of the normal rhythmic beat.

Valvular disease is the faulty activity of the valves of the heart. **Carditis** is an infection of the heart muscle itself – the pumping mechanism. **Endocarditis** is the infection of the sack surrounding the heart, particularly after heart surgery and where the immune system is compromised.

Cardiac arrest is when the heart literally stops beating. Because the oxygen-rich blood does not reach the brain, the person collapses and loses consciousness.

Congestive heart failure is a chronic collection of fluid around and in the heart, as well as in the ankles and feet, and it is accompanied by laboured breathing after even a little exercise.

For all these conditions, there needs to be complete dedication to follow a healthy diet, to lose the excess weight, to stop smoking and drinking alcohol, and to drink more water.

The danger foods

No red meat in any form and avoid all processed foods, fried foods, especially meats, sausages, polony, salami, ham, bacon and biltong, peanut butter, margarine, butter, hydrogenated vegetable oils, cream, fatty foods and heated vegetable oils (especially overheated vegetable oils). Avoiding these foods will help to lower both high cholesterol levels and uric acid levels in a short time. Avoid white flour, cakes, pies, pastries, fast foods, junk foods, chocolate bars and sugar in any form. Change to stevia for sweetness. Also avoid monosodium glutamate (MSG) – an intense flavouring found in many snack foods and also in mixed salts. Do not eat any burnt or charred barbequed foods – these are dangerous to your health. Cut out all alcohol and stop smoking!

The superfoods

Eat smaller, carefully chosen meals. Include coldwater fish like tuna, salmon, mackerel and haddock – these contain the omega 3-fatty acids, which are vital to heart health. Fatty fish has been found to prevent inflammatory conditions in the blood vessels that give rise to plaque formation.

Choose fibre-rich foods which lower total cholesterol like beans, lentils, raspberries, cauliflower, broccoli, turnip greens, Swiss chard, mustard greens and oat bran (add it to home-baked breads and muffins). Also eat whole grains like oats, millet and sesame seeds, which strengthen the cardiovascular system and are rich in lignans (antioxidants) – the soluble fibre in these foods inhibit cholesterol absorption from the diet. Include buckwheat in the diet, which strengthens the capillaries and brinjal (baked, not fried!), which cleans the blood, prevents strokes and haemorrhages and protects the arteries that have been damaged by high cholesterol.

Fresh parsley clears the blood and helps to reduce coagulants in the veins and is an alkaline cleanser – include it in the daily salad. Sunflower seeds and onions help to remove heavy metals and toxins, so eat these often. Globe artichoke served without butter and salt helps to lower cholesterol. Other foods that help to lower cholesterol include barley grains and barley water, bananas, soya beans (they contain lecithin, which controls cholesterol), apples and garlic. Drinking cranberry juice can increase the levels of 'good' or HDL cholesterol and the fruits are high in potent antioxidants. Almonds are a good source of vitamin E and so are organic safflower oils, and this reduces the 'bad' or LDL cholesterol and assist with the dissolving of fibrin, which is a clot-forming protein. Walnuts and hazelnuts have all the correct levels of folic acid and arginine, which increase artery elasticity and reduce cholesterol.

Green and red peppers, celery and cucumber help to lower and normalise blood pressure – include these in the daily salad.

Rye bread (100% rye) is a cleanser and a rejuvenator of the arteries – so eat rye bread daily. Eat foods rich in vitamin C daily (see page 13) – these foods are high in antioxidants that protect the inner lining of the blood vessels. Lettuce is rich in silica, which benefits the arteries, strengthening their walls. Carrots are rich in beta-carotene, which like vitamin C is able to increase the blood vessel elasticity and reduce its spasm.

Avocado is an excellent blood tonic and prevents anaemia. Other blood-building and blood-cleansing foods are beetroot (including the leaves), blackcurrants, blackberries and mung beans. Oysters benefit cardiovascular health and the immune system and blueberries are a tonic for the whole circulatory system. Olive oil is the only oil that is of benefit to the cardiovascular system and should replace all other oils.

Under your doctor's supervision, take a B-complex vitamin supplement – this will help to lower high levels of homocysteine that may have accumulated. It is advisable to have your homocysteine levels checked by your doctor twice yearly.

Caution: Consult with your doctor before you embark on any form of self-diagnosis or self-treatment.

Drink lots of water – a minimum of 6–8 glasses a day is vital.

Tissue Salts: These mineral salts work well with the medication you are on, but do discuss this with your doctor.

Irregular heartbeat: No. 6, 8 and 9 (take 2 of each every half hour until it settles)

Heart palpitations: No. 2, 4, 6 and 8 (take 2 of each every half hour until it settles – not all together in the mouth, but 2 at a time)

Heart tonic: No. 6 and 8 (these two work beautifully together)

High blood pressure: No. 4 and 6; take 2 of each at least twice daily (these will ease the condition *but do not stop your doctor's prescription*)

More Heart Health Tips

Let your dentist check your gums. Interestingly, gingivitis or gum disease is one of the causes of heart disease and the bacteria that infect the gums can travel through the blood to the heart where it can lead to heart attacks and atherosclerosis. So have a dental check-up every 6 months.

Ask your doctor about chelation therapy. This is a medical treatment that has been found to bind or 'chelate' and expel toxic heavy metals, free radicals and deposits of calcium and plaque in the blood vessels out of the body through the urine.

Hawthorn leaves and berries are age-old heart health builders and can be bought in capsule format.

Add finely grated lemon zest to sauces, salads, soups, salad dressings, brown rice or buckwheat. The rich components in the peel, known as polymethoxylated flavones, are excellent heart tonics. A cup of hot water daily with a couple of slices of lemon in it can lower high cholesterol significantly. Also add chopped lemon peel to salads.

Address stress! Take up walking, swimming, yoga or tai chi, meditation and relaxation classes, and have regular calming aromatherapy and kinesiology treatments.

High Cholesterol

Interestingly, there is no cholesterol in plant foods, only in animal products. Even more importantly, cholesterol is needed for healthy cell membranes and as a base for building healthy steroid hormones like oestrogen, progesterone and testosterone. Cholesterol is a fatty component that is transported by lipoproteins in the blood, for example low-density lipoprotein (LDL) and high-density lipoprotein (HDL) and this is what your doctor measures when you get your cholesterol levels checked out. It is not healthy to eat high-cholesterol foods and it is vital to avoid foods that will increase the production of cholesterol within the liver. The aim is to strike a good balance between both LDL and HDL cholesterol and your doctor needs to keep a check on this.

The danger foods

Saturated fats, heated oils and fats, fried foods, processed foods, palm oil, margarine, processed meats particularly salami, fatty meats, fatty bacon, and dairy products, especially cream and full-cream milk. Also avoid sugar, refined carbohydrates

and alcohol. Lack of exercise undermines efforts to build health. Being overweight will add to the danger and stress is very dangerous! So this all needs to be considered and managed.

The superfoods

Whole grains are essential as they are rich in insoluble fibre: millet, oats, buckwheat, brown rice and barley. Also include in the diet: apples, pulses like mung beans, black-eyed beans, chickpeas, lentils, soya beans, also flaxseed (ground with sesame seeds, almonds, walnuts, hazelnuts and pumpkin seeds and sprinkled onto oats porridge), alfalfa sprouts, vegetables like avocado, carrots, onions, artichokes, parsley, buckwheat (sprouts, fresh leaves and flowers), celery, beetroot, sweet green peppers, and lots of fresh fruit like bananas, grapefruit, oranges, pears, prunes, also olives and olive oil and turmeric. Moderate egg consumption (around 3 eggs a week) has little effect upon cholesterol levels. Drinking barley water daily (see recipe on page 135) and eating a big bowl of oats porridge sprinkled with the nuts and seed mixture (see page 26) and served with low-fat milk or plain yoghurt and honey, will 'sop' up high cholesterol.

Ginger, cayenne pepper and fenugreek (leaves and seeds) are all beneficial. Speak to your doctor about supplements: vitamin B-complex, vitamin C and vitamin E (*do not take vitamin E if you are on blood-thinning medication*).

Caution

If you are on statins (cholesterol-lowering drugs) do not eat grapefruit or drink grapefruit juice without your doctor's guidance, as grapefruit will reduce the activity of those enzymes in the liver that are used to metabolise the statin drugs. If they are not metabolised they will remain in the liver.

HIV / AIDS

This is a breakdown of the immune system and it is caused by the **human immunodeficiency virus (HIV)**. People infected with the virus are said to be HIV positive. The virus destroys a type of defence cell that forms part of the body's immune system. The immune system becomes progressively weaker and people with the virus begin to get serious infections like thrush, tuberculosis, pneumonia or certain types of cancer. At this point they are immune deficient and the condition is then called **acquired immunodeficiency syndrome** or **AIDS**.

HIV is usually spread through sexual contact or contact with the blood of an infected person, like shared needles by drug users, shared razors or an accidental needle prick in the case of health workers. Knowledge is your best defence – read up everything that you can find about the disease and *get tested if in any doubt*. Change your lifestyle if you are at risk of contracting HIV.

Symptoms include diarrhoea, swollen lymph nodes, digestive problems, candida, weight loss, skin lesions that are slow to heal, tuberculosis, frequent viral and bacterial infections, constant cough, colds, 'flu, compromised immune system.

The danger foods

The danger foods that compromise the immune system are listed on pages 31 and 240. Avoid food that has been cooked

Caution: Consult with your doctor before you embark on any form of self-diagnosis or self-treatment.

or heated in the microwave and check continuously for food intolerances. Common culprits are gluten (for example in wheat products), dairy products, nuts (especially peanuts), eggs, soya, chocolate and seafood.

The superfoods

The main aim is to boost the immune system. Include in the diet: whole grains, sprouts (especially flaxseed, broccoli, wheat grass and barley grass), green leafy vegetables, red, orange and yellow fruits and vegetables like papayas, oranges, strawberries, mulberries, raspberries, home-grown tomatoes, pumpkins, and so on. Include herbs like parsley, basil, coriander, dandelion, celery and echinacea in the diet. Cabbage, kale, broccoli are immune system boosters – make them into nutritious vegetable soups. Get to know shitake mushrooms (obtainable from Asian shops) and use them in soups and stews. (Hydrate them by soaking in warm water for an hour before cooking.) Drink only water or your own freshly squeezed fruits and vegetables.

Under your doctor's supervision, take a strong multivitamin and lots of vitamin C daily (at least 2 000 mg – take it with a meal).

Tissue Salts: All 12 (take 2 tablets of 'Combin 12' 3 times a day).

Use natural cleaning products in your home; avoid pollution, harmful chemical sprays, air fresheners and perfumes. Become diligent in creating a soothing, stress-free environment.

The thymus gland (found on the flat part of your chest just below the neck) gives a boost to the immune system. Every morning with the flat hand tap it gently – about 30 pats – to stimulate it.

Hives

This is a red itchy rash, often with raised weals, caused by a histamine reaction brought on by a food allergy, a chemical allergy, a plant allergy or even an alcohol allergy. Keep a notebook on when the hives broke out and possible causes.

The danger foods

Peanuts (one of the worst and most dangerous of the allergens), also shellfish, processed meats, eggs, strawberries, alcohol and food additives (colourants, stabilisers, anti-caking agents, etc.) and sometimes citrus fruit, especially oranges, can cause weals in the mouth. Read the labels of processed foods and pre-packed foods – become an informed consumer! – and boost the immune system to fight the inflammation (see page 30).

The superfoods

Apples, pears, melons, papaya, parsley, peas, rice, oats and red onions are considered safe, but make your own lists of what does or does not agree with you. Vitamin C has a strong antihistamine action and pennywort (*Centella asiatica*) will soothe and calm the itch and redness if it is applied as a cooled tea. Apply the juice of bulbinella (*Bulbine frutescens*) to the rash, squeezing it out fresh and frequently, or make a slit in an aloe vera leaf and spread the soothing pulp over the area. Use soaps and washing powders that are free from chemical additives. Tissue Salts: Both No. 4 and 9 will ease the condition (take 2 of each frequently).

Hyperactivity *see* Attention Deficit Disorder

Hyperthyroidism

This is over-activity of the thyroid gland, and ***anything to do with the thyroid needs to be carefully monitored by a specialist***. The thyroid hormones control our metabolism – the rate at which we burn food for energy – and fatigue, exhaustion, insomnia, rapid heartbeat and irritability are some of the symptoms of an over-active thyroid.

The danger foods

Alcohol of any description, tea, coffee (especially instant coffee), chocolate, colas and other carbonated drinks, energy drinks and smoking – all these will push the metabolism into overdrive. Avoid any foods rich in iodine, kelp and sea vegetables, saltwater fish, shellfish and crayfish, as iodine raises thyroid function. Also avoid all sugary foods, refined carbohydrates, processed meats, and dairy foods.

The superfoods

Millet, oats, lettuce, cabbage, broccoli, kale, cauliflower, Brussels sprouts, pulses like chickpeas, beans and lentils, vegetable soups, unsweetened fruit salads, wheat grass and barley grass juice with carrots, apples, pears, beetroot, celery, parsley, buckwheat leaves and flowers. Sprinkle ground almonds, sunflower seeds, flaxseed, pumpkin seeds and sesame seed onto oats porridge served with Bulgarian yoghurt or stir into a fruit smoothie. Snack on fruit or nuts throughout the day or try rice cakes with cucumber and mayonnaise or tomato and chutney.

Follow your doctor's advice on supplements and medications and have your thyroid function checked every 3–6 months.

Tissue Salts: All 12 (take 'Combin 12' up to 3 times a day).

Hypothyroidism

With hypothyroidism there is an under-active thyroid that is not producing sufficient quantities of the hormones that help to control our metabolism, convert food into energy and give us energy and vitality. An under-active thyroid results in constant heavy fatigue, hair loss, slow heart rate, dry skin, cold hands and feet and feeling cold and shivery, brain fog and forgetfulness, weight gain even though there is a poor appetite, constipation, depression and listlessness.

All this can be caused by problems within the thyroid gland itself – not enough hormones or the presence of antibodies within the thyroid that suppress the function of the whole gland. It is believed that lack of exercise, food intolerances, sometimes pregnancy, and disturbances in the endocrine system could add to the problem. ***There is no natural treatment that can clear this up, and you need to consult with an endocrinologist who will prescribe the correct treatment.*** If you are at risk, have your thyroid function checked every 3–6 months.

The danger foods

Make careful lists of the foods that do not agree with you – wheat and wheat products are often top of the list, and shop-bought bread is pure poison to the system. Other grains that contain gluten are rye, barley and oats and these could all be toxic to the thyroid and further suppress its function. Caffeine and dairy products also put stress onto the thyroid – instant coffee and chocolate are the worst – and salty snacks should be avoided too as salt can cause the condition to worsen.

Caution: Consult with your doctor before you embark on any form of self-diagnosis or self-treatment.

Soya, millet, raw cabbage, cauliflower, broccoli and Brussels sprouts should be avoided. Cooked cabbage and cauliflower are usually fine. Beware of sugar, refined carbohydrates, fast foods, processed meats, sweets, cakes and biscuits – all spell trouble for the thyroid. Alcohol and calorie-rich foods must be curbed – it is surprising how we feel better when we eat the good stuff!

The superfoods
Eat lots of fresh fruits, vegetables, seeds, lentils, chickpeas, butter beans, fish, nuts. Make seed mixes and sprinkle on fruit salads or oats (see page 26). Seaweed, like kelp and nori, are excellent as they contain iodine. Ask your doctor about supplements: vitamin C and B-complex, zinc, selenium and magnesium, and be sure to drink enough water daily – at least 6 glasses a day.

Tissue Salts: All 12 are of benefit, taken 2–4 times a day.

Remember, exercise stimulates the whole metabolism, so get a daily dose of vigorous exercise.

The Dangers of Chlorine and Fluoride
Be aware of chemicals like chlorine which is used in swimming pool products, in the cleaning and packaging of fish, fruits and vegetables, and as a bleach and disinfectant in many household cleaners such as laundry bleach, dishwasher soaps, floor tile cleaners and bathroom cleaners. It can be found in tap water to keep it 'clean' and it even has an E number – E295! – which means it is accepted as a food additive. Chlorinated water is linked to several serious illnesses, including cancer of the bladder and the rectum and may also inhibit thyroid function.

Fluoride is another problem as both chlorine and fluoride are chemically similar to iodine and as such can take the place of iodine in the thyroid gland. Fluoride is added to both toothpaste and water to prevent tooth decay but what is extremely worrying is that fluoride is a serious toxin. Although there is little evidence to support that fluoride truly and lastingly supports the structure of the teeth in preventing dental caries, far more alarming is that fluoride is a systemic poison and has been implicated in many illnesses, for example bone fractures and bone pains, diabetes, thyroid ailments, impaired mental development, discolouring the teeth, gastrointestinal reflux and as a suspected oral cancer trigger. Shouldn't we be discussing this with our doctors and dentists?

Hysterectomy
A hysterectomy is the surgical removal of the uterus and a total hysterectomy means that the uterus, the cervix and the ovaries are all removed – and this is a great change for a woman, both mentally and physically. With oestrogen production now quite dramatically reduced, any number of symptoms pertaining to menopause, which has suddenly been put into place, can occur. Hot flushes, palpitations, night sweats, insomnia, irritability, weepiness, and loss of confidence are a few of the symptoms, and with the changes in the woman's body – and sometimes it is a young body, too early for menopause – there is the risk of both osteoporosis and heart disease because of the sudden fall in progesterone and oestrogen. So, at all times be guided by your doctor for hormone replacement therapy and natural treatments. A hysterectomy is usually advised if there is severe and excessive bleeding from the uterus – the monthly menstrual cycle floods so severely there is no other way – and loss of blood can lead to anaemia. Or there are fibroids or cysts on the walls of the uterus, or there is a prolapse of the uterus or severe endometriosis (see page 226).

To regain energy and vitality and to bring the body back to normal again after a hysterectomy, be very careful with everything you put into your mouth.

The danger foods
Smoking, alcohol, sugar, salt and caffeine in any form – most dangerous are the diet colas and the energy drinks. Read every label carefully and beware of additives, which can exacerbate the discomfort, upset the blood sugar and aggravate the menopausal symptoms (see also Menopause on page 246).

The superfoods
Fresh soya and soya products like tofu and tempeh are helpful, but not processed soya – rather use the soya you grow yourself and eat it like green peas. Seaweeds, like kelp and nori, are rich in minerals. The following foods are rich in the essential fatty acids: trout, mackerel, salmon, sardines, sunflower seeds, almonds, pumpkin seeds, sesame seeds, flaxseed and flaxseed oil, hazelnuts, Brazil nuts, chickpeas and lentils. Include lots of green vegetables in the diet, both in soups and in salads, especially fresh lucerne leaves, red clover leaves, amaranth leaves and seeds, dandelion leaves (and roast the root for coffee, see page 231), lettuce, fenugreek leaves and fresh fennel. Eat foods rich in vitamin E to reduce hot flushes (see page 13).

Wheat grass and barley grass juice with fresh carrots, beetroot, lucerne, celery stalks and leaves and apples is vital to increase vitality.

Speak to your doctor about supplements: vitamin D, E, K and B-complex, magnesium and calcium with boron. Probiotics are valuable post-operatively.

Tissue Salts: All 12 are of benefit (take as 'Combin 12', 3–4 times a day).

Start exercising as soon as the surgeon recommends it – walking and later weight-bearing exercises to strengthen the muscles and the bones. Your doctor and physiotherapist will advise you.

Impotence
Lack of sexual desire and erectile dysfunction is caused by a number of factors, including smoking, being on certain medications, B-vitamin deficiencies, diabetes, alcohol, overweight, emotional problems, heart ailments and the biggest of all, intense and daily stress.

The danger foods
Alcohol, sugar, chocolates, sweets, ice-creams, carbonated colas, coffee (worst is instant coffee!), instant foods, processed foods, especially meats like biltong and salty sausages, tinned foods, refined carbohydrates like white bread, white pasta, sugary buns, white rice, white sugar and breakfast cereals with sugar.

The superfoods
Change to a diet rich in vegetables, fruit, oily fish like mackerel, trout, tuna, salmon, sardines (not tinned sardines), snack

Caution: Consult with your doctor before you embark on any form of self-diagnosis or self-treatment.

on unsalted nuts like almonds, cashews, pecans and Brazil nuts. Include avocados for their high levels of vitamins E and B6 and folic acid, which are important for sexual health. Bananas, all kinds of berries, celery, beetroot, chilli, (especially hot chillies, which can be included in stir-fries and sauces) all have aphrodisiac qualities. Celery seeds, leaves and stalks are valuable too as they contain androstenone which is close to testosterone. Cinnamon ground over fruit salads is a superb toner of the kidneys – even the smell boosts alertness and brain function – and garlic, ginger, spinach and gingko biloba are all valuable for sexual health.

Avoid tea and coffee and replace with smoothies or wheat or barley grass juice. Smoothies made with bananas, berries, beetroot, pineapple, kiwifruit, carrots and plain Bulgarian yoghurt are energy giving and very potent. Smoothies give easily accessible vitamins and amino acids that are quickly absorbed. Wheat and barley grass juices with beetroot, celery, carrots, apple, lucerne and parsley will provide stamina (take ½ a glass twice a day). This incredibly vitamin and mineral rich juice is good for adrenal and kidney health too, and acts as a tonic to the prostate gland.

Interestingly, raw chocolate, raw cacao, is thought to promote sexual energy – that is before it is mixed with sugar and milk! Raw cacao nibs are available from health shops and some delicatessens.

Tissue Salts: All 12 (take as 'Combin 12', up to 3 times a day).

Immune System, Weakened

The immune system consists of primarily the red blood cells, the lymphatic system, the bone marrow, the spleen and that marvellous little regulator, the thymus gland. But the entire body, in a state of good health, is part of the whole picture. So building a strong resistance to infection is of primary importance, and diet plays a huge role.

The danger foods

A diet of junk food with sugary snacks, drinks and sweets, ice-creams and refined carbohydrates, like white bread, cakes and biscuits leads to sugar highs and a continuous assault of colds, 'flu, mucus congestion and allergic reactions. Processed foods of every kind, especially processed meats, fast foods, fried foods, artificial sweeteners, salt and salty snacks, alcohol, smoking, late nights, lack of exercise, lack of fresh air and, interestingly, excessive and continuous use of computers, cell phones and microwaves all put a huge strain on an already weakened immune system. Dehydration also plays a role – we drink far too little water daily (6 glasses of plain, pure water is the daily minimum).

More than anything else – learn to avoid sugar in every form, including sucrose, fructose, glucose and too much honey. Replace with stevia for sweetness. Tests showed that ingesting just 100 g of sugar reduced the ability of certain white blood cells to fight infection in less than 30 minutes – and this effect lasted up to 5 hours. These white blood cells or 'neutrophils', which constitute up to 70% of the white blood cells, showed no activity and this means the immune system is compromised. Be diligent – become aware of hidden sugars and look after the thymus gland. It is so susceptible to free radical damage, to stress, to radiation and to drugs – and that means 'recreational drugs' of all kinds – and our bad eating habits, and no one

can do it for you. You have commit to building health and not breaking it down.

Ask your doctor to check you for candida (see page 216), high homocysteine levels and chronic gastrointestinal problems like Crohn's disease and irritable bowel syndrome (see page 222 and 243).

The superfoods

Drastic change is required and to do this you need to do a serious audit of what is in your fridge and store cupboard at this moment, and throw out all the danger foods. Fresh fruits and vegetables are now your lifeline: salads and fruit salads daily with no sugar, no salt or very little salt – herbs like celery, coriander, thyme, oregano, cumin and fresh lemon juice will give the flavour you crave, and at the same time boost the immune system. Fruit and vegetable smoothies and juices like wheat and barley grass with fresh lucerne, parsley, carrots, beetroot, apple, celery, pineapple, radish, ginger and papaya are rich in antioxidants and help to speed recovery after an illness. Make smoothies of all the berries, and add kiwifruit and apples, fresh fruit in season and a good handful of sprouts. Smoothies are an excellent energy food and good for building resistance.

Whole grains like oats, buckwheat, millet, sesame seeds and organically grown wheat are important – it is worth grinding your own grains in a tabletop stone grinder. Pulses are an excellent basic – peas, beans of all kinds, lentils, chickpeas and nuts. These in soups, stews and cooked and served cold with lots of spring onions, garlic, parsley, grated fresh ginger, fresh coriander leaves, celery and a simple dressing of olive oil and lemon juice, become an immune system boost.

Eat adequate, but not excessive, amounts of protein and vary it – fish, chicken, lean mutton, organic lean beef – and always serve with the high-in-carotene fruits and vegetables, all the bright yellow, orange and red fruits and vegetables. The cabbage family – cabbage, cauliflower, broccoli, kale, broccoli sprouts, Brussels sprouts – have tremendous immune-boosting ability, and include mustard leaves, radishes and radish leaves and turnip leaves here too. Jerusalem artichoke is also a valuable addition to immune-boosting soups – add the grated root to the soup pot or a stir-fry. Bake your own bread (see page 35).

Sprouts are 'high-octane fuel' and alfalfa, buckwheat, sunflower seeds, broccoli seeds, fenugreek and chickpea sprouts and organically grown peas with their leafy tips, all are high in their life force energy and excellent for the immune system. Make your own sprouts and grow your own wheat and barley grass for a regular supply (see page 29). Water and herb teas like echinacea, pennywort (Centella asiatica), fennel, ginger, olive leaf, nettle, dandelion, rosehip and lemongrass are essential, and drink at least 6 glasses of plain water every day.

Speak to your doctor about supplements: vitamin C and D, zinc, magnesium, the B-vitamins, probiotics (and eat Bulgarian yoghurt) to keep the intestines in good shape, also garlic and parsley capsules (and eat fresh as well). Deep breathing and exercise are vitally important. Obesity is also associated with impaired immune function, highlighting again the need for regular exercise combined with a healthy diet. Finally, get at least 6 hours of sleep every night – 8 hours is best.

Tissue Salts: No. 1, 4, 5, 6 and 9 (you can also take 'Combin 12', provided you have no implants).

Caution: Consult with your doctor before you embark on any form of self-diagnosis or self-treatment.

Incontinence

A 'leaky bladder' is a source of distress and inconvenience. Causes include prostate problems, gynaecological problems, often after childbirth, obesity, stroke, anxiety and stress, lifting heavy objects, straining with constipation, smoking or merely the ageing process. Spinal injuries, weak pelvic floor muscles or even coughing or sneezing are other triggers of weak bladder control.

The danger foods

Too much salt in the diet is a trigger and so is alcohol and caffeine, especially instant coffee. These put a heavy strain on the kidneys and the constant need to urinate with urgency rules the day! Avoid foods rich in oxalic acid, like Swiss chard, rhubarb, spinach, sorrel, beetroot leaves, asparagus, even eggs – limit these to 2–3 times a week, and soft-boiled eggs are best. Cut down on sugar and avoid fried foods and processed foods. Smoking is a huge NO! Stop smoking today if you want to build health. Incontinence is but one of the many serious health problems induced by smoking, and passive smoking.

The superfoods

All the green vegetables (except spinach, Swiss chard and sorrel); you need all the magnesium and calcium you can get, so include sprouts, fresh lucerne, lettuce, cabbage, broccoli, green herbs like fenugreek leaves, red clover leaves, dandelion leaves, parsley, celery and teas of pennywort (*Centella asiatica*) and stinging nettle. A juice of barley and wheat grass with carrots, lucerne, celery, kiwifruit, parsley, apples, beetroot or pineapple and sprouts like buckwheat, alfalfa and mung beans is a fabulous tonic (try to have a ½ glass daily).

Your aim is to tone, strengthen and revitalise the entire urinary system – so include fish and organic chicken in the diet along with plenty of fruit and vegetables. Increase your intake of vitamins D, B3 and B6, potassium and magnesium under your doctor's supervision. Drink lots of cranberry juice.

Tissue Salts: No. 4 and 11 are immediately helpful (2 tablets of each taken up to 7 times a day); No. 2, 6, 9 and 10 is a valuable treatment for spurts of urine when coughing or sneezing.

Pelvic floor muscle exercises are immensely valuable and I urge you to have a series of treatments to re-educate the pelvic floor.

Indigestion

The world's most common ailment, indigestion is an umbrella term for many discomforts, from heartburn, flatulence, bloating, burping, colic to nausea and even the vomiting of indigestive food. This debilitating condition is caused, it has been established many times over, by eating wrongly! This means eating very spicy, hot or over-flavoured foods, eating fatty foods, overeating, eating with alcohol, eating too quickly or not chewing food well, eating and talking, or eating when highly stressed, emotional or anxious.

The danger foods

Spicy foods, fried foods, fatty foods, especially sausages and processed meats, fast food, packets of crisps and other highly flavoured snacks, and anything containing additives. Become aware of tartrazine and other colourants, flavourants, stabilisers, anti-caking agents, preservatives and the many other chemicals found in processed and long-life foods. Avoid sugary foods, rich creamy sauces, ice-cream, commercial custards, instant desserts and carbonated drinks. Fast food and cold carbonated drinks spell great danger! Caffeine, especially instant coffee, is a no-no, as is all alcohol, not even a sip of wine!

The superfoods

Eat small regular meals and include fresh pineapple (it contains the enzyme bromelain which eases digestion), celery, parsley, asparagus, vegetable soups made with sweet potatoes, pumpkin, carrots, brown rice or barley, fresh peas and pea shoots, lentils or finely shredded fennel bulb. Add finely chopped onions and leeks fried in a little olive oil to give a delicious flavour and use sea salt, lemon juice, thyme, and coriander anise or caraway seed to flavour your soup. Interestingly, a whole butter lettuce finely shredded and added to a soup at the end of the cooking time is an age-old digestive remedy, with chopped fresh parsley sprinkled over the bowl of soup as it is served.

Other easy-to-digest foods include apples, pears, all the berries, papaya, prunes and plums (keep a notebook of all the foods that agree with you.) – eat them in fruit salads or make smoothies or juices.

Drink herbal teas: fennel, chamomile or mint tea made with fresh leaves and flowers – ¼ cup to 1 cup of boiling water, stand 5 minutes, strain and sip slowly. Or aniseed, dill or caraway seed tea – 1 teaspoon seeds in 1 cup of boiling water, stand 5 minutes, stir well and sip slowly. Chew a few seeds too with the tea. Keep a mixture of aniseed, caraway, dill, fennel and cumin seed in a tiny bottle or tin and chew a pinch of seeds every now and then, and keep a little bowl on the dinner table and chew a few seeds before and during the meal.

Two teaspoons of apple cider vinegar in a small glass of warm water is also an excellent digestive sipped before a meal. Don't drink anything during a meal and avoid iced drinks, even on a hot summer's day, and don't drink from a straw as this can introduce air into the digestive system.

A thin slice or two of fresh ginger in a cup of boiling water with a sprig of fresh mint is a natural anti-acidic digestive! No sweetening, just these two ingredients and a good stir – let it stand 5 minutes before drinking. Follow up with 2 tablets each of Tissue Salts No. 2, 8 and 10 and suck them slowly. (This combination also helps projectile vomiting in babies – crush 1 tablet of each and mix with a little water and give it to the baby before each meal, even before breastfeeding.)

Tissue Salts: No. 1, 2, 6, 9 and 10; bruising – No. 2, 8 and 10; nervous indigestion – No. 6, also No. 3 and 12.

Infertility *see* Conception

Inflammation

This is a giant of a word that applies to many things: from invasion of bacteria and viruses and allergic reaction to pollens, foods, bites or stings, to injuries and isolated infections around grazes, wounds or scratches, sore throats like tonsillitis or laryngitis, infected gums like gingivitis, and so on. Inflammation is the body's response to 'attack', one could say, and heat, redness, soreness and even fever and restricted movement, are some of the symptoms. The inflammation can be both external and internal – think of ear infections, bladder infections, cystitis – and often if a condition or illness has a name ending in '-itis' it

Caution: Consult with your doctor before you embark on any form of self-diagnosis or self-treatment.

will mean that inflammation is present. When any inflammatory condition is present there is always stress, tension and anxiety so a speedy response is needed. First let your doctor assess the damage, then be sure you look after the body with a healthy diet to clear up the infection before it becomes a problem.

The danger foods
Refined carbohydrates and sugar, food additives (see page 210), preservatives, artificial sweeteners, all processed foods but especially processed meat, fast foods, instant foods, instant coffee and carbonated cold drinks. Dairy and wheat products can add to the condition.

The superfoods
Eat lots of antioxidant-rich foods: all the berries but blueberries and blackberries in particular, pomegranates, pineapple, peaches, grapes, kiwifruit; foods rich in vitamin C: lemons, oranges, mangoes, cherries (see also page 13); foods rich in zinc (see page 16); ginger; seeds and nuts like pumpkin seeds, flaxseed, sunflower seeds, almonds, macadamias, pecan nuts; and drink wheat and barley grass juice. Make smoothies or juices with apples, bananas, berries, mangoes, carrots, papaya, plums, cherries, watermelon and spanspek and don't forget vegetable smoothies or juices – try carrots with pineapple or carrots, broccoli, celery and beetroot.

There are also essential fats and oils that ease inflammatory conditions so eat oily fish – mackerel, trout, sardines – and olive oil, grape seed oil, sunflower oil, especially if it is cold pressed. Don't forget the water – at least 6–8 glasses of plain water daily – to flush the toxins out of the body and bring the good nutrients into the body. Take extra vitamin C, zinc and probiotics (or eat Bulgarian yoghurt).

Tissue Salts: No. 1, 4, 5 and 7 are your first line of defence; followed a day or two later by 'Combin 12' (unless you have implants). Take 2 of each frequently.

Influenza
A dreaded but common infection, it is usually caused by a virus and its onset can be sudden with fever, feeling hot then cold, sore throat, sneezing, aches, pains and general wretchedness and weakness. If your immune system is weak then 'flu can be severe, turning often into bronchitis – bed rest is vital. The 'flu virus spreads easily and contact with people, stress, shock and lack of sleep can make one susceptible.

The danger foods
Seriously avoid sugar and all refined carbohydrates, so no chocolates, sweets and cakes, colas and other fizzy drinks, energy drinks, fast foods, fried foods, salty foods, processed meats and no fatty foods. In fact, avoid meat altogether at this time. Avoid caffeine and alcohol in every form, and all additives, artificial sweeteners, and no orange-flavoured artificially coloured drinks, not even fresh orange juice as these build up mucus! Even though fresh orange juice is rich in vitamin C, 'flu usually means blocked nose and sinuses and postnasal drip – all of which could be aggravated by orange juice.

The superfoods
Make a vegetable-rich chicken soup (see recipe on page 219), juice fresh vegetables and fruit and make fruit salads with finely grated ginger and a little honey. Add watercress, celery, parsley, radishes, dandelion leaves, mustard leaves and buckwheat leaves to salads, with lemon juice, honey, finely grated ginger and crushed coriander as a salad dressing.

This is a time for clearing out the toxins and herb teas are very helpful: fresh sage leaves with ginger, honey and lemon juice, or try lemon verbena, lemongrass or lemon thyme with honey and ginger. Pour 1 cup of boiling water over ¼ cup fresh herbs, stand 5 minutes, strain and add a squeeze of lemon juice and a touch of honey. Sip slowly.

Ask your doctor to prescribe echinacea or other natural medications, vitamins and minerals. Increase your intake of vitamin C and zinc. Stay in bed.

Tissue Salts: The classic 'flu remedy is No. 1, 4, 5, 9 and 11 (take 2 tablets of each up to 10 times throughout the day). These are also available in a combined tablet and I have also created a natural antibiotic manufactured by Fithealth that works well (see page 18).

Insomnia
Insomnia means sleeplessness and it affects us all at some stage. Life deals many blows and sleepless nights seem to be part of the stress, worry, grief, change and loss. Yet sleep is a vital part of maintaining good health. Lack of sleep takes a huge toll, for example concentration, brain function and alert decision making is impaired, depression gets a foothold and as the much needed repair, rejuvenation and healing takes place when we sleep, without it, we self-destruct.

There are many causes – look at them carefully and try to rectify them at the source: the first is food deficiencies, for example amino-acid deficiencies, too little magnesium in the body, also vitamin deficiencies, especially the B-vitamins (if vitamin B3 is deficient, melatonin, which is the sleep hormone, is affected), so make sure the B-vitamins are included in the daily diet (see pages 11 to 13 for foods rich in the B-vitamins). Other causes are indigestion, cramps, anxiety and certain medications.

The danger foods
One of the greatest problems is sugar, especially at night. Don't be tempted into having mugs of hot chocolate before going to bed, or cakes, sweets or sugary desserts. Caffeine is a stimulant and should be avoided before bedtime – this includes chocolate, colas, cacao, tea and coffee – the worst is instant coffee with sugar and milk or creamer. Avoid alcohol in any form – don't be tempted to have a nightcap. Not only is alcohol a stimulant, it takes a harsh toll on the liver and kidneys and you'll pay for it with increasing severity. Avoid all fatty foods, fried foods and processed and sweetened foods. Your liver and your heart are being put under severe stress.

The superfoods
The secret is to have a fairly light supper no later than 8:30 p.m. Vegetable soups are ideal, especially with green vegetables that are rich in magnesium, or have chicken salad or fish with steamed vegetables like kale, broccoli, cauliflower, green peas (including the tender leafy tops of the pea vine with tendrils), steamed whole radishes, leaves and all, squash and brown rice. Eat lots of lettuce, which has relaxing properties, and snack on magnesium-rich nuts and seeds during the day. Sweet potatoes,

Caution: Consult with your doctor before you embark on any form of self-diagnosis or self-treatment.

millet, buckwheat and buckwheat greens, brown rice, barley and barley water all have sedative effects with the evening meal, and with simple steamed fish or chicken, this becomes a calming end to the day. And don't forget: a bowl of oatmeal porridge with Bulgarian yoghurt, bananas and a sprinkling of ground seeds (see page 26), cinnamon and honey is the age-old calming, soothing and relaxing supper for over-stimulated excitable children and adults.

Exercising during the day will help the sleep pattern, particularly walking. Avoid strenuous exercise just before bed, though, as this will stimulate the adrenal function, increasing the heart rate. So do no strenuous exercise at least 3 hours before going to bed. Watching TV or working on the computer over-stimulates the brain, so avoid these activities close to bedtime.

Try a lavender pillow under the neck for relaxation and add fresh lavender to the bath, soak in it and rub your feet and stiff shoulders with a few drops of essential oil of lavender in a little almond oil or in a chemical-free aqueous cream.

Tissue Salts: The phosphates are all excellent for sleep patterns – they are No. 2, 4, 6, 8 and 10 (take 2 tablets of each at the end of the day every hour before you go to sleep). They are also available combined in a single tablet. In the Fithealth Margaret Roberts Herbal Remedies range we make 'Easy Sleep', a herbal supplement (see page 18).

Irritable Bowel Syndrome

This is an uncomfortable and irritating problem that includes bloating, colic and stomach pain, cramps, flatulence, diarrhoea at times and constipation at other times, and mucus in the stools. The digestive system is under stress and it does not move the food smoothly through the bowels. Sometimes it is moved through too fast and at other times it is moved through too slowly. One causes diarrhoea and the other, the slow movement, causes constipation. Either way it is uncomfortable.

There are several causes and it needs to be diagnosed by your doctor. Check for food intolerances like gluten and dairy products, a deficiency in magnesium, digestive enzymes or hydrochloric acid in the stomach, which aids the digestion. The good bacteria in the bowel might be depleted or you may have candida. All this needs to be established by your doctor.

Irritable bowel syndrome can be greatly eased by looking at the diet, and the irritants in the diet can cause itchiness around the anus, which adds to the discomfort – even an itchy nose, which is not caused by hay fever but by the toxins in the digestive system!

The danger foods

Wheat and dairy products are top of the list, but citrus fruits, even lemon juice, may also cause a reaction; tomatoes, rhubarb, spinach, cabbage, onions, even broccoli and cauliflower sometimes add to the distress of gas and bloatedness, but here bought bread is by far the worst offender. Avoid all forms of sugar as well as artificial sweeteners (replace with stevia), alcohol, coffee, margarine, spicy foods, fatty foods, especially processed meats and high-fat cheeses. Keep a diary and monitor everything that goes into your mouth!

The superfoods

Vegetable broths, steamed bland vegetables like pumpkin, squash, sweet potatoes, peas, potatoes and globe artichokes, buckwheat, brown rice, lentils, sprouted seeds like mung beans, chickpeas and alfalfa. To keep the bowels working smoothly, papaya, figs, prunes, plain Bulgarian yoghurt, grated apples, mashed bananas, rooibos tea, pears, mangoes, dates and all non-acidic fruits.

Try the following herb teas: melissa, peppermint and the other mints, fennel, turmeric, ginger, aniseed, caraway and chamomile tea at night. Add ground flaxseed to smoothies or fruit and yoghurt. Slippery elm is a gentle laxative bought from health stores that tones and comforts – mix it with finely grated apple or warm oatmeal porridge or mix all three together.

Ask your doctor about supplements: vitamin B-complex and vitamin E, magnesium, digestive enzymes and probiotics.

Tissue Salts: No. 2, 6, 8 and 11 (take 2 at a time at least 3 times a day to establish a soothing and gentle calmness within the bowel; lessen the tissue salts as you become more relaxed).

Take your meals in peaceful surroundings and chew your food thoroughly and slowly. Reflexology often helps to relax the stomach and relaxation classes and yoga have been found helpful in many cases. Relaxing after a meal with a hot water bottle over the stomach should it feel uncomfortable, has also proved to be very helpful and soothing.

Jet Lag

This is common with air travel across time zones, which can upset and change the circadian rhythm of the body – night becomes day and hours are lost or gained. The recycled air and the air pressure within the aircraft further tires and upsets the body and a bout of 'flu is not uncommon as one disembarks. If you are planning a long-haul flight, be diligent about building up your immune system to peak heights (see page 30) long before your departure date.

The danger foods

During the flight avoid coffee, carbonated drinks, tea, alcohol of any kind and anything with sugar in it. Ask for water – plain water – and be sure you drink it often throughout the flight. Avoid salted nuts, salty crisps, refined carbohydrates and anything fatty.

The superfoods

Before the flight: One of my most important and sustaining health programmes is a daily ½ a glass of wheat and barley grass juice with apples, carrots, pineapple, beetroot, parsley, celery and fresh lucerne leaves. I drink this diligently every day for at least 15 days before any long-distance flight. I also increase my vitamin C and zinc intake, and make sure I drink enough water to stay hydrated, and I cut down on everything that could compromise the immune system, including the tiniest pinch of sugar!

The day before the flight, eat meals with chicken or turkey, tomatoes, brown rice, fish, bananas, avocadoes, eggs or oats – these tryptophan-rich foods will help you to relax and sleep well once you've landed.

During the flight: Eat carefully and choose salads and fruit salads first if these are offered. I find taking my own little packet of

Caution: Consult with your doctor before you embark on any form of self-diagnosis or self-treatment.

almonds, sunflower seeds, pumpkin seeds, cashew nuts and macadamias help enormously, along with dried, unsweetened apple rings and apricots. These with plenty of water take the strain off the digestive system. Chamomile tea is excellent – take your own teabags and ask the airhostess for a cup of boiling water and make your own.

On arrival don't have a heavy meal. Stick to lots of water and vegetable soups, salads and fruit salads.

Speak to your doctor about supplements: magnesium, vitamin B-complex, vitamin C and zinc.

Tissue Salts: Special tissue salts for easy air travel are No. 2, 6, 8 and 11 (take 2 of each every hour, you'll be astonished at the difference they make). Take them throughout the flight and frequently once you've landed. You'll notice all the fatigue, dizziness and unsettled symptoms you used to feel, disappeared and the journey was an easy one.

Walk around often during the flight, even if it is to the toilet and back, and do feet and leg exercises by moving muscles, tightening and relaxing and circling the feet in both directions. This is essential as it keeps the tissues oxygenated. Use a neck pillow, earplugs and an eye mask if you fly overnight.

Kidney Stones

If you have ever experienced the debilitating pain of a kidney stone you will never forget it. The pain is usually over the kidney area in the middle of the back and can spread over the stomach and intestine area too. It is caused by calcium oxalate build-up, and a bad diet often triggers it, especially ice-cold carbonated drinks! Uric acid builds up to point where a sea of pain seems to completely engulf you. Your doctor must diagnose this condition and you *will* be asked about your diet, so pay attention to what goes into your mouth!

The danger foods

The main offenders are alcohol, carbonated colas and other fizzy drinks, bright orange sweetened juices, sugary cakes, sweets and chocolates. Avoid drinking too much coffee (the worst is instant coffee), anything that contains sugar and refined flour. Eat less meat and avoid all processed meats, fatty meats and sausages, very spicy foods, fried foods and all instant or processed foods. Avoid salt as salt puts a strain on the kidneys by increasing urinary calcium, which increases the risk of kidney stone formation!

Avoid dairy products, black tea, beetroot leaves, chocolates, milkshakes, sorrel salad leaves, rhubarb, figs, plums, prunes, spinach and Swiss chard as these are all high in oxalates and combined with calcium form the start of kidney stones. Also avoid tomatoes, sweet peppers, brinjals, gooseberries and potatoes – all belong to the nightshade family and add to the congestion of the kidneys.

The superfoods

Cranberries and cranberry juice, rye, soya, brown rice, barley and barley water (2 glasses a day – see recipe on page 135), avocadoes, mung beans, kidney beans, parsley, dandelion root tea (see box), sesame seeds, bananas, coconut, watermelon and watermelon juice, fresh grated radish. The following foods contain small amounts of oxalates, eat them in moderation note more than twice a week: all the berries (blueberries, strawberries, raspberries, etc.), members of the cabbage family (broccoli, kale, rocket, mustard greens, turnips, cabbage, cauliflower, Brussels sprouts), sweet potatoes and squash.

Ask your doctor about increased water intake and about supplements: vitamin B6 and magnesium (which is usually 300 to 500 mg daily because magnesium balances the calcium in the body). Check your calcium intake. Take digestive enzymes with meals to ease the digestion.

Drink mint tea and take Tissue Salts No. 2, 10 and 11 (take 2 tablets of each at least 6 times during the day).

Dandelion Root Tea

Dig up the whole plant (use the leaves for salads – they keep well, washed in running water and stored in the fridge in a plastic bag). Chop off the root, wash well, peel with a potato peeler if it is thick and tough, otherwise slice thinly or grate finely. Take about 8 slices or ¼ cup grated root and pour over this 1 cup of boiling water, stand 5 minutes pressing it thoroughly with a teaspoon, strain and sip slowly. Add a little fresh chopped parsley to improve the bitter taste! But this is worth trying as it breaks down the uric acid.

Lactose Intolerance

It is not only babies who are unable to digest the milk sugar lactose. In order to digest lactose, an enzyme known as lactase is needed, and this enzyme is often deficient, resulting in the discomfort of indigestion, flatulence, bloating and often diarrhoea, vomiting and in children, failure to thrive and gain weight and constant fussiness and crying. Lactose intolerance may be due to coeliac disease, colitis, gastroenteritis or it may be a genetic problem.

The danger foods

Avoid all dairy products – processed cheese is one of the most dangerous. Sugar adds to the problem. Avoid all low-fat sweetened yoghurts, not only are they sweetened but in most cases milk powder, which is rich in lactose, is added to give a thicker texture. Butter is in some cases tolerated.

The superfoods

Replace cow's milk with soya milk and eat the following calcium-rich foods: green fresh soya beans and fermented soya products like tofu and tempeh, mackerel and sardines with the bones, oats, green leafy vegetables like cabbage, kale, turnip greens, broccoli and lettuce, okra, chickpeas, sesame seeds, figs (fresh and dried), amaranth, hazelnuts, almonds, Brazil nuts, beans (fresh and dried), alfalfa sprouts and fresh lucerne leaves. Eat magnesium-rich foods to balance the calcium, like Swiss chard, spinach, butter beans, haricot beans, pumpkin seed, avocadoes, brown rice, bananas, seaweed and kelp.

Talk to your doctor about supplements and probiotics, especially *Acidophilus* capsules, which aid the digestion of lactose.

Tissue Salts: Take No. 1, 2, 6, 9 and 10 in drop form (the tablets are in a lactose base); also No. 8 and 12. Take 4 drops of each in a little water.

Drink plenty of water and read labels carefully as lactose appears in many packaged foods. Keep a food diary and note down which foods do and do not agree with you.

Caution: Consult with your doctor before you embark on any form of self-diagnosis or self-treatment.

Liver Damage

The liver is vital for a healthy life and it has so many functions we need to be aware of: detoxification, control of blood sugar and blood cholesterol, absorption of protein and processing of alcohol, to name but a few of its vital functions. Symptoms of liver damage include jaundice, bloatedness, swelling, constipation, diarrhoea, loss of appetite, muscle fatigue, indigestion and nausea. 'Liverishness' is a word my grandmother used when she saw we were nauseous, queasy and felt generally unwell with diarrhoea. The most frequent cause of liver damage is alcohol overdose. Poor diet is another more common cause, especially over-indulgence of rich, fatty foods.

The danger foods

Heated fats, fried foods, cream, all processed and fatty meats, margarine, full-fat dairy products, pastries, instant coffee, creamers, caffeine in all forms, instant foods, refined carbohydrates, sugar, crisps, cakes and pies. Most important of all: **avoid all alcohol of any description.**

The superfoods

Green-coloured foods, especially sprouts, lettuce, spinach, fresh lucerne, buckwheat greens, cabbage and kale as well as wheat grass and barley grass juiced with celery, beetroot, carrot and apple (this is vital every day – ½ a glass mid-morning and ½ a glass mid-afternoon). See also page 29.

Eat lots of fresh fruits, salads and steamed vegetables. Lessen the meat – eat lean mutton only once a week. Where possible, replace meat with fish – steamed or baked without creamy sauces and served with lemon juice.

Add cayenne pepper to foods, lessen the salt and flavour with fresh thyme, oregano, basil, rosemary and coriander (leaves and seeds), eat 5 dandelion leaves every day and drink dandelion root coffee (see page 231). Sprinkle your food with freshly grated ginger and turmeric powder. The vital nutrients in all these amazing foods will help to regenerate the liver cells.

Speak to your doctor about supplements: include milk thistle capsules, digestive enzymes and spirulina.

Tissue Salts: No. 3, 5, 8, 10 and 11 (take 2 of each at least 3 times a day).

Lung Cancer

One of the most common illnesses today, 90% of lung cancer cases is due to smoking and passive smoking. The more you smoke the more likely you are to get lung cancer and you are putting other people's lives in danger too. Air pollution, smoke pollution, tuberculosis and exposure to pesticides, paints, metal dust, petrol and chemical fumes and asbestos are all dangerous for the lungs, and something we tend to forget are dry-cleaning chemicals and chemical cleaning products.

Be aware of a tight chest, wheezing, coughing, breathlessness, chest pains, fatigue, poor appetite, weight loss and phlegm with blood in it, and see your doctor immediately.

The danger foods

Avoid all processed and packaged foods, alcohol in any form, fatty meat, especially fried meats, barbequed meat or meat that is charred on the edges. Avoid saturated fats, full-fat dairy foods, dripping, lard, solid fats, processed meats, trans fats, like block margarine, deep-fried foods and sugar in any form. Limit the number of eggs you eat to no more than 5 a week. Avoid coffee and black tea – replace with rooibos, herb teas and green tea. **If you are a smoker, stop smoking immediately. If you live with a smoker, avoid inhaling second-hand smoke.**

The superfoods

Whole grains, nuts, seeds, tofu, Bulgarian yoghurt, fruit salads, fresh fruits, vegetables, salads, vegetable soups with organically grown vegetables, sprouts, fresh lucerne, parsley, celery. A minimum of 8 fresh fruits and vegetables per day is vital – more is better: apples, tomatoes and onions are rich in antioxidants, particularly a flavonoid called quercetin which is a cancer fighter, and tomatoes also contain lycopene, a powerful phytonutrient which reduces the risk of lung cancer. Freshly squeezed fruit and vegetable juices, wheat grass and barley grass juice daily (see page 29) as well as walnuts, flaxseed, brown rice, peas, beans, lentils and oily fish like mackerel and sardines (twice a week) will boost high-level wellness. Also include foods rich in beta-carotene – berries, carrots, sweet potatoes, squash and pumpkin. It is important to remember that as cholesterol increases so does the risk of lung cancer. Also, as the intake of fruit, vegetables, wheat grass and barley grass juice increases, so the risk of lung cancer decreases.

Drink herb teas like fennel, mint, stinging nettle, ginger, peppermint and lemongrass. Drink at least 6–8 glasses of plain water every single day. Speak to your doctor about supplements: vitamin E, selenium, vitamin B12 and folic acid. See a physiotherapist to teach you about deep breathing exercises and do these with dedication daily. Most of us do not utilise our full lung capacity and with deep and concentrated breathing to expand the lungs a new vitality will emerge.

Tissue Salts: No. 3, 4, 5, 6, 7, 8 and 12 (take 2 of each up to 8 times a day).

Plants That Clean the Air

Choose fresh air away from pollutants and use air-cleaning plants in your home. We have created a great conservatory against the mountain, filled with air-cleaning plants like peace lilies, coffee trees, ferns, pachira nuts, hen and chickens, to name a few. Many visitors with lung ailments come to just sit and relax in there and breathe deeply with great expansion of the lungs and emerge rejuvenated.

Lupus

Lupus is an inflammatory condition, an autoimmune disease in which discomfort, pain and inflammation engulfs the body. It is caused by antibodies produced by the immune system which attack the body. There are two types of lupus: Discoid lupus erythematosus (DLE) is a skin disease that is identified by a red butterfly-shaped rash that covers the nose and the cheeks with often raised yellow lumps on the skin and on the ears. Systemic lupus erythematosus (SLE) often affects the whole body with fatigue, joint pains, a butterfly-shaped red rash over the face and sometimes the scalp, with 'flu-like symptoms, susceptibility to infection, and in really severe cases the kidneys, the lungs and even the brain can be affected.

Caution: Consult with your doctor before you embark on any form of self-diagnosis or self-treatment.

Flare-ups are triggered by continuous stress, viral infections, exhaustion or food allergies and intolerances like gluten, dairy, eggs, yeast, soya and even chocolate! Check for adverse reactions to vitamin K. Lupus is not completely understood as it differs so greatly from person to person, and keeping a diary of foods and symptoms is extremely valuable as food intolerances play a major role. Periods of remission can be considerably lengthened by detoxifying the system, managing stress and seriously avoiding trigger foods. Be guided by your doctor and do everything you can to reduce the inflammation and keep the body in an alkaline state. Eat and drink foods that detoxify, and eliminate any overload on the kidneys, liver and bowel.

The danger foods

Alcohol, in any form, tops the list. Be diligent and don't even allow a sip of wine over the lips as this puts a strain on the kidneys. Do not smoke and avoid passive smoking. Cut out all sugar and refined carbohydrates – avoid white bread, cakes, biscuits, sweets and chocolates. Sugar is a killer – for sweetness only use stevia and a touch of honey. Avoid coffee, tea, carbonated drinks, all processed foods, especially processed meats, tinned foods, anything with food additives (colourants, stabilisers, thickeners, etc.). Any boxed or tinned food, fast food or fried food is pure poison to the lupus sufferer. Take care to avoid foods in the nightshade family: potatoes, tomatoes, brinjals, fruit salad plant, sweet peppers, chillies, and also lucerne and alfalfa sprouts – all these aggravate any inflammatory condition.

The superfoods

You need to get the correct pH balance and fresh fruits and vegetables is the only way to do it. Eat at least 8 portions of fruit and vegetables daily, as these are immune system boosters. A daily salad full of fresh organic ingredients is essential. Where possible, grow your own salad crops – celery, parsley, basil, lettuces, cabbages, kale, broccoli, spinach, dandelion, berries, pumpkins, melons, papayas and lemons. Make soups with lentils, beans, chickpeas, split peas and sweet potatoes, pumpkin, carrots and cabbages. Include oily fish like sardines, salmon, mackerel in the diet as they contain valuable anti-inflammatory oils, or take a good fish oil supplement. Wheat grass and barley grass juiced with beetroot, carrots, apples, celery, parsley, pineapple (½ a glass daily) and your own freshly squeezed fruit juices are the most valuable way of remaining positive, fit, vital and healthy.

Drink at least 6 glasses of water a day and get to know herb teas. Grow your own mints, lemongrass, melissa, chamomile, and so on. Read up about herbs like pennywort (*Centella asiatica*) and sacred basil (*Ocimum tenuiflorum*). These are extraordinary herbs that have been used to treat lupus for centuries.

Speak to your doctor about supplements: magnesium and vitamin E. Use aloe vera juice to soothe the skin.

Tissue Salts: No. 1, 4, 6, 8 and 11; often No. 9 will soothe. Take 2 of each frequently.

Menopause

The 'change of life', as it was once known, is usually experienced around 50 years of age in the average woman, but it can begin far earlier and it is a gradual change. Menopause signals the end of the menstrual cycle and it can last for a few years. Hot flushes, vaginal dryness, night sweats, insomnia, headaches, lack of energy, mood swings, weight gain, depression and osteoporosis are *sometimes*, note sometimes, evident but menopause does *not* have to be a time of negativity, anxiety, fear and upset. It can be a liberating, happy time, too, for it differs in every woman. Comfortingly, with many women it is a gradual change, which we adapt to without undue stress and with the right diet, exercise and appropriate natural hormone replacement therapy, your body adjusts to menopause with ease.

The danger foods

Avoid alcohol, coffee (especially instant coffee) and tea – change to herb teas and rooibos tea. Cut down drastically on sugar, and this means cakes, sweets and chocolates, refined carbohydrates, carbonated drinks and energy drinks, which all lead to weight gain, oestrogen deficiency, overworked adrenal glands, increased bone loss and cardiovascular problems. Too much salt and salty snacks and hot, spicy foods can all trigger hot flushes and add to the discomfort of water retention. Foods high in caffeine, like coffee, ordinary tea and chocolate, contain methylxanthines which are linked to female hormones and can easily cause an imbalance. Alcohol over-stimulates the adrenal glands, upsets blood sugar levels, increases the risk of osteoporosis and disturbs the female hormones even further. Also avoid high-fat dairy (replace with Bulgarian yoghurt) and cut down on red meat and fatty foods (replace with grilled chicken and fish simply served with lemon juice and steamed vegetables).

The superfoods

Basic hormone-balancing foods are the pulses, especially soya beans – eaten fresh like green peas or in the fermented form of tofu, tempeh, miso and soy yoghurt – as well as lentils, beans, split peas and chickpeas. These foods all contain phytoestrogens – plant compounds that can take the place of oestrogen, which is no longer being manufactured by the body. Other foods that show this remarkable effect are flaxseed, parsley, alfalfa sprouts and fresh green lucerne, cashew nuts, pecan nuts, pachira nuts, almonds, hazelnuts, fennel, celery, apple and whole grains. Soya is also rich in calcium, magnesium and protein and may decrease the risk of breast and colon cancer; flaxseed contains omega-3 fats, zinc and lignans; and whole grains are rich in B-vitamins, magnesium, zinc and fibre. Also include in the diet oily fish for omega-3 fats and proteins; pumpkin seeds for zinc, magnesium and essential fatty acids; and shelled raw hemp seeds for the balancing of omega 3, 6 & 9 fats. The cabbage family, especially kale, cabbage, broccoli, mustard greens and turnip greens will protect against breast cancer and heart disease and, as they are rich in calcium, magnesium and folic acid, they build bone health and protect against osteoporosis.

Set up sprouting trays for mung beans, alfalfa, buckwheat, sunflower seeds and sesame seeds and include in the daily salad. Grind a seed mix of pumpkin seeds, sunflower seeds, almonds, sesame seeds and flaxseed to sprinkle over oats porridge every morning, served with Bulgarian yoghurt. Include in the diet green wheat grass juice with barley grass, drink barley water and eat the barley strained from it like rice. Make juices with beetroot, carrots, celery, parsley, apples, wheat grass and barley grass daily. Bake your own whole-wheat bread with added wheat germ, flaxseed and sesame seeds. Your constant aim is to build bones and this

Caution: Consult with your doctor before you embark on any form of self-diagnosis or self-treatment.

A–Z Ailment Chart

is why you *must lessen the red meat and dairy products*, for their saturated fats and because they easily form acid in the diet. In order to neutralise the acid, calcium is leached from the bones. A plant-based diet will not do this.

Helpful Herbs for Menopause

Sage tea (*Salvia officinalis*) helps to reduce night sweats and hot flushes – take 2 cups daily, one just before going to bed.

Red clover tea helps balance oestrogen. Grow your own and eat the leaves and flowers in salads.

Fennel tea flushes toxins out of the body.

Lucerne tea gives energy and vitality.

Oat straw tea builds bones. Grow your own and reap as the grass turns golden (see also page 75).

Gingko biloba rejuvenates the brain!

Chamomile tea at night to help you calm down and sleep.

To make a herb tea: add ¼ cup fresh leaves and sprigs to 1 cup boiling water, stand 5 minutes, strain, sip slowly.

Talk to your doctor the following supplements that could ease menopause symptoms:

- Vitamins C and E reduce hot flushes and vaginal dryness.
- Calcium is essential for bone health and vitamin D is needed to utilise calcium (also get some early morning and late afternoon sunshine onto your skin).
- Vitamin B-complex helps to reduce irritability, anxiety, poor concentration, fatigue and feelings of helplessness.
- Magnesium eases tension, anxiety and mood swings.
- DHEA or dehydroepiandrosterone is an exceptionally valuable supplement that helps to increase the level of oestrogen in the body naturally – but your doctor needs to prescribe it.

Tissue Salts: Take No. 4, 7, 8 and 12 for hot flushes (avoid No. 12 if you have had implants or hip replacements); take No. 4 for night sweats, a florid complexion and swollen feet and hands; No. 2 is a hormone regulator; No. 4 and 6 can be taken for a sudden increase in blood pressure (check with your doctor as well) and for osteoporosis, take No. 2, 9 and 12.

Hormone Replacement Therapy

Hormone Replacement Therapy or HRT looms its big head at this moment. Being 'Mrs Natural' I went the natural route with my doctor watching over me and every now and then trying to convince me to take the newest of the HRT drugs. I refused to take pregnant mare's urine and every time I tried to take any one of the new hormone drugs I got such sore breasts I could not bear it. So he resigned himself to my natural progesterone and oestrogen creams, which I carefully applied and to the diet that I discussed with him and he watched over my easy transition with amazement and never argued again. But I still go for checkups and still use the creams when he sees I need them.

Discuss natural alternatives to HRT with your doctor and be guided by your doctor's advice. The following are some natural menopause treatments: red clover, gingko biloba, black cohosh and Agnus Castus are well-known menopause herbs.

Yam creams, progesterone creams and oestrogen creams are rubbed onto the soft parts of the body – inner arms, inner thighs, under the breasts, arches of the foot, etc.

Ask your doctor to check your thyroid if you show thinning hair, very dry skin and weight gain. Use natural, extra-nourishing skin creams – look at creams enriched with baobab oil, avocado oil or grape seed oil. Find natural shampoos, soaps and body washes that contain plant saponins and oils (we manufacture a range of natural products and can post anywhere). Avoid low-fat diets, in fact avoid diets. Good fats are essential for the production of hormones and skin nourishment. Get outside and build a garden of health. You need the sunlight, the exercise and the interest. Start by planting organically grown salad vegetables and your own vegetables, fruits and herbs. Work in your garden every day and take a brisk daily walk, breathing deeply while you walk. This is the most exciting time of your life – make the most of it.

Metabolic Syndrome

Metabolic syndrome – also sometimes called **Syndrome X** or **Insulin Resistance Syndrome** – is a combination of ailments that increases the risk of developing heart disease and diabetes. It is linked to overweight and obesity and some of the symptoms are high blood pressure, weight gain (especially around the middle), high cholesterol, high blood sugar levels, atherosclerosis, in women often polycystic ovaries and in men prostate problems and prostate cancer.

Diet is the first thing that is questioned and without fail it is revealed that alcohol and a diet high in sugar and refined carbohydrates is linked to insulin resistance, where the body cells become resistant to insulin and the blood insulin and blood glucose levels are much higher than they should be. This is a precursor to type 2 diabetes and can lead to rapid weight gain. The risk of metabolic syndrome increases as you get older, so it is imperative to have regular checkups and to manage your weight and stress levels.

The danger foods

The aim is to keep the insulin levels as low as is possible and this means changing the diet to a carefully watched regime that banishes all sugar, alcohol and salt! Avoid refined carbohydrates, especially white bread, cakes, sweets, chocolate, puddings, biscuits, carbonated drinks, white flour, white rice, white pasta, potatoes, as well as salty foods like crisps, chips, cheesy snacks, biltong, fast foods, processed and instant foods as well as caffeine, so no coffee, tea or colas.

The superfoods

Protein slows down the breakdown of carbohydrates into glucose, so choose lean lightly grilled steak, chicken or fish – cooked with garlic and onions, which helps to break down cholesterol. Protein is also found in legumes and whole grains: oats, lentils, barley and barley water (see recipe on page 135), millet, buckwheat, amaranth, chickpeas and beans, like haricot beans and butter beans.

Sprinkle ground sunflower seeds, flaxseed, almonds, sesame seeds, pumpkin seeds and walnuts over oats porridge every morning for breakfast and over fruit salad (with no sugar) for supper. Include salads of avocado, lettuce, peas and (pea sprigs

A–Z Ailment Chart

Caution: Consult with your doctor before you embark on any form of self-diagnosis or self-treatment.

and tendrils) with pineapple, celery, parsley and cucumber daily. Eat green leafy vegetables like spinach and members of the cabbage family, carrots, beetroot, sweet potatoes, squash, marrows, cherries, mangoes, berries, papaya, figs and apricots (fresh or sun-dried). Grapes are quite high in sugars and so are raisins and dates, so go lightly on those. Make smoothies and vegetable juices, especially a daily wheat grass and barley grass juice with carrots, apples, beetroot and celery (see page 29).

Replace salt with a herb mixture (see page 35) and flavour food with cayenne pepper, black pepper and lemon juice with just a very light grinding of Himalayan rock salt.

Eat regular small meals and lots of salads; leave out bread and flour products – but rye bread and rice cakes can occasionally be a part of the meal.

Talk to your doctor about supplements: coenzyme Q10, vitamin D and vitamin B-complex capsules. Ask about chromium picolinate and magnesium citrate capsules and the correct dose for you.

Tissue Salts: No. 2, 4, 6, 8 and 10 (or take a combination of all 12).

Stop smoking and take daily exercise, in the sunlight to get lots of vitamin D, which helps to improve the insulin reaction in the body.

Migraine

If you have ever had a migraine you will know that there is nothing more debilitating and flattening than the intense and incredible pain that is accompanied by nausea, flashing lights, vomiting, sensitivity to light and blurred vision. Migraines may be linked to stress and anxiety, fluctuating blood sugar levels, poor posture and certain foods, so keeping a food diary is of utmost importance. Dehydration is another trigger, so be sure of drinking at least 6–8 glasses of pure plain water a day. Other possible causes are lack of sleep, grinding the teeth during the night, certain medications or vitamins, noise, bright flashing lights, a neck injury or pressure, constipation, hormonal changes, toxicity and pollution, even inhaling certain scents or fumes like petrol fumes or chemicals like carbon tetrachloride, also avoid smoking or being in a smoker's area. In some cases if you have candida and are stressed, a migraine can really take hold.

The danger foods

The trigger foods differ from person to person so make your own list. The following are common migraine foods: chocolate, alcohol, coffee, especially instant coffee, red wine, beer (because of the yeast), cheese in all its varieties, even cream cheese, processed meats, oranges and naartjies and Chinese foods if MSG has been added (this additive can also affect the lungs with a tight chest and wheezing). Tyramine, an amino acid, is the substance found in all of these foods and along with monosodium glutamate or MSG should be avoided seriously.

Also avoids foods belonging to the nightshade family: potatoes, tomatoes and brinjals, especially if these are cooked. Other possible triggers are wheat products (they contain gluten), salt, yeast and yeast products, and any foods that contain additives like colourants, artificial flavourants, preservatives or stabilisers. So watch out for processed foods, tinned meats, commercial sauces, and so on. Also avoid artificial sweeteners, sugar and all refined carbohydrates and sweetened carbonated drinks.

The superfoods

Seek out magnesium-rich foods like green vegetables, salad greens, dandelion, lucerne, parsley, avocado, watercress, celery, lettuce, spinach, alfalfa sprouts and brown rice. Make fruit and vegetable smoothies and be sure to drink enough water.

Drink herbal teas like chamomile, the mints and pennywort (*Centella asiatica*). Stinging nettle tea is also greatly comforting as it is rich in easily absorbed minerals, as is melissa tea.

Ask your doctor about supplements: magnesium, vitamin B-complex, especially vitamin B6, as well as feverfew capsules.

Tissue Salts: No. 8 and 11 can be taken frequently (suck 2 of each every 10 minutes as soon as you feel a migraine coming on, and with a glass of warm water in between you can often catch and release the severity of it).

Speak to a physiotherapist if you have posture problems, especially with the neck.

Mood Swings

Commonplace, upsetting and affecting everyone around, moodiness seems to be part of everyday life. We all know someone who is so 'out of step' it gets to everyone else and can spoil the day. Depression in various degrees, anger and aggression, uncooperative behaviour, 'otherwise' behaviour, mood swings that happen fast, switching from pleasant to unpleasant in seconds, rudeness, tearfulness and argumentative confrontation is part of it all and everyone else is to blame!

The danger foods

Caffeine – in coffee, tea and colas – is a major trigger and so are additives (artificial flavourants and colourants, stabilisers, etc.), junk foods, chewing gum, coloured cool drinks and *sugar*, especially in children. Chocolate and sweets are quick triggers and also avoid fast foods, fried foods, salty foods and alcohol in every form. Do not overlook the effect of erratic mealtimes, not eating breakfast, constant snacking and watching too much TV, especially in the case of children and teenagers.

The superfoods

Start with sitting down as a family and eating a proper meal together – dinner is a start and it should consist of good-quality, lean protein, three vegetables, salad and fruit for dessert. No ice-cream, cakes or chocolate for dessert! Eat at least 8 portions of fresh fruit and vegetables a day and start the day with a good breakfast. The ideal breakfast is oats porridge with a sprinkling of finely ground seeds and nuts (see page 26) served with milk or plain Bulgarian yoghurt and a drizzle of honey; or scrambled egg on whole-wheat toast with fresh fruit.

Keep healthy snacks on hand: fresh fruit or sun-dried raisins, apple rings, dates, apricots, walnuts, pecan nuts and cashew nuts are rich in natural sugar and the good fats to satisfy the cravings for chocolate, sweets and constant snacking. Or snack on 100% rye bread sandwiches with cheese and tomato or cream cheese and sweet peppers, or hard-boiled egg mashed into homemade mayonnaise.

Squabbling in children can be immediately stopped by a surprise picnic basket of fruit smoothies in easy-to-sip-from fun containers with a sweet treat of chopped nuts and raisins bound with honey in a little cupcake case. Or make your own

Caution: Consult with your doctor before you embark on any form of self-diagnosis or self-treatment.

cupcakes of whole-wheat flour, blueberries, eggs, milk, and stevia to replace the sugar, and top with a little honey and chopped pecan nuts. Become innovative with fruit salads, or offer little tubs of chopped almonds mixed with Bulgarian yoghurt the minute the crying starts or an argument begins.

Do not skip meals and keep the meals wholesome and balanced: vegetables, fruit, and chicken, fish or lean meat for at least one meal a day. Protein is important – do not skip it. Often mood swings are because of a lack of vitamins and the B-vitamins top the list, so speak to your doctor or paediatrician about supplements. A good multivitamin is a positive start and alongside a good breakfast will start the day well.

Drink at least 6–8 glasses of plain water a day – often moodiness is due to dehydration. Herb teas like chamomile, pennywort (*Centella asiatica*) and melissa (lemon balm) are soothing and relaxing. Keep a bowl of rock salt with lavender in it on the corner of the bath for adding to the bath at the end of a bad day. Get regular exercise, like a brisk walk or run in the sunshine, or take the children out to play.

Tissue Salts: No. 2, 6, 9, 11 and 12 and especially No. 8 for temper tantrums. Keep these ready when those tempers flare, and take 2 of each sucked under the tongue. The 'mood lifter' capsule of calming herbs, available in the Fithealth range, has tissue salts included in it, and a capsule or two daily will do much to smooth the way (see page 17).

Mouth Ulcers *see* Canker Sores

Multiple Sclerosis

This is an autoimmune disease that affects the central nervous system, causing the destruction of the myelin sheath around the nerves. It is a gradual deterioration with symptoms like dizziness, tingling in the muscles and muscle weakness, poor coordination, stiffness, slurred speech, fatigue and difficulty in walking. It is thought that stress, poor eating habits, acidity, candida, dehydration, even food intolerances and environmental toxins could all add to the condition or cause it. Alcohol compounds the condition, even drinking alcohol only on occasion.

Improving the diet and lifestyle changes are the most important steps. Gluten and milk, which are common allergens, have been found to play a role in the progression of multiple sclerosis, as does the consumption of saturated fats. Without a doubt a careful diet will be of great benefit.

The danger foods

No margarines, white shortening and hydrogenated oils and fats should be eaten at any time. Avoid meat, eggs, heated fats, fried foods, pastries, all processed meats – sausages, polony, salami, bacon – as these all interfere with the function of the good fats. Foods that contain common allergens such as wheat and gluten products (including rye, oats and barley), dairy products, chocolate, tomatoes, potatoes, soya, yeast products and citrus fruits are to be avoided. Sugar is a serious toxin along with refined carbohydrates like white bread, cakes, biscuits, white pasta and so on, and avoid alcohol, chocolate and caffeine, especially instant coffees. Processed foods and too much salt can put a strain on the kidneys and liver. Avoid these as they all deplete nutrients and create extra toxins.

The superfoods

Green vegetables, fresh in salads or lightly steamed, are high in magnesium and folic acid and should be included in the diet frequently, especially cabbages, kale and broccoli. Include lots of papaya, mango, kiwifruit and berries of all kinds – it is worth growing the new thornless blackberries and also raspberries as they bear prolifically and the leaves make an excellent mineral-rich tea. Add fresh young lucerne leaves to the daily diet and also buckwheat sprouts and young leaves. Grow your own wheat grass and barley grass and have a daily juice of these two superfoods, adding carrots, beetroot, radishes (leaves and all), celery, alfalfa sprouts, apples, parsley, fennel and every now and then some fresh slices of ginger.

Sprinkle ground sunflower seeds, flaxseed, sesame seeds, almonds and pumpkin seeds over fruit salads, oats porridge and plain Bulgarian yoghurt. Eat oil-rich fish three times a week – mackerel, sardines, salmon – and take one teaspoon of cod liver oil daily. Drink at least 2 litres of water a day and replace ordinary tea, and of course coffee, with rooibos tea and herb teas like pennywort (*Centella asiatica*), tulsi or sacred basil (*Ocimum tenuiflorum*) and rose-scented geranium.

Get out into the sunlight every day to boost your vitamin D levels. Talk to your doctor about supplements: folic acid, vitamin B-complex (possibly vitamin B12 injections monthly), vitamins A, C and E, zinc, selenium, coenzyme Q10, and probiotics to help the digestion.

Tissue Salts: All 12 (leave out No. 12 if you have implants). Take frequently, at least 4 times a day.

Use only natural bath and beauty products, petrochemical- and paraben-free cleaning products in the home and natural insect repellents and organic garden products. Find a physiotherapist who will help you with massage therapy, muscle maintenance and hydrotherapy. Exercise is vital, in all forms.

Nail Problems

Brittle nails that break easily, flaking, tearing, and soft, thin nails that grow slowly all indicate deficiency in minerals and vitamins and wrong eating. Add to this the dangers of nail polishes, acetone, nail extensions, and applications of foils and enamels, pigments and lacquers, all of which cause the nail bed to become injured and often destroyed. Young women are the most common victims of a 'beauty' fetish that literally can destroy their nails for life and I am appalled at the nail 'industry' that comes up with more dangerous chemicals by the day.

The danger foods

Fast foods, fried foods, processed foods, carbonated drinks, smoking, coffee, especially instant coffee, coffee creamers and milk substitutes, sugar, cakes, doughnuts, diet drinks, energy drinks, chocolate, sweets and biscuits. Eating junk foods takes a severe toll on our health and appearance. Teenagers beware: you are creating brittle nails – and alongside the nails, brittle hair, teeth and bones!

The superfoods

Top of the list are calcium-rich foods (see page 14), fresh fruits and vegetables. Include Bulgarian yoghurt, lots of green vegetables, and wheat and barley grass juiced with fresh carrots, beetroot, celery, parsley, lucerne and sprouts of all kinds. The fashionable micro-greens are a most delicious way of

Caution: Consult with your doctor before you embark on any form of self-diagnosis or self-treatment.

eating your greens: mustard, buckwheat, radish, kale, cabbage, fenugreek, all in their tiny two-leafed stages are packed with goodness, rich in minerals and enzymes and because of their young and tender growth are worth their weight in gold. Add them to salads, sandwiches, stir-fries and more and get those valuable trace elements into every mouthful. Or juice them with your daily wheat and barley grass energiser.

Speak to your doctor about supplements: vitamin B-complex, vitamin C and E, biotin, zinc, iron, magnesium, selenium, the omega-3 fats, and l-methionine, an important amino acid and antioxidant, are excellent nail strengtheners.

Tissue Salts: No. 2, 7, 9 and 12 (take 2 of each at least 3 times a day).

Healing Nail Oil

This healing oil rubbed into the nails at least twice a day will repair the damage of nail polishes and extensions. Mix 1 teaspoon each of vitamin E oil, rosehip oil and tea tree oil into 3 teaspoons of almond oil. Keep in a dark glass bottle and rub in a drop or two often, working it into and under the nails and the cuticle bed.

Our grandmothers also found digging the nails into the pith of a freshly squeezed lemon revitalised, strengthened and smoothed chipped and flaking nails.

Nausea

Nausea can at times completely overcome us in our day-to-day activity, like morning sickness when you are pregnant or motion sickness when travelling. There is an urge to vomit and a headache, dizziness and intense fatigue take hold and leave a feeling of desperation and helplessness. Migraines can also bring on nausea, as can food poisoning, eating something that disagrees with you, a gastric infection or anorexia.

The danger foods

Fatty foods, processed meats, fried foods, rich creamy foods, spicy food, seafood, too many sugary foods on top of each other. Think of children's parties and the bad tummy aches and the projectile vomiting – an overdose of rich food does nobody any good! Alcohol is another common cause – over-imbibing can lead to alcohol poisoning with intense nausea.

The superfoods

Black, very weak rooibos tea with dry cream crackers will settle a queasy stomach. Chewing pumpkin seeds helps to ease the nausea. Brown rice with a little lemon juice also settles the stomach, or try mashed papaya or papino.

Ginger tea settles the stomach before travelling: boil up 4 thin slices of ginger in 1½ cups of water for 5 minutes, strain, sweeten with a touch of honey and sip slowly. Even eating a few small pieces of crystallised ginger every 10 minutes or so will ease the nausea considerably. (*Caution:* If the nausea has been caused by gallstones avoid taking ginger.) Or try peppermint tea (or melissa tea): ¼ cup fresh peppermint sprigs, pour over this 1 cup boiling water, stand 5 minutes, strain and sip slowly.

Discuss taking magnesium and vitamin B6 supplements with your doctor.

Tissue Salts: No. 4 and 10 are valuable for vomiting; No. 8 and 9 for over-indulging and to release stomach tension; and No. 5 and 11 taken together work wonders (suck 2 of each at the first sign of nausea with a minute or two between so that you hold in your mouth one tissue salt at a time. Repeat every 5–10 minutes).

Obesity

An increasingly worrying health risk is obesity and even more disturbing is obesity in children. The most common cause is wrong eating and lack of exercise. Hormones too play a role, but first and foremost it is lack of exercise – gardening is a good one, really digging, stretching, kneeling, standing up, just moving your body! Better still is jogging, brisk walking, aerobics, running, thai chi, yoga, ball work, dancing, cycling, fitness classes, anything that appeals to you – just do it!

Then there is diet. People today, especially young people, seem to live off a diet of fast foods and junk foods, and food cravings and emotional eating also play a role. Weight gain may also be the result of illnesses such as an under-active thyroid, which controls the metabolic rate. Yo-yo dieting adds to the problem as every fad diet is tried only to gain back all the weight, or more, with the added complication of a metabolism that is now even more sluggish than before!

Losing the weight may seem like a daunting task, so the first step is to cultivate a positive mindset. We need to take ourselves to task and work at discarding the negative thoughts, to set about, one step at a time, clearing away all the heavy stuff and making a turn around. There is no time to waste as obesity increases the risk of these often life-threatening ailments:

- Liver congestion, liver sluggishness and liver toxicity (see page 245); candida (see page 216); diabetes (see page 223); and cardiovascular ailments like high blood pressure, high cholesterol, heart disease, heart attack and stroke (see page 236).

- The excess weight puts a huge strain on the musculo-skeletal system causing backache, spine problems, joint aches, muscle spasms, risk of chronic arthritis (see page 251), gout (see page 234) and chronic pain.

- Respiratory ailments, congested lungs, snoring, sleep apnoea and lack of sleep all are increased as the heart and lungs struggle with the extra weight.

- Female hormone imbalance results in pregnancy weight gain, risk of infertility, menopause weight gain and on top of it intolerable premenstrual tension.

- Bladder incontinence – the extra weight can weaken the bladder valve – and coughing, sneezing, even laughing, cause a spurt of urine and the pressure of the weight over the bladder can cause a slow drip.

- The excess weight puts severe pressure on the veins of the legs and feet, which can lead to varicose veins, pain, contusion leg ulcers that don't heal easily.

- Embarrassing digestive problems like burping, flatulence, colic, bloating, gas and heartburn, caused by the pressure of abdominal fat pushing up burning refluxes, can colour the day and no amount of antacids will clear it up! Gall bladder problems are also increased by excess weight pressing on the gall bladder.

Caution: Consult with your doctor before you embark on any form of self-diagnosis or self-treatment.

- Think about the cancer risk – obesity has been linked to cancer of the uterus, ovaries, breast, colon, and in men the prostate.

Is this list long and serious enough to put your thoughts into gear?

The danger foods

Fast foods and junk foods of every description, coffee, especially instant coffee, sugar, chocolates, pastries, ice-cream, biscuits, sweets, carbonated drinks, energy drinks, fried and fatty foods, processed foods, all instant foods, sweetened breakfast cereals, refined carbohydrates, potatoes, artificial sweeteners, powdered milks and creamers, salty snacks and crisps. All these foods create terrible cravings – you eat one biscuit and crave 10 more! Never satisfied, you constantly binge-eat, which can lead to serious blood sugar highs and overload. Sugar is addictive but there is help at hand – in the form of stevia (see page 197) and health-boosting foods that satisfy that craving for sweets (see below). Alcohol in any form and smoking are out: you need to take a serious look at their deteriorating effect on your body. Interestingly, eating these danger foods actually inhibits your ability to lose weight, and lack of exercise means you are not burning up the calories, and water retention adds to the problem.

The superfoods

Fresh fruit, fresh vegetables, nuts and seeds, whole grains and lean protein should form the basis of your diet – replacing the junk with the good stuff will get rid of the fluid retention and the fat and detoxify the body. Vegetables like sweet potatoes, squash, leafy greens like cabbage, kale and Brussels sprouts, steamed quickly and served with fresh lemon juice and black pepper, brown rice and fish or grilled chicken without the skin, make a filling dinner and fresh fruit for dessert will round it off perfectly.

Snack on a small handful of almonds, Brazil nuts, pecans or raw shelled hemp seeds – all these contain the correct fats – or eat a handful of chickpeas with a touch of rock salt and lemon juice daily. Make smoothies of blueberries, strawberries and papaya, with apple juice every time you crave something sweet. Other delicious combinations are crisp pears and apples with carrots, or plums with apples and beetroot, or pomegranates with mangoes and yoghurt. Note there is *no added sugar*. You don't need it! If you are unable to stop the craving for chocolate, chew a few raw cacao nibs (you can buy them from health shops). Cacao nibs are rich in antioxidants and are sugar-free – is the added sugar and milk solids that make chocolate a danger food.

Have a daily salad – grow your own parsley, lettuce, celery, dandelion leaves, young radishes (leaves and all), rocket, cucumbers, turnip greens, spring onions, young spinach leaves, kale leaves, young lucerne leaves, lots of fennel as well as sprouts (mustard seed, alfalfa, mung beans, sunflower seeds, buckwheat, cress or fenugreek) and micro-greens (these are tiny young seedlings, no longer than your thumb, which are deliciously crisp and packed with nutrients).

The berry fruits, especially blackberries, raspberries and blueberries, are extremely valuable but with no sugar or cream! Apples, carrots, beetroot and celery juiced with wheat grass or barley grass and fresh lucerne with parsley is a magical juice – have it daily and grow your own wheat grass and barley grass for just this purpose (see page 29). Eat oats for breakfast served with

plain Bulgarian yoghurt and a touch of honey and sprinkled with a mixture of ground seeds and nuts (see page 27).

Ginger tea – thin slices of root with boiling water and a touch of honey – gives the metabolism a boost. So make this a daily treat. Drink lots of plain water – 8 glasses minimum a day between meals. Drink it 30 minutes before or after the meal and do not drink water during meals. Having frequent glasses of water helps to rehydrate and flush out toxins; discuss this with your doctor and space the 8 glasses of water throughout the day. Don't be tempted to have a cup of coffee, rather choose herb teas like lemongrass, stinging nettle or mint as they balance the water within the body.

Ask your doctor about supplements: vitamin B-complex, vitamins C and D, coenzyme Q10, digestive enzymes, lecithin, flax oil supplements, amino acid complex tablets, zinc, magnesium and manganese. Garlic, fresh and in capsule form, with parsley is a valuable obesity herb. It actually reduces the absorption of fats by inhibiting an enzyme within the pancreas, and also acts as an appetite suppressant!

Tissue Salts: No. 1, 2 and 9 are especially important, but get to know *all* the Tissue Salts and take them frequently!

Eat small regular meals and chew fennel seeds to aid the digestion. Do not eat a heavy dinner at night. A light meal 2 hours before you go to bed eases the heart, the lungs and the liver. The liver, gall bladder and the kidneys need to set the detoxification process in motion and that happens before midnight.

Oedema *see* Fluid Retention

Osteoarthritis

Osteoarthritis, also known as **degenerative joint disease**, is a type of arthritis that is caused by the breakdown and eventual loss of the cartilage of one or more joints. A disease of old age, the wear and tear of the joints often becomes evident from our late fifties or sixties and, surprisingly, affects more women than men. With the stress on cartilage – knees and ankles are the worst, but also the spine, hips and shoulders – the symptoms are pain, stiffness, swelling, heat, deformity and loss of mobility. Cold and damp seem to make it worse and taking painkillers does not improve the basic condition.

Danger foods

Avoid refined carbohydrates like white bread, buns, cakes, biscuits and sugar in all its forms, chocolate, instant coffee, tea, carbonated drinks, margarine, spreads, mayonnaise, sugary and salty snacks, chips, salted nuts, biltong, crisps and all processed foods. Check your salt intake and avoid saturated fats from dairy and meat, processed meats, especially ham, bacon, sausages, salami and pork products. Even processed chicken and turkey cold meats can affect the condition, as well as fried foods. Tomatoes, brinjals, potatoes, peppers, chillies all belong to the nightshade family and may sometimes cause an acute reaction. Avoid all alcohol, including wine, and in some cases eggs.

The super foods

Eat leafy green vegetables, but avoid spinach and Swiss chard (and also rhubarb), which contain oxalic acid and may add to the pain and stiffness. Foods that contain folic acid and vitamin K are superb for building bone (see page 12 and 14). Replace

Caution: Consult with your doctor before you embark on any form of self-diagnosis or self-treatment.

all breads with 100% pure rye bread and white rice with brown rice. Often arthritis sufferers have a lot of iron and copper in the body and brown rice, rye and millet will help to remove the excess. Also eat fresh pineapple often, as bromelain helps to ease hot, uncomfortable, inflamed areas.

Replace meat with oily fish such as mackerel, salmon, sardines, tuna and pilchards and replace dairy with plain Bulgarian yoghurt. Eat the following foods often: flaxseed, sunflower seeds, lentils, chickpeas, lucerne leaves and sprouts, walnuts, pumpkin seeds, apples, peaches, apricots, grapes, all the berries, lemons, pears, pomegranates – two or three different fruits daily. Eat vegetables daily: salads with dandelion, celery and fresh lucerne, parsley and avocado, baked sweet potatoes, vegetable soups and so on. Wheat grass juice with celery, parsley, carrots, apples and beetroot is hugely comforting. Asparagus with chopped basil and parsley will reduce toxic build-up. Boiled onions and fresh garlic in salads are also excellent.

Make herb teas of pennywort (*Centella asiatica*), burdock, red clover, rosemary, St John's Wort and turmeric. Drink lots of plain water and take supplements of omega-3 essential fats.

Tissue Salts: No. 5, 8, 9 and 12 (do not take silica, No. 12, if you have an implant of any kind, hip replacement, screws, bone plates, etc. It will clear the body of any foreign object.) For acute arthritic pain, take No. 4 and 10 frequently.

Osteoporosis

Osteoporosis is characterised by porous bones, a honeycomb appearance of the bones, and is a very real problem as the bones become weakened, more fragile and easily fractured. It affects a high percentage of usually post-menopausal women, and also a high percentage of men, and the whole skeleton system can be affected.

Oestrogen exerts a strongly protective effect on the density of the bone and when the oestrogen is depleted during and after menopause, there is often an accelerated loss of bone density. The phytoestrogens, although not as strong as oestrogen, definitely have a role to play and soya products become extremely valuable. Interestingly, Chinese women have excellent bone mass due to their high consumption of soya beans and pomegranate, which have compounds that are structurally similar to oestrogen. Bone density is at its highest at around 35 years of age and from then on it declines. We need to be aware of this constantly, especially if there is a thyroid problem. So the younger you begin to build bones consciously the better, and during adolescence and the early twenties it is crucial to eat bone-building foods.

Osteoporosis can be brought on by salty food, too much sugar in the diet, lack of calcium-rich foods and the malabsorption of calcium. Antidepressants, antacids and digestive medication containing aluminium, inflammatory bowel disease, Crohn's disease, coeliac disease and lack of exercise are also implicated.

The danger foods

Topping the list are carbonated drinks – and the colas are the worst. These canned and bottled drinks and diet drinks contain phosphoric acid, which literally leaches out bone minerals. Caffeine – in coffee, tea and chocolate – is the next serious culprit and our love affair with both coffee and chocolate can have serious consequences. Red meat is next on the list and processed meat is the worst. The body's acidity is raised and alkalising bone minerals are drawn from the bones to fight the acidity, risking bone brittleness. Alcohol and smoking, even passive smoking, interferes with the absorption of nutrients in the body, especially calcium and magnesium, which weakens the bones.

Avoid both sugar and salt – we generally use far too much, especially salty snacks, sugary snacks, cakes, sweets, chocolates, biscuits, sugary breakfast cereals, and the worst, the processed meats, like ham, polony, sausages, tinned meats and the vast array of packaged and instant foods. All these spell danger to the bones. Be careful of vegetables and fruits that have a high oxalic content like rhubarb, spinach, Swiss chard, beetroot greens, sorrel, plums, even sour cranberries, and members of the nightshade family in some cases – tomatoes, brinjals, sweet peppers and potatoes.

The superfoods

The good news is we can build up the bones by changing the diet. Top of the list are 6–8 fresh fruits and vegetables daily – the more variety the better! The best are leafy green vegetables like turnip tops, radish leaves, lettuce, broccoli, parsley, rocket, celery, alfalfa sprouts and fresh lucerne sprigs, kale, cabbage, Brussels sprouts and watercress. Find a source of tender micro-greens (tender seedlings of salad plants grown in trays) and grow masses of dandelion to use the leaves for salads, stir-fries, soups or stews, and roast the roots for dandelion 'coffee' (see page 231). Set up a greens garden and have a daily salad with a dressing of olive oil and lemon juice, as well as masses of lightly steamed vegetables. Leafy greens are all rich in magnesium, which helps with calcium absorption, and grow rows of oats.

Substituting meat for tofu or tempeh is a step in the right direction, as a diet low in red meat has been found to be beneficial; free-range chicken or fish twice a week is far better than red meat. Include legumes in the diet daily – all the beans (broad beans, jugo beans, black-eyed beans, haricot beans, butter beans, kidney beans), chickpeas, lentils and split peas. Remember to always soak legumes overnight to remove the phytic acid, which hinders the absorption of calcium, magnesium and zinc. Use exciting dishes of these with chopped mint and thyme and lemon juice as a substitute for meat; and eat sardines often, bones and all.

Snack on bowls of nuts and seeds – pumpkin seeds, sunflower seeds, sesame seeds, flaxseed, almonds, macadamia nuts and cashew nuts. Cooked chickpeas with thyme, celery seeds and coriander seeds make a wonderful substitute for salty crisps and chips. Look out for raw shelled hemp seeds at health shops – these too will become a valuable bone-building food.

Papaya, pineapples, figs, celery, buckwheat greens, lettuce and carrots are all excellent cleansers, digestives and rich in minerals and silica (see box on page 253) – so include these often. Also wheat and barley grass juice is superb for all of us and builds bones beautifully! Sprinkle ground seeds and nuts (see page 26) on oats porridge, plain Bulgarian yoghurt, muesli or fruit salads daily. Have oat straw tea, stinging nettle tea and ginger tea daily, drink lots of water and take digestive enzymes and probiotics to help the digestive process.

Talk to your doctor about supplements: vitamin D, magnesium, calcium, boron, vitamins B12 and K, folic acid and dolomite

Caution: Consult with your doctor before you embark on any form of self-diagnosis or self-treatment.

tablets. Dolomite is valuable for healthy bones, nails, teeth and hair and is also excellent as a heart supplement and calms over-stretched nerves. Dolomite ground from rocks has the perfect calcium and magnesium balance and with vitamin D present, the bones absorb the calcium in dolomite easily. Ask your doctor about vitamin D3 and calcium carbonate for easy absorption. Use natural progesterone and oestrogen creams massaged under the feet – discuss this with your doctor. If you take antidepressants or are gluten intolerant, calcium is not easily absorbed by the bones, so supplements are advisable, but always under your doctor's guidance.

Get out for a good long walk with deep breathing in the sun each day. If your spine is already affected, see a physiotherapist who will guide you on weight bearing exercises as this is of paramount importance. Weightlifting, even in a small way, is valuable, and so is jogging, brisk walking, climbing stairs, yoga exercises and aerobics, but be extra careful and be guided by your doctor if you already have fragile bones.

Tissue Salts: No. 2, 9 and 12 work perfectly together in harmony, each supporting the other. Suck 2 tablets of each, morning and evening – and when you're tired, anxious and stressed take them 3–5 times a day.

A Note About Silica

In addition to taking Tissue Salt No. 12, which is Silica, eating silica-rich foods is also important. All the tall grains are rich in silica – maize, wheat, barley, oats, buckwheat, brown rice – and also chicory, oranges, lettuce, lemons, guavas, apples, quinces, pomegranates, apricots, lentils, carrots, spinach and celery, and don't forget oily fish like mackerel, salmon, trout and sardines! These foods are al rich in vitamins and the essential minerals, and with a daily wheat and barley grass juice with celery, parsley, lucerne, carrots, apple and fresh beetroot, and a cup of oat straw tea, you are well on your way!

Pancreatitis

A distressing and painful disease, pancreatitis is usually caused by blocked ducts into the pancreas as a result of gallstones, medications, injury or high levels of calcium or fats in the blood, deficiencies in antioxidants, even infections, sometimes heredity and also a condition known as oxidative stress, an inflammatory condition. The most common cause of pancreatitis is, however, alcohol abuse. Symptoms include pain, nausea, sometimes vomiting, intense discomfort with a tender, swollen area over the abdomen, dehydration, rapid heartbeat, sometimes jaundice and low blood sugar and low blood pressure.

Chronic pancreatitis is when the pancreas may become scarred after an acute attack and there may be no pain, which may indicate it has stopped working, and the symptoms then are weight loss, the inability to digest food, constant indigestion, anaemia and liver problems, as the role of the pancreas is to produce digestive enzymes that break down carbohydrates, protein and fats from the food we take, and it also produces insulin and glucagons for controlling blood sugar levels. So the pancreas has a vital role to play in the wellness of the entire body. Your doctor needs to diagnose and treat the condition.

The danger foods

Fatty foods, fried foods, fast foods, junk foods, processed meats and saturated fats all put a strain on both the pancreas and the liver, and a diet high in unhealthy fats is the trigger that causes damage to the pancreas. Avoid peanuts, bacon, ham, chips, ice-cream, creamy sauces and desserts, spicy foods, oily dressings, sugar, refined carbohydrates, cakes, pies, sweets, chocolates, artificial sweeteners, carbonated drinks, energy drinks, diet drinks and all processed foods. Fried eggs and bacon and sausages put a huge strain on the pancreas – so avoid greasy breakfasts. Substitute oats porridge, Bulgarian yoghurt and fruit. **Do not drink any alcohol and do not smoke.**

The superfoods

Lecithin granules sprinkled onto breakfast oats porridge will help to emulsify and ease the digestion of fats. Take probiotics and digestive enzymes with every meal. Eat fresh fruit and vegetables as the main part of the meal. Choose foods rich omega-3 fatty acids like mackerel, sardines, trout and salmon. Sunflower seeds, flaxseed, pumpkin seeds, sesame seeds can be ground up with almonds and sprinkled onto oats porridge, fruit salad or plain Bulgarian yoghurt. Brazil nuts, walnuts and avocados are other excellent sources of essential good fats, which are easily digested.

Freshly juiced wheat grass or barley grass with carrots, parsley, celery, fennel leaves, apples and beetroot is an excellent tonic for the pancreas. Grow your own for maximum benefit and also grow your own fresh leaves of red clover, lucerne, fenugreek, dandelion, parsley, celery and fennel.

Dandelion is an extraordinary cleanser and tonic and eating 6 fresh leaves a day in the salad is an excellent liver and blood cleanser or drink dandelion root coffee (see page 231). Eat a variety of vegetables each day, lightly steamed and served with lemon juice and a light grinding of Himalayan rock salt. A little olive oil with lemon juice makes an easily digested salad dressing.

Some sufferers find members of the nightshade family – potatoes, tomatoes, brinjals, green peppers and chillies – difficult to digest, so avoid these if they cause any discomfort. Substitute sweet potatoes, pumpkin, squash and leafy greens, lightly steamed. Eat small regular meals of vegetable soups and salads, and healthy snacks of fruit, sunflower seeds, walnuts and Brazil nuts. These will help to keep the blood sugar levels stable.

Herbal teas – mint, melissa, caraway seed, aniseed and fennel – are all excellent digestives. Have these teas, unsweetened, often. To make the tea: add ¼ cup fresh leaves to 1 cup boiling water, stand 5 minutes, strain and sip slowly. For aniseed, caraway seed, fennel seed or dill seed tea: use 1–2 teaspoons of the seeds, pour over this 1 cup of boiling water, stir well, crushing the seeds, stand 5 minutes, strain, sip slowly and chew a few of the seeds. Also be sure to drink enough water, 6–8 glasses a day is ideal.

Talk to your doctor about supplements: vitamin B-complex, vitamins C, D and E, zinc, chromium, magnesium, manganese, selenium, beta-carotene, probiotics and digestive enzymes, which can be taken with meals.

Tissue Salts: No. 4, 6, 8, 10 and 11. Take 2 of each 6–8 times a day during an attack and 3–4 times a day after it.

Caution: Consult with your doctor before you embark on any form of self-diagnosis or self-treatment.

Parkinson's Disease

Often known as shaking palsy, Parkinson's disease is an imbalance of two chemicals in the brain – dopamine and acetylcholine. Dopamine is responsible for carrying messages from one nerve cell to the next cell and when the brain cannot manufacture sufficient dopamine this degenerative disease emerges. Symptoms include muscle tension or rigidity, stumbling, loss of balance, a typical thumb and fingers action, known as 'pill rolling', tremor in the hands while resting, slurred or impaired speech and a fixed facial expression.

The drug most often prescribed to treat Parkinson's is known as levodopa or L-dopa, but it does have side-effects and needs to be taken under strict doctor's supervision. Note that if you take levodopa you must *not* take vitamin B6. Some doctors suggest taking vitamin B6 alone without levodopa to avoid any side-effects. Talk to your doctor about this; and there are dietary considerations too and new treatments which could be considered.

It is thought that too many toxins, chemicals, medications, drugs and meat from animals reared on antibiotics may be possible causes of Parkinson's disease. Heroin has been found to directly destroy the brain cells that prevent Parkinson's disease.

The danger foods

A chronic poor diet of fast foods, processed foods, fried foods, fatty foods, instant foods, coffee, especially instant coffee, carbonated drinks, artificial sweeteners, sugar, snack foods, ice-cream, junk food, alcohol, refined carbohydrates, white bread, cakes, biscuits and shortenings spell huge danger. Avoid tea and replace with rooibos or herb treas. Avoid smoking or any alcoholic drinks!

Aluminium ingestion may also be implicated in Parkinson's disease. Never use aluminium cooking utensils and pots, deodorants and anything containing lead, and do not *ever* use pots or frying pans that are coated in non-stick Teflon.

The super foods

If you are taking levodopa eat the following foods in moderation (no more than twice weekly), as these are all rich in vitamin B6: bananas, beef, liver, oatmeal, potatoes, peanuts, whole grains and fish. The best foods are raw foods, salads, fruit and seeds, like flaxseed, sunflower seeds, sesame seeds, pecan nuts, almonds, walnuts, broad beans and also sprouted broad beans, which have been found to contain high amounts of L-dopa. Grow your own beans and lettuces, peppers, carrots, beetroot, celery and berries of all descriptions. Keep a notebook of foods that you find helpful and avoid smoking and drinking alcohol – this is utterly destructive to all the good foods you are trying to bring into your diet.

Speak to your doctor about the following supplements:

- Calcium (1 500 mg daily) and magnesium (750 mg daily) – both are needed for nerve stimulation.
- Lecithin (1 tablespoon 3 times a day) helps with the transmission of nerve impulses.
- High potency vitamin B-complex (100 mg 3 times a day with meals). Also ask your doctor about vitamin B6 or pyridoxine injections (up to 1 000 mg weekly or twice weekly), as brain dopamine depends on vitamin B6. *But do **not** take vitamin B6 if you are on levodopa.*

- Vitamin C (3 000–8 000 mg a day) is believed to improve cerebral circulation and is a potent antioxidant and anti-stress vitamin.
- Vitamin E (start with 600 mg a day and increase it slowly up to 1 000 mg a day) is a valuable antioxidant that protects the other vitamins and minerals from free radical destruction.
- Coenzyme Q10, zinc and in some cases iron, are important.
- L-glutamic acid is an amino acid that improves nerve impulses; wheat germ oil contains octocosanol, which revitalises the neuron membranes; and the fatty acids in flaxseed oil may assist with numbness and tingling.
- Include evening primrose oil capsules daily (and grow evening primrose for the flowers and the seeds to sprinkle on fruit salads); also supplements of St John's Wort have proved beneficial to inhibit the enzyme which interferes with the release of dopamine in the brain. Gingko biloba tablets or capsules are taken for memory loss, stroke recovery and Alzheimer's disease and are also found to be helpful in treating Parkinson's disease.

Tissue Salts are of great benefit for the tremors and unsteadiness of Parkinson's disease, particularly No. 12 for slow and difficult thought patterns, restless, jerking and twitching movements and insomnia (do not take if you have implants, hip replacements, plates or screws in the body). Tissue Salt No. 2 helps to foster a positive attitude and Tissue Salts No. 4, 6 and 8 are the particular salts for Parkinson's disease (take 2 of each frequently, gently sucking them together in the mouth). Note that all 12 tissue salts combined in one tablet are available at your chemist, known as 'Combin 12', which makes it easier to take.

Finally, do keep active. Your own positive attitude, an exercise programme of walking in the fresh air and sunlight, tai chi or swimming with supervision, and any activities that stimulate the small motor movements like typing, working with clay, knitting or drawing are very valuable. See a physiotherapist weekly to check your movements, and anything that is difficult to perform needs to be worked at, repeated over and over with attention and positivity. Allow yourself periods of relaxation and join a support group (these can be found in every major city and on the Internet).

Peptic Ulcers

The term 'peptic ulcer' refers to either a stomach ulcer, which is an open wound on the lining of the stomach wall, or a duodenal ulcer, which is a wound in the lining of the intestine. Inflammation caused by acidity, excess stomach acid or insufficient stomach acid affect the mucous membranes that protect the digestive tract. Stomach acid is vital for proper digestion, but the delicate balance is easily upset by stress, tension and anxiety, smoking, drinking alcohol, a diet high in fats and processed foods, aspirin and other medications, missing meals and eating junk foods, drinking sugary high-energy drinks, overindulging and by constantly *chewing gum*!

There is strong evidence that the *Helicobacter pylori* bacterium is found in almost all peptic ulcer sufferers if there is insufficient stomach acid in the stomach, and this organism in fact inhibits production of stomach acid, which further aggravates the condition. It interferes with the entire digestive process and

Caution: Consult with your doctor before you embark on any form of self-diagnosis or self-treatment.

the outcome is indigestion and digestive stress, which includes flatulence, burping, sour reflux, colic and bloating. Taking antacids further reduces the stomach acid and creates a perfect environment in which *H. pylori* can thrive – and thrive it does. So this has to be eradicated in order to bring about the healing of that gnawing wound and to bring the stomach acid back to normal and improve the digestive process. This is done by being diligent in eliminating the danger foods.

The danger foods

Eliminate the following completely: alcohol, red meat, sugar (including chocolate, pastries, cakes, sweets and ice-cream), most dairy products, carbonated drinks (colas, diet drinks and energy drinks are pure poison), fried foods, processed foods, especially processed meats, salty and spicy foods, preserves, pickles and piccalilli, chillies and chilli sauces, dips, mayonnaises, curries, oily foods and all fast foods (no takeaways at all – hamburgers and chips are lethal, as are hot dogs and hot spicy sauces). Tea and coffee, especially instant coffee, will only increase the damage – avoid completely. Avoid very hot and very cold foods, as these will intensify the pain. Stop smoking and seriously change your lifestyle to reduce stress, tension and upsets. Finally, never put chewing gum in your mouth again! The action of chewing and swallowing saliva sends a message to the stomach to increase acid production and when the anticipated food fails to arrive, the excess acid starts to eat away at the stomach lining. Chewing gum is a sure way of inviting an ulcer!

The superfoods

The following advice does not sound appetising but it is one of the quickest remedies to heal a peptic ulcer: make a juice of organic cabbage leaves, carrots and wheat grass. The best proportion is 1 cup wheat grass, 3 cups cabbage leaves and 2 carrots. Take this 2–3 times a day. These three foods are easily digested and are excellent healers. You can add a sweet apple to improve the taste.

Eat sweet potatoes, squash, pumpkin, vegetable soups, avocados mashed with a touch of lemon juice and a touch of Himalayan rock salt, and make fruit smoothies with papaya, apples and bananas. Cooked millet and brown rice will soothe and coat the stomach. Make nut butters by putting almonds, cashew nuts, pecan nuts or walnuts in a liquidiser with a little olive oil. Use this as a spread on rye bread. This will get the essential fatty acids into the body without irritation.

Sip a glass of water 30 minutes before a meal. Drink melissa tea, chamomile tea and mint tea throughout the day – ¼ cup fresh leaves to 1 cup boiling water, stand 5 minutes, strain and sip slowly. They soothe the mucous membranes beautifully.

Eat Bulgarian yoghurt and take probiotics. Ask your doctor about L-glutamine powder (it is an excellent digestive soother), vitamin C to help to eradicate the *H. pylori*, and *Acidophilus* supplements to repopulate the stomach.

Tissue Salts: No. 3, 4, 6, 8 and 10 (take 2 of each – suck 2 of No. 3 with each of the other numbers in turn).

Chewing your food well will help to alkalise it, and being calm and relaxed while eating keeps the general acidity down.

Periodontal Disease

Periodontal disease affects the teeth, gums and jawbone and symptoms include inflammation around the gums, swollen sore gums often with bleeding and ultimately loss of the teeth. Plaque on the teeth, abscesses, halitosis, loose teeth and infection in the bone add to the condition. But even more serious, osteoporosis, heart disease and diabetes could be part of the picture. Grinding of the teeth during sleep, smoking, alcohol abuse, not cleaning the teeth properly and continuous snacking on sugary foods, drinking sugary drinks all the time and a diet high in refined carbohydrates are some of the causes.

The danger foods

Sugar and refined carbohydrates are the main culprits, so avoid all sugar and sugary foods, sweets, especially toffees and hard sweets, chocolates, sweet biscuits, pastries, carbonated drinks, cakes, white bread and potato crisps. Avoid alcohol and smoking – these encourage the build-up of plaque. Avoid citrus fruits as the juice can soften the tooth enamel. A ban needs to be put on to allowing children to drink fizzy drinks and having sweets every day. The phosphoric acid in the fizzy drinks eats away at the enamel of the teeth and the sugar-loving bacteria thrive in the moist crevices between the teeth, leading to decay.

The superfoods

Rethink the diet – choose vegetables and fruits like fresh carrot sticks, apples, celery sticks, crisp fresh pears and melons to chew on daily to clean the teeth and strengthen the gums. Eat raw almonds, berries, pomegranates (chew the seeds), green vegetables and fresh salads daily with celery, parsley, chickpeas, lettuce, fennel, green peppers, pineapple and kiwifruit. Oats porridge with sesame seeds is rich in calcium, so include these daily in the diet. Drink lots of water.

Speak to your doctor about supplements: vitamins B, C and D, bioflavonoids, calcium with boron, zinc and magnesium.

Tissue Salts: No. Take No. 1, 2, 3 and 6 for bleeding gums; No. 3, 4, 7 and 12 for infection; No. 1, 2 and 4 for inflamed gums; No. 5 and 6 for spongy gums; No. 3, 4, 7, 9 and 12 for mouth ulcers, abscesses and boils. (Leave out No. 12 if you have implants.)

A sea salt rinse daily helps to strengthen the gums and clear infections: 1–2 teaspoons of coarse non-iodated sea salt mixed into 1 cup of warm water. Swish around the mouth and spit out.

Tea tree oil will help to clear away gingivitis on the gums and soothe swollen, sore areas: 10 drops in ½ a cup of warm water, swish out in the mouth a little at a time and spit out.

Floss daily and brush your teeth after every meal using a non-fluoride toothpaste (available from health shops). Visit your dentist for regular 3 or 6 monthly check-ups and see an oral hygienist every month or two if necessary.

Piles *see* Varicose Veins and Haemorrhoids

Pneumonia

Pneumonia is a serious inflammatory condition of the respiratory system, often preceded by bronchitis or a viral, bacterial or fungal infection. Those most at risk have a weakened immune system or suffer from malnutrition, and even pollution can affect the lungs. Smokers are at risk, as are diabetics, people who are HIV-positive or suffer from cardiovascular disease. Symptoms are high temperature, difficulty in breathing, coughing up of phlegm, congested lungs, chest pains, muscular aches and pains, joint pains, sweating, shivering and distress.

Caution: Consult with your doctor before you embark on any form of self-diagnosis or self-treatment.

Usually hospitalisation is required and your doctor must immediately be consulted and will advise the proper treatment. Once recovery sets in and nursing can begin at home, it is imperative to be extra careful of the diet.

The danger foods

Milk and dairy products, especially sweetened chocolate milk, ice-cream, custards and milky puddings – all these will increase the amount of mucus in the lungs. Refined carbohydrates, white rice, white flour – breads, cakes, biscuits – are dangerous at this time, as is sugar. Avoid tea, coffee, especially instant coffee, alcohol in any form and smoking, even passive smoking. Salted and sugary snacks must be completely eliminated as these all suppress the immune system even further. Cut down on red meat and eliminate all fast foods, fried foods and all processed foods – anything that has been tinned, packaged or altered in any way, or that has been sugared or salted.

The superfoods

Fresh fruit and vegetables should be the mainstay of the diet. Choose those rich in beta-carotenes like carrots, pumpkins, beetroot, apricots, berries, peaches, papaya, apples, kiwifruit.

A daily juice of wheat grass and barley grass with parsley, celery, carrots, beetroot, pineapple and apples acts as a valuable tonic. Make vegetable soups with lots of cleansing herbs and vegetables – sweet potatoes and their leaves, celery, parsley, asparagus, cabbage, cauliflower, kale, spinach, beetroot greens, turnip greens, pumpkin, squash and tips of the vines of pumpkins and su-su. Seek out greens of all kinds for a daily salad and add carrots, chickpeas, fresh lucerne and lemon juice. Use only non-iodated sea salt or Himalayan rock salt crystals.

Drink lots of water and take a vitamin C supplement.

Tissue Salts: No. 2 helps to clear mucus and for postnasal drip take No. 1, 2 and 9. Take No. 4 for fever.

Consult your doctor at all times and be watchful of everything you eat. You want to build health and clear infection and, above all, strengthen the immune system (see also page 240).

Pregnancy

The best years to fall pregnant are between 20 and 30, but in today's high-pressured, career-driven world many women choose to become pregnant between 30 and 40. Whatever time you choose, proper nutrition is hugely important to boost fertility and reproductive health in general. It is vitally important that you watch your diet vigilantly for the entire duration of your pregnancy to safeguard not only your own health but also that of your baby. See also the section on Conception on page 220.

The danger foods

Alcohol in any form, not even a sip – any doctor will tell you alcohol and babies do not go together. Smoking is an absolute *no*! Smoking has an impact on your oestrogen levels, even passive smoking – lowered oestrogen reduces fertility, so be vigilant.

Avoid sugar and refined carbohydrates, carbonated drinks, diet drinks, bottled and boxed fruit juice, in fact, during the time the only drinks you should consider are water and rooibos tea or your own smoothies and juices made from fresh fruit and vegetables, and wheat and barley grass. Avoid fats and margarines, caffeine in any form, especially instant coffee, and any fast foods, fatty fried foods, rich creamy desserts, chocolates and all processed foods, especially processed meats, sausages, cold meats and hams, bacon and pickled meats, and condiments. Keep a food list of what causes indigestion and discomfort.

Be careful of anything that has peanuts in it (especially if anyone in the family has a nut allergy). Peanuts are a serious allergy food, as are shellfish and shark meat. It is safest to avoid most fish during this time, except tuna, trout, mackerel and sardines and then have only one of them and not more than once a week. Also avoid cheeses, raw eggs or even lightly boiled eggs, mayonnaises that contain raw eggs, salad dressings and desserts with raw eggs, and also chicken livers, liver, kidneys and other offal. All these could contain harmful bacteria that could make you ill, like salmonella, or toxins like traces of mercury.

During conception and early pregnancy balancing the hormones are vital, so become aware of environmental pollution, food that has been treated with pesticides and insecticides, harmful cleaning materials and plastics. Also be aware of and avoid essential oil, not even in your bath, and avoid perfumes and highly perfumed body creams and soaps.

The superfoods

For both fertility and a healthy pregnancy aim for 6–8 servings of different fruits and vegetables every day. Seek out organic fruits and vegetables wherever you can find them. Make a list of the fruits, salads and vegetables you enjoy, like papaya, berries, peaches, persimmons, kiwifruit, grapes, quinces, pineapples, apples, bananas, and the favourite vegetables like carrots, squash, sweet potatoes, the occasional baked potato, broccoli, mealies, cauliflower, celery and so on.

Try this vegetable soup made with chickpeas, soaked overnight then added to the soup. Fry onions and leeks to give a good taste, add chopped celery, grated carrot, the soaked chickpeas, lentils, grated sweet potatoes, grated pumpkin, fresh peas and thinly shredded cabbage, baby spinach leaves, turnip leaves and a little grated turnip, and kale leaves. Top up with water or chicken stock. Do not add the salt until the soup is thoroughly cooked and the chickpeas tender. Add the juice of 3–4 lemons, a little grated ginger, chopped parsley just before serving and a little honey or apricot jam to round off the taste. Only once the soup is ready, stir in non-iodated sea salt. Avoid pepper, chillies, tomatoes and potatoes at the early stage. Once your pregnancy is well underway you can add chopped sweet peppers, potatoes and tomatoes. Keep a diary of foods.

Make sure you include enough protein in your diet and remember, not only meat is a protein! Look at this list: nuts, sprouted seeds, haricot beans, butter beans, white beans, black beans, black-eyed beans, split peas, soya beans, barley grass, wheat grass, plain yoghurt, milk, eggs, chicken, and also brown rice, buckwheat, millet, sunflower seeds, avocados, lentils and pumpkin seeds. Avoid too much red meat and if you do have it, have it very lean and stewed, not fried or highly flavoured. Mutton is best at this stage. Oily fish like sardines, tuna, trout and mackerel is valuable for healthy hormones. Ask your fishmonger for sardines and fry them quickly in a little sunflower oil and serve with brown rice and lemon juice – but only once a week. But watch over your protein intake: 'eating for two' is not always a good thing – be guided by your doctor. Protein is vital, however, especially in the third term of pregnancy.

Watch your fluid balance and drink water, the purest and safest you can find. Filtered water is essential – avoid water in plastic bottles, which may leach toxins.

Herb teas are comforting for morning sickness – peppermint, a tiny grating of ginger every now and then, and chamomile tea are soothing to the digestion – but always talk to your doctor first. Some young mothers do not like the taste of herb teas, so a squeeze of lemon juice in hot water sipped slowly is helpful. See also the section on Nausea on page 250.

During pregnancy many women have food cravings, mostly for salty or spicy foods, sometimes for peaches or mushrooms or one of mine was for pomegranates and papayas. Interestingly, if you include a wide range of foods, especially fresh fruits and vegetables, you'll most likely not have the cravings.

Speak to your doctor about vitamins and minerals and include these foods in the diet to build both your own health and the baby's health:

- Calcium – found in Bulgarian yoghurt, fish, broccoli, cabbage, kale
- Magnesium – found in green leafy vegetables, nuts, brown rice, sunflower seeds
- Zinc – found in pumpkin seeds, whole grains, sun-dried fruit (avoid dried fruit preserved with sulphur – dry your own)
- Iron – found in eggs, seaweed, prunes, fish, stinging nettle tea, dark green vegetables like baby spinach and the dark green outer leaves of the cabbage
- Folic acid – found in green beans, peas, asparagus
- Selenium – found in tuna, herring, mackerel, garlic, broccoli, seaweed and nuts like Brazil nuts, cashews, macadamia nuts, walnuts and pecan nuts
- Manganese – found in seaweed, nuts, whole grains, beans, broad beans, pulses
- The essential fatty acids – found in sunflower seeds, flaxseed, almonds, sesame seeds, pumpkin seeds
- Vitamin A – found in carrots, tomatoes, pumpkin, cabbage, spinach
- Vitamin B-complex – found in lentils, brown rice, avocados, eggs, sardines, chickpeas
- Vitamin E – found in nuts, seeds, olives, wheat germ, avocados
- For your vitamin D requirement be sure you get some early morning and late afternoon sunlight.

Tissue Salts: For morning sickness and nausea take No. 2, 4, 9 and 10; No. 2 and 8 help healthy bone development in the baby; No. 9 eases haemorrhoids and No. 11 subdues vomiting – but always consult your doctor first before you try anything.

Premenstrual Syndrome

Premenstrual syndrome or PMS is a very real, very tense time of the month for many women. The symptoms vary from woman to woman but all can be eased with understanding what happens to our bodies. Menstruation is a monthly cycle and with it, in the frantic pace of day-to-day living, comes tension, anxiety and often the feeling of not being able to cope, irritability, mood swings, cravings for chocolate, coffee, sweets, cakes and all the 'bad things' for a few days leading up to the period. In more serious cases there is depression, weepiness, helplessness, forgetfulness and confusion, as well as the discomfort of tender breasts, water retention, weight gain and general despair. In some women it is a dark and desperate time of the month that lasts a few days. Natural hormonal imbalance can be blamed, and added to it stress and liver problems. 'Life depends upon the liver' is an old saying, and a liver loaded with toxins can be one of the causes of PMS.

The danger foods

Foods high in sugar and salt should be eliminated to ease the load on the liver. Cut down on red meat – and here we need to really rethink our intake of red meat: most of the meat we buy today is full of hormones, even steroids, antibiotics and an array of growth stimulants and additives that are added to the diet of the cattle that we often do not even think about. For a woman this can contribute to hormonal imbalance, so avoid red meat for 7–10 days before the period is due.

Avoid all carbonated drinks, especially energy drinks and colas, tea and sweetened fruit juices – all these further disrupt hormone levels and with chocolate or salty junk food snacks, the mood swings can be intolerable. Dairy products with saturated fats can also add to the hormonal imbalance – so avoid these before and during the period. Look carefully at what you eat and keep a food diary, and add to it every month.

The superfoods

Replacing sugary and salty foods with fresh fruit, nuts, seeds, tofu, fresh vegetables and salads, will literally give you the positive feeling of being able to cope and, as an added bonus, the weight drops away, leaving you fit and vibrant. Include magnesium-rich foods daily – lots of pulses, lentils, chickpeas, sprouted alfalfa and mung beans, and avocado. Make vegetable soups of black-eyed beans, lentils, split peas, spinach, kale, cabbage, fresh lucerne sprigs, buckwheat, green squash, su-su and lots of carrots, turnip leaves and radishes, leaves included. You will come to rely on these energy-building soups. Vary the ingredients daily.

Eating ground sunflower seeds, flaxseed, pumpkin seeds, sesame seeds and almonds sprinkled over oats porridge (the non-instant kind), fruit salad or plain Bulgarian yoghurt every day helps to balance hormones, removes toxins and gives an energy boost. Eat brown rice, millet, and fish, like mackerel, sardines, salmon and trout to replace the meat. Buckwheat flour pancakes, sunflower seeds and sunflower oil are rich in vitamin E, which helps breast tenderness. Asparagus – fresh and green – boiled until tender and served with fresh lemon juice, flushes out the bladder and kidneys and eases water retention.

Fennel tea helps to cleanse and has an excellent diuretic action, and celery and parsley and basil, chopped fresh onto salads and added to soups and sprinkled fresh on top of them, have marvellous anti-bloating and diuretic affects. Wheat and barley grass with fresh carrots, lucerne, apples, parsley, celery and beetroot, and a handful of micro-greens like mustard, cress, broccoli, rocket, all juiced together, will give you a head start daily. Learn to make smoothies from all your favourite fruits like watermelon, papaya, kiwifruit, pineapple and berries and ring the changes daily.

Caution: Consult with your doctor before you embark on any form of self-diagnosis or self-treatment.

Talk to your doctor about supplements: vitamin A, vitamin B-complex, vitamin E, flaxseed oil capsules, lecithin granules, milk thistle supplements to protect and cleanse the liver, magnesium and zinc for balancing the hormones and converting the essential fatty acids. Talk to your doctor about the best time to take supplements – before or after the period.

Tissue Salts: Take No. 9 for tearfulness, rage and feelings of helplessness; No. 3, 10, 11 and 12 all eliminate toxins and ease restlessness and agitation; for insomnia No. 2, 3, 4 and 6 are beneficial; No. 6, 8 and 9 are comforting, especially when tempers flare and life gets too pressurised; panic attacks are helped by taking No. 4, 6 and 7; and for moodiness, No. 2 and 8 are valuable. To regulate and to ease menstruation there are tissue salts that fit every part of the cycle, so become familiar with them – they are easily available at every chemist.

For stress release exercise is vital – try walking, tai chi, yoga or swimming, and do deep-breathing exercises to release tension.

Prostate Problems

An enlarged prostate gland is extremely common in men over the age of 45. The symptoms are frequent and often painful intermittent urination that is every man's dread and can send him into a panic. The urine flow becomes weak and hesitant, with the feeling of not emptying the bladder fully. There can be pain or discomfort in the stomach area, and there are a number of causes. One is hormone imbalance – the high testosterone levels of the young man gradually decline, in some sooner than others, and other hormones increase, for example oestrogen, prolactin, dihydro-testosterone, which can induce the enlargement of the prostate. High cholesterol could also play a part and if not monitored could damage the cells of the prostate. If you experience any symptoms, consult your doctor immediately as urine that is not excreted can damage the kidneys and raise toxins in the blood.

It is worth having twice yearly check-ups with your doctor or urologist to ascertain the general health of the kidneys, bladder and prostate. Interestingly, it has been well documented that correct eating with appropriate supplementation under your doctor's supervision, can sometimes correct the condition and certainly alleviate much of the discomfort, and while surgery often seems to be the best option, much can be done to ease the symptoms.

Note that the following lists apply to both prostate enlargement and prostate cancer.

The danger foods

Avoid the danger foods at all costs, especially if you are over 55. It may seem like a huge sacrifice in the beginning, but by watching the diet all sorts of other smaller problems will clear up at the same time. You'll lose the excess weight that built up over the years, have more energy, and become leaner, more vital, more positive and nicer to live and work with!

Start with sugar – those much-loved chocolates, sweets, sugar in the coffee, ice-cream, cake, biscuits and sweetened breakfast cereals all play havoc with your blood sugar levels and invite a number of dread diseases. Replace sugar with stevia (see page 197) and do *not* ever use artificial sweeteners. In addition to sugar, caffeine and alcohol are potent and reliable killers, depleting the body of valuable nutrients, changing the personality and adding weight. Replace coffee, tea and alcohol with rooibos tea without milk and with lemon and a touch of raw honey if you long for sweetness.

Avoid barbequed meat or meat that has been charred or cooked at sizzling temperatures. In fact, avoid all fried meats, especially fatty meat. Eating burned fat or charred meat is literally carcinogenic (cancer forming). Cut down on salt and dairy products and avoid all refined foods – white flour, white rice, white bread, white pasta – as well as processed foods. Return to vegetables, fruits, herb flavourings and whole foods that satisfyingly can replace these.

The superfoods

Eat whole grains like oats, brown rice and millet and lots of carrots, beetroot, celery, parsley, pineapple, apples, fresh lemon juice, salad greens, green mealies, all the green vegetables, avocados, sweet potatoes, onions, garlic and dandelion leaves, also tomatoes, olive oil, pink grapefruit, blueberries, melons, watermelon and Brazil nuts. Add sprouts to salads, especially alfalfa, soya and sunflower seeds. Seek out organic fruits and vegetables or grow your own.

Include oily fish in the diet to replace fatty red meat – mackerel, trout, sardines, tuna and salmon – and also free-range chicken and soya products. Lean meat and chicken that has been lightly grilled, three or four times a week, is good in casseroles, stews and served with steamed vegetables and salads, and fresh fruit for dessert.

For breakfast every morning sprinkle finely ground seeds, like pumpkin seeds (rich in zinc!), flaxseed, sunflower seeds and sesame seeds, and nuts, like almonds and pecans, over oats porridge served with Bulgarian yoghurt and a touch of honey.

Drink wheat grass and barley grass juice with carrots, beetroot, apples, celery, fresh lucerne sprigs, parsley and red clover leaves. Red clover and lucerne are two potent anti-cancer herbs and extremely valuable. This is a most extraordinary anti-cancer treatment that can literally clear the toxins, rejuvenate, revitalise and kick start the entire body into health and wellness.

Drink barley water daily (see recipe on page 135) – 3 glasses a day is ideal, but even just 1 glass mid-morning will do wonders. This flushes out toxins and with fresh lemon juice it helps to keep the flow of urine constant. Barley is a wonderful grain for flushing of the bladder, kidneys and urinary system.

Drink at least 8 glasses of water a day and herb teas of stinging nettle and the silk from inside the husk of the green mealie. Take ¼ cup fresh green mealie silk, pour over this 1 cup of boiling water, stand 5 minutes, strain and sip slowly. This is an excellent and reliable prostate tea that flushes out toxins – drink 2 cups of this daily in the morning and afternoon. Make the stinging nettle tea in the same way.

Talk to your doctor about supplements: extra vitamin D (and spend some time in the sun daily), milk thistle for cleansing the liver and spirulina and kelp tablets to build healthy hormones.

Tissue Salts: No. 1 and 3 taken 3 times a day are excellent for both an enlarged prostate and prostate cancer; No. 4 and 9 taken together are also beneficial and No. 5, 8 and 12 are good for building general health.

Regular exercise is vital as it increases the circulation and oxygen to the area. Swimming is excellent but cycling should be avoided as this can put pressure onto the prostate gland. Hot and cold showers – a 30-second cold shower in between the hot showers – help to increase the circulation to the area. Direct the flow of water to the lower abdomen.

Search out everything organic, even in the soap you use in the shower and the shaving cream you use. (We have developed a skin-softening baobab oil and palm kernel soap-on-a-rope; see our website margaretroberts.co.za)

Psoriasis

Psoriasis is a skin disorder distinguished by reddish, raised, rough patches that have a silvery plaque-like scale and often itchy, hot and irritating lesions. Distressing and difficult to cure, it often appears in the late teens or between the ages of 20 and 30 or even sooner, and it manifests in certain families – so it is considered to be mostly hereditary. Other causes could be from nutrient deficiencies, toxaemia, over-loaded liver, sluggish bowels, incomplete protein digestion, candida, infections, pregnancy and/or hormonal problems, alcohol consumption (for example, certain wines could cause toxaemia), even excess stress could trigger it, as well as over-consumption of animal fats. It can manifest first a dry scaly patch behind the knee or ankle or in the elbow joint or on the scalp, around the genitals and anus and sometimes across areas on the back and even the neck, and it varies in every individual. The actual description of psoriasis is the over-production of skin cells that multiply faster than the normal skin cells, causing flakiness of the skin before the old cells have been shed and doctors are finding today that the diet plays an important role in managing it.

The danger foods

Avoid pork and pork products – ham, bacon, cold meats, processed meats, sausages, spreads, meat pies and bacon bits in biscuits or salads. The nitrates that are added to most pork products are considered to be a trigger. Avoid sugar and refined carbohydrates, cakes, sweets, white flour, cornflour, white rice and any polished grains like barley. Limit the intake of fatty meats – animal fats are a serious trigger – and lessen the consumption of dairy products. Caffeine is another trigger, so delete chocolate, coffee, tea, colas and energy drinks from the diet. Beware of members of the nightshade family – tomatoes, potatoes, brinjals, green and red peppers and paprika. Lessen the eggs in the diet, also citrus and gluten-rich foods like wheat, oats, rye and barley (replace with buckwheat, brown rice and millet).

The superfoods

Salads, smoothies, juices, vegetable soups are going to be lifesavers for you. Include brown rice in the diet as well as the cabbage family – broccoli, cauliflower and kale particularly – as well as artichokes, dandelion, parsley and carrots; make a daily salad with celery, lucerne, radishes and lettuce. Learn to make super smoothies with fruits and vegetables and have them daily. Include mackerel, tuna, herrings, sardines and trout in the diet for the essential omega-3 fats.

Eat foods high in the B-vitamins (see page 11) and ask your doctor about supplements: vitamin B-complex, vitamins A and D, omega-3 oils, zinc and milk thistle supplements to treat the liver. *Do not take vitamin A if you are pregnant.*

Tissue Salts: No. 5, 7 and 9 (take 2 of each, 3–6 times a day).

Try exposing the area to the sun daily, but experiment as in some cases the sun aggravates the condition. Check the soaps and skin creams you use and avoid highly perfumed ones. Manage your stress. Chamomile calming tea may be helpful and yarrow and pennywort (*Centella asiatica*) tea are also beneficial. Keep a food diary and update it often – psoriasis can be controlled!

Raynaud's Disease

This is a condition where there is constriction of the blood vessels in the extremities. The arteries literally 'freeze' into a spasm and the nose, ears, fingers or toes go icy cold, turn white or blue and numb in response to cold. Usually more women are affected than men and during winter it can be particularly distressing. Causes include poor circulation (chilblains are another, separate symptom) and heart disease – arteriosclerosis is considered to be the major cause. Some medications and smoking aggravate the condition, and there is also a link with migraine sufferers. It is of paramount importance to improve the general circulation – and the diet is the place to begin.

The danger foods

Avoid chilled foods, especially during winter – cold drinks, ice-cream and cold foods of any kind. Fried foods, fatty foods and fast foods are pure poison. Alcohol must in every way be avoided as it plays havoc with your body temperature in any kind of weather. Sugar and refined carbohydrates impair the circulation. Replace sugar with fresh or dried stevia leaves (avoid processed stevia). White flour, cakes, sweets, chocolates, white bread, white pasta, white sugar and white rice are all really bad for you, as is anything with caffeine in it – tea, coffee, especially instant coffee, colas and energy drinks. Cut out all carbonated drinks and also bottled fruit drinks (due to their preservatives). Avoid processed foods and check labels for additives like preservatives. Sulphur dioxide and benzoic acid are two dangerous preservatives that must be avoided.

Smoking is an absolute no-no! Do everything you can to stop the habit and avoid passive smoking. Smoking will literally throw you on to a downward spiral and your health will suffer very quickly.

The superfoods

Start by drinking water – fresh, filtered (set up a reliable water filter in your kitchen today!). You need a minimum of 6 glasses a day. Start gradually and work up to a comfortable amount. Have a glass every 2 hours and place a covered jug of water and a glass in a place where you can see it.

Buckwheat contains rutin, which strengthens the walls of the arteries and veins. Grow your own and use the fresh buckwheat leaves and flowers in salads. Dehusked buckwheat and buckwheat flour can be bought from health shops. Include beetroot (and the leaves) in the diet daily. Juice it, grate it into salads with apples – it is an excellent circulatory food, as is parsley, celery, alfalfa sprouts and green fresh lucerne. Grow your own lucerne along with red clover leaves. These are rich in vitamins and minerals and juiced with wheat and barley grass, carrots and apples make a superb circulatory drink.

Learn to make soups with soya beans and lots of green vegetables like peas and pea vine tips, leeks, cabbage, marrows,

Caution: Consult with your doctor before you embark on any form of self-diagnosis or self-treatment.

sweet potatoes, pumpkin and lentils. Add finely grated ginger, mustard leaves, cumin, turmeric – these are warming spices – and add cayenne pepper to rich hot stews and casseroles. Soya beans, tofu and freshly picked green soya beans, lightly steamed, are also excellent additions to the diet. Enjoy oily fish like mackerel, tuna, herring and trout with lots of ground coriander, cumin and ginger. Sardines with avocado and sprouts make a valuable lunch dish.

Sprinkle a mixture of finely ground flaxseed, sunflower seeds, almonds, pumpkin seeds and sesame seeds onto hot oats porridge and add chopped walnuts or macadamia nuts. Have it daily for breakfast, served with warmed Bulgarian yoghurt. Add a few chopped dates or sun-dried sultanas or raisins to give sweetness.

Speak to your doctor about supplements: coenzyme Q10, vitamin B-complex (vitamin B3 is particularly important), gingko biloba and hawthorn capsules.

Tissue Salts: No. 1, 2, 4 and 6 (take 2 of each, 6 times a day).

Pennywort (*Centella asiatica*) is the top circulation herb. Make a tea by adding 3 leaves to a cup of boiling water, stand 5 minutes, strain and sip slowly. Take 1 cup a day and after 2 weeks give it a rest for 2–3 days, then begin again.

Daily exercise – cycling, brisk walking, skipping, tennis, jogging – will get the circulation going, and so will brisk massages with a loofah in a hot bath. It worth going to a physiotherapist weekly to get a deep and invigorating massage to the hands and feet as well as the exercises that will move the circulation. Dress warmly and wear gloves, warm cotton or woollen socks, vests and thermal underwear during winter.

Rheumatoid Arthritis

Debilitating and painful, rheumatoid arthritis is a chronic autoimmune condition that leads to inflammation of the joints and surrounding tissues. Symptoms are fever, fatigue, pain in the small joints of the hands, wrists, ankles and feet, which swell and become red and over time may become disfigured. The causes vary from a hereditary gene to adrenal weakness and overload, to toxaemia, to deficiencies within the diet, to liver dysfunction, chronic stress and anxiety, and even chronic constipation can add to the condition.

Ask your doctor to test for vitamin deficiencies like the B-vitamins, vitamin D, zinc and the essential fatty acids. Today's treatment of rheumatoid arthritis is so different and so much more effective and doctors agree it begins with the diet. Interestingly, going vegetarian, even fully vegan, is one of the most effective treatments and many patients can verify remarkable recovery after leaving meat, fish and dairy products completely out of their diets!

The danger foods

Meat is a serious trigger – pork, beef, even mutton – also cow's milk, cheese and cream cheese, even yoghurt. Next come gluten-rich foods – wheat, oats and rye. By deleting everything that has gluten in it eases the pain and inflammation and sorts out the bowel beautifully. Pay attention to this: some sufferers even include mealies in this list. The citrus fruits are next on the list – all of them, including lemon and orange juice. Then for some rheumatoid arthritis cases the nightshade family has proved to be a problem. Lessen potatoes, tomatoes, brinjals,

sweet peppers, paprika and chillies. Some say the pain is intensified when eating these vegetables.

Avoid coffee, especially instant coffee, malt, sugar, junk foods and processed foods with additives such as artificial colourings and sweeteners, also fizzy drinks, colas, diet drinks, energy drinks, cakes, biscuits, pies, fries and fast foods. Microwaved food, too, is out – you really cannot afford to expose your body for even a moment to microwave energy, or eat irradiated food.

Keep a food diary and be aware of exactly what is going into your mouth – every mouthful needs to be as pure, as natural and as health building as is possible.

The superfoods

A constantly changing selection of organic fruits and vegetables, packed with antioxidants, vitamins and minerals, is vital for wellness. The berries are particularly beneficial, as are all the red and yellow fruits and vegetables you can find. Experiment with juices, smoothies, salads and soups. A nut and seed sprinkle (see page 26) is an energy booster. Use flaxseed, almonds, hazelnuts, cashews or pecan nuts with sesame seeds, sunflower seeds and pumpkin seeds. Sprinkle over fruit salads of papaya and mashed berries and mangoes or peaches, nectarines, apricots or whatever is in season.

Green vegetables – Cabbage, kale, broccoli and Brussels sprouts – are extremely valuable in the daily diet. Extract wheat grass and barley grass juice with carrots, celery, cabbage, apples and pineapple. Olive oil and avocado in salads and oily fish – sardines, mackerel, trout and herring, eaten three times a week – are rich in omega-3 oils, which have important anti-inflammatory properties. Eat free-range organic chicken twice a week and add turmeric to brown rice or to chicken and vegetable stews – it too has anti-inflammatory properties. Make soups and stews with a variety of beans, chickpeas and sprouts and drink herb teas made of pennywort (*Centella asiatica*), melissa, mint, and ginger and honey often.

Eat foods that are rich in vitamins B, D and E daily (see pages 11–13) and speak to your doctor about supplements: vitamin B12 injections, extra vitamin B5, flax oil, fish oil – like cod liver oil – and borage oil. Have your doctor check for low stomach acid and take probiotics and glutamine powder to help the digestive process.

Tissue Salts: No. 4 and 10 are comforting, and so is the antispasmodic No. 8. Rheumatoid arthritis sufferers also benefit from No. 1 and No. 12 for flexibility. Take 2 of each frequently.

See a physiotherapist on a regular basis for massages and exercise and add a dash of apple cider vinegar to your bath water – its soothing, anti-acid action eases the pain considerably.

Rosacea

Rosacea or rose rash is a chronic flush of red, rough, uneven skin that spreads across the cheeks, nose and chin. It can affect both men and women of all ages and it can even come out in raised welts, spots and rashes. Causes are varied and it is persistent and irritating. It can be a sign of liver toxicity, hormonal imbalance, alcohol, lactose intolerance or digestive problems triggered by certain foods like spicy hot foods, pork products, caffeine, even parasites. In some cases it is hereditary and stress and anxiety play a role, even being in the hot sunlight can trigger a rash. It is important to try and pinpoint the cause, especially if it is food intolerance, and to eliminate the triggers one by one.

Caution: Consult with your doctor before you embark on any form of self-diagnosis or self-treatment.

The danger foods

The dairy foods are a good start to eliminate, then the trans fatty acids – these are often problem foods and are included in cakes, pies, fast foods, fried foods, margarines and shortenings, and pastries. Avoid refined carbohydrates: white bread and buns, biscuits, doughnuts, and foods high in sugar – iced cakes, cupcakes, syrups and dressings, even spreads, mayonnaises and many processed foods! Also avoid carbonated drinks, packaged fruit juices and citrus drinks.

The superfoods

Radically change the diet to mainly fresh vegetables and fruits to cleanse the liver: celery, parsley, cabbage, broccoli, squash, and green salads with only fresh lemon juice as a dressing. Have one meal a day consisting only of a large mixed salad. For example, include watercress, lettuce, avocados, spring onions, cucumbers, finely grated carrots, thinly shredded fennel root, cabbage, sprouts and lots of chopped celery and parsley. Make fruit salads with pineapple, kiwifruit, berries, papayas, mangoes, litchis, cherries, pomegranate seeds, and sprinkle with ground flaxseed, almonds, sesame seeds and sunflower seeds.

Make vegetable soups with fresh lucerne and red clover leaves, grated pumpkin and sweet potato, green peas and pea shoots, green beans and lots of cabbage and kale. Replace red meat with chicken and legumes, like lentils and chickpeas.

Avoid tea and coffee and replace with herb teas like mint tea, stinging nettle tea, chamomile tea, weak rooibos tea with fresh lemon juice or just hot water with fresh lemon juice. The aim is to clear the liver and to flush the body of toxins – so drink lots of water as well.

Talk to your doctor about supplements: vitamin C to act as an inflammatory and vitamin B-complex (avoid niacin or vitamin B3 on its own as this can cause flushing) and milk thistle capsules to clear the liver. Avoid treating the condition with antibiotics: rather use a good diet to clear it up.

Tissue Salts: No. 4 and 10 ease the redness and irritation; and take No. 9 as well if there is itchiness.

Be careful of the soaps you use on the face as well as the creams – make your own soothing healing cream (see box) or order it ready made (see our website, www.margaretroberts.co.za).

Soothing Healing Cream

Simmer 1 cup of pennywort (*Centella asiatica*) leaves with ½ cup calendula petals in 1 cup of pure aqueous cream in a double boiler for 20 minutes. (Dry the winter-flowering calendulas for all year round use.) Strain and add 3 teaspoons of vitamin E oil (this acts as a natural preservative). Apply as a soothing healing skin cream. To treat dry skin, add 2–4 teaspoons almond oil and/or 2–4 teaspoons flaxseed oil. This will become your treasured beauty product.

Schizophrenia

This condition varies in symptoms such as depression, angry outbursts, withdrawal from society, feelings of despair, paranoia, behaviour that is demanding and unreasonable, even hallucinations. Causes vary too, such as head injury, intense stress (see page 266), biochemical abnormalities such as excessively high zinc and copper levels or nutrient deficiencies, food intolerances and environmental toxins. Some medications can also affect the patient, even extra-high histamine levels or a family history of mental health problems. Everything needs to be carefully discussed with the doctor, and medical treatment is advised. But to complement the treatment it is imperative to change the diet and build up nutritional deficiencies. Blood sugar levels need to be kept stable, as this can cause mood swings and alter the chemistry of the brain.

The danger foods

Sugar and refined carbohydrates, processed foods and instant foods, all junk foods, fast foods, fried foods, carbonated drinks, colas, energy drinks, diet drinks, alcohol in any form, and also caffeine, so avoid coffee, especially instant coffee, and tea – substitute rooibos tea. Other dangers are recreational drugs, living the high life on the go with constant partying, over-exposure to noise and lights, drinking and smoking.

The superfoods

Choose everything whole, fresh, unprocessed. Eat fruits, vegetables, nuts, seeds – fresh is best – so include daily fruit salads, salads and soups prepared from a variety of fresh vegetables with no sauces or additives. Drink freshly squeezed fruit juices, smoothies and lots of water. Make carrot, apple, celery, beetroot juices with wheat grass and barley grass. Grow your own sprouts like alfalfa, mung beans, cress and mustard and add them to the daily salad with avocado, pineapple, radishes and lots of lettuce, watercress, parsley, fennel, celery and dandelion leaves. Oats porridge sprinkled with a nut and seed mix (see page 26) and served with Bulgarian yoghurt and a touch of honey or a few seedless raisins makes a sustaining breakfast.

Include in the diet lean white meat like grilled chicken, steamed vegetables, especially green leafy vegetables, foods rich in vitamin E (see page 13) to protect the brain, boiled eggs, oily fish like salmon, trout, mackerel, sardines, as well as chickpeas, green peas, lentils and beans, like butter beans and haricot beans, as well as foods rich in vitamin B and magnesium (see page 11 and 15).

Be aware of potential allergens in foods, such as nuts and fish and avoid all processed sauces, condiments and flavourings. Make your own with herbs and spices and use only sea salt, lemon juice and natural herb flavourings.

Tissue Salts, especially the phosphates, will ease tension and anxiety; No. 2, 4, 6, 8, 10 and 11 are good for temper flare-ups, and take No. 2 and 6 to ease night terrors and calm and soothe (take 2 of each frequently).

Scoliosis

Although spinal curvature can be detected at birth, it often becomes evident in small children during growth spurts (juvenile scoliosis) or during the teenage years (adolescent scoliosis). Get your child to stand in front of you, feet together, arms hanging at the sides, and check the spine, the level of the shoulders – one not higher than the other – and run your finger down the spine. Sometimes there is pain and often you can trace the sideways curve. This must be seen to by a doctor

Caution: Consult with your doctor before you embark on any form of self-diagnosis or self-treatment.

and a programme of corrective exercises needs to be followed, along with attention to the diet and avoiding carrying heavy school bags, even playing a musical instrument like the violin that requires holding a position to one side. Causes are often found to be mineral deficiencies such as lack of vitamins B, D and E, manganese and magnesium, or a diet too high in sugar – and this is often the most common cause.

The danger foods
Avoid the following foods that impair muscle and bone development: sugar and refined carbohydrates, white bread, white rice, white pasta, white flour, cakes, pies, biscuits, condensed milk so loved by children, ice-creams, instant coffee, sugary cereals, fast foods, fried foods, junk foods, sweets, chocolates, crisps, fried chips and the most dangerous of all, the carbonated drinks – the colas, the energy drinks, the brightly coloured sugary tinned drinks so loved by young people.

And surprisingly alcohol! Young children think it is clever to drink and teenage alcoholism is on the rise. During the growth years alcohol can do great damage to the liver and kidneys and it weakens the muscles that hold the spine in place. It is vital to address this for the future.

The superfoods
Eat fresh vegetables and fruit in abundance and drink at least 6 glasses of plain water throughout the day.

Vegetable soups with chickpeas, butter beans, haricot beans, black-eyed beans, lentils or split peas and lots of grated carrots, onions, kale or thinly shredded cabbage, pumpkin or sweet potatoes, parsley, celery, spinach, and even broccoli or cauliflower, finely chopped and with their thinly shredded leaves, will nourish the bones and the muscles and keep the liver and kidneys working well. Do not flavour the soup with sauces and stock cubes. Rather fry the onions in olive oil and add sea salt as the cooking time ends, with chopped thyme and crushed coriander seeds and a little homemade chutney and lots of freshly squeezed lemon juice mixed with a touch of honey.

The daily salad is extremely important – include avocados, asparagus, dandelion leaves, soya beans and tofu, along with fennel, celery, lettuce, cucumber and sprouts. Many young people rely on bread as a daily staple, so be diligent in searching out wholesome unadulterated breads made with brown flour or rye, free from preservatives, stabilisers and anti-caking agents, or better still bake your own (see page 35). Eat oily fish – sardines, trout or mackerel – a few times a week and lessen the red meat.

Sprinkle a seed and nut mix (see page 26), about a tablespoon daily, over oats porridge to build bones and muscles and provide energy. Almonds, hazelnuts, walnuts, pecan nuts and cooked chickpeas make healthy snacks. Substitute sugar with stevia and occasionally honey, and replace sweets and desserts with smoothies made with fresh fruit like melons and pineapple, apples and papayas, berries and kiwifruit – any combination of whatever fruit is in season – and, if liked, mix with Bulgarian yoghurt.

Try the following herb teas: mint tea, especially peppermint tea at exam times, lemongrass tea, pennywort (*Centella asiatica*) tea and sacred basil (*Ocimum tenuifolium*). Pour 1 cup of boiling water over ¼ cup fresh herbs, stand 5 minutes and strain. Sip slowly, unsweetened. These are valuable and strengthening.

Eat foods rich in vitamins D and E and talk to your doctor about supplements: vitamin B-complex, vitamins D and E, magnesium, zinc and omega-3 fatty acids.

Tissue Salts: Take a combination of all 12 in one tablet.

Join a Pilates class or an exercise class and learn deep breathing exercises. There is much that can change and much to be positive about!

Shingles

Shingles is caused by *Herpes zoster*, the same virus that causes chicken pox, and anyone who has had chicken pox harbours it in the body, where it lies dormant until something triggers it. Then it flares up into the dreaded shingles, or in the case of *Herpes simplex* into fever blisters. Shingles is seriously painful and debilitating and affects the nerve endings, starting with a rash, blisters, tenderness, painful itching and feverishness. It can affect the skin over the rib cage, abdomen, along the spine or even the face, and the intense pain can continue for many weeks. The pain can continue once the blisters have formed scabs and healed and the condition needs to be treated by the doctor as it can have long-lasting and serious effects if left untreated.

Keeping the immune system in good shape keeps it at bay, but shingles can take hold when the whole body is deficient in certain nutrients or weakened by severe and long-lasting stress, by chemotherapy or by shock. The aim is therefore to improve and fortify the immune system, to keep the body alkaline and to build wellness, reduce nervous tension and to generally boost the whole system (see also page 240).

The danger foods
Fast foods, fatty foods and fried foods do nothing to improve the immune system. Also lessen the sugar, saturated fats and caffeine – all of them break down health. Avoid foods rich in arginine – wheat, wheat germ and wheat products, carob, chocolate, soya beans, sesame seeds and gelatine. In some cases coconut, peanuts, fish and even pineapple may intensify the attack. So become aware of what you eat and keep a food diary. Avoid pastries, jams, jellies and sweets, especially those made with gelatine and sugars. Read the labels carefully and avoid all flavourants, additives, stabilisers and too much sugar – they break down the immune system.

The superfoods
Wheat and barley grass juice with fresh lucerne, parsley, celery, carrots and apples is excellent. Chicken and fish are good choices too. You need to build alkalinity – so include lots of smoothies made with fresh fruits and vegetables and salads with chickpeas and sprouts, especially mung bean and alfalfa sprouts.

Speak to your doctor about supplements: vitamins C, D, E and B-complex, zinc, echinacea tablets and spirulina.

Tissue Salts: A comforting formula for shingles sufferers is No. 6, 8 and 9 (take 2 tablets of each 6–10 times a day); at night take 2 tablets each of No. 2, 4, 5, 6 and 9 (take No. 5, 6 and 9 together and after 10 minutes take No. 2 and 4 together; you can take this 2–3 times during the night should you wake).

Herb teas are helpful to drink and to wash with: chamomile, melissa and sacred basil are excellent, especially last thing at night. I also put warmed tea of any one of these herbs into a

A–Z Ailment Chart

spritz bottle with 4 crushed tissue salts of No. 8 (Mag.Phos) and No. 9 (Nat.Mur). Sprayed very gently over the area they immediately soothe. Apply a good healing cream to the sores frequently – we make one with calendula, pennywort and chickweed, which we can post anywhere.

A little dab of lavender essential oil with tea tree oil on the sores often helps them to dry out, but go very carefully first. Oats with fresh lavender tied in a soft cotton bag can be used as a sponge in the bath – the oats soothes beautifully and the lavender helps the healing.

Sinusitis

Sinusitis is inflammation of the sinus cavities, which causes the nasal passages to become congested and the head to ache. Postnasal drip leads to coughs, discharge, fever, discomfort, with often a throbbing headache, and a runny nose and a feeling of fatigue and pure wretchedness. It can be caused by several things and if it recurs frequently it needs to be seriously investigated in order to correct it. Food allergies, like peanuts, brinjals, wheat, etc., and swimming in chlorine-treated swimming pools are common causes, but heaters, underfloor heating, air-conditioners, environmental pollution, smoking and passive smoking, constant 'flu or colds, nutrient deficiencies, especially zinc, poor eating habits and food intolerances like dairy foods and eggs all add to the problem. It is worth keeping a careful diary on everything you eat, for just a mouthful of the wrong food may trigger a flare-up.

The danger foods

The aim here is to strengthen the body's immunity. Avoid caffeine in all forms, which means coffee, especially instant coffee, tea, colas, energy drinks, chocolate and chocolate cakes and, in the case of sinusitis, the 'lethal' combination of chocolate and coffee! Also avoid sugar and refined carbohydrates, cakes, biscuits, pies, baked tarts, as well as fried foods, fatty foods, all forms of alcohol, processed foods, especially processed meats, unhealthy oils and fats (see page 33), instant foods and anything microwaved. Consider gluten and other food intolerances and avoid wheat and dairy products and nuts. Replace sugar with stevia and literally change the diet to only fresh fruits and vegetables to completely get rid of the toxic build-up.

The superfoods

Start with increasing your daily water consumption and drink 6–8 glasses of water, not teas, flavoured waters or energy drinks, just *plain* water and do not drink it with ice or chilled as this makes the sinuses ache! Stock up on fresh vegetables like carrots, celery, parsley, radishes, cabbage, broccoli, watercress, turnips, sweet potatoes, pumpkin, squashes, tomatoes – especially cherry tomatoes – baby spinach, fennel and all the salad greens you can find. Start your own salad garden and grow as much as you can organically. Chickpeas, lentils, black-eyed beans, green beans and green peas are excellent, and only have chicken or white fish like hake – avoid red meat. Make chickpea fritters with spring onions, leeks and garlic, and have vegetable soups and broths and smoothies daily. Grate fresh ginger into salad dressings with lemon juice. Horseradish will greatly reduce mucus, so grow your own and grate the root into salads and soups. Like onions, it will make your eyes water and your nose run which, in the case of blocked sinuses, is helpful!

Eat fruit salads daily and squeeze your own fresh fruit juices and add wheat grass and barley grass juice to the daily diet (see page 29). Grow your own and diligently drink at least ½ a glass of the juice with pineapple, carrot, beetroot, parsley and celery every day.

Herb teas of fresh sage or thyme or basil (especially sacred basil) and garden violets (both flowers and the leaves) help to drain the sinuses and clear up the mucus. Pour 1 cup of boiling water over ¼ cup fresh herb of your choice (always select one herb at a time – do not mix them). Stand 5 minutes, strain and sip slowly. Drink unsweetened, but add a little lemon juice if liked.

Talk to your doctor about supplements, especially vitamins A, B, C and D to strengthen the immune system. One of my most successful capsules is the one called 'Sinus and Hay Fever' which contains Tissue Salts No. 7 and 9, violet leaf powder, lemon, bioflavonoids, mullein leaves and pantothenic acid (vitamin B5) and it is available from most pharmacies.

Tissue Salts: Take No. 2 for aching sinuses, No. 3 and 7 for blocked sinuses, No. 5 and 9 for sinusitis and No. 4 and No. 9 for allergic sinusitis (suck 2 of each frequently; taken every half hour or every 20 minutes it will quickly ease the pain, the headache and the watery misery and after 3 or 4 doses you will feel considerably better).

Steam at least 3 times throughout the day: Pour boiling water into a large bowl, add drops of tea tree oil or eucalyptus oil and cover your head over the bowl with a towel. Keep the eyes tightly closed and inhale through the nose for as long as the steam rises. (Avoid steaming if you have thread veins on the nose.) A handkerchief with a few drops of tea tree oil held under the nose also helps. Also add tea tree oil to a hot bath and inhale the steam through the nose. Hot facial compresses of a face cloth wrung out in hot water to which a few drops of tea tree oil or eucalyptus oil have been added can be greatly comforting to aching sinuses.

Deep breathing exercises are extremely helpful and it is worth visiting a physiotherapist for this, as well as going for walks in unpolluted air away from heavy traffic.

Skin Problems

The skin is a true mirror of health. A poor diet deprives the skin of many essential nutrients so that deficiencies in our diet show up first on the skin. The skin cells are constantly being renewed and the outer cells are sloughed off – a few million of them daily! These outer cells have absorbed waste, pollution and shed easily, making the skin one of our most important organs of elimination alongside the kidneys, the bowels and the lungs.

Acne and problem skin

Pimples, infected blackheads and red spots usually affect teenagers and are often due to a hormone imbalance. Oiliness and enlarged pores are often due to overactive sebaceous glands, not cleansing the skin properly and the wrong diet. Allergies to some foods, for example milk, may also come into play.

The danger foods

Fatty foods, refined sugar and white flour, white bread, cakes, sweets, chocolate, fast foods like hot dogs, hamburgers and

Caution: Consult with your doctor before you embark on any form of self-diagnosis or self-treatment.

chips, commercial tomato sauces, mustard sauces, eggs (especially fried), alcohol, smoking and carbonated drinks (the real enemy of healthy skin) and all sweetened, processed and instant foods.

The superfoods

Drink water: 6–8 glasses of plain water a day. Twice a day, drink a glass of water with 2 teaspoons apple cider vinegar added (and add a dash of apple cider vinegar to the rinsing water after washing the face). Increase your intake of fresh fruit and green leafy vegetables. A salad with dandelion, fennel and celery with lemon juice twice daily is vital. Include sprouts, sunflower seeds, sesame seeds and chickpeas in the diet. Replace red meat with chicken, steamed or grilled, and served with brown rice and fresh lemon juice. Extract your own wheat grass juice with carrots, celery, parsley, apple and beetroot. Take vitamin supplements: vitamins A, C and B-complex, especially vitamin B6. Eat plain Bulgarian yoghurt to introduce probiotics to the digestive tract.

Use oats soaked in warm water as a facial scrub and use fresh mashed strawberry or pineapple as a cleansing mask.

Dry Skin

Chapping, thickening, itchiness – the natural skin barrier is put under stress by many factors and our polluted world has a lot to do with it! Worse is winter when the atmosphere dries out to a brittleness and the cold seems to retard the flow of the skin's natural oils. Dry skin is now a concern even in tiny babies. Dry skin can be caused by poor diet, excessive dieting, pollution and age – as we get older the skin becomes dryer and thinner and cracks, and it flakes and bleeds easily. Hormones also play a role as well as thyroid conditions, but most of all we need to really consider our diet.

The danger foods

First is too much tea, coffee and alcohol. Rather drink herb teas and rooibos tea and avoid all carbonated drinks, diet drinks, energy drinks, sugar, spices and also excess salt as too much salt causes skin puffiness, even swellings in the soft skin around the eyes and nose. Lessen dairy and meat – especially processed meats – refined foods and fried foods. Do not smoke – this coarsens the skin, adding to pollution damage.

Chemicals in every form damage the skin – carefully read the labels and use only natural skin products that are free from petrochemicals, parabens, stabilisers, perfumes and other chemicals. Look at the 'E' numbers in foods – many have detrimental effects on dry skin (see also page 210).

The superfoods

Antioxidant foods like berries, yellow and red fruits and vegetables, broccoli, green leafy vegetables, avocado all help in the production of collagen and new cells, reduce puffiness and rejuvenate the skin. The essential fatty acids are vital: omega-3 fatty acids as well as monounsaturated oils which are found in flaxseed and flaxseed oil, almonds and almond oil, olive oil, pumpkin seeds, millet and fish like salmon, tuna and mackerel.

Include lots of fresh vegetables – raw in salads or lightly steamed – in the diet. Have fruit salads daily and be adventurous: try pineapple and guavas, granadillas and mangoes, pomegranates and pears, and serve with Bulgarian yoghurt and ground seeds

and nuts. Just changing your diet to wholesome vegetables, fruits and whole grains (bake your own bread – see page 35) will soon have your skin glowing.

Drink lots of pure plain water – at least 6 glasses a day and be sure you eat fibre-rich foods, as keeping your digestive system regular is vital. No skin can cope with toxic waste, so eat brown rice, beans, peas, lentils, papaya, prunes, millet and oats (the non-instant kind). The cabbage family is an excellent cleanser and a hydrator, so include kale, cabbage and cauliflower, broccoli frequently, as well as radishes, turnips, watercress, peaches, plums, apricots, mangoes and strawberries. Extract your own fresh wheat grass and barley grass juice with fresh lucerne, celery, carrots, beetroot and apples daily. Take flaxseed oil and evening primrose oil in supplement form daily.

Take lots of exercise and be sure you cleanse the skin daily using pure soaps and creams that have no chemicals in them. (We have developed a superb soap made only of palm kernel oils and baobab oil with vitamin E oil, and a basic aqueous cream free of any chemicals, stabilisers and harsh emulsifiers. We post countrywide and we are dedicated to continuing these formulas.) Always protect your skin with an appropriate sun factor cream when you are outside.

Use almond oil with baobab oil as a massage oil after the bath and avoid taking long hot showers and baths – soaking in hot water leaches out the protecting oils on the skin. If you add a little almond oil or olive oil to the bath you'll find a great improvement, especially if you add a few drops of vitamin E oil.

Skin Cream for Extra Dry Skin

Make your own skin cream and use it lavishly:

1 cup of pure aqueous cream
2 teaspoons vitamin E oil
1 teaspoon evening primrose oil
2 teaspoons baobab oil (if you can find it, otherwise leave it out)
2 teaspoons olive oil
2 teaspoons avocado oil
3 teaspoons almond oil

Add everything together and whisk gently for 5 minutes. Store in a sterilised jar and use lavishly all over the body, concentrating on the very dry areas like legs and feet. Do this after the bath each night and wear cotton pyjamas.

Oily skin

Oily skin or **seborrhoea** is red inflamed, oily, or even scaly patches that form on the skin and scalp. The oil-secreting glands produce an oily substance called sebum, and in babies this is known as 'cradle cap'. Seborrhoea is often the result of the body eliminating waste through the skin and the diet needs to be watched, as food intolerance may be a trigger. Other possible causes are yeast overgrowth, nutrient deficiencies, particularly vitamins A and B and biotin, or even a poor diet. In the case of babies with cradle cap the mother may be eating fast foods or fatty foods, which then come through her milk. Overactive sebaceous glands are common in teenagers and young adults, but can even appear in the forties and are a source of much distress. Luckily the problem can be addressed by changing the diet, so keep a food diary and note the foods that exacerbate the condition in a red pen at the back of the diary!

The danger foods

The usual suspects are sugar and refined carbohydrates. This includes white bread, white rolls, cakes, biscuits, sugary buns, fancy breads, pancakes, doughnuts, chocolates and sweets, sugary breakfast cereals, colas, energy drinks, and carbonated drinks in any form, even fizzy vitamin drinks. Also avoid diet drinks, artificial sweeteners, coffee, especially instant coffee, and chocolate drinks. Avoid all processed foods and watch out especially for foods that contain tartrazine, which is found in many orange and red coloured drinks and foods.

Processed and saturated fats are real danger foods for this condition. Processed meats, dairy products (except plain Bulgarian yoghurt), bacon, ham, sausages and meat pies, need to be avoided diligently. Salty crisps, chips, orange-coloured cheesy puffs are pure poison – just a handful will raise the red sore spotty oily area overnight. Also look at gluten-rich foods such as wheat, oats, barley and rye (see also page 218) as doctors link gluten intolerance to seborrhoeic dermatitis and seborrhoea.

The superfoods

Your greatest skin cleanser is daily servings of fresh fruit, fresh vegetables and freshly juiced wheat and barley grass (this is the green grass from wheat and barley, and not the gluten-rich seed) with carrots, parsley, celery, apples and beetroot. Fresh green salads with lettuce, cucumber, lucerne sprigs, rocket, radishes, baby spinach, chickpeas, parsley, celery and grated carrots, dressed with lemon juice only, is a magnificent cleanser to the whole system. Make smoothies with fresh fruit like mango and papaya and carrots, or peaches and apples and pineapple, or pears and carrots and celery – create your own exciting combinations. Eat lots of yellow, orange and red fruit, like the berries, papayas, mangoes, nectarines, loquats, peaches, pomegranates, and so on, for their beta-carotene. Kiwifruit, cucumber, parsley and celery are particularly delicious 'skin cleansers' and should be eaten often (kiwifruit can also be applied to the skin as a face mask where it acts as a deep cleanser directly on the skin!).

Include fish, especially mackerel and sardines, and chicken in the diet and eat lean mutton or beef occasionally. Sunflower seeds, sesame seeds, flaxseed, pumpkin seeds, brown rice, millet and buckwheat (including the leaves and flowers) are all excellent skin conditioners. Make vegetable soups with grated carrots, chickpeas, lentils, leeks, onions, thinly shredded cabbage, celery, and lots of parsley; and fresh lucerne sprigs, sweet potato, pumpkin or squash, peas and pea shoots, finely chopped spinach, radishes, turnips and their leaves can all be added. Use thyme, oregano, celery seeds and coriander seeds as a flavouring to lessen the salt.

Apple cider vinegar is a fabulous standby both as a drink (2 teaspoons in a glass of water daily) and a added to the rinsing water after you have washed your face or shampooed your hair. Dab apple cider vinegar onto the hot red inflamed areas too (test first and dilute in water if necessary). Use plain Bulgarian yoghurt to cleanse the face too every now and then – keep it on as a face mask for 15 minutes, then rinse off with warm water.

Tissue Salts: No. 7 is a skin lubricator; take No. 1 and 12 for dry cracked skin and No. 9 for oily patches on the face; No. 12 reduces wrinkles and No. 7 removes age spots while No. 2, 7 and 10 are superb rejuvenators (take all three together) and for thin white scaly patches No. 9 is excellent.

Sore Throat and Tonsillitis

This is a common ailment and often the beginning of 'flu, a cold or a streptococcal infection, so check with your doctor quickly should it become feverish and you feel wretched. Other possible causes are over-using the voice, stress, glandular fever, general low immunity, zinc deficiency or even an allergic reaction.

The danger foods

Avoid sugar and refined carbohydrates: white bread, cakes, sweets, chocolates, carbonated drinks and colas, as all these will compromise the immune system. Dairy products are potentially mucous forming – so avoid these for now. Avoid all fried foods, fatty foods, margarines, fast foods, instant foods and processed foods – these are packed with harmful chemicals. Alcohol and iced drinks in any form are a danger to health! Not even a hot toddy will help at this stage.

The superfoods

Soups, vegetable broths and salads are the most comforting foods along with fruit smoothies and juices you have made yourself. Include in the soups finely grated and shredded carrots, cabbage, broccoli, sweet potatoes, leeks, onions, garlic, celery, chickpeas, lentils, pumpkin, parsley, squashes, turnips and turnip greens, radishes (including the leaves) and fennel. Flavour with thyme and coriander and lots of lemon juice and use a good chicken stock as a base. Serve with chopped fresh parsley. (Avoid eating the soup with bread as wheat products may exacerbate the problem.)

Salads can be delicious with mustard greens, sprouts, pineapple, green peppers, avocado, lettuce, cucumber, celery, dandelion leaves, parsley, thyme and lemon juice. Pineapple is excellent for the throat, so use it as a base for smoothies along with apples, carrots, mangoes, granadillas or whatever fruit is in season.

Drink plenty of water and take immune-boosting vitamins and minerals. For tonsillitis include echinacea, elderberry, vitamin C and zinc. If there are recurrent tonsillitis attacks check your child's diet – sugar and too much milk may be the culprit.

For a sore throat, sage tea is excellent – ¼ cup fresh sage leaves to 1 cup of boiling water, stand 5 minutes and strain. Squeeze in a good 1 tablespoon of lemon juice and sweeten with a little honey and sip slowly, holding it in the mouth and let it trickle down the throat gradually. Immediately take 1 000 mg of vitamin C and a zinc tablet. A sore throat can also be eased by gargling with ½ a glass warm water to which a teaspoon of non-iodated coarse sea salt or Himalayan rock salt crystals have been added, along with 2–3 drops of tea tree oil.

Tissue Salts: No. 3, 4 and 7 are excellent for a sore throat (suck 2 of each every hour); for swollen tonsils take No. 2 and 5 (suck 2 of each every hour or every half hour). At the first sign of a sore throat, suck No. 1 with No. 4 every half hour. This often eases it, and gargle with 1 teaspoon salt in ½ glass warm water or 2 teaspoons apple cider vinegar in ½ glass of warm water.

Caution: Consult with your doctor before you embark on any form of self-diagnosis or self-treatment.

Stress

A modern-day 'illness', stress is a crippling and debilitating condition that plays havoc with our health, our relationships and our work! And it is well nigh impossible to avoid. It is said: 'If you're alive, you're stressed to some degree!'

This is what stress does to us: It upsets the digestion causing heartburn, colic, digestive disturbances and constipation. It elicits a 'fight or flight' response, flooding the bloodstream with the stress hormones, cortisol and adrenaline which are there to help you respond to emergencies, shock, fear, running for your life, reacting to a terrifying situation. With chronic stress, this response happens several times a day and the damage to the body is considerable. Toxins flood into the body, blood sugar levels rise, the heart rate increases, blood vessels constrict, breathing is fast and you are in a state of supreme tension. This is when heart attacks, strokes and burst blood vessels occur.

Stress can cause clogged, constricted arteries, elevated blood pressure, headaches of debilitating proportions, chest constriction and shallow breathing, stomach ulcers, and it places so great a load on the endocrine system that it actually impairs our immune response and so can trigger serious illness.

We need to ease the stress in our lives just to survive. We need to find ways to nurture ourselves, our children and our families, and we need to create a refuge, a space where we can repair ourselves, calm ourselves and find ways of changing what we possibly can.

The danger foods

Top of the list are alcohol and caffeine. It has been proven that caffeine intake heightens anxiety, so this means coffee, tea, chocolate, colas and energy drinks are out! Both alcohol and caffeine over-stimulate the adrenal glands, and the stress hormones, now out of control, disturb the metabolism and give rise to accelerated heartbeat, tremors, agitation, nervousness, a rise in blood pressure, perspiration and acute irritation.

Next, cut down on sugar. Fast foods, snack foods, cakes, carbonated drinks, sweets, sugared desserts, ice-cream and, of course, sugar in the coffee, create irritability, poor concentration, flaring tempers and 'heaviness of heart' – depression, anxiety and palpitations.

Salt is another enemy and salty snacks, crisps, biltong, salty cheeses and extra salt added to food all increase the blood pressure. Also avoid processed foods with monosodium glutamate (MSG) and other additives like artificial colourants, flavourants, anti-caking agents and stabilisers – especially those bright orange cheesy snacks so loved by children. Read the labels and shun flavoured sauces, dressings and sprinkles. Use herbs and spices to flavour foods and make your own salt-free flavourant (see page 35).

Finally, avoid saturated fats and trans fats. The list includes full-fat dairy products, fried meats, fatty sausages, margarines, shortenings, fatty bacon, ham, fried foods, fast foods, junk foods, chips fried in oil and over-heated oils. Both the salt and the fats increase the load on the adrenal glands and the liver and put strain on the digestive system, which only adds to the stress levels.

The superfoods

Stock your cupboards and fridge with these superfoods: Avocados are rich in minerals, especially sodium and potassium, and it is one of the top foods for combating fatigue and stress.

Serve it on whole-wheat or rye toast with a squeeze of lemon juice as a snack or light lunch.

Leafy green vegetables: parsley, spinach, broccoli, fenugreek leaves, red clover leaves, lucerne leaves, mustard leaves, turnip leaves, young coriander leaves, lettuce, cabbage, kale, celery (leaves and stalks), peas (pods, leaves and vine tips), as well as spring onions, garlic, baby beetroot, green asparagus, cucumber, green baby seedlings like radishes, baby lettuce, mustard lettuce, wheat grass and barley grass juice and sprouts (especially mung beans, alfalfa, mustard and cress). Include the tips of pumpkin, squash and su-su vines, lightly steamed, and make a fabulous green salad daily. Dress with lemon juice only.

Snack on almonds, pecan nuts, walnuts, sun-dried raisins and sultanas, dried figs, apple rings, sunflower seeds and pumpkin seeds. Eat brown rice, lentils and chickpeas regularly. Sprinkle a mixture of ground sesame seeds, flaxseed, sunflower seeds and almonds over fruit salads, stir-fries, salads or plain Bulgarian yoghurt.

The berries are extremely valuable. Grow your own and dry them or mash them into a pulp and spread on a baking sheet to dry for snacks. A smoothie made with banana, cinnamon, honey and cashew nuts or almonds with raspberries is a real stress-buster. Have mango, peach, flaxseed and pecan nut smoothies when you're dying for a cup of coffee and learn to make your own wheat grass juice with parsley, celery, carrot and beetroot.

Drink at least 6–8 glasses of water a day and get to know herb teas. A soothing cup of mint, melissa, chamomile, sacred basil, ginger, aniseed, lemon verbena or elderflower tea will go a long way in unsnarling the tension and the fury, fear and shakiness. Pour 1 cup of boiling water over ¼ cup fresh herb – any one of the above list. Stand 5 minutes, strain and sip slowly.

Speak to your doctor about supplements: vitamin B-complex, selenium, vitamins D, C and E, calcium, iron and phosphorus. All these boost the whole system, lift the mood and balance the hormones.

Tissue Salts: No. 2, 4 and 6 are my little lifesavers when I'm not coping. Take them all together, 2 of each, and keep taking them to ease tension before it becomes unmanageable.

Put on soft music with a beat slower than your heartbeat and add fragrant, relaxing oils to the bath – rose, neroli, jasmine or lavender (but only a few drops and not at all if you are pregnant). Visit a reputable kinesiologist who will show you how to use 'stress taps' to literally break down the tension in the body. Deep breathing is vital, calming and hugely beneficial. Concentrate on it and slow your pace to accommodate the deep, slow breaths.

Swelling *see* Fluid Retention

Ulcerative Colitis

Like irritable bowel syndrome and Crohn's disease, this is a painful inflammatory condition of the large intestine. Symptoms are fever, griping pains, painful bowel movements with gas, flatulence, bloating and explosive diarrhoea, often with blood in it, as well as constipation. There is often weight loss and extreme lassitude, the rectum may have fissures in it and anaemia may be present with fatigue and depression. Ulcers can form in the bowel lining and high acidity is part of the problem. The

Caution: Consult with your doctor before you embark on any form of self-diagnosis or self-treatment.

condition needs to be diagnosed by a doctor, as often the intense pain can be due to appendicitis and any rectal bleeding and abscesses will require immediate medical attention.

Many causes can lead to this condition, ranging from food allergies to stress, especially emotional stress, high sugar intake, dairy intolerance, low immunity and bacterial infection, parasites and liver problems. Once the condition has been diagnosed and treatment is in place, much can be done by eating correctly and being aware of what to eat for maximum benefit.

The danger foods
The 'killer foods' for this condition are sugar, junk food, fast foods, fried food, hamburgers, chips, spicy foods, cakes, biscuits, white bread, white rolls, white pasta, pizza, coffee, especially instant coffee, tea, drinking chocolate, milkshakes and even certain fruit juices. Surprisingly, raw food should also be avoided as it adds to the irritation in the bowel. Learn to lightly steam or poach vegetables and fruits.

Caffeine is to be seriously avoided and colas and carbonated drinks will send you into a spiral of pain, gas and bloating discomfort. Never chew chewing gum!

The superfoods
Vegetable soups and broths with chicken are vital to provide essential vitamins and minerals. Go lightly on seasoning, rather use herbs like celery, mint, caraway seeds, aniseed, fennel and melissa, all of which are digestive herbs. Chicken, fish and turkey are the best 'meats' for ulcerative colitis, and white fish, like hake, is best of all – not fried but rather poached or steamed.

Oats porridge (not the instant kind), puréed if needed and served with a little honey and plain Bulgarian yoghurt, is an excellent choice for breakfast. For variety add mashed banana or figs. When figs are not in season, soak dried figs overnight and include them every couple of days in the breakfast oats porridge.

Peel fruits like apples, pears and peaches and include fruits and vegetables in the form of freshly squeezed juices and smoothies. Try apple and banana, or apple and papaya, or pear and carrot – keep experimenting. Keep a food diary and introduce new foods every now and then, little by little!

Melissa (also known as lemon balm) is a lemon-flavoured mint and the best of all digestive herbs. Grow your own and have it as a tea daily – ¼ cup fresh sprigs to 1 cup boiling water, stand 5 minutes, strain and sip slowly unsweetened. Peppermint teas and mint teas are also wonderful digestives and soothe and heal the ulcers and act as a tonic for the whole bowel.

Flaxseed tea is proving to be very helpful. In a pestle and mortar, crush 1 tablespoon of flaxseeds lightly. Pour over this 1 cup of boiling water and leave overnight. Next morning strain and drink the 'tea' or add it to an apple smoothie.

Speak to your doctor about supplements: a good multivitamin is essential, as you need the best nutrition possible, and ask about extra B-vitamins, magnesium, zinc, the omega-3 oils and probiotics. Find out about iron injections, as anaemia is often a side-effect of the blood loss and the diarrhoea. Slippery elm powder is greatly comforting as a soothing treatment for constipation and the bowel in general.

Tissue Salts: No. 8, 10 and 11 will ease the pain of indigestion (take 2 of each daily) and No. 3 and 10 are excellent for bowel ulcers (take 2 of each dissolved in the mouth together).

Underweight
Some people are naturally thin and remain so no matter what they eat, but any unexplained weight loss must be investigated by your doctor. Possible causes are anorexia, diabetes, cancer, AIDS or other underlying health problems, even stress, shock and grief. Parasites or an imbalance in the intestinal flora can lead to severe weight loss, as nutrients cannot be absorbed. An over-active thyroid also plays a role in weight loss, as does liver function. Crohn's disease, ulcerative colitis, diverticulitis and candida can add to the condition (see the individual entries for these ailments).

The danger foods
The big no-no is caffeine in any form – coffee, especially instant coffee, tea (change to herb teas and rooibos), carbonated cola drinks, in fact all carbonated drinks are dangerous to this condition. Chocolate with coffee speeds up the metabolism and quickly depletes nutrients in the body. Avoid processed foods, especially meats, fried foods like chips and sausages, and sugar in all its many forms (change to stevia or to honey).

The superfoods
Start with sprouts, which are just packed with essential nutrients – alfalfa, mung beans, red clover, fenugreek, buckwheat, sunflower seeds, mustard seeds. Grow borders of fenugreek and buckwheat, as they are filled with fabulous vitamins and minerals and can be picked daily for salads – and make that daily salad a priority.

Smoothies are a safe and natural way of building health – make your own combinations and be adventurous, for example: banana, papaya and mango is richly satisfying; pears and apples with orange is refreshing and energising; strawberries with pomegranates and pineapple is revitalising; carrots and sprouts like alfalfa and sunflower seeds with apple and pineapple give you the kick start mid-afternoon. Add plain Bulgarian yoghurt and even almonds, cashew nuts, macadamia nuts or pecan nuts to fruity smoothies to give you that sustaining strength you need.

Include whole grains, legumes and seeds in the diet: brown rice, millet, oats, rye, buckwheat, chickpeas, lentils, sesame seeds, flaxseed, sunflower seeds, as well as avocados, oily fish and, olive oil and lots of fresh vegetables and fruits in the diet. For breakfast every day, sprinkle a finely ground seed and nut mix (see page 26) over oats porridge, served with Bulgarian yoghurt or warm full-cream milk and a little honey.

Include celery, fennel, dill, caraway seeds, aniseed, ginger, melissa and the mints – all aid digestion and if you lessen the salt and the pepper you will find these herbs flavour the food beautifully.

Try eating 6 small meals a day using the superfoods – for example, a fruit smoothie of your choice and an open sandwich with avocado and sprouts on rye bread; or a bowl of vegetable soup with homemade rye bread and cream cheese; or a quick stir-fry using vegetables and fish.

Talk to your doctor about supplements: zinc, magnesium, amino acids and probiotics are all valuable.

Tissue Salts: All 12 (take 'Combin 12', up to 8 times a day).

Urticaria *see* Hives

Varicose Veins and Haemorrhoids
These are contused, often raised, veins that most often occur in the legs, the rectum and the anus. They become weak spots

Caution: Consult with your doctor before you embark on any form of self-diagnosis or self-treatment.

due to the malfunction of the minute one-way valves within the walls of the veins which return the blood to the heart. Blood then collects in certain areas, often causing throbbing discomfort or a dull ache and can be exacerbated by standing, or long periods of sitting and keeping the legs crossed. The condition is aggravated by lack of exercise, overweight, poor circulation, liver overload, a diet high in fats and sugars and low in fibre, laxative abuse, and even pregnancy.

The danger foods
The most important factor is to diligently remove from you diet *all* refined foods, fast foods and processed foods (read the labels and avoid all additives: preservatives, stabilisers, colourants, anti-caking agents and flavourants of any description). Cut out sugar, cakes, pies, pastries, sweets, alcohol, dairy products, caffeine (present in tea, coffee, colas, energy drinks and chocolate) and alcohol – all these exacerbate the condition.

The superfoods
Fresh fruits, vegetables and salads daily top the list! The antioxidants in fruits and vegetables tone and strengthen the walls of the veins and arteries, boosting the circulation. Stinging nettle, both as a tea and eaten as a spinach, is excellent as is amaranth, lucerne, flaxseed, all the berries, grapefruit juice, pomegranate juice, celery, parsley, baby spinach, marrows, pumpkin, squashes, melons, nectarines, green and red peppers, fresh green buckwheat, grapes, cherries, apricots, tomatoes, plums, pears, red rosehips, mangoes, papaya, loquats, onions, garlic, spring onions, sprouts, especially alfalfa, buckwheat, sunflower and mustard greens. Eat dandelion greens, turnip greens, radish leaves and radishes, as well as beetroot (steam the leaves as spinach). Eat prunes and papaya daily to ease constipation, and be sure to drink 6–8 glasses of water daily. Make herb teas of pennywort (*Centella asiatica),* stinging nettle, melissa or mint, and drink them unsweetened. (The cooled pennywort tea also makes a soothing lotion and wash.)

Speak to your doctor about supplements: vitamin B-complex and vitamin C, lecithin, selenium, zinc, coenzyme Q10, beta-carotene, bioflavonoids and milk thistle for a congested liver.

Tissue Salts: No. 1, 3 and 4 (take 2 of each, 4 times a day).

Haemorrhoid Cream

In a double boiler simmer 1 cup of fresh pennywort (*Centella asiatica*) leaves in one cup of pure aqueous cream with ½ cup fresh lucerne sprigs. Stir frequently, pressing out the juices of the herbs. Strain and add 3 teaspoons of vitamin E oil and 1 tablespoon of witch hazel. Also add the above tissue salts – 4 of each crushed finely into the cream. Mix well. Spoon into sterilised jars and keep the excess in the fridge. Apply frequently. This cream allows the haemorrhoids to slip back into the rectum.

Worms

Surprisingly, worms are more common in the intestinal tract than we would think! And we can pick them up from many sources, including from processed meats, from eating meat and fish that is undercooked, from our pets and from poor hygiene. When we say 'worms' it includes wire worms, roundworms, pinworms and tapeworms, and the symptoms are restlessness at night when the worms are at their most active, abdominal discomfort, rectal and anal itching, cravings for sweet things, loss of appetite and, in some cases, constant hunger, diarrhoea, anaemia, weight loss, and sometimes worms or larvae are visible in the stool. Check your children regularly for sometimes there are no obvious symptoms!

Parasites in any form can lead to severe anaemia and susceptibility to other infections as the immune system can be compromised. Your doctor will advise you on the de-worming procedure. If you have pets, your vet will advise you on a regular de-worming programme. Most important of all is washing the hands always before eating, after going to the toilet and when you have stroked your pets!

The danger foods
A diet high in sugar, refined carbohydrates, processed foods, meat and dairy foods creates a climate in which worms can thrive. Avoid processed meats, fish, poultry and rare beef or mutton, or pork or bacon that is not fully cooked. Gluten build-up is another breeding ground as worms thrive in mucus-rich environment, so avoid anything that contains gluten – wheat and wheat products, rye, oats, barley – as well as dairy foods, eggs and citrus fruits. White bread and white rolls and sugary buns and doughnuts are the worst, and even very sweet fruits are full of the sugars that worms love – the only two they don't like are pineapples and figs!

The superfoods
Foods with anti-worm properties include figs, pumpkin seeds, raw onions, garlic and pineapple, especially the core of the pineapple. A juice of wheat grass, barley grass, lucerne, parsley and celery with carrots, beetroot and pineapple makes an excellent de-worming drink. Dandelion leaves, bitter and strong, added to this have an excellent effect on the worms. Finely chopped raw garlic added to pumpkin seeds is an excellent remedy and should be taken first thing in the morning for 10 days. Take 1 teaspoon of each, mixed together, washed down with a cup of hot melissa tea.

Aloe vera juice, made by liquidising the inner 'fillet' of the leaf (carefully remove all of the skin – you only want the soft gel from inside the leaf) with an equal quantity of fresh pineapple is an ancient folk remedy. Take 2 tablespoons full on an empty stomach first thing in the morning and then again last thing at night.

Colon cleansing seeds, like sesame seeds, fenugreek seeds and flaxseed, mixed with fresh thyme for its antibacterial properties and turmeric powder – a teaspoon of each – makes a de-worming mixture that can be eaten with mashed papaya and figs (dried figs soaked overnight in warm water can be taken when no fresh figs are in season). A rinse for fruits and vegetables can be made from grapefruit seed extract and tea tree oil – mix 10 drops of each in 2 litres of warm water and wash fruits and vegetables in it carefully.

Wash bed linen, towels, underclothes and socks in hot water, rinse twice in hot water and dry on a line out in the sun. Use a tea tree spritz to spray mattresses and bedside carpets: boil up 2 cups of tea tree sprigs in 4 litres of water with 4 cups of khakibos sprigs or marigold leaves for 20 minutes. Cool, strain, add 20 drops tea tree oil.

Speak to your doctor about de-worming tablets, vitamin and mineral supplements and probiotics.

Tissue Salts: No. 10 and 11 are helpful taken 6 times a day.

Caution: Consult with your doctor before you embark on any form of self-diagnosis or self-treatment.

Index

Index

Index